MEDICAL RISKS

MEDICAL RISKS

1991 Compend of Mortality and Morbidity

A Compilation of Reference Articles
Published in the
"Journal of Insurance Medicine" of
The American Academy of Insurance Medicine

Richard B. Singer, M.D.
Editor

Michael W. Kita, M.D.
Associate Editor

John R. Avery
Managing Editor

PRAEGER

Westport, Connecticut
London

Library of Congress Cataloging-in-Publication Data

Medical risks : 1991 compend of mortality and morbidity / Richard B.
  Singer, editor; Michael W. Kita, associate editor; John R. Avery,
  managing editor.
        p.   cm.
  "A compilation of reference articles published in the Journal of
insurance medicine, of the American Academy of Insurance Medicine".
  Includes bibliographical references and index.
  ISBN 0-275-94553-7 (alk. paper)
  1. Mortality. 2. Death—Causes. 3. Mortality—Research—
Methodology.   I. Singer, Richard B.   II. Kita, Michael W.
III. Avery, John R.   IV. Journal of insurance medicine (New York,
N.Y.)
RA407.M4 1994
614.4'2—dc20   94-18560

British Library Cataloguing in Publication Data is available.

Library of Congress Catalog Card Number: 94-18560
ISBN: 0-275-94553-7

First published in 1994

Praeger Publishers, 88 Post Road West, Westport, CT 06881
An imprint of Greenwood Publishing Group, Inc.

Printed in the United States of America

The paper used in this book complies with the
Permanent Paper Standard issued by the National
Information Standards Organization (Z39.48-1984).

10 9 8 7 6 5 4 3 2 1

CONTENTS

* See Chapter 5 and Appendix (Chapter 5) for explanation of codes.

CONTENTS (continued)

* See Chapter 5 and Appendix (Chapter 5) for explanation of codes.

CONTENTS (continued)

* See Chapter 5 and Appendix (Chapter 5) for explanation of codes.

CONTENTS (continued)

* See Chapter 5 and Appendix (Chapter 5) for explanation of codes.

CONTENTS (continued)

* See Chapter 5 and Appendix (Chapter 5) for explanation of codes.

ACKNOWLEDGMENTS

The Editors extend grateful thanks to various members of the American Academy of Insurance Medicine (AAIM) who provided crucial support for the sponsorship of the preparation of this *1991 Compend* volume by the Academy. These members include: W. John Elder, M.D., President of AAIM and Editor of the *Journal of Insurance Medicine*, 1991; John P. Carey, M.D., President of AAIM, 1992; William J. Baker, M.D., Secretary of AAIM, 1991; members of the Executive Council of AAIM who approved the project at their May, 1991 meeting; the members of the Committee on Mortality and Morbidity of AAIM and its respective Chairmen (David Wesley, M.D., 1990, David E. Artzerounian, M.D., 1991, and W. John Elder, M.D., 1991-92); Roger H. Butz, M.D., current Editor of the *Journal of Insurance Medicine*; and other members who have given their assistance.

One indispensable feature of the project was the financial support of the desktop publishing work needed to prepare the master copy for the publisher. For this the Editors are grateful to the Chairman and members of the Board of Directors of MIB, Inc. (Medical Information Bureau), who approved inclusion of the project in the MIB's research activities at their June, 1991 meeting, and to Neil M. Day, President and Chief Executive Officer of the MIB, who approved the budget and schedule of the MIB's Center for Medico-Actuarial Statistics (CMAS), where the desktop publishing work was carried out. We greatly appreciate the expertise and hard work of the CMAS Director, John R. Avery and his staff, including Joseph E. Hilton, Kathleen McGrath, and Lauretta G. Ray.

The Editors extend their thanks to all of the Contributors, not only for their initiative in writing their material, but also for generously giving permission for its republication in this volume. Special thanks are due Robert K. Palmer, M.D., and Richard E. Braun, M.D., for the time expended on their respective major contributions, previoulsy unpublished and prepared or rewritten for this *Compend*.

We also thank Dan Eades, Editor, for his assistance in shepherding the volume to publication through Praeger Publishers.

Finally, the Editor wishes to express his personal appreciation for the unstinting support given by his colleagues and friends, Michael W. Kita, M.D., Associate Editor, and John R. Avery, Managing Editor, in bringing our AAIM project to a successful completion.

CONTRIBUTORS

William H. Alexander, M.D.
Vice President and Medical Director
Great West Life Assurance Company
Financial Services Division
Englewood, Colorado

John R. Avery
Director, Center for Medico-Actuarial Statistics
MIB, Inc.
Westwood, Massachusetts

Richard L. Bergstrom, F.S.A.
Consulting Actuary
Milliman & Robertson, Inc.
Seattle, Washington

Richard E. Braun, M.D.
Medical Director
Lincoln National Risk Management, Inc.
Fort Wayne, Indiana

Arthur E. Brown, M.D.
Vice President-Medical, Selection and Issue (Retired)
New England Mutual Life Insurance Company
Boston, Massachusetts

Robert A. Bruce, M.D., F.A.C.C.
University of Washington
Seattle, Washington

Roger H. Butz, M.D., M.P.H.
Editor
Journal of Insurance Medicine, AAIM
Kenmore, Washington

Ole Zeuthen Dalgaard, M.D., Ph.D.
Consultant Physician
TRYG Insurance Life Pension International
Skodsborg, Denmark

Arthur W. DeTore, M.D.
Vice President and Medical Director
Lincoln National Risk Management, Inc.
Fort Wayne, Indiana

M. Irené Ferrer, M.D.
Consultant in Cardiology
Metropolitan Life Insurance Company
New York, New York

Manfred Fessel, Dipl. Math., F.I.T.
Vice President
Medico-Actuarial Research and Statistics
Swiss Reinsurance Company
Zurich, Switzerland

Daniel M. Hays, M.D.
Professor of Surgery and Pediatrics
Children's Hospital of Los Angeles
University of Southern California School of Medicine
Los Angeles, California

John R. Iacovino, M.D.
Vice President and Medical Director
New York Life Insurance Company
New York, New York

Michael W. Kita, M.D.
Vice President and Chief Medical Director
UNUM Life Insurance Company
Portland, Maine

Edward A. Lew, F.S.A.
Consulting Actuary
Punta Gorda, Florida

B. Ross Mackenzie, M.D., F.R.C.P(C), F.A.C.C.
Vice President and Chief Medical Director
Sun Life Assurance Company of Canada
Toronto, Canada

Robert K. Palmer, M.D.
Vice President and Chief Medical Director
North American Reassurance Company
New York, New York
(Former Assist. V. P. and Medical Director
Connecticut General Life Insurance Company
Bloomfield, Connecticut)

Frank I. Pitkin, M.D.
Senior Medical Director (Retired)
New England Mutual Life Insurance Company
Boston, Massachusetts

Robert J. Pokorski, M.D.
Vice President, Medical Research
North American Reassurance Company
Westport, Connecticut
(Former Medical Director
Lincoln National Life Insurance Company
Fort Wayne, Indiana)

John H. Reardon, M.D.
Associate Medical Director
Transamerica Occidental Life Insurance Company
Los Angeles, California

Ferris J. Siber, M.D.
Senior Associate Medical Director (Retired)
New England Mutual Life Insurance Company
Boston, Massachusetts

Richard B. Singer, M.D.
Consultant to the
American Academy of Insurance Medicine (AAIM)
Falmouth, Maine
(Director of Medical Research
2nd Vice President, Retired
New England Mutual Life Insurance Company
Boston, Massachusetts)

Robert L. Stout, Ph.D.
President
Clinical Reference Laboratory, Inc.
Kansas City, Missouri

Orrin S. Tovson, F.S.A.
Research Actuary
American United Life Insurance Company
Indianapolis, Indiana

PART I

CHAPTER TEXT

CHAPTER 1

INTRODUCTION

Richard B. Singer, M.D.

Background and Purpose

Mortality studies on policyholders with specific medical risks have been conducted by life insurance companies for about a century, starting with the Specialized Mortality Investigation, published by the Actuarial Society of America in 1903.[1] Such studies, often made on a cooperative intercompany basis, have been carried out for the purpose of aiding the underwriting selection process: to determine which risks can be included in the limits of mortality for standard insurance, which risks are insurable with an extra premium, and which are uninsurable because the excess mortality is too large. Insurance studies, valuable as they are, have never been adequate to meet all the needs of medical directors and lay underwriters responsible for the risk selection process: they have always been limited in number, and limited in providing little or no experience as a guide in such common risks among applicants as a history of cancer after apparently successful operation, or a history of myocardial infarction (MI) with good recovery.

Following World War II mortality follow-up studies of other segments of the general or patient population began to appear in the medical literature in increasing numbers. Aware of this, a few interested members of the Association of Life Insurance Medical Directors of America (ALIMDA)* proposed to the Executive Council of that professional organization that results of such non-insurance studies be described and that tables of comparative mortality should be constructed as a useful supplement to the insurance studies. After a favorable report from a feasibility study, the Executive Council of ALIMDA agreed in 1966 to sponsor preparation of a reference volume to contain "abstracts" of this sort, organized into a short text containing sections for References, Subjects Studied, Follow-up, Results, Comment, and usually two or more tables of comparative mortality and survival. Funds were raised and an ad hoc committee was appointed to complete the project. Several actuaries were invited to participate in the work of preparation, and after

some delays at the outset a retired actuary, the late Mr. Louis Levinson, F.S.A., was engaged to serve as Project Director and Co-editor. The Society of Actuaries co-sponsored the project by providing funds needed to complete the final years of work. In 1976 the committee sent to a medical publisher a reference volume of nearly 800 pages, with chapter text and about 200 mortality abstracts, mostly drawn from results in the medical literature rather than insurance studies.[2] The committee and editors expressed the hope that the volume would prove to be a useful reference to a wide variety of physicians, clinical investigators and epidemiologists outside the life insurance field. Additional background on the design and use of mortality abstracts, and the life table methodology employed, is given in the first three chapters of the volume.[2]

Although the Liaison Committee of ALIMDA and the Society of Actuaries agreed that work should be started on a successor volume as soon as feasible, the production of this was not achieved until a monograph twice as large was published in 1990.[3] This was prepared under the supervision of a joint committee of actuaries and medical directors, with Mr. Edward A. Lew, F.S.A., as Project Director. ALIMDA and the Society of Actuaries again served as sponsors, and funding was arranged through the MIB, Inc. (Medical Information Bureau), a service organization for the life insurance industry.[4] A research unit of the MIB, the Center for Medico-Actuarial Statistics, prepared numerous drafts and final copies of the text and tables, comprising 1,600 pages.

During the past decade there have been other developments with respect to both insurance mortality studies and mortality abstracts. Three massive mortality studies sponsored by the Society of Actuaries and ALIMDA have been published,[5-7] and a special study of atrial fibrillation in policyholders, a study with data submitted by a record 393 life insurance companies.[8] In addition, mortality abstracts and related articles have been published in the *Journal of Insurance Medicine,* the official journal of ALIMDA. The accumulation of abstracts and articles since the cutoff date for processing material for the *1990 Medical Risks* has grown to the point at which ALIMDA's Mortality and Morbidity Committee has considered it desirable to collect this material for publication in a small

---

* ALIMDA was renamed in 1991 as the American Academy of Insurance Medicine (AAIM). Almost all of the material in this book was prepared before 1991. The acronym ALIMDA is therefore retained in most instances.

volume as an up-to-date reference supplement to the large studies cited above.

Nature of Contents

The mortality abstracts have been prepared in the standard format to be found in the two *Medical Risks* monographs.[2,3] Other articles presenting comparative mortality results of current interest have been included without any attempt to transform them into the standard abstract format. This collection is therefore heterogeneous in nature, with each piece signed by the original contributor. It does not provide comprehensive coverage over the entire spectrum of diseases, nor does it provide in-depth analysis of mortality in a single area, such as bypass surgery, a feature of the abstract design in the last *Medical Risks* book.[3] However, a commentary chapter serves to orient the reader on the relation of each article or abstract to other results recently published and cited above.

One subject area has received a clear focus in this volume: aspects of methodology that are discussed often as a new presentation, or in considerably greater detail than in the material cited above.[2-7] Chapter 2 contains the official text of the course initially developed for the benefit of ALIMDA members in 1977 and now one of the courses sponsored by the Board of Insurance Medicine. Additional topics in Chapter 3 include applications of computer technology to life insurance medicine, the conversion of mortality ratios for underwriting use when population or other tables are used to derive expected mortality, the subject of comparative morbidity as an analogue of comparative mortality, and two articles on the application of statistical methods to the evaluation of results of laboratory tests.

Chapter 4 contains a two-part set of guidelines, first for the evaluation of follow-up articles as a suitable source for a mortality abstract, and then for the methods used to analyze the results in a suitable article, and methods for converting them into the desired tables of comparative mortality. This is new material going into much greater detail than the methodology of Chapter 2, and has not appeared until one of the 1991 issues of the *Journal of Insurance Medicine*. It should also be useful to physician-readers as an aid in the interpretation of the results of published follow-up studies.

A new classification system for mortality abstracts and related articles is described in Chapter 5. This has a pragmatic purpose: a consistent method of coding the abstracts and mortality articles in this volume, and in future issues of the *Journal of Insurance Medicine* and other ALIMDA publications. The editors also intend to

prepare a cumulative index of mortality results, including abstracts, published since 1951, and starting with the *1951 Impairment Study*.[9] A uniform coding system will be needed for this subject index.

How to Use This Volume

Mortality abstracts and mortality articles not dealing with methodology are in the later portion of this volume, following the numbered chapters. They appear in the order of the Subject Classification code (Chapter 5). Readers may locate a particular abstract or mortality article in any one of several different ways: on the list in Part II of the Table of Contents arranged in the order of the classification code, from mention in the Commentary text of Chapter 6, and from the subject index. There is also an author index for contributors, together with a list of source articles used in the abstracts, by first author, in alphabetical order.

The Table of Contents outlines the subjects covered in the six chapters of the initial text portion of the volume, although it should be noted that some mortality data are given in Chapters 2 and 3, as examples of the results to be derived from follow-up studies. Chapter 1 should be read with care by readers who are unfamiliar with the concept of mortality abstracts as utilized in the two large reference monographs cited above.[2,3] Those who desire a simplified step by step development of life table methodology as used in mortality abstract tables should pay special attention to Chapter 2. The reference material includes extracts from U.S. Life Tables, and a table of 90% and 95% confidence limits based on the number of observed deaths and Poisson distributions for the tabular numbers. In Chapter 3 will be found a variety of articles on methodology in the subject area of mortality. These are discussed in the preceding section of this chapter.

In Chapter 4 the authors carry forward the application of life table methodology to many of the practical problems encountered by all workers in this area who are called upon (a) to make a critical evaluation of follow-up articles, or (b) to adapt the results to tables of comparative mortality of the type used in mortality abstracts. This discussion is more detailed than that contained in either of the reference monographs.[2,3] As noted above, it is new material, of potential interest to all physicians interested in follow-up articles and the interpretation of the published results.

The Classification System described in Chapter 5 should be understood by all readers because it is the basis for the coding and arrangement of the abstracts and articles, not only in this volume, but in future issues of the *Journal of Insurance Medicine* and any future compends of this nature. The editors intend to use the classification and coding system for a comprehensive index of all mortality/morbidity abstracts and related mortality results published from 1951 to 1990 and contained in the sources cited in Chapter 5. Such individual results not previously collected in this period carry a K source code. The letter L has been set aside for any important source articles published prior to 1960. For the decade 1991-99, a letter M source code will be used for the individual abstracts and articles to be published in the *Journal of Insurance Medicine*, or in any future compends similar to this volume. Preparation of this comprehensive index has already begun. It is the hope of the editors that such an index will be very useful to all scientists interested in mortality and morbidity results from follow-up studies, regardless of their specialty. Since the 1991 publication draft of this article, the coding system has been revised and expanded. The revised basic list, including all 3-digit codes used in this volume, is given in the Appendix to Chapter 5.

Chapter 6 contains a commentary on the heterogenous abstracts and articles that is intended to provide a common perspective. In the reference monographs[2,3] this was accomplished through a series of chapters, each devoted to a particular disease or risk area. Numbers are not sufficient in this volume to warrant more than a single chapter of commentary, but the purpose is similar.

The Subject Index contains three types of entries to assist the reader in different ways. The first type gives the page number or a range of page numbers. The second type gives the acronym "cd" immediately followed by the 3-digit code number of the disease or other item in the Classification Code. The number of entries far exceeds the number in the expanded list on pages 104-107, the Appendix of Chapter 5. The third type of entry is a freely paraphrased title of each abstract and article in Part II. These are distinguished by the characteristic complete code arrangement: the 3-digit Classification code, the capital letter K for the source, and the unique identifier, a single digit. An example would be 338K1 for the Mortality Abstract on the ". . . Aspirin Component of the Physicians' Health Study." After the main heading of the paraphrased title and the complete code, the initial page number is given in parentheses to facilitate location of the Abstract or Article. This arrangement of the Subject Index, it is hoped, will enhance its usefulness to the reader.

[Note: Very recently a comprehensive description has been published about the work of the Center for Medico-Actuarial Statistics.[10]]

REFERENCES

1. *Specialized Mortality Investigation* (Compiled and published by the Actuarial Society of America, predecessor of the Society of Actuaries, 1903).

2. R. B. Singer, L. Levinson, eds., *Medical Risks: Patterns of Mortality and Survival* (Lexington, MA, Lexington Books, 1976).

3. E. A. Lew, J. Gajewski, eds., *Medical Risks: Trends in Mortality by Age and Time Elapsed* (New York, Praeger, 1990).

4. P. S. Entmacher, "Medical Information Bureau," *JAMA*, 233 (1975): 1370-72.

5. *Build Study 1979* (Boston, Soc. Actuaries and Assoc. Life Ins. Med. Dir. Amer., 1980).

6. *Blood Pressure Study 1979* (Boston, Soc. Actuaries and Assoc. Life Ins. Med. Dir. Amer., 1980).

7. *Medical Impairment Study 1983, Volume I* (Boston, Soc. Actuaries and Assoc. Life Ins. Med. Dir. Amer., 1986).

8. J. Gajewski, R. B. Singer, "A Mortality Study of Atrial Fibrillation in an Insured Population," *JAMA*, 245 (1981): 1540-44.

9. *1951 Impairment Study* (Compiled and published by the Society of Actuaries, 1954).

10. J. R. Avery, "Center for Medico-Actuarial Statistics of MIB, Inc.," *J. Ins. Med.*, 24 (1992): 117-25.

CHAPTER 2

MORTALITY METHODOLOGY AND ANALYSIS SEMINAR

*Text Sponsored by The American Academy of Insurance Medicine
and the Board of Insurance Medicine
(Revised, December 1992)*

Robert J. Pokorski, M.D.

INTRODUCTION
Abstract

Equity is one of the basic tenets of private insurance, i.e., each member of a risk group must pay premiums that are commensurate with the risk presented by that group. The goal of this course is to determine the magnitude of that risk for a group of medically impaired individuals by applying life table methodology to articles taken from the clinical literature.

Throughout the following discussion, it is important to remember that most of the calculations are being performed in order to determine two parameters: mortality ratio (MR) and excess death rate (EDR). Very detailed calculations are shown in order to exemplify all of the steps needed to develop a complete mortality table. In the vast majority of cases, however, the calculations in this paper are much more extensive than those that would be required on a day-to-day basis in order to extract useful mortality data from a clinical or insurance article.

Course Materials

The course materials consist of:

(1) Introduction

(2) Narrative: a detailed discussion of Mortality Methodology and Analysis

(3) Glossary of Symbols and Definitions

(4) Examples 1 and 2

(5) U.S. Population Life Tables used for Examples 1 and 2 (see pages 21-34).

(6) Suggested Rules for "Rounding Off" and Number of Significant Digits for Mortality Monograph Tables.

(7) Confidence Limits Table

Source: R. J. Pokorski, "Mortality Methodology and Analysis Seminar," *J. Ins. Med.*, 20, no. 4 (1988): 20-45. Reproduced with permission of author and publisher.

Suggested Study Pattern

(1) Briefly review the Suggested Rules for "Rounding Off" and Number of Significant Digits for Mortality Monograph Tables, the Confidence Limits Table, the U.S. Population Life Tables used for Examples 1 and 2, and the Glossary of Symbols and Definitions.

(2) Carefully read the narrative.

(3) Work through Examples 1 and 2.

Calculator/ECG Calipers/Millimeter Ruler

A calculator that can extract roots such as $\sqrt[x]{y}$ is essential for this course in order to determine geometric average annual survival rates. It will have a y^x key and an "inverse function (INV)" key. As an example, it must be able to perform this calculation: $\sqrt[5]{0.9765} = 0.9953$ (after rounding off). ECG calipers and a millimeter ruler are also needed in order to accurately measure cumulative survival from a survival curve.

Additional Information

A detailed discussion of mortality methodology is also in Chapter 2 of *Medical Risks: Patterns of Mortality and Survival*.

NARRATIVE: MORTALITY METHODOLOGY AND ANALYSIS

I. INTERVALS, TIME, AND DURATION OF FOLLOW-UP

Interval of Follow-up (i)

An interval of follow-up, designated i, is one of a series of successive periods of time during which mortality is studied. Intervals are numbered sequentially as 1, 2, 3, etc. There are 5 intervals in Example 1 and 7 intervals in Example 2.

Intervals are sometimes combined in order to obtain average annual rates as, for instance, in Examples 1 and

2, where the data from intervals 1 and 2, 3 to 5, and 1 to 5 are combined. There is no established rule that dictates when this should be done; it is somewhat arbitrary and at the discretion of the individual performing the mortality analysis. Most commonly, annual data from the first 5 years of a study are combined and averaged in order to compare it to the average annual results experienced for years 5-10, 10-15, etc.

A subscript, designated i, is often used in definitions to refer to any one of a number of intervals. For example, E_i (see discussion below) would refer to the number of individuals exposed to the risk of death during an interval i that is not otherwise specified.

Time (t) and Duration (Δt) of Follow-up

The symbol t refers to the amount of time that has passed between the beginning of follow-up and the beginning of an interval. The time at the beginning of the interval is therefore designated t, the duration (length) of the interval is Δt (Δ is the Greek letter delta), and the end of the interval is designated $t+\Delta t$. Both t and Δt are generally measured in years but other time units may also be used depending on the purpose of the mortality analysis and the nature of the data available.

In Example 2, for instance, interval 3 begins at 2 years (t = 2 years), has a duration of 1 year (Δt = 1 year), and ends at 3 years ($t+\Delta t$ = 3 years). Likewise, interval 6 begins at 5 years (t = 5 years), has a duration of 5 years (Δt = 5 years), and ends at 10 years ($t+\Delta t$ = 10 years). The end of any interval is obviously the same point in time as the beginning of the next interval, e.g., 3 years marks both the end of interval 3 ($t+\Delta t$ = 3 years) and the beginning of interval 4 (t = 3 years).

II. OBSERVED DATA

Number of Living Entrants (ℓ)

The number of entrants (individuals) alive at the beginning of an interval is designated ℓ (the cursive lower case letter l). For any interval, ℓ is equal to the number of individuals alive at the end of the preceding interval, i.e., $\ell_i = \ell_{i-1} - w_{i-1} - d_{i-1}$. In Example 1, ℓ_2 (the number of entrants alive at the beginning of interval 2) is equal to $\ell_1 - w_1 - d_1 = 1000-5-47 = 948$.

Number of Observed Deaths (d)

The number of deaths observed during an interval is designated d. In Example 1, d_4 (the number of observed deaths during interval 4) is 21. The number d may not always be available because study results are sometimes given only as survival curves without any tabular results for d, ℓ, w (entrants withdrawn alive), or E (entrants exposed to risk of death).

Entrants Lost to Follow-up (u) or Withdrawn (w)

The symbol w is used to designate the combined total of the entrants who are lost to follow-up or withdrawn alive from the study. Occasionally, a study may provide very detailed data that lists both the subjects who are lost to follow-up and those who are withdrawn. The symbol w is used in this case to represent the cases who are withdrawn, and u is the designation for those who are untraced or lost to follow-up. In the majority of medical studies, however, such detailed data are unavailable, and w will generally refer to the total number of entrants that are lost to follow-up and withdrawn. In Example 1, w_3 (the combined total of those entrants that are lost to follow-up or who are withdrawn alive from the study during interval 3) is 3.

Entrants Exposed to Risk of Death (E)

The number of entrants who are exposed to the risk of death during an interval is designated E. E corrects for the subjects that are lost to follow-up or withdrawn. Since it is usually not known exactly when these cases were lost or withdrawn, it is assumed that they exit the study in the middle of the interval. E is therefore equal to the number of individuals alive at the beginning of the interval minus one-half the number of withdrawn or lost entrants, i.e., $E = \ell - w/2$. If no subjects are lost to follow-up or withdrawn from the study, w = 0, and $E = \ell$. For those studies that list both the cases that were lost to follow-up and those that were withdrawn, E would be calculated as $E = \ell - (u+w)/2$.

The exposure, E, is always expressed in person-years. If the interval of follow-up is 1 year, E is simple $\ell - w/2$, as in Example 1, where E_2 (the number of entrants exposed to the risk of death in interval 2) = $\ell_2 - w_2/2 = 948 - 4/2 = 946$. For intervals (or combinations of intervals) of follow-up that are longer than 1 year, E is determined by summing the annual E values. For instance, the total exposure E in Example 1 for the combined intervals 3, 4, and 5 is given by $E = E_3 + E_4 + E_5 = 902.5 + 866.0 + 842.0 = 2610.5$. If the interval of follow-up is less than 1 year, exposure is expressed in person-years by multiplying the number of individuals exposed to the risk of death within the interval by the duration, in years, of the interval, e.g., the exposure E of 60 individuals exposed to the risk of death for 3 months is 60(0.25) = 15 person-years, and the exposure of 1000 individuals exposed to the risk of death for 1 day is (1000)(0.0027) = 2.7 person-years.

The symbol ΣE (the Greek letter sigma) is used to indicate the total number of entrants exposed to the risk of death in a series of successive intervals. ΣE is equal to the sum of the exposure within the individual intervals beginning with interval 1 and ending with interval i, i.e.,

$$\Sigma E = E_1 + E_2 + E_3 \ldots E_i$$

Since the exposure in each individual interval (E_1, E_2, E_3, etc.) is always expressed in person-years, total exposure ΣE is also expressed in person-years.

When performing a mortality analysis, the survival curve graphs and the Methods section of the published article should always be examined with care to see if follow-up begins at the customary starting point (when observed cumulative survival P = 1.000) or at some later duration that excludes early deaths. This is because it is desirable to separate the early experience from the long-term experience when acute or early mortality is much higher than subsequent long-term mortality.

The consequences of this type of adjustment can be dramatic. For instance, if a study graphs the long-term survival in a cohort that has suffered a myocardial infarction, the overall 5-year survival will reflect both the high mortality during the first 30 days following the infarction as well as the mortality of those that survived the infarction and were discharged from the hospital. If the early mortality is not excluded from analysis, the 5-year mortality rate (as well as the average annual mortality rate that is derived from the 5-year rate) will be markedly biased upward. Later text will discuss this concept in greater detail.

Number Exposed to Risk (NER)

When duration is less than 1 year, the number of entrants exposed to the risk of death is designated NER, which is calculated in the same way as exposure, i.e., NER = ℓ = w/2. For example, if 500 patients with acute myocardial infarction (MI) survive 1 month, and w = 10 in the 11-month balance of the first year, then NER = 500–10/2 = 495. However, NER must be adjusted to convert to E in *patient-years* in the following way:

$$E = (11/12)(NER) = (11/12)(495) = 453.8 \text{ pt.-yrs.}$$

This is because the duration of exposure was only 11 months or 11/12 year. When early mortality is very high, as in MI or stroke, or with major surgical procedures, it is customary to exclude early deaths (within 1 month or less) from the long-term follow-up experience. In this example, the mortality rate as d/NER is an *interval* rate, for 11 months, but as d/E the rate is an *annualized* rate, based on the experience of the last 11 months of the first year of follow-up.

Observed Interval Mortality Rate (q_i) and Interval Survival Rate (p_i)

The observed interval mortality rate q is the death rate observed among those exposed to the risk of death during that interval: $q_i = d_i/E_i$. Observed interval survival rate p_i is the survival rate observed among those exposed to the risk of death during that interval. Because mortality and survival rates are complementary functions (their sum is

equal to 1), p = 1–q. Both q and p are usually expressed as a decimal but may be given as a percent, or the number of deaths or survivors, respectively, per 1000 individuals exposed to the risk of death.

For intervals with a duration of 1 year, the interval mortality and survival rates are obviously also annual rates, such as in Example 1, where q_2 (the observed interval mortality rate during the 1 year duration of interval 2) is calculated as:

$$q_2 = d_2/E_2 = 40/946.0 = 0.0423$$

Correspondingly, the survival rate p_2 is given by:

$$p_2 = 1-q_2 = 1-0.0423 = 0.9577$$

If the intervals are shorter than 1 year, NER must be adjusted as described above in order to derive an annualized mortality rate, but the interval mortality rate (q_i) is needed in order to derive p_i and P for an observed survival curve. The duration of the intervals need not be uniform. If intervals are longer than 1 year, the interval mortality rate (q_i) should be derived as ($1-p_i$), from P values in the survival curves or detailed annual life table data.

The interval survival and mortality rates are the rates experienced during the *entire* duration of the interval. In Example 2, q_6 and p_6 represent the mortality and survival rates, respectively, for the entire 5-year duration of interval 6. If annual (yearly) rather than interval rates were needed, they could be derived as a geometric or aggregate average annual rate as discussed below.

Observed Cumulative Survival Rate (P) and Cumulative Mortality Rate (Q)

Observed cumulative survival rate P after any duration of follow-up t is the proportion of those who are still surviving at any given point in time to those exposed to the risk of death from the beginning of the study. The cumulative survival rate is equal to the product of each of the interval survival rates: P = $(p_1)(p_2)(p_3)$. . .(p_t). Observed cumulative mortality rate Q is the complement of P, i.e., Q = 1–P. In Example 1, P_3 (the observed cumulative survival rate at the end of interval 3) is given by:

$$P_3 = (p_1)(p_2)(p_3) = (0.9529)(0.9577)(0.9612) = 0.8772$$

Q_3 is calculated as the complement of P:

$$Q_3 = 1-P_3 = 1-0.8772 = 0.1228$$

A cumulative survival rate is encountered very commonly in the medical literature. For instance, if a study reports a "5-year survival of 75%," this is equivalent to stating that the cumulative survival rate P after 5 years of follow-up is 0.75 or 75%.

Once the cumulative survival rates at the beginning and end of an interval are known, the interval survival rate can be determined if it is not already known. By simply restating the above formula, it is apparent that the interval survival rate p_i is equal to the cumulative survival rate at the end of the interval in question ($P_{t+\Delta t}$) divided by the cumulative survival rate at the end of the prior interval (P_t), i.e.,

$$p_i = P_{t+\Delta t}/P_t$$

For instance, in Example 2, p_6 (the interval survival rate during the 5-year duration of interval 6) is equal to P_6 (the cumulative survival rate at the end of interval 6) divided by P_5 (the cumulative survival rate at the end of interval 5), or

$$p_6 = P_6/P_5 = 0.735/0.840 = 0.875$$

This method of determining the interval survival rate is often used if only cumulative survival data are available for mortality analysis, as, for example, in a medical study such as Example 2 in which all of the given data are displayed graphically in a cumulative survival curve.

Observed Average Annual Survival Rate ($\check{p}$, $\bar{p}$) and Mortality Rate ($\check{q}$, $\bar{q}$)

As discussed above, the interval mortality and survival rates refer to rates that are experienced during the *entire* duration of that interval. But it is often necessary to know the corresponding average mortality and survival rates for a one-year period of time within that interval. These rates are known as average annual survival and mortality rates.

Average annual survival and mortality rates are commonly used if (1) the data in the study being analyzed cover a period of time that is longer (or, rarely, shorter) than 1 year, such as the 5-year duration of interval 6 in Example 2, or, (2) the data from several intervals have been combined in order to obtain average annual rates, such as the combination of intervals 1 and 2, 3 to 5, or 1 to 5 in Example 2.

There are two types of average annual mortality and survival rates: aggregate and geometric.

The aggregate average annual mortality rate, designated $\bar{q}$, is derived by dividing the sum of the deaths Σd over the duration of exposure by the total number of individuals exposed to the risk of death ΣE, i.e.,

$$\bar{q} = \Sigma d/\Sigma E$$

The aggregate average annual survival rate, designated $\bar{p}$, is the complement of $\bar{q}$: $\bar{p} = 1-\bar{q}$

In Example 1, for instance, the aggregate average annual mortality rate for the combined intervals 1 and 2 is:

$$\bar{q} = 87/1943.5 = 0.0448$$

For the combined intervals 3 to 5 this rate is:

$$\bar{q} = 70/2610.5 = 0.0268$$

For combined intervals 1 to 5 the mean is:

$$\bar{q} = 157/4554.0 = 0.0345$$

The corresponding aggregate average annual survival rates are, respectively, 0.9552, 0.9732, and 0.9655.

The geometric average annual survival rate $\check{p}$ is calculated with Δt as the root (where Δt = the number of years within the interval) of the interval survival rate p_i, ie.,

$$\check{p} = \sqrt[\Delta t]{p_i} = \sqrt[\Delta t]{P_{t+\Delta t}/P_t}$$

Note that it is necessary to first know the interval survival rate before this calculation can be performed. As discussed above, the interval survival rate p_i may already be known or it may be necessary to first derive it from the cumulative survival rates. The geometric average annual mortality rate $\check{q}$ is the complement of $\check{p}$: $\check{q} = 1-\check{p}$.

In Example 2, the geometric average annual survival rate for the combined intervals 1 and 2 is:

$$\check{p} = \sqrt[2]{0.915} = 0.957$$

For the combined intervals 3 to 5 the annual rate is:

$$\check{p} = \sqrt[3]{0.840/0.915} = \sqrt[3]{0.918} = 0.972$$

For interval 6 the annual rate is:

$$\check{p} = \sqrt[5]{0.735/0.840} = \sqrt[5]{0.875} = 0.974$$

The corresponding geometric average annual mortality rates are the complements of the survival rates, or 0.043, 0.028, and 0.026, respectively.

There are often differences between the aggregate and geometric average annual rates. These differences are due to different methods of weighting with respect to the exposures, deaths, and annual rates. In life insurance studies, it is customary to use the aggregate average annual mortality rates when they can be calculated because these give mortality rates that are weighted by exposure. Aggregate rates tend to give higher mortality results when the mortality and exposure are highest in the first year or two, as, for example, in studies addressing the annual mortality within the first 5 years following a myocardial infarction or surgery for a serious malignancy. Aggregate average annual rates can generally be determined if the medical study being analyzed has a table that lists exposure and deaths on an annual basis. If this detailed information is not available, geometric average annual rates are derived instead. It is often necessary to determine geometric rather than aggregate average rates for medical studies in which the only data available are in the form of survival curves.

Note that an average annual mortality rate cannot be determined by simply dividing the cumulative mortality rate by the number of years in the interval Δt. In other words, $Q/\Delta t$ is an incorrect method for determining the average annual mortality rate. Average annual mortality must be determined as an aggregate or geometric average rate as discussed above.

III. EXPECTED DATA

Expected mortality and survival data that are obtained from a standard mortality table are always identified with the prime (') symbol in order to differentiate them from observed data. The term "standard" in this case refers to any of the mortality tables that are used to obtain expected data (such as those discussed below) and not to "standard" insurance.

Number of Expected Deaths (d')

The number of expected deaths, designated d', during an interval is derived by multiplying the expected annual mortality rate (q') by the number of individuals exposed to the risk of death (E), i.e., $d' = q'E$. In Example 1, d'_4 (the number of expected deaths during interval 4) is equal to $q'_4 E_4 = 0.0101(866.0) = 8.75$.

Expected Mortality Rate (q') and Survival Rate (p')

The expected annual mortality rate, designated q', is the death rate expected among those exposed to the risk of death during that annual interval. It is always obtained from one of the "standard" mortality tables that list the annual expected mortality rate by age for the group from whom it was derived. All of the other expected data are derived from q'. Expected annual survival rate (p') is the survival rate expected among those exposed to the risk of death during that interval. The rate p' is the complement of q', i.e., $p' = 1 - q'$.

Annual q' is a very important value because it is the "standard" mortality rate against which the subjects in the study being analyzed are compared. Several basic factors must be considered when choosing q': (1) the type of mortality table that should be used, and (2) the age, sex, and race of the study participants.

Type of Mortality Tables

There are five different types of basic mortality tables: Population, Cohort, Group Insurance, Individual Insurance, and Annuity. The rate q' is obtained from whichever of these basic tables is most appropriate for the group being analyzed, i.e., q' is taken from a mortality table that was developed from a group of individuals that had similar characteristics to the study group being analyzed.

Population mortality tables provide expected mortality data for the general population. They have the highest mortality rates since place of residence is usually the only selection criterion used, and all lives—standard, substandard, uninsurable, and dying—are included. Since most articles in the medical literature are based on subjects taken from the general population, q' is usually obtained from this type of table. The population table chosen should be appropriate for the group being studied. For example, q' is obtained from a United States Life Table if the study was based on a United States population.

Regional or state population tables may also be used if applicable.

Cohort tables are occasionally used in mortality analysis. These tables list the mortality in the cohort from which the impaired group was drawn as a sample. The expected mortality rates in the Framingham Study, for example, would be obtained from a cohort mortality table for the Framingham study population.

The rate q' may be obtained from a group insurance table in certain circumstances. Group insurance tables show somewhat lower mortality rates than corresponding population tables because one additional selection factor is used in the populace involved in group insurance: all of the people are actively at work. This eliminates many of the very highly impaired lives incorporated in a mortality table for the general population.

Individual insurance tables, i.e., Basic Select and Ultimate Tables are constructed from data on standard lives only and show lower mortality rates than either population or group insurance tables. This is because the underwriting process has largely eliminated the substandard and uninsurable lives. (Commissioner's Standard Ordinary Tables—CSO Tables—are used to determine reserves and cash values, and they should not be used as an "expected" table in the analysis of comparative mortality.) Annuity tables show still lower mortality rates since the inherent selection process involved—self-selection by the annuitant—is a very effective one. The use of individual insurance and annuity tables is generally limited to mortality studies performed on groups that had been issued insurance, or occasionally for other series for which they are suitable standards. These tables are seldom used in the mortality analysis of an article taken from the clinical literature.

Population Life Tables

The basic feature of a population life table is the annual mortality rate q'_x. A subscript is used to identify the age to which it applies. For instance, q'_{40} represents the mortality rate expected for all individuals between their 40th and 41st birthdays. The subscript i may also be used to designate a specific interval, e.g., q'_3 refers to the expected mortality rate during interval 3.

The following remarks specifically concern the use of United States Population Life Tables. These concepts are also applicable to other "standard" mortality tables.

There are two types of United States Life Tables.

Decennial United States Life Tables (refer to 1979-81 U.S. Life Tables following the narrative) are highly accurate life tables that are published every ten years. They provide annual population mortality and survival data that represent an average for a three-year period such as 1959-61, 1969-71, or 1979-81. Decennial Life Tables are very easy to use since q' is simply listed in separate tables by sex, age, and race. With respect to sex, q' is obtained from the "Life Table For Males" if all (or the great majority) of the study participants were male, from the "Life Table For Females" if all (or the great majority) of the study participants were female, and from the "Life Table For The Total Population" if the study participants were fairly equally divided between males and females, or if the sex distribution is unknown but presumed to be fairly equally divided. The appropriate table for race should also be used if this information is provided in the medical study. The rate q' should be obtained from this type of table whenever possible. A Decennial Table was used to determine all the values for q' in Examples 1 and 2.

Abridged United States Life Tables (refer to 1974 U.S. Life Table following the narrative) are published yearly. They are somewhat less accurate than the Decennial Life Tables and slightly more difficult to use because q' values must be derived. In order to determine the annual q', the annual p' is first derived from the specific mortality table entitled "Number of Survivors at Single Years of Age, Out of 100,000 Born Alive, by Race and Sex: United States." For any age x, the expected annual survival rate p'_x is equal to the ratio of the number of individuals who are alive at the end of that year (who are now x+1 years old) to the number who were alive at the beginning of that year (who were x years old then).

For example, consider a study performed between 1973-75 that tracked the 5-year survival rate of a group of impaired males with an age range of 45-54 and a mean age of 50. For intervals 1, 2, and 3 of the table below, p'_x is determined from the 1974 United States Population Life Table (refer to 1974 U.S. Life Table following the narrative). For the purposes of this example, assume that the average attained age of the group increases by one year with the passage of each calendar year.

The expected survival rate p'_1 during the 1-year duration of interval 1 is equal to the ratio of the number of males alive at age 51 to the number alive at age 50:

$$p'_1 = 86,401/87,182 = 0.9910$$

The mortality rate q'_1 is the complement of p'_1:

$$q'_1 = 1-p'_1 = 1-0.9910 = 0.0090$$

The expected survival rate p'_2 for the 1-year duration of interval 2 is the ratio of the number of males alive at age 52 to the number alive at age 51:

$$p'_2 = 85,563/86,401 = 0.9903$$

Again, q'_2 is derived as the complement of p'_2:

$$q'_2 = 1-p'_2 = 1-0.9903 = 0.0097$$

The expected survival rate p'_3 for the 3-year duration of interval 3 is the ratio of the number of males alive at age 55 to the number alive at age 52, and q'_3 are derived:

$$p'_3 = 82,615/85,563 = 0.9655$$
$$q'_3 = 1-p'_3 = 1-0.9655 = 0.0345$$

Note that q'_3 is so much larger than q'_1 or q'_2 because q'_3 represents the expected mortality rate for a three-year rather than a one-year duration; it is an *interval* rate.

Derivation of q'_1, q'_2, and q'_3 from 1974 U.S. Life Table For Males

No	Interval Start-End	Estimated Age at Start	Interval Survival Rate	Interval Mortality Rate
i	t to t+Δt	x_i	p'	q'
1	0-1 yr	50	0.9910	0.0090
2	1-2	51	0.9903	0.0097
3	2-5	52	0.9655	0.0345

The rate q' is always obtained from the population life table that is most representative of the expected mortality rate during the period of time when the study was being performed. For example, a 1979-81 U.S. Life Table could be used if the study analyzed U.S. subjects and spanned or significantly overlapped the years 1978-83. If the study was performed between 1973-77, however, it would be better to use the 1975 U.S. Life Table.

Age, Sex, and Race of the Study Participants

As noted earlier, the basic factors that must be considered when choosing q' are the type of mortality table that should be used and the age, sex, and race of the study participants. It is usually fairly easy to choose the proper mortality table, but it is often very difficult to determine the expected mortality rate q' if there are insufficient data regarding the age and sex (and, less commonly, race) distribution of the entrants.

Suppose that the medical study being analyzed does not provide a detailed age/sex distribution of the participants. It does, however, state that the mean (average) age of the group at the beginning of the study is x. How is q' determined? Can q' for the first year of the study (duration 0-1 year) be estimated solely on the basis of the mean age x of the group? Possibly. The answer to this question depends on the age range among the entrants. If there is a fairly narrow age range (10 years or less), the q' for the entire group could be based on the median (middle) age within the range. For example, if the study evaluated a group with an age range of 45-54, the central age of 50 could be used as the basis for the first-year q', i.e., the expected mortality rate for the entire group would be q'_{50}. The second-year q' would then be q'_{51}, the third-year q' would be q'_{52}, and so on.

If, however, there is a wide age range among the entrants, q' cannot be estimated solely on the basis of the mean age. In this situation, such a practice could potentially lead to serious errors because (1) a first-year q' based solely on mean age invariably underestimates the mean q' (the average q' for the entire group that is weighted for the age/sex distribution of all entrants; this is discussed in detail below), and (2) the mean age of the entire group would actually increase by less than 1 year with the passage of each calendar year.

Consider a study performed between 1977-82 to determine the 5-year survival among males and females with a certain type of cancer. We are told that the study participants all lived in the United States and ranged in age from 17 to 82 with a mean age of 51. A detailed age/sex distribution of the subjects is not provided.

What is the appropriate first-year q'? The 1979-81 U.S. Life Table For The Total Population is consulted. Is it q'_{51} (0.0064)? No. Regardless of the nature of the impairment (and, for that matter, even if there was no impairment and the subjects were all healthy), the older individuals would die at a greater rate than the younger individuals and the mean q' for this group (if it could be determined) would be somewhat greater than 0.0064. But how much greater?

Suppose that one year has passed. What is the appropriate second-year q'? Is it q'_{52} (0.0070)? Once again, the answer is "no." Although one full year has passed and all of the survivors are indeed one year older, the mean age of the group is now actually less than 52 because of a disproportionately greater death rate among the older individuals.

It is apparent from this example that some assumptions are often required when choosing q' if the article that is being analyzed does not contain sufficiently detailed data. A few practical rules will be suggested during the course that will tend to minimize the error in these situations.

Mean q'

If the medical study does contain more detailed data about the age, sex, and race distribution of the participants, the accuracy of the mortality analysis can be markedly increased by determining the mean q'. Mean q' is the average mortality rate experienced by the entire group that is weighted for the age and sex distribution of all of the study participants. The mean q' reflects the expected mortality much more accurately than a q' based solely on mean age, and it should always be determined if the data are available.

Consider once again the 5-year survival study discussed above that was performed between 1977-82. The entrants ranged in age from 17-82 and had a mean age

of 51. But more detailed data have now been obtained. For each of the five years of the study, we are told the age and sex distribution of the subjects exposed to the risk of death. The data for the first year (duration 0-1 year) listed in Table 003K2-1 are used to calculate first-year mean q', as shown below.

TABLE 003K2-1

AGE/SEX EXPOSURE, DURATION 0-1 YEAR

	Male	Female
Age <30	17	9
30-39	96	87
40-49	158	163
50-59	244	201
60-69	106	114
70 up	37	42
All ages	658	616

In Table 003K2-2 (on page 11) Fraction of Total, F, refers to the percentage of the entire group that is formed by a certain age category. For example, males age 60-69 account for 16.1% (106/658 = 0.161) of the entire group of males.

Central Group Age x_c, is always the median (middle) age within an age range if there are an odd number of years in the age range, or the age 1 year above the "median" age within an age range if there are an even number of years in the age range. If the lower and upper limits of the age distribution are unknown as in the "<30" and "70 up" ranges, generally assume an age 5 years younger and older, respectively, as a central age for this group, i.e., assumes 25 and 74 in this example.

Average Group Mortality Rate is the q' that corresponds to the central age. For males age 40-49, the average group mortality rate based on a central age of 45 is q'_{45}, which is 0.0048.

Age Factor, (x)(F), is a calculation which yields a mean age for the group. 51.4 is the mean age of the combined male + female group.

No. of Deaths Expected, d', and Exposure, E, are self-explanatory. Mean q' is calculated by dividing the sum of the expected deaths by the sum of the exposure. For example, the mean q' for females is:

$$q' = \Sigma d'/\Sigma E = 4.73/616 = 0.0077$$

As indicated by Table 003K2-2, the mean q' for duration 0-1 year is 0.0138 for males, 0.0077 for females, and 0.0108 for males + females combined. These mean q' values are used as the expected mortality rate when constructing a mortality table for duration 0-1 year. Depending on the intent of the mortality analysis, comparative mortality and survival experience could be calculated for males, females, or males + females combined. Mean q' is derived in a similar manner for each of the subsequent years (data not shown), i.e., durations 1-2, 2-3, 3-4, and 4-5 years.

Observe that the mean q′ of 0.0108 for males + females combined for duration 0-1 year approximately corresponds to q'_{57} in the 1979-81 U.S. Life Table For The Total Population. q'_{57} in this table is actually 0.0106. In other words, the expected mortality rate among the study participants for duration 0-1 year is similar to that which would be expected if the entire group was composed of individuals that were all age 57. Note: if the study being analyzed had not provided a complete age/sex distribution for each year of the study, subsequent q′ values would be estimated by advancing the age corresponding to mean q′ by one year with the passage of each successive year of the study. For example, since the mean q′ for males + females combined at the beginning of duration 0-1 approximately corresponds to q'_{57}, the q′ for duration 0-1 would be the mean q′ of 0.0108 (not q'_{57}), the q′ for duration 1-2 years would be q'_{58} (0.0115), the q′ for duration 2-3 years would be q'_{59} (0.0125), and so on.

Return once again to the two situations discussed in the paragraphs above. In the first instance, the age/sex distribution of the study participants was not provided and the first-year q′ was based solely on the mean age of the group: the mean age was 51 and q'_{51} from the 1979-81

Life Table For The Total Population was 0.0064. In the second case, the complete age/sex distribution was available and the mean q′ for duration 0-1 year was calculated: for males + females combined, mean q′ = 0.0108 which approximately corresponds to q'_{57}. If 0.0064 rather than 0.0108 were used to estimate q′, the actual expected mortality rate would have been underestimated by 41% [100 (0.0108–0.0064)/0.0108] and the mortality ratio and excess death rate for this impairment would have been markedly overestimated.

Expected Interval and Cumulative Rates (q'_i, p'_i, Q', P')

In population life tables with complete annual data, w = 0, and the interval mortality rate for any set of consecutive years starting at age x may be derived from the table as $q'_i = \Sigma d'/\ell_x$. In the population life table, P starting at birth may be obtained at any age as ℓ_x/100,000 (the cohort consists of 100,000 persons born alive). P′ starting at age x is calculated as $\ell_{x+\Delta x}/\ell_x$, and the corresponding Q′ as (1–P′).

Expected Average Annual Survival Rate ($\breve{p}'$, $\bar{p}'$) and Mortality Rate ($\breve{q}'$, $\bar{q}'$)

Expected geometric average annual survival and mortality rates are also derived in the same way as the

TABLE 003K2-2
CALCULATION OF MEAN q′,
DURATION 0-1 YEAR

Sex/age Category	Exposure Patient-Yrs E	Fraction of Total F	Average Group Mort. Rate * q′	No. of Deaths Expected d′ = q′E	Central Group Age x_C	Age Factor (x)(F)
Males						
Age <30	17	0.026	0.0020	0.03	25	0.6
30-39	96	0.146	0.0022	0.21	35	5.1
40-49	158	0.240	0.0048	0.76	45	10.8
50-59	244	0.371	0.0121	2.95	55	20.4
60-69	106	0.161	0.0282	2.99	65	10.5
70 up	37	0.056	0.0574	2.12	74	4.1
All ages	658	1.000	0.0138*	9.06	–	51.5
Females						
Age <30	9	0.015	0.0007	0.01	25	0.4
30-39	87	0.141	0.0010	0.09	35	4.9
40-49	163	0.265	0.0026	0.42	45	11.0
50-59	201	0.326	0.0063	1.27	55	17.9
60-69	114	0.185	0.0143	1.63	65	12.0
70 up	42	0.068	0.0311	1.31	74	5.0
All ages	616	1.000	0.0077*	4.73	–	51.2
All ages						
Male	658	0.516	0.0138	9.06	–	26.6
Female	616	0.484	0.0077	4.73	–	24.8
Male + Female	1,274	1.000	0.0108**	13.79	–	51.4

* Basis of expected mortality: 1979-81 U.S. Life Tables For Males and Females separately.

** 0.0138, 0.0077, and 0.0108 are the mean q′ values for males, females, and males + females combined, respectively, for duration 0-1 year.

observed geometric average annual survival and mortality rates: $\check{p}' = \sqrt[\Delta t]{p'_i} = \sqrt[\Delta t]{P'_{t+\Delta t}/P'_t}$ and $\check{q}' = 1-\check{p}'$.

Likewise, expected aggregate average survival and mortality rates are determined in the same manner as the observed aggregate average annual survival and mortality rates: $\bar{q}' = \Sigma d'/\Sigma E$, and $\bar{p}' = 1-\bar{q}'$.

IV. COMPARATIVE MORTALITY AND SURVIVAL FUNCTIONS

Mortality Ratio (MR)

Within an interval of any duration, the mortality ratio, designated MR, is the ratio of the number of deaths observed to the number of deaths expected. The ratio is a decimal that is multiplied by 100 to obtain a percent: $MR = 100d/d'$. Since $q = d/E$ and $q' = d'/E$, this formula may also be restated as $MR = 100q/q'$. As an actuarial practice, MR is expressed as the ratio of observed to expected deaths ($MR = 100d/d'$) when the required data are available rather than as the ratio of observed to expected mortality rates ($MR = 100q/q'$), but the mortality ratios are identical regardless of which of these two formulas is used.

In Example 1, the MR (after rounding off) for interval 2 is:

$$MR = 100(q_2/q'_2) = 100(0.0423/0.0085) = 500\%$$

Or, by using the ratio of d and d', we get the same result:

$$MR = 100(d_2/d'_2) = 100(40/8.04) = 500\%$$

Since the duration of interval 2 is 1 year, the interval MR is also an annual MR in this case.

For the combined intervals 3 to 5 in Example 1, the interval MR (the MR for the entire duration covered by intervals 3 to 5) is calculated as:

$$MR = 100(q_{3-5}/q'_{3-5}) = 100(0.0776/0.0301) = 260\%$$

This is slightly lower than the MR if d and d' are used:

$$MR = 100 (d_{3-5}/d'_{3-5}) = 100(70/26.40) = 265\%$$

In this case the two mortality ratios are not equal: the interval rate is slightly lower, just as $MR = 100(Q/Q')$ is lower than an aggregate mean annual MR.

But what if we wanted to know the annual (as opposed to interval) MR? The mortality ratio would be calculated as either an aggregate or geometric MR. The aggregate average $MR = 100(\bar{q}/\bar{q}')$. For the combined intervals 3 to 5 in Example 1, we would get:

$$MR = 100(\bar{q}_{3-5}/\bar{q}'_{3-5}) = 100(0.0268/0.0101) = 265\%$$

i.e., the aggregate average annual MR experienced during this 3-year interval is 265%. This is identical to the MR derived as $100(\Sigma d/\Sigma d')$:

$$MR = 100(70/26.40) = 265\%$$

The geometric average annual $MR = 100(\check{q}/\check{q}')$. For the combined intervals 3 to 5 in Example 1, this gives:

$$MR = 100(\check{q}_{3-5}/\check{q}'_{3-5}) = 100(0.0266/0.0101) = 265\%$$

Since the aggregate rates are weighted by exposure, an aggregate average annual MR should always be derived rather than a geometric average annual MR if the data are available. The mortality ratio may also be calculated as a cumulative mortality ratio: $MR = 100Q/Q'$.

Survival Ratio (SR)

Survival ratios, designated SR, may be derived in a similar fashion.

The cumulative $SR = 100P/P'$. This is the most commonly used survival ratio. It is also known as the "relative survival rate" and it is often encountered in the clinical literature, especially in cancer studies. In Example 1, the cumulative SR for intervals 1 to 5 is calculated as:

$$SR = 100P_5/P'_5 = 100(0.8416/0.9542) = 88.2\%$$

Other survival ratios that may be calculated include the interval survival ratio ($SR = 100p/p'_i$), the aggregate average annual survival ratio ($SR = 100\bar{p}/\bar{p}'$), and the geometric average annual survival ratio ($SR = 100\check{p}/\check{p}'$).

Excess Death Rate (EDR)

The excess death rate (EDR) is the number of extra deaths that occur per 1000 individuals exposed to the risk of death per year. In each of the formulas below, the difference between the number of observed and expected deaths or the death rates is multiplied by 1000 to eliminate the decimal.

If the duration of the interval is one year, then:

$$EDR = 1000(d-d')/E = 1000(q-q')$$

For the 1-year duration of interval 3 in Example 1:

$$EDR = 1000(d_3-d'_3)/E_3 = 1000(35-8.30)/902.5 = 30$$

This is also equal to:

$$EDR = 1000(q_3-q'_3) = 1000(0.0388-0.0092) = 30$$

Thus, 30 extra deaths occur per 1000 individuals exposed to the risk of death per year.

For an interval or combination of intervals that have a duration greater than 1 year, we have:

$$EDR = 1000(\Sigma d - \Sigma d')/\Sigma E$$

In Example 1, the EDR for the 3-year duration covered by the combined intervals 3 to 5 is:

$$EDR = 1000 (\Sigma d_{3-5}-\Sigma d'_{3-5})/\Sigma E_{3-5}$$
$$= 1000(70-26.40)/2610.5 = 17$$

Thus, 17 extra deaths occur per 1000 individuals exposed to the risk of death per year (not per 3 years).

EDR may also be calculated from aggregate or geometric average annual rates per 1000.

The aggregate average EDR = $1000(\bar{q}-\bar{q}')$. Note that since $\bar{q} = \Sigma d/\Sigma E$ and $\bar{q}' = \Sigma d'/\Sigma E$, this formula may be rewritten as:

$$EDR = 1000[(\Sigma d/\Sigma E)-(\Sigma d'/\Sigma E)] = 1000(\Sigma d-\Sigma d')/\Sigma E$$

which is the same formula used in the paragraph above to calculate EDR for an interval or combination of intervals that have a duration greater than 1 year.

Geometric average EDR = $1000(\check{q}-\check{q}')$. The geometric average EDR for the 5-year duration of interval 6 in Example 2 is:

$$1000(\check{q}_6-\check{q}'_6) = 1000(0.026-0.0143) = 12$$

In other words, 12 extra deaths occur per 1000 individuals exposed to the risk of death per year (not per 5 years).

GLOSSARY OF SYMBOLS AND DEFINITIONS

Symbol   **Definition or Formula**

i   Interval of follow-up. One of a series of successive periods of time during which mortality is studied.

t   Time. The amount of time that has passed between the beginning of follow-up and the beginning of an interval.

Δt Duration of follow-up. The duration (length) of an interval of follow-up.

Observed data

ℓ   Number of living entrants. The number of individuals alive at the beginning of an interval. For any interval, ℓ_i is equal to the number of individuals alive at the end of the preceding interval.

$$\ell_i = \ell_{i-1}-w_{i-1}-d_{i-1}$$

d   Number of observed deaths. The number of deaths observed during an interval.

w   Entrants withdrawn during an interval. w is usually used to designate the combined total of the entrants withdrawn alive (w) from the study or lost (untraced) (u) to follow-up.

u   Entrants lost to follow-up (untraced) during an interval.

E   Entrants exposed to risk of death. The number of individuals who are exposed to the risk of death during an interval.

$$E = \ell-(u+w)/2$$

E is always expressed in person-years.

NER Number exposed to risk. The number of entrants that are exposed to the risk of death during an interval that has a duration less than 1 year.

$$NER = \ell-w/2$$

q   Observed mortality rate. The death rate observed among those exposed to the risk of death during that year or interval.

$$q = d/E \text{ (annual rate)}$$
$$q_i = d_i/E_i \text{ (interval rate)}$$

p   Observed survival rate. The survival rate observed among those exposed to the risk of death during that interval. p = 1−q (annual rate). For interval survival rate, p_i, see below and on page 6.

P   Observed cumulative survival rate. The proportion of those observed to have survived after any duration of follow-up t to those exposed to the risk of death from the beginning of the study.

$$P_t = (p_1)(p_2)(p_3)...(p_t)$$

This formula may be rewritten as $p_i = P_{t+\Delta t}/P_t$, i.e., the interval survival rate p_i is equal to the cumulative survival rate at the end of the interval in question ($P_{t+\Delta t}$) divided by the cumulative survival rate at the end of the prior interval (P_t).

Q   Observed cumulative mortality rate. The proportion of those observed to have died after any duration of follow-up t to those exposed to the risk of death from the beginning of the study.

$$Q = 1-P$$

If w = 0, then $Q = \Sigma d/\ell_1$.

$\bar{q}$ Observed aggregate average annual mortality rate $\bar{q}$ is equal to the sum of the deaths, Σd, over the duration of exposure divided by the total number of entrants exposed to the risk of death, ΣE, during that interval.

$$\bar{q} = \Sigma d/\Sigma E$$

$\bar{p}$ Observed aggregate average annual survival rate.

$$\bar{p} = 1-\bar{q}$$

$\check{p}$ Observed geometric average annual survival rate $\check{p}$ utilizes the root Δt (where Δt = the number of years within the interval) of the interval survival rate, p_i.

$$\check{p} = \sqrt[\Delta t]{p_i} = \sqrt[\Delta t]{P_{t+\Delta t}/P_t}$$

$\check{q}$ Observed geometric average annual mortality rate.

$$\check{q} = 1-\check{p}$$

Expected data

q' Expected annual mortality rates (q') are ordinarily taken directly from the population or other life table used as a standard (only rarely are expected data available in an article from the medical literature). The interval mortality rate (q'_i) may be derived from the life table by more than one method (see page 11). In the Abridged U.S. Life Tables for mortality rates, these are tabulated as 5-year interval rates.

d′ Number of expected deaths. The number of deaths expected during an interval.

$$d' = q'E$$

Values of d′ are ordinarily calculated on an annual basis, with $\Sigma d'$ for longer intervals.

p′ Expected interval survival rate. The survival rate expected among those exposed to the risk of death during that interval.

$$p' = 1-q'$$

(either annual or a period of other than 1 year—see page 11).

P′ Expected cumulative survival rate. The proportion of those expected to have survived after any duration of follow-up t to those exposed to the risk of death from the beginning of the study.

$$P'_t = (p'_1)(p'_2)(p'_3)\ldots(p'_t)$$

As with the observed interval survival rate, the interval p'_i may be calculated in the same way.

$$p'_i = P'_{t+\Delta t}/P'_t$$

Q′ Expected cumulative mortality rate. The proportion of those expected to have died after any duration of follow-up t to those exposed to the risk of death from the beginning of the study.

$$Q' = 1-P'$$

q̄′ Expected aggregate average annual mortality rate q̄′ is equal to the sum of the deaths, $\Sigma d'$, over the duration of exposure divided by the total number of entrants exposed to the risk of death, ΣE, during that interval each year.

$$\bar{q}' = \Sigma d'/\Sigma E$$

p̄′ Expected aggregate average annual survival rate.

$$\bar{p}' = 1-\bar{q}'$$

p̌′ Expected geometric average annual survival rate p̌′ is calculated with Δt as the root (where Δt = the number of years within the interval) of the interval survival rate, p'_i.

$$\check{p}' = \sqrt[\Delta t]{p'_i} = \sqrt[\Delta t]{P'_{t+\Delta t}/P'_t}$$

q̌′ Expected geometric average annual mortality rate.

$$\check{q}' = 1-\check{p}'$$

Comparative mortality and survival functions

MR Mortality ratio. The ratio of the number of deaths observed to the number of deaths expected. For any interval or combination of intervals:

$$MR = 100d/d' = 100q/q'$$

The mortality ratio may also be calculated as an aggregate average (MR = $100\bar{q}/\bar{q}'$), or a geometric average (MR = $100\check{q}/\check{q}'$), or as a cumulative ratio (MR = $100Q/Q'$).

SR Survival ratio. The ratio of the number of survivors observed to the number of survivors expected. For any interval or combination of intervals:

$$SR = 100p/p'$$

The survival ratio may also be calculated as a geometric average (SR = $100\check{p}/\check{p}'$), an aggregate average (SR = $100\bar{p}/\bar{p}'$), or a cumulative ratio (SR = $100P/P'$).

EDR Excess death rate. The number of extra deaths that occur per 1000 individuals exposed to the risk of death per year. For an interval with a duration of 1 year, EDR is calculated as shown.

$$EDR = 1000(d-d')/E = 1000(q-q')$$

For an interval or combination of intervals that have a duration greater than 1 year, the calculation is similar.

$$EDR = 1000(\Sigma d-\Sigma d')/\Sigma E$$

EDR may also be calculated as an aggregate average (EDR = $1000[\bar{q}-\bar{q}']$) or a geometric average (EDR = $1000[\check{q}-\check{q}']$).

EXAMPLE 1

Example 1 is based on a study performed on United States subjects between 1977-82. Some 1000 males with a medical impairment were followed for 5 years after the completion of treatment. The age of the participants ranged from 45-54 with a mean age of 50. Because no subsequent information about the mean age was provided, it is assumed that the mean age of the group increases by one year with the passage of each calendar year.

	Interval	Entrants	Withdrawn	Deaths
No.	Start-End			
i	t to t+Δt	ℓ	w	d
1	0-1 yr.	1000	5	47
2	1-2		4	40
3	2-3		3	35
4	3-4		0	21
5	4-5		6	14

DEVELOPMENT OF DATA FOR INTERVALS 1,2,3,4, AND 5

Observed Data and Rates (Annual and Cumulative)

Step 1—Enter the number of observed deaths (d) and the number of entrants withdrawn (w) for each interval in the appropriate locations in the table (all of the calculations described below have already been made for you).

Step 2—Calculate the number of living entrants ℓ for each interval. For example,

$$\ell_2 = \ell_1 - w_1 - d_1 = 1000 - 5 - 47 = 948$$

Step 3—Calculate the exposure (E) for each interval. For example,

$$E_1 = \ell_1 - w_1/2 = 1000 - 5/2 = 997.5$$

Step 4—Calculate the observed interval mortality rate (q) for each annual interval. For example,

$$q_1 = d_1/E_1 = 47/997.5 = 0.0471$$

Step 5—Calculate the observed interval survival rate (p) for each annual interval. For example,

$$p_1 = 1 - q_1 = 1 - 0.0471 = 0.9529$$

Step 6—Calculate the observed cumulative survival rate (P) at the end of each interval. For example,

$$P_2 = p_1 p_2 = (0.9529)(0.9577) = 0.9126$$

Step 7—Calculate the observed cumulative mortality rate (Q) at the end of each interval. For example,

$$Q_2 = 1 - P_2 = 1 - 0.9126 = 0.0874$$

Expected Data and Rates

Step 1—Enter the exposure (E) for each interval in the appropriate locations in the table of EXPECTED RATES, page 17.

Step 2—Obtain the expected interval mortality rate (q') for each interval from the appropriate life table. Since the study was performed on United States males and spanned the years 1977-82, q' is obtained from the 1979-81 U.S. Life Table For Males. We are told that the mean age of the participants was 50, but no subsequent age data are provided. Because there is a fairly narrow age range among the subjects, it is assumed that the mean age of the group increases by one year with the passage of each calendar year, i.e., the mean age for intervals 1 through 5 will be, respectively, 50, 51, 52, 53, and 54. Consult the 1979-81 U.S. Life Tables For Males and obtain q'_{50} (rounded to the fourth decimal place) for interval 1 (0.0078), q'_{51} for interval 2 (0.0085), q'_{52} for interval 3 (0.0092), q'_{53} for interval 4 (0.0101), and q'_{54} for interval 5 (0.0111). Enter q' in the table of EXPECTED RATES, page 17.

Step 3—Calculate the number of expected deaths (d') for each interval. For example,

$$d'_1 = q'_1 E_1 = (0.0078)(997.5) = 7.78$$

Step 4—Calculate the expected interval survival rate (p') for each interval. For example,

$$p'_1 = 1 - q'_1 = 1 - 0.0078 = 0.9922$$

Step 5—Calculate the expected cumulative survival rate (P') for each interval. For example,

$$P'_3 = p'_1 p'_2 p'_3 = (0.9922)(0.9915)(0.9908) = 0.9747$$

Note that P'_3 may also be calculated as

$$P'_3 = P'_2 p'_3 = (0.9838)(0.9908) = 0.9747$$

Step 6—Calculate the expected cumulative mortality rate (Q') for each interval. For example,

$$Q'_2 = 1 - P'_2 = 1 - 0.9838 = 0.0162$$

DEVELOPMENT OF DATA FOR THE COMBINED INTERVALS 1 AND 2, 3 TO 5, AND 1 TO 5

Observed Data and Rates

Step 1—Enter the number of living entrants (ℓ) for each combination of intervals in the appropriate locations in the table on page 16.

Step 2—Calculate the total exposure (ΣE) for each combination of intervals. For example,

$$E_{1-2} = E_1 + E_2 = 997.5 + 946.0 = 1943.5$$

Step 3—Calculate the total number of observed deaths (d) for each combination of intervals. For example,

$$d_{1-2} = d_1 + d_2 = 47 + 40 = 87$$

Step 4—Calculate the observed interval survival rates, p_{1-2} as P_2, and p_{3-5} as P_5/P_2.

Step 5—Calculate the observed interval mortality rates:
$$q_{1\text{-}2} = 1 - p_{1\text{-}2} \text{ and } q_{3\text{-}5} = 1 - p_{3\text{-}5}$$
Step 6—Copy P_2 and P_5 in the appropriate locations in the table for intervals 1-2, 3-5, and 1-5.

Step 7—Copy Q_2 and Q_5 in the appropriate locations in the table for intervals 1-2, 3-5, and 1-5.

Step 8—Calculate the observed aggregate average annual mortality rate ($\bar{q}$) for each combination of intervals. For example,
$$\bar{q}_{1\text{-}2} = d_{1\text{-}2}/E_{1\text{-}2} = 87/1943.5 = 0.0448$$
Step 9—Calculate the observed aggregate average annual survival rate ($\bar{p}$) for each combination of intervals. For example,
$$\bar{p}_{1\text{-}2} = 1 - \bar{q}_{1\text{-}2} = 1 - 0.0448 = 0.9552$$
Step 10—Calculate the observed geometric average annual survival rate ($\check{p}$) for each combination on intervals, as shown herewith.
$$\check{p}_{1\text{-}2} = \sqrt[2]{p_{1\text{-}2}} = \sqrt[2]{0.9126} = 0.9553$$
$$\check{p}_{3\text{-}5} = \sqrt[3]{p_{3\text{-}5}} = \sqrt[3]{0.9222} = 0.9734$$
$$\check{p}_{1\text{-}5} = \sqrt[5]{p_{1\text{-}5}} = \sqrt[5]{0.8416} = 0.9661$$
Step 11—Calculate the observed geometric average annual mortality rate ($\check{q}$) for each combination of intervals. For example,
$$\check{q}_{1\text{-}2} = 1 - \check{p}_{1\text{-}2} = 1 - 0.9553 = 0.0447$$

Expected Data and Rates

Step 1—Enter the total exposure (E) for each combination of intervals in the appropriate locations in the table.

Step 2—Calculate the total number of expected deaths (d') for each combination in intervals. For example,
$$d'_{1\text{-}2} = d'_1 + d'_2 = 7.78 + 8.04 = 15.82$$
Step 3—Calculate the expected interval survival rate (p') for each combination of intervals. For example,
$$p'_{1\text{-}2} = p'_1 p'_2 = (0.9922)(0.9915) = 0.9838$$
$$p'_{3\text{-}5} = p'_3 p'_4 p'_5 = (0.9908)(0.9899)(0.9889) = 0.9699$$
$$p_{1\text{-}5} = p'_1 p'_2 p'_3 p'_4 p'_5 = P'_5 = 0.9542$$
Step 4—Calculate the expected interval mortality rate (q') for each combination of intervals. For example,
$$q'_{1\text{-}2} = 1 - p'_{1\text{-}2} = 1 - 0.9838 = 0.0162$$
Step 5—Calculate the expected cumulative survival rate (P') for each combination of intervals. For example,
$$P'_2 = p'_{1\text{-}2} = 0.9838$$
$$P'_5 = p'_{1\text{-}5} = 0.9542$$
Step 6—Calculate the expected cumulative mortality rate (Q') for each combination of intervals. For example,
$$Q'_2 = 1 - P'_2 = 1 - 0.9838 = 0.0162$$
Step 7, 8, 9, 10—Calculate the expected aggregate average annual mortality rates ($\bar{q}'$) and survival rates ($\bar{p}'$), and the expected geometric average annual survival rates ($\check{p}'$) and mortality rates ($\check{q}'$) in the same manner as the corresponding observed values.

Comparative Experience

Use the appropriate formulas to calculate the mortality ratios, survival ratios, and excess death rates for each interval and combination of intervals.

EXAMPLE 1— TABLES

OBSERVED DATA

Interval No.	Interval Start-End	Entrants	Withdrawn	Exposure Person-Yrs	Deaths (Observed)
i	t to t+Δt	ℓ	w	E	d
1	0-1 yr.	1,000	5	997.5	47
2	1-2	948	4	946.0	40
3	2-3	904	3	902.5	35
4	3-4	866	0	866.0	21
5	4-5	845	6	842.0	14
1 and 2	0-2	1,000	9	1,943.5	87
3 to 5	2-5	904	9	2,610.5	70
1 to 5	0-5	1,000	18	4,554.0	157

OBSERVED RATES

	Mortality Rate				Survival Rate			
	Interval	Cumulative	Geo. Ave. Ann.	Agg. Ave. Ann.	Interval	Cumulative	Geo. Ave. Ann.	Agg. Ave. Ann.
	q_i	Q	$\check{q}$	$\bar{q}$	p_i	P	$\check{p}$	$\bar{p}$
1	0.0471	0.0471	—	—	0.9529	0.9529	—	—
2	0.0423	0.0874	—	—	0.9577	0.9126	—	—
3	0.0388	0.1228	—	—	0.9612	0.8772	—	—
4	0.0242	0.1440	—	—	0.9758	0.8560	—	—
5	0.0166	0.1582	—	—	0.9834	0.8418	—	—
1 and 2	0.0874	0.0874	0.0447	0.0448	0.9126	0.9126	0.9553	0.9552
3 to 5	0.0776	0.1582	0.0266	0.0268	0.9224	0.8418	0.9734	0.9732
1 to 5	0.1582	0.1582	0.0339	0.0345	0.8418	0.8418	0.9661	0.9655

EXAMPLE 1— TABLES (continued)

EXPECTED RATES

Interval No.	Start-End	Observed Exposure Person-Yrs.	Expected Deaths	Mortality Rate				Survival Rate			
				Interval	Cumulative	Geo. Ave. Ann.	Agg. Ave. Ann.	Interval	Cumulative	Geo. Ave. Ann.	Agg. Ave. Ann.
i	t to t+Δt	E	d'	q'_i*	Q'	$\breve{q}'$	$\bar{q}'$	p'_i	P'	$\breve{p}'$	$\bar{p}'$
1	0-1 yr.	997.5	7.78	0.0078	0.0078	—	—	0.9922	0.9922	—	—
2	1-2	946.0	8.04	0.0085	0.0162	—	—	0.9915	0.9838	—	—
3	2-3	902.5	8.30	0.0092	0.0253	—	—	0.9908	0.9747	—	—
4	3-4	866.0	8.75	0.0101	0.0351	—	—	0.9899	0.9649	—	—
5	4-5	842.0	9.35	0.0111	0.0458	—	—	0.9889	0.9542	—	—
1 and 2	0-2	1,943.5	15.82	0.0162	0.0162	0.0081	0.0081	0.9838	0.9838	0.9919	0.9919
3 to 5	2-5	2,610.5	26.40	0.0301	0.0458	0.0101	0.0101	0.9699	0.9542	0.9899	0.9899
1 to 5	0-5	4,554.0	42.22	0.0458	0.0458	0.0093	0.0093	0.9542	0.9542	0.9907	0.9907

* Basis of expected mortality: 1979-81 U.S. Life Table For Total Males (annual rates, intervals 1-5).

COMPARATIVE EXPERIENCE

Interval No.	Start-End	Mortality Ratios				Survival Ratios				Excess Death Rate		
		Interval	Geo. Ave. Ann.	Agg. Ave. Ann.	Cumulative	Interval	Geo. Ave. Ann.	Agg. Ave. Ann.	Cumulative	Interval	Geo. Ave. Ann.	Agg. Ave. Ann.
i	t to t+Δt	100d/d'	$100\breve{q}/\breve{q}'$	$100\bar{q}/\bar{q}'$	100Q/Q'	$100p_i/p'_i$	$100\breve{p}/\breve{p}'$	$100\bar{p}/\bar{p}'$	100P/P'	$1000(q_i-q'_i)$	$1000(\breve{q}-\breve{q}')$	$1000(\bar{q}-\bar{q}')$
1	0-1 yr.	605	—	—	605	96.0	—	—	96.0	39	—	—
2	1-2	500	—	—	540	96.6	—	—	92.8	34	—	—
3	2-3	420	—	—	485	97.0	—	—	90.0	30	—	—
4	3-4	240	—	—	410	98.6	—	—	88.7	14	—	—
5	4-5	150	—	—	345	99.4	—	—	88.2	6	—	—
1 and 2	0-2	550	550	550	540	92.8	96.3	96.3	92.8	—	37	37
3 to 5	2-5	265	265	265	345	95.1	98.3	98.3	88.2	—	17	17
1 to 5	0-5	370	365	370	345	88.2	97.5	97.5	88.2	—	25	25

EXAMPLE 2

Example 2 is based on the data from the graph on page 18. The study was performed on United States subjects and spanned the years 1973-87. Some 1,000 males with a medical impairment were followed for 15 years after the completion of treatment. The age of the participants ranged from 45-54 with a mean age of 50. Because no detailed data about the age of the group were provided, it is assumed that the mean age of the group increases by one year with the passage of each calendar year.

In this graph, 0 to 60 percent survival has been omitted, and 60 to 100 percent survival is drawn to proper scale. Graphic presentations of data in medical studies frequently use this technique in order to reduce graph size and highlight changes in survival or mortality.

Table 003K2-3 is now developed. It lists the percent survival at year 0 and at the end of intervals 1 (1 year), 2 (2 years), 3 (3 years), 4 (4 years), 5 (5 years), 6 (10 years), and 7 (15 years). This table is constructed in the following fashion with the use of calipers and a millimeter ruler. Note: the measurements in Table 003K-3 were determined from the original graph for Example 2 used in the Mortality Methodology and Analysis Seminar and not from the graph reproduced on page 18.

At year 0, there are 75.0 millimeters along the vertical axis between 0.60 (60 percent survival) and 1.00 (100 percent survival). This 75.0 millimeters corresponds to 0.40 or a 40 percent survival. When this 0.40 is added to the 0.60 (60%) from that portion of the graph that is not drawn to scale, the survival is 1.000 or 100 percent.

At the 1 year point on the horizontal axis (the end of interval 1), there are 66.4 vertical millimeters between 0.60 and the curve. In order to determine the percent survival x corresponding to this 66.4 millimeters, a proportion is used: the ratio of 0.40 to 75.0 mm. is equal to the ratio x to 66.4 mm.: 0.40/75.0 = x/66.4, or x = 0.355. The sum 0.60 (from the portion of the graph that is not drawn to scale) +0.355 = 0.955, ie., the survival at the end of 1 year, is 0.955 or 95.5 percent. The survival rates for the subsequent years are computed in the same fashion.

TABLE 003K2-3

DURATION SINCE COMPLETION OF TREATMENT (YEARS)

Year	Millimeters Between 60-100%	Decimal*	Decimal + 0.60
0	75.0	0.400	1.000
1	66.4	0.355	0.955
2	59.0	0.315	0.915
3	51.6	0.275	0.875
4	47.8	0.255	0.855
5	45.0	0.240	0.840
10	25.4	0.135	0.735
15	10.4	0.055	0.655

* Each of these cumulative survival rates has been measured to three decimal places and rounded to the nearest 0.005.

Note: by convention, the cumulative survival rate (P) on a graph is measured in this manner to three decimal places and then rounded to the nearest 0.005. This is done because measurements from a graph are generally only accurate to two decimal places since errors and inaccuracies of scale often occur during the preparation and photo copying of graphs, and it is also technically difficult to measure the graph more accurately. For example, P_1 (the cumulative survival rate at the end of year 1) can be measured to approximately 0.354 (your measure-

ment will probably be slightly different), this is rounded to 0.355, and 0.355 (rather than 0.354) is entered in the appropriate location in the table. Subsequent calculations in the table are rounded to the nearest 0.001 as exemplified by the steps below. This procedure (measuring P to three decimal places, rounding to the nearest 0.005, and rounding subsequent calculations to the nearest 0.001) should generally be used whenever data are measured from a graph. Since inaccuracies are inevitable in these situations, it is always preferable to obtain three-decimal place data from a table or the text if it is available.

DEVELOPMENT OF DATA FOR INTERVALS 1, 2, 3, 4, 5, 6, AND 7

Observed Data and Rates

Step 1—Determine the observed cumulative survival rate (P) for each interval from the cumulative survival curve on the graph (all of these measurements and calculations have been given in Table 003K2-3).

Step 2—Calculate the observed cumulative mortality rate Q for each interval. For example,

$$Q_2 = 1-P_2 = 1-0.915 = 0.085$$

Step 3—Calculate the observed interval survival rate (p_i) for each interval. For example,

$$p_1 = P_1 = 0.955$$
$$p_2 = P_2/P_1 = 0.915/0.955 = 0.958$$
$$p_6 = P_6/P_5 = 0.735/0.840 = 0.875$$
$$p_7 = P_7/P_6 = 0.655/0.735 = 0.891$$

15-YEAR CUMULATIVE SURVIVAL

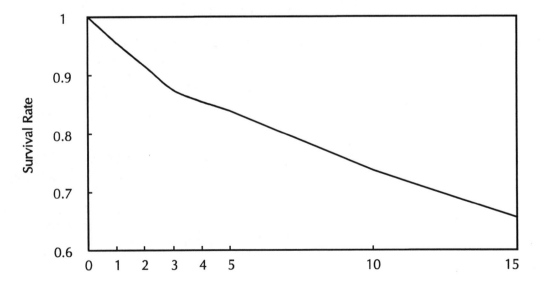

Duration Since Completion of Treatment (Years)

Step 4—Calculate the observed interval mortality rate (q_i) for each interval. For example,

$$q_2 = 1-p_2 = 1-0.958 = 0.042$$

Step 5—Calculate the observed geometric average annual survival rate $(\breve{p})$ for intervals 6 and 7. For example,

$$\breve{p}_6 = \sqrt[5]{p_6} = \sqrt[5]{0.875} = 0.974$$

Step 6—Calculate the observed geometric average annual mortality rate $(\breve{q})$ for intervals 6 and 7. For example,

$$\breve{q}_6 = 1-\breve{p}_6 = 1-0.974 = 0.026$$

Expected Data and Rates

Step 1—Obtain the expected annual mortality rate (q') for intervals 1-5 from the appropriate life table. Since the study was performed on United States males and spanned the years 1972-87, q' is obtained from the 1979-81 U.S. Life Table For Males. We are told that the mean age of the participants was 50, but no subsequent age data are provided. Because there is a fairly narrow age range among the subjects, it is assumed that the mean age of the group increases by one year with the passage of each calendar year, i.e., the mean age for intervals 1 thru 5 will be, respectively, 50, 51, 52, 53, and 54. Consult the 1979-81 U.S. Life Table For Males and obtain q'_{50} (rounded to the fourth decimal place) for interval 1 (0.0078), q'_{51} for interval 2 (0.0085), q'_{52} for interval 3 (0.0092), q'_{53} for interval 4 (0.0101), and q'_{54} for interval 5 (0.0111).

Step 2—Calculate the expected interval survival rate (p') for intervals 1-5. For example,

$$p'_1 = 1-q'_1 = 1-0.0078 = 0.9922$$

Step 3—Calculate the expected interval survival rate (p'_i) for intervals 6 and 7. Since it is assumed that the mean age of the group increases by one year with the passage of each calendar year, the mean age of the group at the beginning of intervals 6 and 7 is, respectively, 55 and 60. Consult the 1979-81 U.S. Population Life Table For Males. p'_6 is equal to the ratio of the number of males alive at age 60 to the number alive at age 55, i.e., 79,012/84,936 = 0.9303. p'_7 is equal to the ratio of the number of males alive at age 65 to the number alive at age 60, i.e., 70,646/79,012 = 0.8941.

Step 4—Calculate the expected interval mortality rate (q'_i) for intervals 6 and 7. For example,

$$q'_6 = 1-p'_6 = 1-0.9303 = 0.0697$$

Step 5—Calculate the expected cumulative survival rate (P') at the end of each interval. For example,

$$P'_3 = p'_1p'_2p'_3 = (0.9922)(0.9915)(0.9908) = 0.9747$$

Note that P'_3 may also be calculated as

$$P'_3 = P'_2p'_3 \ (0.9838)(0.9908) = 0.9747$$

Likewise,

$$P'_6 = P'_5p'_6 = (0.9542)(0.9303) = 0.8877$$

and

$$P'_7 = P'_6p'_7 = (0.8877)(0.8941) = 0.7937$$

Step 6—Calculate the expected cumulative mortality rate (Q') at the end of each interval. For example,

$$Q'_2 = 1-P'_2 = 1-0.9838 = 0.0162$$

Step 7 and 8—For intervals 6 and 7, calculate the expected geometric average annual survival and mortality rates, $\breve{p}'$ and $\breve{q}'$, respectively, in the same manner as the corresponding observed values.

DEVELOPMENT OF DATA FOR THE COMBINED INTERVALS 1 AND 2, 3 TO 5, AND 1 TO 5

Observed Data and Rates

Step 1—Obtain the observed cumulative survival rate (P) for each combination of intervals from the annual data above and enter it in the appropriate locations in the table. For example,

$$P_{1-2} = P_2 = 0.915$$
$$P_{3-5} = P_{1-5} = P_5 = 0.840$$

Step 2—Calculate the observed cumulative mortality rate (Q) for each combination of intervals in the appropriate locations in the table. For example,

$$Q_{1-2} = 1-P_{1-2} = 1-0.915 = 0.085$$

Step 3—Calculate the observed interval survival rate (p_i) for each combination of intervals. For example,

$$p_{1-2} = P_2 = 0.915$$
$$p_{1-5} = P_5 = 0.840$$
$$p_{3-5} = P_5/P_2 = 0.840/0.915 = 0.918$$

Step 4—Calculate the observed interval mortality rate (q_i) for each combination of intervals. For example,

$$q_{1-2} = 1-p_{1-2} = 1-0.915 = 0.085$$

Step 5—Calculate the observed geometric average annual survival rate $(\breve{p})$ for each combination of intervals. For example,

$$\breve{p}_{1-2} = \sqrt[2]{p_{1-2}} = \sqrt[2]{0.915} = 0.957$$
$$\breve{p}_{3-5} = \sqrt[3]{P_5} = \sqrt[3]{0.840} = 0.972$$
$$\breve{p}_{1-5} = \sqrt[5]{p_{1-5}} = \sqrt[5]{0.840} = 0.966$$

Step 6—Calculate the observed geometric average annual mortality rate $(\breve{q})$ for each combination of intervals. For example,

$$\breve{q}_{1-2} = 1-\breve{p}_{1-2} = 1-0.957 = 0.043$$

Expected Data and Rates

Step 1—Obtain the expected cumulative survival rate (P') for each combination of intervals from the annual data above and enter in the appropriate locations in the table.

Step 2—Calculate the expected cumulative mortality rate (Q') for each combination of intervals. For example,

$$Q'_{1-2} = 1-P'_{1-2} = 1-0.9838 = 0.0162$$

Step 3,4—Calculate the expected interval survival and mortality rates, p'_i and q'_i, respectively, in the same manner as the corresponding observed values.

Step 5,6—Calculate the expected geometric average annual survival and mortality rates, $\check{p}'$ and $\check{q}'$, respectively, in the same manner as the corresponding observed values.

Comparative Experience

Use the appropriate formulas to calculate the mortality ratios, survival ratios, and excess death rates for each interval and combination of intervals.

EXAMPLE 2—TABLES

OBSERVED RATES / EXPECTED RATES

No. i	Interval Start-End t to t+Δt	Cumulative P	Interval p_i	Geo. Ave. Ann. $\check{p}$	Cumulative Q	Interval q_i	Geo. Ave. Ann. $\check{q}$	Cumulative P'	Interval p'_i	Geo. Ave. Ann. $\check{p}'$	Cumulative Q'	Interval q'_i*	Geo. Ave. Ann. $\check{q}'$
1	0-1yr.	0.955	0.955	—	0.045	0.045	—	0.9922	0.9922	—	0.0078	0.0078	—
2	1-2	0.915	0.958	—	0.085	0.042	—	0.9838	0.9915	—	0.0162	0.0085	—
3	2-3	0.875	0.956	—	0.125	0.044	—	0.9747	0.9908	—	0.0253	0.0092	—
4	3-4	0.855	0.977	—	0.145	0.023	—	0.9649	0.9899	—	0.0351	0.0101	—
5	4-5	0.840	0.982	—	0.160	0.018	—	0.9542	0.9889	—	0.0458	0.0111	—
1 and 2	0-2	0.915	0.915	0.957	0.085	0.085	0.043	0.9838	0.9838	0.9919	0.0162	0.0162	0.0081
3 to 5	2-5	0.840	0.918	0.972	0.160	0.082	0.028	0.9542	0.9699	0.9899	0.0458	0.0301	0.0101
1 to 5	0-5	0.840	0.840	0.966	0.160	0.160	0.034	0.9542	0.9542	0.9907	0.0458	0.0458	0.0093
6	5-10	0.735	0.875	0.974	0.265	0.125	0.026	0.8877	0.9303	0.9857	0.1123	0.0697	0.0143
7	10-15	0.655	0.891	0.977	0.345	0.109	0.023	0.7937	0.8941	0.9779	0.2063	0.1059	0.0221

*Basis of expected mortality: 1979-81 U.S. Life Tables For Total Males.

COMPARATIVE EXPERIENCE

No. i	Interval Start-End t to t+Δt	Mortality Ratios Interval $100q_i/q'_i$	Mortality Ratios Geo. Ave. Ann. $100\check{q}/\check{q}'$	Mortality Ratios Cumulative $100Q/Q'$	Survival Ratios Interval $100p_i/p'_i$	Survival Ratios Geo. Ave. Ann. $100\check{p}/\check{p}'$	Survival Ratios Cumulative $100P/P'$	Excess Death Rate Interval $1000(q_i-q'_i)$	Excess Death Rate Geo. Ave. Ann. $1000(\check{q}-\check{q}')$
1	0-1 yr.	575	—	575	96.3	—	96.2	37	—
2	1-2	495	—	525	96.6	—	93.0	34	—
3	2-3	480	—	495	96.5	—	89.8	35	—
4	3-4	230	—	415	98.7	—	88.6	13	—
5	4-5	162	—	350	99.3	—	88.0	7	—
1 and 2	0-2	525	530	525	93.0	96.5	93.0	—	35
3 to 5	2-5	270	280	350	94.6	98.2	88.0	—	18
1 to 5	0-5	350	365	350	88.0	97.5	88.0	—	25
6	5-10	179	182	235	94.0	98.8	82.8	—	12
7	10-15	103	104	167	99.7	99.9	82.5	—	1

TABLE 5-2. Number of Survivors at Single Years of Age, Out of 100,000 Born Alive, by Color and Sex: United States, 1974

AGE	TOTAL			WHITE			ALL OTHER		
	BOTH SEXES	MALE	FEMALE	BOTH SEXES	MALE	FEMALE	BOTH SEXES	MALE	FEMALE
0	100,000	100,000	100,000	100,000	100,000	100,000	100,000	100,000	100,000
1	98,325	98,126	98,535	98,510	98,318	98,714	97,511	97,272	97,759
2	98,228	98,017	98,450	98,421	98,216	98,638	97,378	97,130	97,636
3	98,152	97,933	98,382	98,352	98,139	98,577	97,269	97,013	97,535
4	98,090	97,865	98,326	98,296	98,077	98,527	97,179	96,916	97,453
5	98,038	97,808	98,280	98,249	98,025	98,426	97,104	96,830	97,387
6	97,993	97,756	98,242	98,207	97,977	98,451	97,041	96,757	97,334
7	97,953	97,708	98,209	98,169	97,932	98,420	96,987	96,493	97,290
8	97,916	97,663	98,180	98,134	97,890	98,393	96,940	96,636	97,254
9	97,883	97,623	98,154	98,102	97,852	98,368	96,900	96,586	97,223
10	97,853	97,588	98,131	98,074	97,818	98,345	96,864	96,542	97,195
11	97,826	97,557	98,109	98,048	97,789	98,323	96,831	96,502	97,168
12	97,799	97,526	98,086	98,022	97,760	98,301	96,797	96,461	97,141
13	97,767	97,487	98,060	97,991	97,723	98,276	96,758	96,413	97,111
14	97,723	97,431	98,030	97,949	97,668	98,247	96,708	96,348	97,076
15	97,663	97,350	97,993	97,891	97,588	98,211	96,643	96,260	97,035
16	97,586	97,241	97,949	97,815	97,481	98,168	96,561	96,146	96,986
17	97,492	97,107	97,898	97,722	97,348	98,118	96,462	96,006	96,929
18	97,384	96,951	97,841	97,616	97,194	98,063	96,343	95,835	96,862
19	97,267	96,779	97,780	97,503	97,027	98,005	96,202	95,628	96,785
20	97,144	96,595	97,718	97,387	96,853	97,947	96,037	95,384	96,698
21	97,015	96,401	97,655	97,268	96,673	97,890	95,848	96,099	96,599
22	96,880	96,197	97,590	97,146	96,487	97,833	95,635	94,776	96,488
23	96,742	95,987	97,523	97,023	96,299	97,775	95,403	94,423	96,368
24	96,603	95,778	97,455	96,901	96,115	97,717	95,160	94,052	96,241
25	96,467	95,575	97,385	96,782	95,937	97,657	94,910	93,672	96,108
26	96,334	95,380	97,313	96,666	95,768	97,596	94,655	93,286	95,971
27	96,203	95,191	97,240	96,554	95,607	97,533	94,394	92,892	95,827
28	96,073	95,007	97,164	96,443	95,451	97,469	94,126	92,491	95,676
29	95,942	94,823	97,085	96,332	95,297	97,402	93,850	92,080	95,517
30	95,807	94,637	97,002	96,219	95,142	97,332	93,564	91,659	95,349
31	95,668	94,447	96,914	96,103	94,985	97,259	93,267	91,227	95,171
32	95,524	94,253	96,821	95,984	94,825	97,181	92,959	90,784	94,981
33	95,374	94,052	96,721	95,860	94,661	97,098	92,637	90,327	94,779
34	95,217	93,844	96,614	95,730	94,490	97,009	92,300	89,852	94,562
35	95,051	93,626	96,499	95,592	94,310	96,913	91,944	89,356	94,330
36	94,875	93,395	96,375	95,445	94,119	96,809	91,568	88,836	94,081
37	94,686	93,149	96,241	95,287	93,915	96,696	91,170	88,290	93,813
38	94,482	92,887	96,094	95,115	93,695	96,573	90,748	87,717	93,522
39	94,261	92,606	95,933	94,928	93,458	96,437	90,297	87,114	93,203

TABLE 5-2. Number of Survivors at Single Years of Age, Out of 100,000 Born Alive, by Color and Sex: United States, 1974

AGE	TOTAL			WHITE			ALL OTHER		
	BOTH SEXES	MALE	FEMALE	BOTH SEXES	MALE	FEMALE	BOTH SEXES	MALE	FEMALE
40	94,021	92,303	95,755	94,724	93,201	96,286	89,815	86,480	92,853
41	93,760	91,976	95,558	94,501	92,922	96,120	89,299	85,813	92,469
42	93,475	91,622	95,342	94,257	92,618	95,936	88,746	85,110	92,049
43	93,163	91,235	95,105	93,987	92,282	95,734	88,155	84,366	91,595
44	92,820	90,807	94,846	93,686	91,905	95,511	87,524	83,576	91,109
45	92,442	90,333	94,565	93,351	91,481	95,265	86,851	82,735	90,592
46	92,027	89,807	94,259	92,978	91,005	94,994	86,133	81,840	90,043
47	91,572	89,227	93,926	92,565	90,475	94,697	85,368	80,889	89,459
48	91,077	88,595	93,567	92,112	89,892	94,374	84,555	79,882	88,837
49	90,544	87,913	93,181	91,622	89,259	94,026	83,691	78,818	88,171
50	89,972	87,182	92,767	91,095	88,578	93,652	82,755	77,698	87,458
51	89,360	86,401	92,323	90,529	87,848	93,251	81,805	76,522	86,694
52	88,703	85,563	91,846	89,920	87,061	92,819	80,779	75,287	85,878
53	87,995	84,660	91,334	89,260	86,209	92,353	79,693	73,984	85,011
54	87,229	83,680	90,782	88,542	85,279	91,847	78,539	72,600	84,094
55	86,398	82,615	90,186	87,758	84,262	91,297	77,313	71,126	83,126
56	85,499	81,460	89,544	86,904	83,154	90,699	76,015	69,559	82,111
57	84,529	80,215	88,854	85,978	81,953	90,052	74,646	67,906	81,044
58	83,484	78,874	88,110	84,976	80,653	89,352	73,207	66,178	79,916
59	82,359	77,432	87,308	83,893	79,248	88,596	71,698	64,391	78,713
60	81,149	75,886	86,444	82,724	77,734	87,781	70,121	62,559	77,426
61	79,850	74,233	85,510	81,465	76,107	86,901	68,468	60,682	76,039
62	78,460	72,474	84,503	80,115	74,368	85,953	66,741	58,760	74,556
63	76,985	70,612	83,430	78,676	72,519	84,939	64,965	56,806	73,010
64	75,433	68,654	82,299	77,154	70,564	83,864	63,174	54,833	71,449
65	73,810	66,604	81,114	75,553	68,507	82,728	61,387	52,851	69,901
66	72,120	64,469	79,876	73,872	66,350	81,529	59,631	50,877	68,396
67	70,355	62,248	78,572	72,107	64,096	80,255	57,889	48,905	66,910
68	68,500	59,935	77,179	70,247	61,743	78,890	56,087	46,893	65,344
69	66,532	57,522	75,664	68,278	59,290	77,410	54,124	44,783	63,564
70	64,437	55,005	74,003	66,191	56,737	75,797	51,933	42,537	61,482
71	62,214	52,391	72,190	63,988	54,093	74,049	49,488	40,143	59,060
72	59,870	49,691	70,226	61,673	51,308	72,161	46,834	37,632	56,352
73	57,407	46,916	68,104	59,237	48,565	70,113	44,064	35,067	53,475
74	54,829	44,080	65,817	56,670	45,687	67,881	41,309	32,533	50,597
75	52,144	41,198	63,364	53,969	42,743	65,450	38,669	30,097	47,841
76	49,362	38,287	60,748	51,141	39,748	62,819	36,186	27,790	45,262
77	46,498	35,365	57,977	48,202	36,722	60,000	33,855	25,615	42,841
78	43,568	32,454	55,065	45,175	33,692	57,011	31,642	23,558	40,529
79	40,593	29,576	52,029	42,087	30,687	53,877	29,509	21,601	38,267
80	37,595	26,757	48,887	38,966	27,737	50,623	27,431	19,736	36,017
81	34,598	24,025	45,659	35,840	24,873	47,271	25,408	17,969	33,770
82	31,630	21,410	42,367	32,736	22,126	43,845	23,465	16,325	31,550
83	28,720	18,946	39,036	29,862	19,529	40,364	21,658	14,845	29,421
84	25,899	16,687	35,690	26,703	17,113	36,847	20,069	13,588	27,479
85	23,201	14,611	32,358	23,826	14,912	33,311	18,806	12,630	25,856

TABLE 1
LIFE TABLE FOR THE TOTAL POPULATION
UNITED STATES, 1979-81

AGE INTERVAL	PROPORTION DYING	OF 100,000 BORN ALIVE		STATIONARY POPULATION		AVERAGE REMAINING LIFETIME
PERIOD OF LIFE BETWEEN TWO AGES	PROPORTION OF PERSONS ALIVE AT BEGINNING OF AGE INTERVAL DYING DURING INTERVAL	NUMBER LIVING AT BEGINNING OF AGE INTERVAL	NUMBER DYING DURING AGE INTERVAL	IN THE AGE INTERVAL	IN THIS AND ALL SUBSEQUENT AGE INTERVALS	AVERAGE NUMBER OF YEARS OF LIFE REMAINING AT BEGINNING OF AGE INTERVAL
(1)	(2)	(3)	(4)	(5)	(6)	(7)
x to $x+t$	$_tq_x$	ℓ_x	$_td_x$	$_tL_x$	T_x	$\overset{\circ}{e}_x$
DAYS						
0-1	0.00463	100,000	463	273	7,387,758	73.88
1-7	0.00246	99,537	245	1,635	7,387,485	74.22
7-28	0.00139	99,292	138	5,708	7,385,850	74.38
28-365	0.00418	99,154	414	91,357	7,380,142	74.43
YEARS						
0-1	0.01260	100,000	1,260	98,973	7,387,758	73.88
1-2	0.00093	98,740	92	98,694	7,288,785	73.82
2-3	0.00065	98,648	64	98,617	7,190,091	72.89
3-4	0.00050	98,584	49	98,560	7,091,474	71.93
4-5	0.00040	98,535	40	98,515	6,992,914	70.97
5-6	0.00037	98,495	36	98,477	6,894,399	70.00
6-7	0.00033	98,459	33	98,442	6,795,922	69.02
7-8	0.00030	98,426	30	98,412	6,697,480	68.05
8-9	0.00027	98,396	26	98,383	6,599,068	67.07
9-10	0.00023	98,370	23	98,358	6,500,685	66.08
10-11	0.00020	98,347	19	98,338	6,402,327	65.10
11-12	0.00019	98,328	19	98,319	6,303,989	64.11
12-13	0.00025	98,309	24	98,297	6,205,670	63.12
13-14	0.00037	98,285	37	98,266	6,107,373	62.14
14-15	0.00053	98,248	52	98,222	6,009,107	61.16
15-16	0.00069	98,196	67	98,163	5,910,885	60.19
16-17	0.00083	98,129	82	98,087	5,812,722	59.24
17-18	0.00095	98,047	94	98,000	5,714,635	58.28
18-19	0.00105	97,953	102	97,902	5,616,635	57.34
19-20	0.00112	97,851	110	97,796	5,518,733	56.40
20-21	0.00120	97,741	118	97,682	5,420,937	55.46
21-22	0.00127	97,623	124	97,561	5,323,255	54.53
22-23	0.00132	97,499	129	97,435	5,225,694	53.60
23-24	0.00134	97,370	130	97,306	5,128,259	52.67
24-25	0.00133	97,240	130	97,175	5,030,953	51.74
25-26	0.00132	97,110	128	97,046	4,933,778	50.81
26-27	0.00131	96,982	126	96,919	4,836,732	49.87
27-28	0.00130	96,856	126	96,793	4,739,813	48.94
28-29	0.00130	96,730	126	96,667	4,643,020	48.00
29-30	0.00131	96,604	127	96,541	4,546,353	47.06

AGE INTERVAL	PROPORTION DYING	OF 100,000 BORN ALIVE		STATIONARY POPULATION		AVERAGE REMAINING LIFETIME
PERIOD OF LIFE BETWEEN TWO AGES	PROPORTION OF PERSONS ALIVE AT BEGINNING OF AGE INTERVAL DYING DURING INTERVAL	NUMBER LIVING AT BEGINNING OF AGE INTERVAL	NUMBER DYING DURING AGE INTERVAL	IN THE AGE INTERVAL	IN THIS AND ALL SUBSEQUENT AGE INTERVALS	AVERAGE NUMBER OF YEARS OF LIFE REMAINING AT BEGINNING OF AGE INTERVAL
(1)	(2)	(3)	(4)	(5)	(6)	(7)
x to $x+t$	$_tq_x$	ℓ_x	$_td_x$	$_tL_x$	T_x	$\mathring{e}_x$
30-31	0.00133	96,477	127	96,414	4,449,812	46.12
31-32	0.00134	96,350	130	96,284	4,353,398	45.18
32-33	0.00137	96,220	132	96,155	4,257,114	44.24
33-34	0.00142	96,088	137	96,019	4,160,959	43.30
34-35	0.00150	95,951	143	95,880	4,064,940	42.36
35-36	0.00159	95,808	153	95,731	3,969,060	41.43
36-37	0.00170	95,655	163	95,574	3,873,329	40.49
37-38	0.00183	95,492	175	95,404	3,777,755	39.56
38-39	0.00197	95,317	188	95,224	3,682,351	36.63
39-40	0.00213	95,129	203	95,027	3,587,127	37.71
40-41	0.00232	94,926	220	94,817	3,492,100	36.79
41-42	0.00254	94,706	241	94,585	3,397,283	35.87
42-43	0.00279	94,465	264	94,334	3,302,698	34.96
43-44	0.00306	94,201	288	94,057	3,208,364	34.06
44-45	0.00335	93,913	314	93,756	3,114,307	33.16
45-46	0.00366	93,599	343	93,427	3,020,551	32.27
46-47	0.00401	93,256	374	93,069	2,927,124	31.39
47-48	0.00442	92,882	410	92,677	2,634,055	30.51
48-49	0.00488	92,472	451	92,246	2,741,378	29.65
49-50	0.00538	92,021	495	91,773	2,649,132	26.79
50-51	0.00589	91,526	540	91,256	2,557,359	27.94
51-52	0.00642	90,986	584	90,695	2,466,103	27.10
52-53	0.00699	90,402	631	90,086	2,375,408	26.28
53-54	0.00761	89,771	684	89,430	2,285,322	25.46
54-55	0.00830	89,087	739	88,717	2,195,892	24.65
55-56	0.00902	88,348	797	87,950	2,107,175	23.85
56-57	0.00978	87,551	856	87,122	2,019,225	23.06
57-58	0.01059	86,695	919	86,236	1,932,103	22.29
58-59	0.01151	85,776	987	85,283	1,845,867	21.52
59-60	0.01254	84,789	1,063	84,258	1,760,584	20.76
60-61	0.01368	83,726	1,145	83,153	1,676,326	20.02
61-62	0.01493	82,581	1,233	81,965	1,593,173	19.29
62-63	0.01628	81,348	1,324	80,686	1,511,208	18.58
63-64	0.01767	80,024	1,415	79,316	1,430,522	17.88
64-65	0.01911	78,609	1,502	77,859	1,351,206	17.19

TABLE 1 (continued)
LIFE TABLE FOR THE TOTAL POPULATION
UNITED STATES, 1979-81

AGE INTERVAL	PROPORTION DYING	OF 100,000 BORN ALIVE		STATIONARY POPULATION		AVERAGE REMAINING LIFETIME
PERIOD OF LIFE BETWEEN TWO AGES	PROPORTION OF PERSONS ALIVE AT BEGINNING OF AGE INTERVAL DYING DURING INTERVAL	NUMBER LIVING AT BEGINNING OF AGE INTERVAL	NUMBER DYING DURING AGE INTERVAL	IN THE AGE INTERVAL	IN THIS AND ALL SUBSEQUENT AGE INTERVALS	AVERAGE NUMBER OF YEARS OF LIFE REMAINING AT BEGINNING OF AGE INTERVAL
(1)	(2)	(3)	(4)	(5)	(6)	(7)
x to $x+t$	$_tq_x$	ℓ_x	$_td_x$	$_tL_x$	T_x	$\overset{\circ}{e}_x$
65-66	0.02059	77,107	1,587	76,314	1,273,347	16.51
66-67	0.02216	75,520	1,674	74,683	1,197,033	15.85
67-68	0.02389	73,846	1,764	72,964	1,122,350	15.20
68-69	0.02585	72,082	1,864	71,150	1,049,386	14.56
69-70	0.02806	70,218	1,970	69,233	978,236	13.93
70-71	0.03052	68,248	2,083	67,206	909,003	13.32
71-72	0.03315	66,165	2,193	65,069	841,797	12.72
72-73	0.03593	63,972	2,299	62,823	776,728	12.14
73-74	0.03882	61,673	2,394	60,476	713,905	11.58
74-75	0.04184	59,279	2,480	58,039	653,429	11.02
75-76	0.04507	56,799	2,560	55,520	595,390	10.48
76-77	0.04867	54,239	2,640	52,919	539,870	9.95
77-78	0.05274	51,599	2,721	50,238	486,951	9.44
78-79	0.05742	48,878	2,807	47,475	436,713	8.93
79-80	0.06277	46,071	2,891	44,626	389,238	8.45
80-81	0.06882	43,180	2,972	41,694	344,612	7.98
81-82	0.07552	40,208	3,036	38,689	302,918	7.53
82-83	0.08278	37,172	3,077	35,634	264,229	7.11
83-84	0.09041	34,095	3,083	32,553	228,595	6.70
84-85	0.09842	31,012	3,052	29,486	196,042	6.32
85-86	0.10725	27,960	2,999	26,461	166,556	5.96
86-87	0.11712	24,961	2,923	23,500	140,095	5.61
87-88	0.12717	22,038	2,803	20,636	116,595	5.29
88-89	0.13708	19,235	2,637	17,917	95,959	4.99
89-90	0.14728	16,598	2,444	15,376	78,042	4.70
90-91	0.15868	14,154	2,246	13,031	62,666	4.43
91-92	0.17169	11,908	2,045	10,886	49,635	4.17
92-93	0.18570	9,863	1,831	8,948	38,749	3.93
93-94	0.20023	8,032	1,608	7,228	29,801	3.71
94-95	0.21495	6,424	1,381	5,733	22,573	3.51
95-96	0.22976	5,043	1,159	4,463	16,840	3.34
96-97	0.24338	3,884	945	3,412	12,377	3.19
97-98	0.25637	2,939	754	2,562	8,965	3.05
98-99	0.26868	2,185	587	1,892	6,403	2.93
99-100	0.28030	1,598	448	1,374	4,511	2.82

TABLE 1 (continued)
LIFE TABLE FOR THE TOTAL POPULATION
UNITED STATES, 1979-81

AGE INTERVAL	PROPORTION DYING	OF 100,000 BORN ALIVE		STATIONARY POPULATION		AVERAGE REMAINING LIFETIME
PERIOD OF LIFE BETWEEN TWO AGES	PROPORTION OF PERSONS ALIVE AT BEGINNING OF AGE INTERVAL DYING DURING INTERVAL	NUMBER LIVING AT BEGINNING OF AGE INTERVAL	NUMBER DYING DURING AGE INTERVAL	IN THE AGE INTERVAL	IN THIS AND ALL SUBSEQUENT AGE INTERVALS	AVERAGE NUMBER OF YEARS OF LIFE REMAINING AT BEGINNING OF AGE INTERVAL
(1)	(2)	(3)	(4)	(5)	(6)	(7)
x to $x+t$	$_tq_x$	ℓ_x	$_td_x$	$_tL_x$	T_x	$\overset{\circ}{e}_x$
100-101	0.29120	1,150	335	983	3,137	2.73
101-102	0.30139	815	245	692	2,154	2.64
102-103	0.31089	570	177	481	1,462	2.57
103-104	0.31970	393	126	330	981	2.50
104-105	0.32786	267	88	223	651	2.44
105-106	0.33539	179	60	150	428	2.38
106-107	0.34233	119	41	99	278	2.33
107-108	0.34870	78	27	64	179	2.29
108-109	0.35453	51	18	42	115	2.24
109-110	0.35988	33	12	27	73	2.20

TABLE 2
LIFE TABLE FOR MALES
UNITED STATES, 1979-81

AGE INTERVAL	PROPORTION DYING	OF 100,000 BORN ALIVE		STATIONARY POPULATION		AVERAGE REMAINING LIFETIME
PERIOD OF LIFE BETWEEN TWO AGES	PROPORTION OF PERSONS ALIVE AT BEGINNING OF AGE INTERVAL DYING DURING INTERVAL	NUMBER LIVING AT BEGINNING OF AGE INTERVAL	NUMBER DYING DURING AGE INTERVAL	IN THE AGE INTERVAL	IN THIS AND ALL SUBSEQUENT AGE INTERVALS	AVERAGE NUMBER OF YEARS OF LIFE REMAINING AT BEGINNING OF AGE INTERVAL
(1)	(2)	(3)	(4)	(5)	(6)	(7)
x to $x+t$	$_tq_x$	ℓ_x	$_td_x$	$_tL_x$	T_x	$\overset{\circ}{e}_x$
DAYS						
0-1	0.00503	100,000	503	273	7,011,493	70.11
1-7	0.00278	99,497	277	1,633	7,011,220	70.47
7-28	0.00152	99,220	150	5,705	7,009,587	70.65
28-365	0.00467	99,070	463	91,256	7,003,882	70.70
YEARS						
0-1	0.01393	100,000	1,393	98,867	7,011,493	70.11
1-2	0.00101	98,607	99	98,557	6,912,626	70.10
2-3	0.00073	98,508	72	98,472	6,814,069	69.17
3-4	0.00058	98,436	57	98,408	6,715,597	68.22
4-5	0.00047	98,379	46	98,356	6,617,189	67.26
5-6	0.00042	98,333	42	98,312	6,518,833	66.29
6-7	0.00039	98,291	39	98,272	6,420,521	65.32
7-8	0.00036	98,252	35	98,234	6,322,249	64.35
8-9	0.00032	98,217	31	98,202	6,224,015	63.37
9-10	0.00026	98,186	26	98,173	6,125,813	62.39
10-11	0.00021	98,160	21	98,150	6,027,640	61.41
11-12	0.00021	98,139	20	98,129	5,929,490	60.42
12-13	0.00030	98,119	29	98,104	5,831,361	59.43
13-14	0.00048	98,090	47	98,066	5,733,257	58.45
14-15	0.00072	98,043	71	98,008	5,635,191	57.48
15-16	0.00096	97,972	94	97,925	5,537,183	56.52
16-17	0.00118	97,878	116	97,820	5,439,258	55.57
17-18	0.00137	97,762	134	97,695	5,341,438	54.64
18-19	0.00153	97,628	149	97,554	5,243,743	53.71
19-20	0.00167	97,479	163	97,398	5,146,189	52.79
20-21	0.00181	97,316	175	97,228	5,048,791	51.88
21-22	0.00194	97,141	189	97,047	4,951,563	50.97
22-23	0.00203	96,952	196	96,854	4,854,516	50.07
23-24	0.00205	96,756	199	96,656	4,757,662	49.17
24-25	0.00203	96,557	196	96,459	4,661,006	48.27
25-26	0.00199	96,361	192	96,265	4,564,547	47.37
26-27	0.00196	96,169	189	96,074	4,468,282	46.46
27-28	0.00193	95,980	185	95,888	4,372,208	45.55
28-29	0.00191	95,795	183	95,704	4,276,320	44.64
29-30	0.00191	95,612	182	95,521	4,180,616	43.72

TABLE 2 (continued)
LIFE TABLE FOR MALES
UNITED STATES, 1979-81

AGE INTERVAL	PROPORTION DYING	OF 100,000 BORN ALIVE		STATIONARY POPULATION		AVERAGE REMAINING LIFETIME
PERIOD OF LIFE BETWEEN TWO AGES	PROPORTION OF PERSONS ALIVE AT BEGINNING OF AGE INTERVAL DYING DURING INTERVAL	NUMBER LIVING AT BEGINNING OF AGE INTERVAL	NUMBER DYING DURING AGE INTERVAL	IN THE AGE INTERVAL	IN THIS AND ALL SUBSEQUENT AGE INTERVALS	AVERAGE NUMBER OF YEARS OF LIFE REMAINING AT BEGINNING OF AGE INTERVAL
(1)	(2)	(3)	(4)	(5)	(6)	(7)
x to $x+t$	$_tq_x$	ℓ_x	$_td_x$	$_tL_x$	T_x	$\overset{\circ}{e}_x$
30-31	0.00191	95,430	183	95,338	4,085,095	42.81
31-32	0.00191	95,247	181	95,157	3,989,757	41.89
32-33	0.00193	95,066	184	94,974	3,894,600	40.97
33-34	0.00198	94,882	187	94,789	3,799,626	40.05
34-35	0.00205	94,695	194	94,597	3,704,837	39.12
35-36	0.00216	94,501	204	94,399	3,610,240	38.20
36-37	0.00229	94,297	216	94,189	3,515,841	37.28
37-38	0.00244	94,081	229	93,967	3,421,652	36.37
38-39	0.00261	93,852	245	93,729	3,327,685	35.46
39-40	0.00280	93,607	262	93,477	3,233,956	34.55
40-41	0.00303	93,345	283	93,203	3,140,479	33.64
41-42	0.00332	93,062	308	92,908	3,047,276	32.74
42-43	0.00363	92,754	337	92,586	2,954,363	31.85
43-44	0.00398	92,417	368	92,232	2,861,752	30.97
44-45	0.00435	92,049	400	91,849	2,769,550	30.09
45-46	0.00476	91,649	436	91,431	2,677,701	29.22
46-47	0.00522	91,213	476	90,975	2,566,270	28.35
47-48	0.00576	90,737	523	90,475	2,495,295	27.50
48-49	0.00638	90,214	575	89,927	2,404,820	26.66
49-50	0.00705	89,639	632	89,323	2,314,893	25.82
50-51	0.00775	89,007	690	88,662	2,225,570	25.00
51-52	0.00846	88,317	747	87,944	2,136,908	24.20
52-53	0.00924	87,570	809	87,166	2,048,964	23.40
53-54	0.01010	86,761	876	86,323	1,961,798	22.61
54-55	0.01105	85,885	949	85,410	1,875,475	21.84
55-56	0.01206	84,936	1,024	84,424	1,790,065	21.08
56-57	0.01310	83,912	1,099	83,362	1,705,641	20.33
57-58	0.01423	82,813	1,179	82,224	1,622,279	19.59
58-59	0.01549	81,634	1,264	81,002	1,540,055	18.87
59-60	0.01690	80,370	1,358	79,691	1,459,053	18.15
60-61	0.01846	79,012	1,459	78,282	1,379,362	17.46
61-62	0.02016	77,553	1,563	76,772	1,301,080	16.78
62-63	0.02201	75,990	1,673	75,154	1,224,308	16.11
63-64	0.02398	74,317	1,782	73,426	1,149,154	15.46
64-65	0.02604	72,535	1,889	71,591	1,075,728	14.83

TABLE 2 (continued)
LIFE TABLE FOR MALES
UNITED STATES, 1979-81

AGE INTERVAL	PROPORTION DYING	OF 100,000 BORN ALIVE		STATIONARY POPULATION		AVERAGE REMAINING LIFETIME
PERIOD OF LIFE BETWEEN TWO AGES	PROPORTION OF PERSONS ALIVE AT BEGINNING OF AGE INTERVAL DYING DURING INTERVAL	NUMBER LIVING AT BEGINNING OF AGE INTERVAL	NUMBER DYING DURING AGE INTERVAL	IN THE AGE INTERVAL	IN THIS AND ALL SUBSEQUENT AGE INTERVALS	AVERAGE NUMBER OF YEARS OF LIFE REMAINING AT BEGINNING OF AGE INTERVAL
(1)	(2)	(3)	(4)	(5)	(6)	(7)
x to $x+t$	$_tq_x$	ℓ_x	$_td_x$	$_tL_x$	T_x	$\overset{\circ}{e}_x$
65-66	0.02817	70,646	1,990	69,651	1,004,137	14.21
66-67	0.03044	68,656	2,090	67,611	934,486	13.61
67-68	0.03289	66,566	2,189	65,472	866,875	13.02
68-69	0.03563	64,377	2,294	63,229	801,403	12.45
69-70	0.03868	62,083	2,402	60,883	738,174	11.89
70-71	0.04207	59,681	2,510	58,426	677,291	11.35
71-72	0.04571	57,171	2,614	55,864	618,865	10.82
72-73	0.04951	54,557	2,701	53,206	563,001	10.32
73-74	0.05338	51,856	2,768	50,472	509,795	9.83
74-75	0.05736	49,088	2,816	47,680	459,323	9.36
75-76	0.06167	46,272	2,853	44,846	411,643	8.90
76-77	0.06647	43,419	2,886	41,975	366,797	8.45
77-78	0.07170	40,533	2,907	39,080	324,822	8.01
78-79	0.07740	37,626	2,912	36,170	285,742	7.59
79-80	0.08365	34,714	2,904	33,262	249,572	7.19
80-81	0.09069	31,810	2,885	30,368	216,310	6.80
81-82	0.09859	28,925	2,851	27,499	185,942	6.43
82-83	0.10708	26,074	2,792	24,678	158,443	6.08
83-84	0.11579	23,282	2,696	21,933	133,765	5.75
84-85	0.12463	20,586	2,566	19,303	111,832	5.43
85-86	0.13419	18,020	2,418	16,812	92,529	5.13
86-87	0.14479	15,602	2,259	14,472	75,717	4.85
87-88	0.15554	13,343	2,075	12,306	61,245	4.59
88-89	0.16618	11,268	1,873	10,331	48,939	4.34
89-90	0.17700	9,395	1,663	8,564	38,608	4.11
90-91	0.18848	7,732	1,457	7,004	30,044	3.89
91-92	0.20125	6,275	1,263	5,643	23,040	3.67
92-93	0.21542	5,012	1,080	4,472	17,397	3.47
93-94	0.23080	3,932	907	3,479	12,925	3.29
94-95	0.24641	3,025	746	2,652	9,446	3.12
95-96	0.26149	2,279	596	1,982	6,794	2.98
96-97	0.27438	1,683	461	1,452	4,812	2.86
97-98	0.28654	1,222	351	1,046	3,360	2.75
98-99	0.29797	871	259	742	2,314	2.65
99-100	0.30867	612	189	517	1,572	2.57

TABLE 2 (continued)
LIFE TABLE FOR MALES
UNITED STATES, 1979-81

AGE INTERVAL	PROPORTION DYING	OF 100,000 BORN ALIVE		STATIONARY POPULATION		AVERAGE REMAINING LIFETIME
PERIOD OF LIFE BETWEEN TWO AGES	PROPORTION OF PERSONS ALIVE AT BEGINNING OF AGE INTERVAL DYING DURING INTERVAL	NUMBER LIVING AT BEGINNING OF AGE INTERVAL	NUMBER DYING DURING AGE INTERVAL	IN THE AGE INTERVAL	IN THIS AND ALL SUBSEQUENT AGE INTERVALS	AVERAGE NUMBER OF YEARS OF LIFE REMAINING AT BEGINNING OF AGE INTERVAL
(1)	(2)	(3)	(4)	(5)	(6)	(7)
x to $x+t$	$_tq_x$	ℓ_x	$_td_x$	$_tL_x$	T_x	$\overset{\circ}{e}_x$
100-101	0.31865	423	135	356	1,055	2.49
101-102	0.32792	233	94	241	699	2.43
102-103	0.33650	146	65	161	458	2.36
103-104	0.34443	120	45	106	297	2.31
104-105	0.35174	84	20	70	191	2.26
105-106	0.35845	55	20	45	121	2.22
106-107	0.36461	35	13	23	76	2.13
107-108	0.37024	22	3	19	48	2.14
108-109	0.37539	14	5	11	29	2.10
109-110	0.38009	7	4	7	18	2.07

TABLE 3
LIFE TABLE FOR FEMALES
UNITED STATES, 1979-81

AGE INTERVAL	PROPORTION DYING	OF 100,000 BORN ALIVE		STATIONARY POPULATION		AVERAGE REMAINING LIFETIME
PERIOD OF LIFE BETWEEN TWO AGES	PROPORTION OF PERSONS ALIVE AT BEGINNING OF AGE INTERVAL DYING DURING INTERVAL	NUMBER LIVING AT BEGINNING OF AGE INTERVAL	NUMBER DYING DURING AGE INTERVAL	IN THE AGE INTERVAL	IN THIS AND ALL SUBSEQUENT AGE INTERVALS	AVERAGE NUMBER OF YEARS OF LIFE REMAINING AT BEGINNING OF AGE INTERVAL
(1)	(2)	(3)	(4)	(5)	(6)	(7)
x to $x+t$	$_tq_x$	ℓ_x	$_td_x$	$_tL_x$	T_x	$\overset{\circ}{e}_x$
DAYS						
0-1	0.00421	100,000	421	273	7,762,496	77.62
1-7	0.00212	99,579	211	1,636	7,762,223	77.95
7-28	0.00126	99,368	124	5,713	7,760,587	78.10
28-365	0.00366	99,244	364	91,463	7,754,874	78.14
YEARS						
0-1	0.01120	100,000	1,120	99,085	7,762,496	77.62
1-2	0.00086	98,880	84	98,838	7,663,411	77.50
2-3	0.00056	98,796	56	98,768	7,564,573	76.57
3-4	0.00042	98,740	41	98,720	7,465,805	75.61
4-5	0.00033	98,699	33	98,682	7,367,085	74.64
5-6	0.00031	98,666	30	98,651	7,268,403	73.67
6-7	0.00027	98,636	27	98,623	7,169,752	72.69
7-8	0.00024	98,609	24	98,596	7,071,129	71.71
8-9	0.00022	98,585	22	98,575	6,972,533	70.73
9-10	0.00019	98,563	19	98,553	6,873,958	69.74
10-11	0.00018	98,544	17	98,536	6,775,405	68.75
11-12	0.00018	98,527	18	98,518	6,676,869	67.77
12-13	0.00020	98,509	20	98,499	6,578,351	66.78
13-14	0.00026	98,489	25	98,477	6,479,852	65.79
14-15	0.00033	98,464	32	98,448	6,381,375	64.81
15-16	0.00040	98,432	40	98,411	6,282,927	63.83
16-17	0.00047	98,392	46	98,369	6,184,516	62.86
17-18	0.00052	98,346	52	98,320	6,086,147	61.89
18-19	0.00055	98,294	54	98,267	5,987,827	60.92
19-20	0.00057	98,240	56	98,212	5,889,560	59.95
20-21	0.00058	98,184	57	98,156	5,791,348	58.98
21-22	0.00060	98,127	59	98,097	5,693,192	58.02
22-23	0.00062	98,068	61	98,037	5,595,095	57.05
23-24	0.00063	98,007	61	97,977	5,497,058	56.09
24-25	0.00064	97,946	63	97,914	5,399,081	55.12
25-26	0.00065	97,883	63	97,851	5,301,167	54.16
26-27	0.00066	97,820	65	97,788	5,203,316	53.19
27-28	0.00067	97,755	66	97,722	5,105,528	52.23
28-29	0.00070	97,689	68	97,655	5,007,806	51.26
29-30	0.00072	97,621	70	97,586	4,910,151	50.30

31

TABLE 3 (continued)
LIFE TABLE FOR FEMALES
UNITED STATES, 1979-81

AGE INTERVAL	PROPORTION DYING	OF 100,000 BORN ALIVE		STATIONARY POPULATION		AVERAGE REMAINING LIFETIME
PERIOD OF LIFE BETWEEN TWO AGES	PROPORTION OF PERSONS ALIVE AT BEGINNING OF AGE INTERVAL DYING DURING INTERVAL	NUMBER LIVING AT BEGINNING OF AGE INTERVAL	NUMBER DYING DURING AGE INTERVAL	IN THE AGE INTERVAL	IN THIS AND ALL SUBSEQUENT AGE INTERVALS	AVERAGE NUMBER OF YEARS OF LIFE REMAINING AT BEGINNING OF AGE INTERVAL
(1)	(2)	(3)	(4)	(5)	(6)	(7)
x to $x+t$	$_tq_x$	ℓ_x	$_td_x$	$_tL_x$	T_x	$\overset{\circ}{e}_x$
30-31	0.00075	97,551	74	97,514	4,812,565	49.33
31-32	0.00079	97,477	77	97,439	4,715,051	48.37
32-33	0.00083	97,400	81	97,360	4,617,612	47.41
33-34	0.00089	97,319	86	97,276	4,520,252	46.45
34-35	0.00096	97,233	93	97,186	4,422,976	45.49
35-36	0.00104	97,140	101	97,089	4,325,790	44.53
36-37	0.00114	97,039	111	96,984	4,228,701	43.58
37-38	0.00125	96,928	121	96,868	4,131,717	42.63
38-39	0.00137	96,807	132	96,741	4,034,849	41.68
39-40	0.00149	96,675	144	96,603	3,938,108	40.74
40-41	0.00163	96,531	157	96,452	3,841,505	39.80
41-42	0.00180	96,374	174	96,287	3,745,053	38.86
42-43	0.00199	96,200	191	96,104	3,648,766	37.93
43-44	0.00218	96,009	210	95,904	3,552,662	37.00
44-45	0.00239	95,799	229	95,684	3,456,758	36.08
45-46	0.00262	95,570	250	95,445	3,361,074	35.17
46-47	0.00286	95,320	273	95,184	3,265,629	34.26
47-48	0.00315	95,047	299	94,897	3,170,445	33.36
48-49	0.00347	94,748	329	94,584	3,075,548	32.46
49-50	0.00381	94,419	359	94,239	2,980,964	31.57
50-51	0.00416	94,060	391	93,864	2,886,725	30.69
51-52	0.00452	93,669	424	93,457	2,792,861	29.82
52-53	0.00490	93,245	457	93,017	2,699,404	28.95
53-54	0.00532	92,788	494	92,541	2,606,387	28.09
54-55	0.00578	92,294	534	92,028	2,513,846	27.24
55-56	0.00627	91,760	575	91,472	2,421,818	26.39
56-57	0.00678	91,185	618	90,876	2,330,346	25.56
57-58	0.00733	90,567	664	90,235	2,239,470	24.73
58-59	0.00796	89,903	716	89,545	2,149,235	23.91
59-60	0.00867	89,187	773	88,800	2,059,690	23.09
60-61	0.00947	88,414	837	87,996	1,970,890	22.29
61-62	0.01035	87,577	907	87,123	1,882,894	21.50
62-63	0.01129	86,670	979	86,181	1,795,771	20.72
63-64	0.01226	85,691	1,050	85,166	1,709,590	19.95
64-65	0.01325	84,641	1,121	84,081	1,624,424	19.19

TABLE 3 (continued)
LIFE TABLE FOR FEMALES
UNITED STATES, 1979-81

AGE INTERVAL	PROPORTION DYING	OF 100,000 BORN ALIVE		STATIONARY POPULATION		AVERAGE REMAINING LIFETIME
PERIOD OF LIFE BETWEEN TWO AGES	PROPORTION OF PERSONS ALIVE AT BEGINNING OF AGE INTERVAL DYING DURING INTERVAL	NUMBER LIVING AT BEGINNING OF AGE INTERVAL	NUMBER DYING DURING AGE INTERVAL	IN THE AGE INTERVAL	IN THIS AND ALL SUBSEQUENT AGE INTERVALS	AVERAGE NUMBER OF YEARS OF LIFE REMAINING AT BEGINNING OF AGE INTERVAL
(1)	(2)	(3)	(4)	(5)	(6)	(7)
x to $x+t$	$_tq_x$	ℓ_x	$_td_x$	$_tL_x$	T_x	$\mathring{e}_x$
65-66	0.01427	83,520	1,192	82,923	1,540,343	18.44
66-67	0.01538	82,328	1,267	81,695	1,457,420	17.70
67-68	0.01664	81,061	1,349	80,387	1,375,725	16.97
68-69	0.01811	79,712	1,443	78,990	1,295,338	16.25
69-70	0.01980	78,269	1,549	77,495	1,216,348	15.54
70-71	0.02169	76,720	1,665	75,887	1,138,853	14.84
71-72	0.02375	75,055	1,782	74,164	1,062,966	14.16
72-73	0.02600	73,273	1,905	72,321	988,802	13.49
73-74	0.02842	71,368	2,028	70,354	916,481	12.84
74-75	0.03106	69,340	2,154	68,263	846,127	12.20
75-76	0.03388	67,186	2,276	66,048	777,864	11.58
76-77	0.03704	64,910	2,404	63,707	711,816	10.97
77-78	0.04073	62,506	2,546	61,233	648,109	10.37
78-79	0.04515	59,960	2,707	58,607	586,876	9.79
79-80	0.05033	57,253	2,881	55,812	528,269	9.23
80-81	0.05622	54,372	3,057	52,844	472,457	8.69
81-82	0.06269	51,315	3,217	49,706	419,613	8.18
82-83	0.06973	48,098	3,354	46,422	369,907	7.69
83-84	0.07722	44,744	3,455	43,016	323,485	7.23
84-85	0.08519	41,289	3,517	39,531	280,469	6.79
85-86	0.09409	37,772	3,554	35,995	240,938	6.38
86-87	0.10405	34,218	3,561	32,437	204,943	5.99
87-88	0.11420	30,657	3,501	28,907	172,506	5.63
88-89	0.12427	27,156	3,374	25,469	143,599	5.29
89-90	0.13471	23,782	3,204	22,180	118,130	4.97
90-91	0.14461	20,578	3,017	19,069	95,950	4.66
91-92	0.16024	17,561	2,814	16,154	76,881	4.38
92-93	0.17460	14,747	2,575	13,459	60,727	4.12
93-94	0.18904	12,172	2,301	11,022	47,268	3.88
94-95	0.20348	9,871	2,009	8,867	36,246	3.67
95-96	0.21823	7,862	1,715	7,004	27,379	3.48
96-97	0.23221	6,147	1,428	5,433	20,375	3.31
97-98	0.24560	4,719	1,159	4,140	14,942	3.17
98-99	0.25834	3,560	919	3,101	10,802	3.03
99-100	0.27040	2,641	714	2,283	7,701	2.92

TABLE 3 (continued)
LIFE TABLE FOR FEMALES
UNITED STATES, 1979-81

AGE INTERVAL	PROPORTION DYING	OF 100,000 BORN ALIVE		STATIONARY POPULATION		AVERAGE REMAINING LIFETIME
PERIOD OF LIFE BETWEEN TWO AGES	PROPORTION OF PERSONS ALIVE AT BEGINNING OF AGE INTERVAL DYING DURING INTERVAL	NUMBER LIVING AT BEGINNING OF AGE INTERVAL	NUMBER DYING DURING AGE INTERVAL	IN THE AGE INTERVAL	IN THIS AND ALL SUBSEQUENT AGE INTERVALS	AVERAGE NUMBER OF YEARS OF LIFE REMAINING AT BEGINNING OF AGE INTERVAL
(1)	(2)	(3)	(4)	(5)	(6)	(7)
x to $x+t$	$_tq_x$	ℓ_x	$_td_x$	$_tL_x$	T_x	$\overset{\circ}{e}_x$
100-101	0.28176	1,927	543	1,655	5,418	2.81
101-102	0.29242	1,384	405	1,182	3,763	2.72
102-103	0.30237	979	296	831	2,581	2.64
103-104	0.31163	683	213	577	1,750	2.56
104-105	0.32023	470	150	394	1,173	2.50
105-106	0.32817	320	105	268	779	2.44
106-107	0.33550	215	72	178	511	2.38
107-108	0.34224	143	49	119	333	2.33
108-109	0.34843	94	33	77	214	2.28
109-110	0.35411	61	22	50	137	2.24

SUGGESTED RULES FOR "ROUNDING OFF" AND NUMBER OF SIGNIFICANT DIGITS FOR MORTALITY MONOGRAPH TABLES

Variable	Range of Values	Significant Digits	Examples
Observed deaths, d	0 up	1	5, 11, 23
Expected deaths, d'	0.000 to 0.199	0.001	0.001
	0.20 to 9.99	0.01	0.21, 5.73
	10.0 to 99.9	0.1	11.2, 57.3
	100 to 999	1	112, 573
Exposure, E	0 to 100	0.1	34.5
	100 to 9,999	1	345, 3,452
Observed Mort. Rate, q or Q	0.000 to 1.000	0.001	0.001, 0.112
Observed Surv. Rate, p or P	1.000 to 0.000	0.001	0.989, 0.888
Expected Mort. Rate, q' or Q'	0.00000 to 0.00199	0.00001	0.00011
	0.0020 to 1.000	0.0001	0.0072
Expected Surv. Rate, p' or P'	1.0000 to 0.0000	0.0001	0.9993, 0.9928
Mortality Ratio, MR	0 to 199%	1%	112%
	200 to 995%	5%	575%
	1,000 to 1,990%	10%	1,120%
	2,000 to 9,950%	100%	5,800%
	10,000 to 19,900	100%	11,200%
	20,000 up	1000%	58,000%
Survival Ratio, SR	100.0 to 0.0%	0.1%	98.6%, 57.5%
Excess Death Rate, EDR	<0 to 1000	1	−1, 11, 112

Note 1. In worksheets an additional significant figure may be carried, if it is feasible to do so.

Note 2. Rounding off will be done at the final stage of table preparation. If two values of a variable should happen to differ slightly after calculation from two different sets of rounded-off data appearing in the table, they should be equalized.

Note 3. With "20" as a division point for number of significant digits in many of the variables, it may be that a column of results will contain data with differing numbers of digits, e.g. d' = 0.172, 0.26, 5.90, 17.2. This inconsistency must be accepted if the appearance of unwarranted precision is to be avoided in critical parts of the tables.

CONFIDENCE LIMITS BASED ON NUMBER OF
OBSERVED DEATHS—POISSON DISTRIBUTION[*]

Deaths Observed d	LIMITS WITH RESPECT TO d				LIMITS AS A RATIO OF d			
	95% Limits		90% Limits		95% limits		90% limits	
	Lower LL	Upper UL	Lower LL	Upper UL	Lower LL	Upper UL	Lower LL	Upper UL
3	0.6	8.8	0.8	7.8	0.21	2.93	0.27	2.60
4	1.1	10.2	1.4	9.2	0.27	2.56	0.34	2.29
5	1.6	11.7	2.0	10.5	0.32	2.33	0.39	2.10
6	2.2	13.1	2.6	11.8	0.37	2.18	0.44	1.97
7	2.8	14.4	3.3	13.1	0.40	2.06	0.47	1.88
8	3.5	15.8	4.0	14.4	0.43	1.97	0.50	1.80
9	4.1	17.1	4.7	15.7	0.46	1.90	0.52	1.74
10	4.8	18.4	5.4	17.0	0.48	1.84	0.54	1.70
11	5.5	19.7	6.2	18.2	0.50	1.79	0.56	1.66
12	6.2	21.0	6.9	19.4	0.52	1.75	0.58	1.62
13	6.9	22.2	7.7	20.7	0.53	1.71	0.59	1.59
14	7.7	23.5	8.5	21.9	0.55	1.68	0.61	1.56
15	8.4	24.7	9.2	23.1	0.56	1.65	0.62	1.54
16	9.1	26.0	10.0	24.3	0.57	1.62	0.63	1.52
17	9.9	27.2	10.8	25.5	0.58	1.60	0.64	1.50
18	10.7	28.4	11.6	26.7	0.59	1.58	0.64	1.48
19	11.4	29.7	12.4	27.9	0.60	1.56	0.65	1.47
20	12.2	30.9	13.3	29.1	0.61	1.54	0.66	1.46
22	13.8	33.3	14.9	31.4	0.63	1.51	0.68	1.43
24	15.4	35.7	16.5	33.8	0.64	1.49	0.69	1.41
26	17.0	38.1	18.2	36.1	0.65	1.47	0.70	1.39
28	18.6	40.5	19.9	38.4	0.66	1.45	0.71	1.37
30	20.2	42.8	21.6	40.7	0.67	1.43	0.72	1.36
32	21.9	45.2	23.3	43.0	0.68	1.41	0.73	1.34
34	23.5	47.5	25.0	45.3	0.69	1.40	0.74	1.33
36	25.2	49.8	26.7	47.5	0.70	1.38	0.74	1.32
38	26.9	52.2	28.5	49.8	0.71	1.37	0.75	1.31
40	28.6	54.5	30.2	52.1	0.72	1.36	0.76	1.30
45	32.8	60.2	34.6	57.7	0.73	1.34	0.77	1.28
50	37.1	65.9	39.0	63.3	0.74	1.32	0.78	1.27
55	41.4	71.6	43.4	68.9	0.75	1.30	0.79	1.25
60	45.8	77.2	47.9	74.4	0.76	1.29	0.80	1.24
65	50.2	82.8	52.3	79.9	0.77	1.27	0.80	1.23
70	54.6	88.4	56.8	85.4	0.78	1.26	0.81	1.22
75	59.0	94.0	61.3	90.9	0.79	1.25	0.82	1.21
80	63.4	99.6	65.9	96.4	0.79	1.24	0.82	1.20
85	67.9	105.1	70.4	101.8	0.80	1.24	0.83	1.20
90	72.4	110.6	75.0	107.2	0.80	1.23	0.83	1.19
95	76.9	116.1	79.6	112.7	0.81	1.22	0.84	1.19
100	81.4	121.6	84.1	118.1	0.81	1.22	0.84	1.18

[*]The confidence limits have been calculated in accordance with the traditional formula and definition of confidence interval for the Poisson distribution, as described in *Distributions in Statistics: Discrete Distributions*, by N.L. Johnson and S. Kotz. Boston, Houghton, Mifflin & Co. (1969). We are indebted to Dr. Robert A. Lew for his assistance in the preparation of this table. When d exceeds 100, an approximation of the confidence limits that is satisfactory for most purposes can be obtained by assuming a normal distribution. The formula is: 95% limits = $d \pm 1.96 \sqrt{d}$, 90% limits = $d \pm 1.65 \sqrt{d}$.

N. B. TO obtain the lower confidence limits, LL, for a mortality ratio, MR, or a mortality rate q, multiply MR or q by the appropriate LL factor in the right-hand portion of the table. The upper confidence limits, UL, for MR or q may similarly be computed by multiplying MR or q by the appropriate UL factor from the right-hand part of the table.

CHAPTER 3

MEDICAL INFORMATICS IN INSURANCE MEDICINE
AN INTRODUCTION TO COMPUTERS FOR INSURANCE MEDICAL DIRECTORS
Arthur W. DeTore, M.D.

Introduction

"Data! data! data!" he cried impatiently. "I can't make brick without clay."[1]

Although these words were spoken by a fictional hero, the master detective Sherlock Holmes, they express a sentiment which is frequently felt by many physicians today. This issue was examined by Covell et al. in the *Annals of Internal Medicine*. They looked at the information needs of medical practitioners in their office practice and whether those needs were being met on a day-to-day basis. What they found was that the information needs were great, but they were not being met in a satisfactory way because 70% of these needs were not satisfied.[2]

A considerable component of this problem is the amount of information necessary to practice medicine today because of the explosion of medical knowledge. David Sackett of McMasters has commented on this situation:

". . . the biomedical literature is expanding at a compound rate of 6% to 7% per year. Thus, from the time you start medical school until you are established in practice 10 or 12 years later, the biomedical literature will have doubled! During your professional career it may increase tenfold! How can anyone keep up?

". . . To put it in an even more depressing way, if you were all caught up now, and read one article every day from the subsequently published medical journals, by this time next year you would be 55 centuries behind in your reading."[3]

This phenomenon is a reflection in the medical field of what is happening in all areas of knowledge. Some general evidence of this is the expansion of the Library of Congress. From 1933 to 1966, the Library of Congress is said to have doubled. It doubled again from 1967 to 1979, and is expected to double again by the end of 1987.[4]

As these comments indicate, today the traditional approaches for physicians to access and stay current with information are not adequate.

Thus, new approaches to information management in medicine have become necessary which has led to the development of a new specialty, Medical Informatics.

Medical Informatics

Medical Informatics has been defined as the basic science of computers in medicine, dealing with the exchange of information through computer-based systems.[5] It arose from the need for better information management in medicine, and the development of computer technology (also called information technology or informatics) to fulfill that need.

The concept of Medical Informatics is only a subset of a much greater awareness of the importance of information in today's society. In his book, *Megatrends*, John Naisbitt states that one of the ten major transformations taking place within our society is a shift from an Industrial society to an information society. This transformation has become possible because of the development of information technology. Naisbitt holds that the computer is to the information age, what mechanization was to the industrial revolution.[6] Information technology provides the actual tool which can manipulate and disseminate information in new, more effective ways. Medical informatics is the discipline involved with the use of these tools for dealing with medical information.

Significance of Medical Informatics in Medicine Today

Although relatively new, there is evidence to suggest that the importance of Medical Informatics is increasing. The World Health Organization has developed a division of Information Systems Support which is promoting the role of Medical Informatics in developing countries.[5] The American Medical Association included Medical Informatics in its "Specialty Review" issue for the first time in 1986.[7] The American College of Cardiology has a standing committee on Computer Applications and has recently offered a series of articles on computer applications for cardiologists.[8]

A recent book review of Harrison's *Principles of Internal Medicine* and Stein's *Internal Medicine* published in the *New England Journal of Medicine*, questioned the place of textbooks as a source of information in today's practice of medicine by stating, "The first question, it seems to me, concerns the purpose of encyclopedic books. Are specific information needs best satisfied

Source: A. W. DeTore, "Medical Informatics in Insurance Medicine— An Introduction to Computers for Insurance Medical Directors," *J. Ins. Med.*, 20, no. 1 (1988): 3-9. Reproduced with permission of author and publisher.

by a complete textbook of medicine or by a computer search system?"[9] All of these developments point to increasing importance in Medical Informatics in the medical community.

The Importance of Medical Informatics in Insurance Medicine

In insurance medicine, a key element of the insurance industry, information management is vital because of the importance of data in the industry. As described in the Life Office Management Association's text, *Systems and Data Processing in Insurance Companies*:

"What the production line is to the manufacturer, the data processing system is to an insurer. Its raw materials are data: data on mortality, morbidity, interest, and loss experience, from which the products are designed; data on policy applicants, on which underwriting is based; data on pertinent events throughout the life of the policy for which service is required. Thus, data occupies an inherently critical place in the operations of an insurance company."[10]

Hence, in an industry whose main resource is information, information technology and its specific subset dealing with medicine, Medical Informatics is crucial, especially to the medical director whose ultimate responsibility is the quality of medical information from which strategic planning and day-to-day decisions are made.

Information Technology

The foundation of Medical Informatics is information technology (i.e., computers and computer systems) which will be briefly reviewed here. For a more technical coverage of the subject, the *Journal of the American College of Cardiology* has recently published a thorough review on information technology as it relates to Medical Informatics.[11]

Computers are machines which receive, process, store, and deliver information. To do this, a computer needs two components, hardware and software. Hardware, as the name implies, is the mechanical and electronic component. Software is the instructions for the hardware.[12]

Computer Hardware

An interesting analogy about hardware has been made by computer scientist Alan Kay, who said that computers are to computing as instruments are to music.[13] Hardware has structures for each of its four functions: input devices, the central processing unit (or CPU), memory, and output devices. Input devices accept information. The most familiar input device is the keyboard. Other input devices include the mouse (which allows information to be moved around a screen without using the keyboard), light pens (which can point directly to the screen to change information), optical scanners, and

devices for data entry directly from other machinery.[14] The CPU actually processes information. The size of the CPU determines the speed with which the computer works, and the amount of information which it can handle, sometimes referred to as the "computing power." Memory stores information. Depending upon the amount, this may be done by internal memory or may require an external data storage device such as magnetic tape, magnetic disk, or the new plastic compact disk (usually called a CD). One CD can hold over half a billion characters of data, equivalent to 275,000 pages of typed text.[15] Output devices deliver information to the user or another computer. The most common output device is the Video Display Terminal (VDT) which displays information as words or graphics. Other output devices include printers, voice simulation devices, and monitors.

Hardware is often classified by its physical size, its internal memory capacity, its computing power, and the number of simultaneous users. Microcomputers (also called micros, personal computers, or PCs), are generally small enough to fit on the top of a desk and have a single user. Their computing power and memory are limited to performing computational tasks for an individual or a small group. On the other end of the spectrum are mainframe computers. They generally require a climate-controlled room for themselves, have multiple simultaneous users, and have tremendous computing power. Minicomputers are those which fall in between. The distinctions between small minicomputers and microcomputers, as well as between large minicomputers and mainframe computers are sometimes difficult to make.[12]

Computer Software

Software is the instructions for the hardware. It is termed "software" because it takes a general machine (the hardware) and by changing its internal workings, converts it to a task-specific machine (the software).[16] Software can be classified into several basic categories: operating systems, programming languages, and application software.[12] The operating system coordinates the general flow of information within the computer. Returning to a music metaphor, the operating system is the instructions on how to play the instrument. There could be no computing without an operating system as one could not play music without knowing how to play an instrument.

A programming language insures that the information which the programmer wants to convey to the computer is the same as the information which the machine receives. Within the music metaphor, if the computer is the instrument, a programming language is writing music for that instrument. If the music is written properly, then anyone who knows how to play the instrument (i.e., has the correct operating system) can play the song correctly.

Application software refers to programs (sets of instructions) written to perform a specific task such as word processing, interpreting an ECG, or working with a spreadsheet. Each of these applications is like a separate "song" from all the "music" which the computer could be instructed to play.

Computer Systems

The previous discussion has dealt with the components of a single computer. Frequently, a computer is not used in isolation ("stand alone"), but is integrated into a larger system. Computer systems require another component of information technology called Telecommunications. This technology is designed to link computers to pass information. The telecommunication link may be as simple as connecting a microcomputer to a mainframe computer through telephone lines by a modem (a device that MOdulates and DEModulates electrical information). More complex technology is necessary to connect groups or networks of microcomputers (called a Local Area Network or LAN) or networking information among multiple microcomputers and mainframes.

Areas of Applications of Medical Informatics

Areas of patient care to which Medical Informatics has been applied include medical history taking, medical records, medical data base information retrieval, test performance, test result retrieval, decision support, patient monitoring, medical education, quality assurance and utilization review, medical research, and medical office and financial management. Each will be briefly reviewed with special emphasis on the aspects most useful to medical directors (Table 001K1-1).

TABLE 001K1-1

Areas of Applications of Medical Informatics

1. Medical History Taking
2. Medical Records
3. Medical Data Base Information Retrieval
4. Test Performance
5. Test Result Retrieval
6. Decision Support
7. Patient Monitoring
8. Medical Education
9. Quality Assurance and Utilization Review
10. Medical Research
11. Financial Management
12. Office Management
13. Word Processing
14. Electronic Mail

Medical History Taking

Projects to program a computer to take a medical history have been in existence since the early 1960s.[18] Most of these early efforts were directed toward histories in subspecialty areas such as allergy and neurology. Some of the programs had limited success.[19] Since that time, research has been directed toward programs to take a full medical history. Currently, in the Fourth Annual Medical Software Buyer's Guide in *M.D. Computing* (an official journal of the American Association for Medical Systems and Information) several programs are listed as available for medical history taking.[20] However, definitive studies demonstrating the accuracy and efficacy of medical history programs are not presently available.

There is one area of computerized history taking of special interest to medical directors: computerized insurance applications. This would make available to the field programs to capture the entire application, including the medical history, and transmit it to the home office for initial processing to decrease turn-around time. This could be seen as a strategic tool. As Gary Wilson, a senior systems analyst for Massachusetts Mutual stated for a *Best's Review* article on new technology, "Right now, every time you have to go back to the customer, you lower the probability that you are going to close the sale. Whereas, if you bring all the information you need to one sitting, and a laptop (portable microcomputer) can help you do that, then I think there are some long term advantages."[21] Such a scenario is developing today. For example, within the same article, Robert Brumm, director of systems consulting for Aid Association for Lutherans (AAL), stated that half of AAL's sales force is currently equipped with laptops.[21]

Medical Records

For clinicians as well as for medical directors, the traditional paper-based medical record is the major source of medical information on an individual. However, its disorganization and nonstandard format make it a poor source of continually changing information.

Because of its limitations, the paper system has been held directly responsible for many failures in the quality of medical care delivered, especially in the area of medication administration.[22]

Computerized medical record systems have the advantage of not being held to the sequence and organization used in recording the data, and not being contained in one fixed physical form. Therefore, computerized medical information can be available to multiple users at one time and can be organized in any sequence or format to fit the needs of the users.[23] Several studies have suggested that by resolving these problems, the quality of medical care can be improved by computerized medical record systems.[24,25]

Although the direct patient care aspect of computerized medical records may not be beneficial to insurance medical directors, these systems would markedly improve the access and quality of medical information on individuals for claims, underwriting, quality assessment, and utilization review.

Medical Data Base Information Retrieval

Computerized retrieval of information from large data bases, especially the medical literature, is an area of Medical Informatics which has been rapidly expanding. It is currently changing the way in which the medical community accesses information.[26]

The National Library of Medicine's data base of over five million citations and abstracts can be accessed with a microcomputer, a modem, a printer, and the appropriate software. This can be accomplished in several ways. Existing hardware can be adapted by subscribing to the appropriate software service and connecting by modem to the National Library of Medicine's computer or all the necessary equipment can be leased from a software vendor. The subject to be researched is input and the abstracts from the appropriate articles will be extracted from the National Library of Medicine's data bank. The different software packages available to do this vary in their expense and ease of use. They have been reviewed recently in the *Annals of Internal Medicine*.[27]

Services also are available in which the full text of articles, rather than just the abstracts, are retrievable. With these data bases, although more than the abstract is available, the number of journals in the data base is not as great as that available from the National Library of Medicine.[28]

There are anecdotes of the utility of these services to clinicians, including a letter to the *New England Journal of Medicine* in which a surgeon relates consulting a computer for information in the middle of a procedure because of a surprise finding on a frozen section from a biopsy of an abdominal mass.[29]

On a larger scale, these systems are generally utilized once implemented. In a study of computer use at the Beth Israel Hospital in Boston, during a one week period, 752 hospital personnel performed 1,423 bibliographic searches.[30] More importantly, these systems are believed to be capable of supplying many of the information needs of medical practitioners. In a national survey, 90% of responding physicians thought a computer data base would improve their access to information in the literature, and 85% thought it would improve their overall practice of medicine.[31]

As well as the data base of the medical literature, there are other specific medical data bases available which can be searched by computer. These include information on AIDS (AIDS Update), drug evaluations (AMA/NED Drug Evaluation), epidemiology (CDC Information Service), Medicare (Medicare Eligibility Database), oncology (the National Institute of Health's Physician Data Query [PDR]), rare diseases (the Rare Disease Database), and other topics.[25]

This ability to search medical data bases by computer is an essential tool for insurance medical directors seeking information for underwriting, claims, technology assessment, quality assurance, utilization review, or other research.

Test Performance

Prior to the 1950s most laboratory procedures were performed manually. By the 1960s automated processes were being coupled with computers to increase efficiency in production and data reporting. The sophistication of computerized laboratory medicine has continued to increase and incorporate new areas of testing such as immunology and medical genetics.[32] Furthermore, computerization is expanding into other areas of test performance, especially diagnostic imaging.

In imaging, the first major step came with the advent of computerized tomographic scanning. This trend has continued such that computers are now used routinely in imaging, most significantly in cardiovascular imaging including echocardiography, digital angiography, radionuclide imaging, positron emission tomography, and nuclear magnetic resonance imaging.[33] Medical directors must become familiar with these advances as information to review for underwriting becomes more complex and they are called upon to do technology assessment, quality assurance work, and utilization review.

Test Result Retrieval

Computerized retrieval is a way to improve access of test results. A study done to examine the usage of a system in a hospital setting showed that 818 patient care providers used a common registry of 539,000 patients to access laboratory data over 16,000 times in a one-week period. Further, of 545 hospital workers polled, 81% said that the computer system made their work more accurate, and 83% said that it made their work quicker.[30]

Information on improving physician performance with a retrieval system is limited but does suggest the approach is helpful. At the Regenstreif Health Center in Indianapolis, a controlled trial was undertaken to determine the effect of computerized test result retrieval on outpatient test ordering. Presenting physicians with previous test results reduced the ordering of tests by 13%. This trend disappeared when computer terminals were turned off.[34] The advantages of this approach appear to be speed of access of information, the ability to flag abnormal results, and tracking test results to reveal trends.

Another method to increase access to test results is Telepathology. This is practicing pathology at a distance by visualizing an image on a video monitor rather than viewing a specimen directly through a microscope. The advantages of Telepathology are rapid access to the services of a remote pathologist and immediate long-distance consultations among pathologists.[35] Teleradiology utilizes the same technology in a similar methodology for diagnostic imaging.[36]

Some commercial laboratories offer medical directors computerized test result retrieval with the flagging of abnormal results by direct access from their mainframe computer. After information has been retrieved, it can be stored on data bases to track overall usage, trends, and for research. Telepathology and Teleradiology may become available to medical directors in the future to review specimens and images for underwriting or claims.

Decision Support

Computer systems are able to bring together an individual's clinical information, laboratory information, and information on the clinical condition from the medical literature as well as decision support software to assist in problem solving.

Shortliffe recently reviewed computer programs for decision support. In his article, he defines a medical decision-support system as any program designed to help health professionals make clinical decisions, and he differentiates three types of decision support tools: those for information management, those for focusing attention, and those for patient specific consultation.[37] The first two of these have been discussed above. The third involves programs designed to assist in the work-up, diagnosis and/or management of a patient. These programs may be created with traditional programming using statistical or decision analysis techniques, or with the new technology of expert systems.

Expert systems (also called knowledge-based systems) are a development of artificial intelligence (AI), the branch of computer science which deals with creating programs to perform tasks which if done by a person would require intelligence.[12]

Expert systems are programs designed to solve problems in a particular area (called a domain) using factual and procedural knowledge derived from human experts, in a nonprocedural way (i.e., not programmed in a step by step fashion) to simulate human reasoning. These systems are different than conventional programs in that they can function with a variety of different initial data (they are said to be "data driven"); and they can handle uncertain and incomplete information because of programmed "rules of thumb" (heuristics).[12] They have three major components; the knowledge base, the inference engine, and the user interface. The knowledge base contains the "book knowledge" on the domain. The inference engine contains the "know how" to actually use the "book knowledge" to solve problems. The user interface allows the person using the system (the user) to interact with the expert system.

Medical expert systems have been written to interpret pulmonary function tests;[38] solve clinical pathological conferences in internal medicine;[39] determine appropriate chemotherapy for certain cancers;[40] diagnose rheumatological disease;[41] and evaluate patients with suspected transient ischemic attacks.[42]

Although the performance of some of these systems has been excellent, as discussed in a recent editorial in the *New England Journal of Medicine*, more development is necessary before such systems are used routinely in clinical medicine.[43]

However, within the insurance industry, expert system development has been more successful. The most useful area for expert systems of interest to insurance medical directors has been underwriting where currently expert systems can perform screening functions but are also capable of decision assistance in medical underwriting. A system to do actual case underwriting of complex medical impairments has already been developed and is being implemented in some companies. Similar systems will soon be available for claims evaluation as well.

Patient Monitoring

Computers can be used to monitor direct patient information in acutely ill patients. Intensive Care Units utilize monitoring equipment which can be connected to computers which monitor, store, and display physiological data such as arrhythmias, blood pressure, cardiac output, and other hemodynamic parameters. Further, through telecommunications, these monitoring computers can be linked with laboratory retrieval systems, data bases of clinical and pharmacological information, and decision support systems to consolidate information and assist in patient management.[44]

The merging of information technology with advances in biotechnology is leading to even more sophisticated monitor devices called biosensors. These are a new class of medical devices for real-time, on-line quantitative biochemical monitoring of patients. They utilize a biological molecule (e.g.,antibody, enzyme, or receptor) as a sensing or signal-transducing element in a microelectronic system to monitor physiological changes.[45] At this time, biosensor technology is still emerging although computer monitoring of arrhythmias and hemodynamic parameters is done routinely in Critical Care Units. Even though the direct patient care aspects of computerized monitoring devices do not impact upon the daily practice of medical directors, they must maintain a current familiarity with the technology for effective claims and utilization review.

Medical Education

Medical Informatics can be applied to medical education on several levels. Computer-based training can be a useful tool in undergraduate medical education because it combines audio-visuals with programmed logic and user interactions to individualize the educational experience. Also, computers can be used for more sophisticated testing by tracing decision-making. Currently, the National Board of Medical Examiners has a project utilizing a computer-based testing system to grade residents on thought processes to replace the patient management problems in Part III of the National Medical Boards by 1989.[46]

Computers are also being seen as an integral part of continuing medical education for practicing physicians. Relevant, practice-linked continuing medical education programs can be developed by allowing better analysis of the educational needs of practitioners as well as increasing access to educational material and introducing new formats of instruction.[47] In insurance medicine, computers can help medical directors with their own continuing medical education and enhance the educational process of underwriters and claims personnel.

Quality Assurance and Utilization Review

Computers can be useful in the process of quality assurance or utilization review by improving access to information; performing statistical correlations, and, in the future, actually assessing standards of care and performing the utilization review with expert systems. At this time, however, only the initial steps can be taken by computers. There is suggestive information from several studies that computer-assisted quality assurance systems can improve short term health outcomes, decrease medical costs, and improve physician documentation.[48,49] It will have to be seen with more extensive studies if this proves to be universally true. If so, as the need to control costs continues and insurance companies play a more important role in this process, medical directors will be called upon for control and support of these systems.

Medical Research

Because of their ability to handle massive amounts of data, computers have become indispensable tools for medical research. Large multicenter studies are impossible without data banks, telecommunication, and computing facilities. As well as managing data bases and performing statistical analysis, computers are doing "re-cord linkage" by combining different types of data bases such as treatment data bases and cancer registries to develop new perspectives on data.[50] Some researchers even believe that computers, data base management techniques, and artificial intelligence approaches will actually help develop new theories in biology and medicine.[51]

This development of new data perspectives by computer analysis has been done with insurance claims data bases. Two recent articles have appeared concerning the use of claims information for medical research. One examined claims data to evaluate health care outcomes,[52] while the other discussed the use of claims data to set health promotion goals.[53] There are many other possible uses of these data bases with which medical directors need to be familiar in order to maximize their contribution to their companies.

Financial Management, Office Management, Word Processing, and Electronic Mail

The use of computers for financial management, office management, word processing and electronic mail in medical settings are areas which involve the use of the computer more as a general business tool rather than as a specific medical tool. Such applications are becoming very commonplace in patient care settings such as hospitals and physician's offices.[25]

An area of specific interest to medical directors is networking the financial management systems of providers to the claims processing of the insurance companies to ease processing of claims and decrease turn around time. Systems to do this are available today.[54] In the future, accessing medical information for underwriting may be possible in a similar fashion.

Integration of Medical Informatics with Other Information Systems

Within the hospital and other patient care environments, even though many of the applications discussed above could be run on isolated personal computers, there are those who feel that the applications of Medical Informatics should not be "stand alone" applications, but rather, should be integrated into the larger medical information management systems to insure that the medical as well as administrative aspects of these systems are well developed.[55]

Further, as discussed at the College of American Pathologists Foundation Conference on new technology in January 1987, physicians should not be passive observers of this process of insuring patient-centered rather than financially-centered medical informations systems. There is an increasing recognition of the need for physician-level medical information specialists to serve as medical institution chief information officers (medical

CIO's) assuming responsibility for collecting, maintaining, and processing patient care-related data.[22]

This is even more important in the insurance industry. As discussed above, because of the importance of data in the insurance industry, especially medical data, medical directors must become more aware of Medical Informatics and its role in information systems. With important new medical issues like AIDS and its impact upon insurance, where medical information strongly affects business, medical directors must become medical CIO's to coordinate the use of medical knowledge and Medical Informatics with corporate information systems for the company's strategic advantage.

This is not the first time this message has been conveyed to medical directors. Dr. Warren Kleinsasser delivered a similar message in a recent essay on the future of Insurance Medicine,

> "The new breed of insurance medical specialist must also have a working relationship with computerization. This will evolve both from the development of computerized underwriting, issues, and claims processes, and from the need to develop quickly the support information required to underwrite new and changing disorders and diseases and to aid in claims evaluations . . . Familiarity with computers may also enable the medical director to take relevant information from these searches and translate it quickly, via tailor-made computer programs into relevant actuarial data. This capability should have a significant impact on one's company's abilities to function in an era of increasing pricing competition in which the realistic pricing of substandard or rated business may play a pivotal role in company profitability."[56]

REFERENCES

1. A. C. Doyle, "The Copper Beeches," *The Adventures of Sherlock Holmes* (New York, Harper & Brothers, 1892).

2. D. G. Covell, G. C. Uman , P. R. Manning, "Information Needs in Office Practice: Are They Being Met?" *Ann. Intern. Med.,* 103 (1985): 596-99.

3. D. L. Sackett, R. B. Haynes, P. Tugwell, "How to read a Clinical Journal," *Clinical Epidemiology: A Basic Science for Clinical Medicine* (Boston, Little Brown and Company, 1985), pp. 285-319.

4. F. W. McFarlan, J. L. McKenney, *Corporate Information Systems Management: The Issues Facing Senior Executives* (Homewood, IL, R. D. Irwin, 1983).

5. J. R. Beck, "Who Takes Lead in Promoting Medical Informatics," *Comp. News Physic.,* (July 1986): C-10.

6. J. Naisbitt, *Megatrends: Ten New Directions Transforming Our Lives* (New York, Warner Books, 1984).

7. D. A. B. Lindberg, "Medical Informatics and Computers In Medicine," *JAMA,* 256 (1986): 2120-22.

8. E. A. Geiser, D. J. Skorton, eds., "Seminar on Computer Applications for the Cardiologist, Introduction," *J. Am. Coll. Cardiol.,* 8 (1986): 930-32.

9. G. N. Burrow, "Book Reviews," *N. Engl. J. Med.,* 317 (1987): 987-88.

10. C. H. Cissley, *Systems and Data Processing in Insurance Companies,* Revised Edition (Atlanta, GA, FLMI Insurance Education Program, Life Management Institute, LOMA 1, 1982).

11. J. R. Cox, Jr., C. Zeelenberg, "Computer Technology: State of the Art and Future Trends," *J. Am. Coll. Cardiol.,* 9 (1987): 204-14.

12. M. Williamson, *Artificial Intelligence for Microcomputers* (New York, Brady Communications Company, Inc., 1986).

13. A. Kay, "Computer Software," *Sci. Am.,* 251 (1984): 53.

14. F. M. Mims, III, ed., *Consumers Guide: Easy to Understand Guide to Home Computers* (USA Publications International, 1982).

15. R. K. Wertz, "CD-ROM, A New Advance in Medical Information Retrieval," *JAMA,* 256 (1986): 3376-78.

16. L. G. Tesler, "Programming Languages," *Sci. Am.,* 251 (1984): 70-78.

17. W. S. Davis, *Computers and Business Information Processing* (Reading, MA, Addison-Wesley Publishing Company, 1981).

18. W. V. Slack, "A History of Computerized Medical Interviews," *MD Comp.,* 1 (1984): 52-59.

19. D. S. Bana, A. Leviton, W. V. Slack, D. E. Geer, J. R. Graham, "Use of a Computerized Data Base in a Headache Clinic," *Headache,* 21 (1981): 72-74.

20. R. A. Polacsek, "The Fourth Annual Medical Software Buyer's Guide," *MD Comp.,* 4 (1987): 23-135.

21. B. T. Benham, "The Promise of Technology," *Best's Rev.,* 88 (1987): 40-46.

22. R. A. Korpman, "Using the Computer to Optimize Human Performance in Health Care Delivery," *Arch. Pathol. Lab. Med.,* 111 (1987): 637-45.

23. G. O. Barnett, "The Application of Computer-Based Medical-Record Systems in Ambulatory Practice," *N. Engl. J. Med.,* 310 (1984): 1643-50.

24. Q. E. Whiting-O'Keefe, D. W. Simborg, W. V. Epstein, A. Warger, "A Computerized Summary Medical Record System Can Provide More Information Than the Standard Medical Record," *JAMA,* 254 (1985): 1185-92.

25. S. Ridgway, "Computers Leap Beyond Billing to Patient Care," *Med. World News,* 22 (1987): 30-40.

26. J. Zylke, "Medical Libraries Undergoing Dramatic Changes (Medical News)," *JAMA,* 258 (1987): 3216.

27. R. B. Haynes, K. A. McKibbon, D. Fitzgerald, G. H. Guyatt, C. J. Walker, D. L. Sackett, "How to Keep Up With the Medical Literature: V. Access by Personal Computer to the Medical Literature," *Ann. Intern. Med.,* 105 (1986): 810-24.

28. M. F. Collen, C. D. Flagle, "Full-Text Medical Literature Retrieval by Computer," *JAMA,* 254 (1985): 2768-74.

29. N. Sohon, R. D. Robbins, "Computer-Assisted Surgery (Letter)," *N. Engl. J. Med.,* 312 (1985): 924.

30. H. L. Bleich, R. F. Beckley, G. L. Horowitz, et al., "Clinical Computing in a Teaching Hospital," *N. Engl. J. Med.,* 312 (1985): 756-64.

31. J. Singer, H. S. Sacks, F. Lucente, et al., "Physician's Attitudes Toward Applications of Computer Data Base Systems," *JAMA,* 249 (1983): 1610-14.

32. W. W. McLendon, "Technological Revolutions in Modern Pathology and Laboratory Medicine," *Arch. Pathol. Lab. Med.,* 111 (1987): 581-83.

33. S. M. Collins, D. J. Skorton, "Computers in Cardiac Imaging," *J. Am. Coll. Cardiol.,* 9 (1987): 669-77.

34. W. M. Tierney, C. J. McDonald, D. K. Martin, S. L. Hui, M. P. Rogers, "Computerized Display of Past Test Results," *Ann. Intern. Med.,* 107 (1987): 569-74.

35. R. S. Weinstein, K. J. Bloom, L. S. Rozek, "Telepathology and the Networking of Pathology Diagnostic Services," *Arch. Pathol. Lab. Med.,* 111 (1987): 646-52.

36. J. N. Gitlin, "Teleradiology," *Radiol. Clin. North Am.,* 24 (1986): 55-68.

37. E. H. Shortliffe, "Computer Programs to Support Clinical Decision Making," *JAMA,* 258 (1987): 61-66.

38. J. S. Aikins, J. C. Kunz, E. H. Shortliffe, R. J. Fallat, "PUFF, An Expert System for Interpretation of Pulmonary Function Data," *Comput. Biomed. Res.,* 16 (1983): 199-208.

39. R. A. Miller, H. E. Pople, Jr., J. D. Myers, "INTERNIST-I, An Experimental Computer-Based Diagnostic Consultant for General Internal Medicine," *N. Engl. J. Med.,* 307 (1982): 468-76.

40. D. H. Hickman, E. H. Shortliffe, M. S. Bischoff, A. C. Scott, C. D. Jacobs, "The Treatment Advice of a Cancer Chemotherapy Protocol Advisor," *Ann. Intern. Med.,* 103 (1985): 928-36.

41. L. C. Kingsland, III, D. A. B. Lindberg, G. C. Sharp, "Anatomy of a Knowledge-Based Consultant System: AI/RHEUM.," *MD Comp.,* 3 (1986): 18-26.

42. J. A. Reggia, D. R. Tabb, T. R. Price, M. Banko, R. Hebel, "Computer-Aided Assessment of Transient Ischemic Attacks," *Arch. Neurol.,* 41 (1984): 1248-54.

43. W. B. Schwartz, R. S. Patil, P. Szolovits, "Artificial Intelligence in Medicine: Where Do We Stand? (Editorial)," *N. Engl. J. Med.,* 316 (1987): 685-88.

44. R. M. Gardner, B. J. West, T. A. Pryor, K. G. Larson, H. R. Warner, T. P. Clemmer, J. F. Orme, Jr., "Computer-Based ICU Data Acquistion as an Aid to Clinical Decision-Making," *Crit. Care Med.,* 10 (1982): 823-30.

45. K. W. Hunter, Jr., "Technological Advances in Bedside Monitoring: Biosensors," *Arch. Pathol. Lab. Med.,* 111 (1987): 633-36.

46. C. A. Hinz, "Computer Tests Track Decisions in Making," *Am. Med. News,* 6 (March): 1.

47. P. R. Manning, D. W. Petit, "The Past, Present, and Future of Continuing Medical Education," *JAMA,* 258 (1987): 3542-46.

48. M. Lenauer, B. Posner, R. K. Stone, J. Hughes, R. B. Halpern, J. O'Brien, "Effects of the Pediatric Protocol System on Ambulatory Care in New York City Municipal Hospitals (Abstract)," *Med. Decis. Making,* 6 (1986): 267.

49. R. B. Haynes, C. J. Walker, "Computer-Aided Quality Assurance," *Arch. Intern. Med.,* 147 (1987): 1297-1301.

50. M. L. Johnson, "Record Linkage," *Arch. Dermatol.,* 122 (1986): 1383-84.

51. H. J. Morowitz, "Past, Present, Future," *Hosp. Prac.,* 22 (1987): 209-13.

52. J. E. Wennberg, N. Roos, L. Sola, A. Schori, R. Jaffe, "Use of Claims Data Systems to Evaluate Health Care Outcomes," *JAMA,* 257 (1987): 933-36.

53. T. M. Wicker, M. Samuelson, "Using Claims Data to Set Health Promotion Goals," *Bus. and Health,* 4 (1987): 28-31.

54. H. Meyer, "Electronic Processing: New System Speeds Up Bill Collections," *Am. Med. News,* 6 (March 1987): 10.

55. B. A. Friedman, J. B. Martin, "Hospital Information Systems: The Physician's Role," *JAMA,* 257 (1987): 1792.

56. W. L. Kleinsasser, "Insurance Medicine — The Future," *J. Ins. Med.,* 17 (1986): 8-10.

THE EVALUATION OF ABNORMAL LABORATORY RESULTS

Arthur W. DeTore, M.D.

"You can . . . never foretell what any one man will do, but you can say with precision what an average number will be up to. Individuals vary, but percentages remain constant."[1]

Sherlock Holmes was describing a situation with which Medical Directors must deal on a daily basis. Ultimately, the job of the Medical Director is to assist in the risk classification process; i.e., "foretelling" into what risk group or "average number" an individual should be assigned for mortality. In order to do this, the Medical Director must understand the statistical principles underlying standard mortality and then develop a consistent approach to determining an individual's increase in mortality.

Once a medical impairment has been identified in an individual, to classify the risk, the impairment can be conceptually categorized as one that is correlated with a single pathological entity such as cystic fibrosis or one that represents an abnormality such as elevated liver enzymes which may be caused by a number of underlying pathological conditions.

Determining appropriate ratings for the first type of impairment is generally straightforward (though not always easy). If studies of insured populations with the impairment exist, then the mortality of those with the impairment can be compared to the mortality of a standard insured population to determine the degree of substandard mortality. If no insurance mortality studies exist, then studies from the medical literature may be found and the mortality methodology can be applied.[2] Once the assumed mortality is adjusted for an appropriate mortality benchmark, ratings can be determined. If there are no studies because of the rarity of the disease, then experience with a more common impairment with a similar pathophysiology may be chosen to make a reasonable "guesstimate" by analogy. For many impairments of this type, the background research has been done and is presented in underwriting manuals. The task then becomes matching the proposed insured's characteristics to those of the appropriate section of the manual to determine the ratings.

With the second type of impairment, the situation is more complex because the underlying pathological condition causing the abnormality is not known. In some cases, such as certain electrocardiographic findings (which may be normal variants or caused by cardiac disease), there are adequate insurance studies on those isolated abnormalities (e.g., minor T wave changes) to be able to determine a rating.[2] If no studies of insured lives exist, it is unusual to find a study from the medical literature to analyze because most medical studies look at specific diseases and not isolated abnormalities.

If there are no clinical or insurance mortality studies available on a given abnormality, such as an isolated elevated Gamma-Glutamyl Transpeptidase (GGTP) result, then Medical Directors must have an approach to analyze these abnormalities. Although this analysis may be used for physical exam findings (e.g., rhonchi) or findings on paraclinical data (e.g., X-ray abnormalities), the evaluation of abnormal laboratory results will be the main topic of this discussion.

The approach requires answers to several questions:

1. Is the result abnormal?
2. What is the significance of the abnormality?
3. What should be done about the abnormality?

Although "abnormal" can be defined in many ways, the initial consideration is if the result lies outside the "normal range" for the laboratory performing the test. The reference value of normal that accompanies most laboratory tests is the range of test results within two standard deviations around the mean test value in a population without disease.[3]

This definition has limitations because it assumes that laboratory values follow a "normal" or Gaussian distribution. Although this assumption is generally not valid, using the "normal range" does serve as a reasonable starting point.[4] If the result falls outside these limits then the Medical Director must proceed to answer the next two questions.

This involves examining the specific test on multiple levels:

1. Analytic level
2. Diagnostic level
3. Operational level
4. Decision Making level[5]

Source: A. W. DeTore, "The Evaluation of Abnormal Laboratory Results," *J. Ins. Med.*, 20, no. 2 (1988): 5-9. Reproduced with permission of author and publisher.

The analytic level is concerned with the technical factors of the test's performance. On the analytic level, two variables are important, precision and accuracy. They determine the reliability of the number. Precision refers to the agreement between repeated measurements performed in the same way. It measures test reproducibility so that precise tests have little variation if measurement of the same sample is repeated. Accuracy of a test represents agreement between the measured quantity and the true value.[6]

Imprecision is caused by random error. This may arise from small changes in procedure; innate diurnal changes in metabolism; or age, sex, and race differences. Inaccuracy is caused by systematic error, i.e., error that can be attributed to a specific etiology such as the laboratory instrumentation, reagents, specimen labeling, or interfering substances. A laboratory test must be precise to be accurate. However, accuracy is not required for precision, that is, the same result may be obtained on repeated testing, but have no relationship to the true value. These types of errors are additive and produce the overall analytic variability.[7]

Further, there is a "multiplier effect" if many tests are done at one time. Independently, each test has a 95% chance of being normal (this is the range of the mean and 2 standard deviations). For n number of tests the probability that a completely normal person will have all normal results on all n tests is the probability of one test being normal times the probability of the next text being normal, i.e., 0.95 times 0.95 n times or 0.95 to the nth power. This means that if there are 20 tests there is a 36% probability that all tests will be normal.[8]

To help decide if an abnormal result is due to analytic variability, the test must be examined on the diagnostic and operational levels. The diagnostic aspects of a test are its sensitivity and specificity. The sensitivity is the likelihood of a positive test result in a person with a disease. The specificity of a test is the likelihood of a negative test result in a person without disease.[9] These can only be determined if the test has been subjected to an independent "blind" comparison with a "gold standard" of diagnosis.[4] Further, the population in which the test has been evaluated must be explicitly defined to avoid problems of spectrum bias in which the reference population is different (e.g., hospitalized patients) than the population in which the test is being performed (e.g., ambulatory population).[10]

Sensitivity and specificity are excellent indices of the diagnostic aspects of a test. Likelihood ratios (sensitivity/1–specificity) are another useful index. They express the odds (probability of event/1–probability of event) that a given level of diagnostic test result would be expected in a person with the underlying disease. For example, the

sensitivity of an abnormal stress test (one with greater than 1 mm. of ST depression) indicating greater than 70% narrowing of at least one coronary artery is often given as about 65%. The likelihood ratio of an abnormal stress test with 1-1.49 mm. of ST depression is 2.1 to 1, which means that these results are 2.1 times more likely to come from people with coronary artery disease than from people without coronary artery disease. The likelihood ratio of a test with greater than 2.5 mm. ST depression is 39 to 1.[11]

Although the diagnostic analysis of test results adds to the understanding of interpreting abnormalities because it tells how well the test performs in the presence or absence of disease (i.e., how often the person with disease will have a positive test and how often the person without disease will have a negative test), it really only deals with the situation in which there is already knowledge of the presence or absence of the underlying disease. Because the Medical Director has only an abnormal test result with which to deal, the test must next be examined on the operational level which tells how often a person with a positive test has disease and how often a person with a negative test does not have disease.

On the operational level, two indices are important, the predictive value positive and the predictive value negative. The predictive value positive is the probability of a disease being present if a test result is positive. The predictive value negative is the probability of a disease being absent if a test result is negative.[9] These are calculated from the sensitivity and specificity (or the likelihood ratios) of the test, the prevalence of the disease, and the prevalence of the test abnormality. This can be determined by using Bayes' theorem.[12]

Bayes' theorem states that the probability of a disease, given an abnormal test result, is equal to the probability of the test being abnormal in the diseased population, multiplied by the prevalence of the disease divided by the prevalence of abnormal test results in the normal and diseased populations. One formula for the predictive value positive is:

$$\frac{(\text{prevalence}) \times (\text{sensitivity})}{(\text{prevalence}) \times (\text{sensitivity}) + (1-\text{prevalence}) \times (1-\text{specificity})}[13]$$

The predictive value negative has a corresponding formula. There are several other ways of expressing formulas for Bayes' theorem including calculations which can be done with likelihood ratios.[4]

Once the test has been examined on the operational level and the predictive value positive and negative have been calculated using Bayes' theorem, the Medical Director has an idea of the significance of the abnormality, i.e., the probability that the test result indicates disease and is not due to analytic variability or is otherwise falsely positive. However, for risk classification, the final question, "What should be done about the abnormality?" must be answered by working on the decision making level. This involves the Medical Director determining and explicitly weighing the consequences of true positive and negative results versus false positive and negative results in terms of mortality and cost. An explicit cost-benefit analysis needs to be done. Decision Analysis, a quantitative technique for making decisions about complex problems in situations of uncertainty, is an effective way to do this.[14]

Here, an example case will be developed to demonstrate the entire process by determining the best course of action to take in a case with an isolated laboratory abnormality. The underwriter presents to the Medical Director a case for $100,000 on a 55-year-old male. There are no problems with the financial underwriting, inspection report, or examination. He is without complaints, and has no known history of alcohol abuse, alcoholism, or liver disease. The only abnormality is a Gamma-Glutamyl Transpeptidase (GGTP) result of 210 U/L on a routine blood chemistry profile.

As discussed above, the first question, "Is the result abnormal?" must be answered. A recent reference text for laboratory medicine lists the "normal range" for GGTP for adult males to be 9-69 units/L.[15] Further, the reference laboratory at which the test was performed (Home Office Reference Laboratory) lists 2-65 U/L as their "usual clinical range." Since the result falls outside that range, it can be considered "abnormal" and the other questions need to be answered.

Next, "What is the significance of the abnormality?" Reviewing the test on the various levels, it can be seen that the analytical aspects of the GGTP have been well studied.[16] It is a test with a well-defined conventional methodology which can be readily performed in most laboratories.

On a diagnostic level, what is its sensitivity and specificity? To answer this, the Medical Director must decide which disease is being considered. In this example, it will be assumed that liver disease due to alcohol is the important underlying disorder. The sensitivity of GGTP for alcoholic liver disease (define against the "gold standard" of liver biopsy) was 87.7%.[17] In that study the population was hospitalized patients which may have led to some spectrum bias. However, in another study from an ambulatory population with alcoholic liver disease (which also used liver biopsy as the "gold standard") the sensitivity was 52% using the cutoff value of 200 U/L. The specificity of GGTP was found to be 85%.[18]

Operationally, as stated above, to calculate the predictive value positive with Bayes' theorem, the prevalence of alcoholic liver disease needs to be known. The National Institute on Alcohol Abuse and Alcoholism estimates that 13% of the adult population (21% of the males) is composed of heavy drinkers — defined as drinking more than 60 drinks a month.[19] However, only about 10% of the population reach the stage of alcohol abuse — defined as medical, social, and occupational complications caused by high (greater than seven drinks a day) alcohol intake.[20] Liver biopsy studies correlated with alcohol consumption has demonstrated that 60% of people ingesting this much alcohol will have alcoholic liver disease.[21] For the insured population who drinks enough to be at risk for liver disease, this estimate will be decreased to 5%. (Since the prevalence of alcoholic liver disease in the insured population is not known, it is estimated to be 5%. The reasonableness of this estimate will be tested later.)

Using these numbers in the formula for Bayes' theorem given above, the predictive value of the GGTP for alcoholic liver disease is 15.4% [(0.05) x(0.52)/(0.05) x(0.52)+(0.95)x(0.15)]. That is, 15.4% of those with an elevated GGTP will have alcoholic liver disease (which conversely means that 84.6% of those with an elevated GGTP will not have alcoholic liver disease).

Now, since the significance of the abnormality is known, as asked above, "What should be done about the abnormality?" According to the previous analysis, there is only a 15.4% chance that the proposed insured has alcoholic liver disease. How can that information be used to decide what should be done with this application? The test must be examined on the decision making level using Decision Analysis. This involves five steps:

1. Determine the possible options and their consequences for decision making.
2. Determine the chance events and their probabilites within each option.
3. Quantify the results of each option.
4. Calculate the value of each option.
5. Determine the best option and the changes in the options with changes in the probabilities.[14]

To do this, the problem is dissected and then structured as a decision tree in which each branch looks at the choices and chance events which may occur. Each branch is then evaluated to determine the best option.

Here, there are three options: take the case standard (i.e., ignore the GGTP result assuming it is an analytic error or falsely positive because the predictive value is too low); rate the case because of the possibility of alcoholic liver disease; or decline the case because of the possibility of liver disease. These are the main branches of the tree. Each branch has different possible uncertain events which can be represented as further branches. If the case is taken standard, then the chance event is that

FIGURE 001K2-1

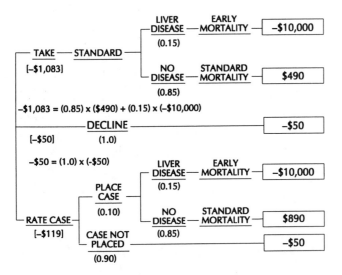

FIGURE 001K2-1

$$-\$119 = (0.9) \times (-\$50) + (0.1) \times [(0.85) \times (\$890) + (0.15) \times (-\$10,000)]$$

the elevated GGTP is due to alcoholic liver disease which will lead to early mortality. If the case is rated, then the chance events are the same as before, as well as the chance that a rated case will not be placed in an asymptomatic person. All this can be depicted in the decision tree. (See Fig. 001K2-1)

To determine the probabilities, some assumptions must be made. The main assumption is that the primary disease of concern is alcoholic liver disease. (There may be other diseases which cause the elevated GGTP, but for this analysis, they are considered of less importance.)

Further, what is the consequence of having alcoholic liver disease; i.e., what is the mortality (all causes) of drinking enough alcohol to cause liver disease? The 1983 Medical Impairment Study showed that for the impairment of alcohol abuse, the standard mortality was 199%, the highest mortality ratio for any standard risk category in the study! For the minimally and moderately substandard groups, the mortality ratios were 207% and 284% respectively.[22] Therefore, in the analysis, the mortality ratio for alcohol abuse will be estimated as 200%. (It could be argued that the mortality ratio of 200% is too low for those with alcohol abuse and liver disease. The reasonableness of this assumption will be examined later in the analysis.)

The last assumption for the analysis is that if the case is rated (table D) for the elevated GGTP, in an asymptomatic individual without an admitted history of alcohol abuse, there is only a one in ten chance that the case will be placed. (Once again, the reasonableness of this assumption will be examined also.)

Next, the explicit consequences for each option need to be determined. What is the consequence of early mortality on a $100,000 policy if the proposed insured does have liver disease? This can be estimated as a loss of $100,000 (the mortality cost "unanticipated" by premium revenue when a 55-year-old male with a mortality ratio of 200% is misclassified as a standard risk) (*personal communication*, J. Mast). The expected profit of a standard case would be about $490 for a standard case and $890 for a case rated table D (*personal communication,* D. Becker).

Each of these figures can be inserted into the tree and then by following a formula, $V = b \times (u3) + (1-b) \times [a \times (u2) + (1-a) \times (u1)]$, on each major branch, the value of each option can be calculated. (See Fig. 001K1-2) In Decision Analysis, this is called "folding back the tree." The calculations show that the first option, taking the case standard, has a value of −$1,083 (i.e., a loss of $1,083). The second option, declining the case has a value of −$50 (i.e., the loss of $50 to review the case). The third option, rating the case, has a value of −$119 (i.e., a loss of $119). (See Fig. 001K1-1) In this situation, as there is no way to make a profit since all the final values are negative, it is clear that the best option is to decline the case because this minimizes the loss.

FIGURE 001K2-2

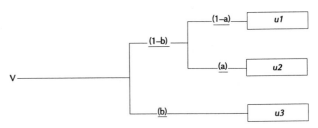

$$v = b \times (u3) + (1-b) \times [a \times (u2) + (1-a) \times u1]$$

To complete the Decision Analysis, the assumptions and probabilities need to be analyzed to see how much the decision would change if they were altered. This is called a sensitivity analysis because it determines how sensitive the decision is to the assumptions and probabilities. The results of the sensitivity analysis show that if the other assumptions are kept constant, the predictive value of the elevated GGTP would have to be less than 5% (i.e., only 5% of those with an elevated GGTP actually have liver disease) before it is advantageous to take the case standard! For this to happen, either the prevalence of heavy drinkers in the insured population would have to be less than 1.5%; or the specificity of the test would have to be less than 15%.

What about the assumption of the mortality ratio for an individual with a history of alcohol abuse and liver disease, is 200% reasonable (i.e., how much would the decision change with a different estimate)? Since there is a loss on all options when calculating with a mortality ratio of 200%, with a higher mortality ratio, the "unanticipated" mortality loss would be even greater. Therefore, the final decision to decline the case would stay the same. If the prevalence, sensitivity and specificity are kept the same, then a mortality ratio of greater than 150% would result in a loss.

Futher, if the chances of placing a rated policy are greater than one in ten, and are increased to a fifty-fifty chance (50%), then the value of the option to rate the case at table D would be a loss of $397. There could also be a greater chance of antiselection with an increased number of "asymptomatic" people accepting rated cases. So, declining the case would still be the best option.

Hence, for a wide range of values, the same decision holds, that is, the option which maximizes profitability (the best decision) for the case is to decline. In a competitive environment, there may be other considerations for the underwriter to make a "business decision" to "take the case" Standard (i.e., take a loss of $1,083). But the role of the Medical Director, as stated above, is to assist in the risk classification and not necessarily make the final decision.

In theory several more complex analyses could be done. The best cutoff to define an "elevated" GGTP level could be examined by using Receiver Operating Characteristic (ROC) curves which graph the tradeoffs of sensitivity and specificity for different cutoff levels.[14] A family of decision trees using a series of cutoffs with different likelihood ratios could be created. Other causes of elevated liver function tests (such as hepatitis or tumors) could be included as well as analyses for other liver function tests (e.g., SGOT). However, for the above case, they would not add substantially to the above analysis.

In summary, by answering several key questions and by approaching abnormal laboratory test results on the analytic, diagnostic, operational, and decision making levels using probability theory, Bayes' theorem, and Decision Analysis, Medical Directors can further assist underwriters in the evaluation of cases with isolated laboratory abnormalities. Although this methodology appears complex, with the improvements in information Technology, especially artificial intelligence, it can be programmed and distributed to underwriters and Medical Directors.[23]

[I am indebted to the members of the Medical, Underwriting Research and Development, and Actuarial Departments of Lincoln National Life Insurance Company, especially Jess Mast, for assistance.]

REFERENCES

1. A. C. Doyle, *The Sign of Four* (London, Ward Lock, 1890).

2. R. B. Singer, L. Levinson, eds., *Medical Risks: Patterns of Mortality and Survival* (Lexington, MA, Lexington Books, 1976).

3. J. S. Schwartz, "Understanding Laboratory Test Results," *Med. Clin. North Am.*, 71 (1987): 639-52.

4. D. L. Sackett, R. B. Haynes, P. Tugwell, "How to read a Clinical Journal," *Clinical Epidemiology: A Basic Science for Clinical Medicine* (Boston, Little Brown and Company, 1985), pp. 285-319.

5. J. B. McCabe, "Decision Making in Laboratory Test Studies," *Emerg. Med. Clin. North Am.*, 4 (1986): 1-14.

6. R. Robinson, *Clinical Chemistry and Automation: A Study in Laboratory Proficiency* (Baltimore, MD, Williams and Wilkins, 1971).

7. P. Rausmussen, "Use of the Laboratory in Patient Management," *Am. Fam. Prac.*, 35 (1987): 214-23.

8. R. D. Cebul, J. R. Beck, "Applications in Ambulatory Screening and Preadmission Testing of Adults," *Biochem. Profiles*, 106 (1987): 403-13.

9. H. C. Sox, "Probability Theory in the Use of Diagnostic Tests," *Ann. Intern. Med.*, 104 (1986): 60-66.

10. D. F. Ransohoff, A. R. Feinstein, "Problems of Spectrum and Bias in Evaluating the Efficacy of Diagnostic Tests," *N. Engl. J. Med.*, 299 (1978): 926-30.

11. G. A. Diamond, J. S. Forrester, "Analysis of Probability as an Aid in the Clinical Diagnosis of Coronary Artery Disease," *N. Engl. J. Med.*, 300 (1979): 1350-58.

12. T. Bayes, "An Essay Toward Solving a Problem in the Doctrine of Chances," *Philos. Trans. R. Soc. Lond.*, 53 (1763): 370-75.

13. R. H. Fletcher, S. W. Fletcher, E. H. Wagner, *Clinical Epidemiology: The Essentials* (Baltimore, MD, Williams and Wilkins, 1982).

14. M. C. Weinstein, H. V. Fineberg, *Clinical Decision Analysis* (Philadelphia, W. B. Saunders Company, 1980).

15. J. Wallach, *Interpretation of Diagnostic Tests: A Synopsis of Laboratory Medicine* (Boston, Little Brown and Company, 1986).

16. D. M. Goldberg, "Structural, Functional, and Clinical Aspects of Gamma-Glutamyltransferase. CRC Critical Reviews," *Clin. Lab. Sci.,* 12 (1980): 1-58.

17. A. J. Levi, D. M. Chalmers, "Recognition of Alcoholic Liver Disease in a District General Hospital," *Gut,* 19 (1978): 521-25.

18. J. Erickson, P. Staun Olsen, A. C. Thomsen, "Gamma-Glutamyltranspeptidase, Aspartate Aminotransferase, and Erythrocyte Mean Corpustular Volume as Indicators of Alcohol Consumption in Liver Disease," *Scand. J. Gastroenterol.,* 19 (1984): 813-19.

19. W. B. Clark, L. Midanik, "Alcohol Use and Alcohol Problems Among U.S. Adults: Results of the 1979 National Survey, in Alcohol Consumption and Related Problems," *Alcohol and Health Monograph 1* (Rockville, MD, National Institute on Alcohol Abuse and Alcoholism, 1982).

20. G. E. Vaillant, *The Natural History of Alcoholism* (Cambridge, MA, Harvard University Press, 1983).

21. W. K. Lelbach, "Leberschaden bei Chronischem Alcoholismus," *Acta. Hepatosplenol.,* 14 (1967): 9-39.

22. Medical Impairment Study Committee, "1983 Medical Impairment Study: Provisional Results," *J. Ins. Med.,* 14 (1983): 8-23.

23. A. W. DeTore, "Medical Informatics in Insurance Medicine: An Introduction to Computers for Insurance Medical Directors," *J. Ins. Med.,* 20, no.1 (1988): 3-9.

USE OF PROBABILITY THEORY TO EVALUATE COST EFFECTIVENESS OF LABORATORY TESTS IN INSURANCE MEDICINE

John R. Iacovino, M.D.

As technology advances, new laboratory tests are spawned to improve diagnostic efficiency. These tests are marketed to insurance companies by their laboratories which, on occasion, do not consider the problems unique to insurance testing. In order to respond to marketing pressures, the medical director must evaluate two factors. First, whether the new test, which is almost always developed for clinical use, is useful for screening populations where disease prevalence is low. An example is fructosamine. It has clinical utility, but what is its role in screening for glucose intolerance in a low prevalence population? Second, is the test cost effective? The evaluation of the latter factor will be the basis of this paper.

Our emphasis should not be on cost per test but cost per new individual correctly diagnosed and, most importantly in insurance medicine, accurately underwritten.

In addition to correctly underwritten cases, the medical director requires tools to evaluate the percentage of overrated and underrated cases as both will affect profitability of their company. Those overrated will not likely take their policies; those underrated will take their toll at claim time.

Figure 001K3-1 is a 2x2 table illustrating the possible underwriting results on testing a population with and without a disease.

Box (a) True positives — correctly underwritten cases
Box (d) True negatives — correctly underwritten cases
Box (c) False positives — overrated cases
Box (b) False negatives— underrated cases

The sensitivity (Sn) and specificity (Sp) of a test will yield the proportion of individuals in each of the four preceding underwriting groups.

Sensitivity (Sn) — the proportion of those diseased, who have a positive test.

$$\frac{a}{a+b}$$

FIGURE 001K3-1
2x2 table illustrating underwriting possibilities

	Disease	
	Present	**Absent**
Positive **Test** **Negative**	Number of individuals diseased and who have a positive test (a)	Number of individuals without disease who have a positive test (c)
	Number of individuals diseased and who have a negative test (b)	Number of individuals without a disease who have a negative test (d)

Specificity (Sp) — the proportion of those disease-free, who have a negative test.

$$\frac{d}{c+d}$$

Sn and Sp are independent of the prevalence of disease in a population; they are a measure of the test itself. However, when one wishes to calculate the number of individuals in a tested group, disease prevalence must be considered.

Another way to evaluate a test is the use of predictive values. The proportion and, if prevalence is considered, the number of correctly underwritten individuals can be predicted through their use.

Positive Predictive Value (PPV) — the proportion of those with a positive test who are diseased.

$$\frac{a}{a+c}$$

Negative Predictive Value (NPV) — the proportion of those with a negative test who are disease-free.

$$\frac{d}{b+d}$$

Several laboratories offer to reflex various apolipoproteins from predetermined levels of HDL and cholesterol or their ratio. The medical director must decide: a) Is this cost effective? and b) What will be the underwriting implication? To answer these, facts must be blended with assumptions. The facts are Sn, Sp and cost of the reflex

Source: J. R. Iacovino, "Use of Probability Theory to Evaluate Cost Effectiveness of Laboratory Tests in Insurance Medicine," *J. Ins. Med.,* 21 (1989): 200-2. Reproduced with permission of author and publisher.

tests; all are available from the laboratory. The assumptions are the responsibility of the medical director and include: a) At what levels do I want to reflex the HDL and cholesterol? and b) What is the prevalence of the disease, for which I am testing, in the population?

The assumptions are difficult! The medical director, not the laboratory, should determine the appropriate reflex levels predicated on their company's marketing, agency and financial goals and constraints. If the reflex level is too low, costs will increase since more reflex testing will be generated. This diminishes cost effectiveness. Also if the reflex level is too low, you may classify too many individuals abnormal, resulting in a marketing and agency revolt. The medical director must keep the number of rated and declined cases within a given range if a product is to be successfully marketed. Various degrees of mortality must be accepted; this is considered in the actuarial pricing. Conversely, if you set the reflex too high, you will not diagnose enough individuals to be cost effective. Additionally, you will underrate too many individuals; however, marketing and agency will love you.

Let us proceed to determine the cost effectiveness of a reflex test.

The facts are the Sn and Sp. For the HDL/cholesterol ratio which is superior to the cholesterol alone in predicting mortality, the Sn is 0.71 and the Sp is 0.87. The calculations use a cohort of 1,000 proposed insureds. The reflex level is established to identify only the worst 10% of the population at risk. Remember, if we go lower, we risk rating too many individuals with the potential loss of business. Figure 001K3-2 shows the underwriting results.

FIGURE 001K3-2
HDL/Cholesterol underwriting result

		Disease	
		+	−
Test	+	71	117
	−	29	783
		100	900

From the preceding figure, the following underwriting results are obtained:
- Correctly underwritten 85%
- Overrated 12%
- Underrated 3%

The HDL/cholesterol ratio with its relatively low sensitivity (0.71) coupled with a low risk population (0.10) will yield more false positive than true positive results. The PPV would be only 38%; the NPV is 96%. Combining these, we would correctly underwrite 85% of those tested by the HDL/cholesterol ratio alone.

The laboratory will automatically reflex *all* our "positive" HDL/cholesterol ratios above a preset level, despite false positives comprising 62% of the total positives. There is no way to separate the true from false positives.

I have elected to use the ApoA1/ApoB ratio for the reflex test. Its Sn and Sp are considerably better than for ApoA1 alone. Assume the laboratory charges $8.00 per reflex test. Up front, this will cost $1,500 *per 1,000* blood samples tested (188 positives x $8.00). Is this cost justified? For the ApoA1/ApoB ratio the Sn is 0.87 and Sp 0.80. We will assume (guess) the disease prevalence is now 85% in those reflexed (recall we took the top 10% of abnormals yet due to the low specificity had more false positives than true positives). The total number of reflexed tests is 188. Eighty five percent of those we assume are diseased, so we have 160 diseased and 28 nondiseased. This underwriting result is illustrated in Figure 001K3-3.

FIGURE 001K3-3
ApoA1/ApoB ratio reflexed underwriting result

		Disease	
		+	−
Test	+	140	6
	−	20	22
		160	28

From the above 2x2 table, we have the following results on these 188 tests.
- Correctly underwritten 86%
- Overrated 3%
- Underrated 11%

For those original positives reflexed by the ApoA1/ApoB ratio, the PPV is 96% and the NPV is 52%. We have nearly as many false negatives as true negatives due to the relatively low specificity (0.80) of the test.

Finally, we must assimilate all the results from the original and the reflex test groups (Figure 001K3-4).

FIGURE 001K3-4
HDL/Cholesterol and ApoA1/ApoB ratio combined underwriting result

		Disease	
		+	−
Test	+	140	6
	−	49	805

- Correctly underwritten 94%
- Overrated 1%
- Underrated 5%

The PPV for our entire initially tested and reflexed group is 96%, the NPV is 94%.

The following (Table 001K3-1) summarizes the results of testing.

TABLE 001K3-1

Summary of Test Results (1,000 tested individuals)

	True Pos.	True Neg.	False Pos.	False Neg.
Original group tested (1,000)	71	783	117	29
Result of positive tests reflex	(188)	140	22	6
Final outcome of original group tested (1,000)	140	805	6	49
Net change from reflex testing	+69	+22	–111	+20

Discussion

Laboratory costs are dramatically escalating as testing limits, necessitated by the AIDS epidemic, continue to drop. There may come a time in the not distant future, when we test all applicants for insurance. Facing this expense, medical directors must become involved in the financial planning of their company to help maintain increasingly thin profit margins. By the use of probability theory, we can make informed financial decisions to strengthen our importance in our companies.

Sn and Sp are determined by testing diseased and nondiseased reference or gold-standard populations. Their calculation is independent of the prevalence of disease. However, when used to determine cost effectiveness, disease prevalence must be considered. Prevalence is estimated both by knowledge of disease and the company's agency and marketing needs. Each medical director must derive their own prevalence assumptions.

Prevalence can profoundly affect the underwriting outcome of a particular test depending on its Sn and Sp. A test with a low sensitivity in a low prevalence population carries the risk of excessive false positives; cases which will be overrated or declined. Conversely, a low specificity carries the risk of excessive false negatives; cases which will be underrated with subsequent exces-sive mortality. Given the same Sn and Sp, these disparities narrow as the prevalence increases.

The purpose of reflexing the HDL/cholesterol ratio is to use a test of higher sensitivity to identify highest risks in the abnormal or high risk group; a secondary gain is the removal, via a higher specificity, from the reflex group of those not at highest risk. However, those removed are not necessarily low risk; we cannot rate every abnormal risk.

Initially, we identified 71 true positives (those presumed at highest risk) through our basic testing profile. After reflexing all 188 positives, we had 140 true positives for a net gain of 69 true positives out of our original 1,000 tested individuals (Table 001K3-1).

Per 1,000 tests, we spent $1,500 to identify an additional 69 true positives and 22 true negatives. In actuality, the 22 true negatives are not clinical true negatives. They were derived from our original 188 positives (71 true, 117 false); those initially identified as high risk. As discussed, for marketing reasons, we are unable to rate all abnormals in a group. With the new cholesterol normal limits we could theoretically rate up to 25% of our insurance buying population — this is clearly not acceptable. We must cull out of this large group those individuals at highest risk, in this case the reflexed true positives. Therefore, the number of new *correctly underwritten tests* is not the 91 total true test results but only the 69 true positives. The cost per 1,000 per new correctly underwritten test with the preceding assumption would be $21.75. Additionally, we generated 20 more false negatives per 1,000 that would be underrated.

Mitigating this $21.75 cost per new correctly underwritten test per 1,000 is our false positives (overrated cases) are reduced by 111.

The difficult question to be answered in this reflex scenario is whether the net gain of 69 additional correctly underwritten tests per 1,000 at a cost of $21.75 each, is cost effective in view of its potential mortality savings.

In summary, we have examined a methodology to evaluate the cost effectiveness of laboratory tests. Each medical director must use both objectivity and subjectivity to arrive at a decision which is consistent with their company's goals.

REFERENCES

1. R. K. Riegelman, "Diagnostic Discrimination of Test," *Studying a Study and Testing a Test — How to Read the Medical Literature* (Boston, Little Brown and Company, 1981).

2. Home Office Reference Laboratory, *Laboratory Bulletin*, 88-06.

3. W. P. Castelli, R. J. Garrison, P. W. F. Wilson, R. D. Abbott, S. Kalousdian, W. B. Kannel, "Incidence of Coronary Heart Disease and Lipoprotein Cholesterol Levels — The Framingham Study," *JAMA,* 256 (1986): 2835-39.

4. D. J. Gordon, J. L. Probstfield, R. J. Garrison, J. D. Neaton, W. P. Castelli, J. D. Knoke, D. R. Jacobs, S. Bangdiwala, H. A. Tyroler, "High-Density Lipoprotein Cholesterol and Cardiovascular Disease — Four Prospective American Studies," *Circulation,* 79 (1989): 8-15.

5. R. C. Elser, "Apolipoproteins, Lipoproteins and Coronary Heart Disease," *Roche Labtrends,* 2 (1988): 1-8.

6. H. K. Naito, "The Clinical Significance of Apolipoprotein Measurements," *J. Clin. Immunoassay,* 9 (1986): 11-20.

DRAWING CONCLUSIONS FROM TEST RESULTS

Michael W. Kita, M.D.

Some of the terminology surrounding the interpretation of laboratory tests is a little esoteric and subject to confusion. But for underwriters, medical directors and others who use such data, the basic concepts and probability principles are really fairly simple.

Let's take a hypothetical case. The applicant is a 50 year-old executive who applies to your company, Few-Hoops Life Insurance Company, for a $2,000,000 life policy. On his application, he notes a recent "false positive" treadmill. An Attending Physician's Statement also notes that treadmill result and reports that "he has perhaps a 20 to 90% chance of coronary artery disease (CAD)." The case is a rush. What do you do?

Well, you *could* consider issuing standard since the risk might be small — after all, it could be a "false positive" — but the uncertainty element makes you nervous. You might rate for coronary artery disease; but maybe it isn't, and maybe you'll lose the case. You could rate Table D (as a "don't know" hedge), but that's not very scientific. You could *reject the applicant* since this might even be unstable angina. You could *reject the test* results, but that would be risky, too. You could *repeat the test* — the size of the case might justify it — but that would create delay and could be perceived by the applicant as *one hoop too many* to jump through. Or, you could consider the statistical logic behind the AP's statement.

When the attending physician said that the chance was 20 to 90% for coronary disease, why the broad span? Was he being clever or ridiculous? Actually, he was being Bayesian. Bayes' theorem is a way of expressing the likelihood that a disease is present, given a positive test result for it. It is an expression of "conditional probability."

In All Probability

Probability should be familiar, not mysterious to any of us, since it is merely the expression of the likelihood of something happening, expressed on a scale of 0 to 1 (0% to 100%). Probability is simply a means of "quantitatively expressing uncertainty or risk." We live in a world in which we deal with uncertainty and probability all the

FIGURE 001K4-1

Evaluative Process

Population prevalence

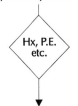

"Effective prevalence" (prior probability)

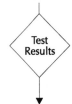

Disease likelihood (post-test probability)

time — 30% chance of rain, 10% chance the airline will be late, 50% chance that your cholesterol level will lead to a heart attack in your lifetime. In the medical and insurance world, we have coined some unique expressions to connote our estimates of the perceived degree of uncertainty — terms like "consistent with," "suggestive of," "essentially normal," "borderline standard," and "send it to Reinsurance."

"Conditional probability" is simply the likelihood of something being the case *given that* something *else* is already the case. In other words, **conditional probability** statements would include the following: a) the likelihood of having a positive test result, given the presence of a disease, and b) the likelihood of having a disease, given a positive test result. Note that "a" and "b" are not the same thing: "a" describes the **sensitivity** of a test, and "b" the **predictive value of a positive test** result. These concepts will be explained and developed further in a little bit.

Look at Figure 001K4-1. What the evaluative process of deciding the significance of a test result actually is, is a process of *revising probabilities*. In the absence of other information, you can begin with the general population prevalence for a disease or condition, assuming that the

Source: M. W. Kita, "Drawing Conclusions from Test Results," *J. Ins. Med.*, 22 (1990): 270-78. Reproduced with permission of author and publisher.

person could reasonably belong to that population. For heart disease, you could start with published findings of Framingham studies, American Heart Association data, or other such measurements. This will give the probability of disease for an applicant walking in off the street. Then, in light of the relevant *history* and *physical exam* (conducted by a physician as part of his diagnostic process, or as part of an application for insurance), the initial "population prevalence" is modified to come up with an "effective prevalence" based on the totality of information at hand. This effective prevalence becomes the "prior probability" of disease, i.e., the probability of disease prior to conducting the next diagnostic test.

After the test is done, its result is factored into an estimation of disease likelihood and a "post-test probability" of disease (or posterior probability) is calculated.

Expected Variation

In order to understand test results, it is important to be aware of the several sources of *expected* variation — including *biologic* variation, *sample* variation and *analytic* variation.

Biologic variation refers to variability of test results due to age, sex, diurnal variation, pregnancy, fasting state and other such *biologic* factors, *Sample* variation refers to the variability caused by specimen-handling (spun or unspun, "time in the tube," exposure to heat or cold, etc.) and processing. *Analytic* variation refers to variability due to test methodology (e.g., type of assay) and the inherent accuracy and precision of the technique. (*Accuracy* refers to the degree to which the lab result is identical to the *actual* or *absolute* value [e.g., when compared to a known "standard"] and *precision* refers to the *reproducibility* of a test result on repetitive runs.)

For a given test, the person attempting to interpret the test result needs to factor in *all* such sources of variation known to him in order to interpret a test result as *abnormal*, and then to judge whether the abnormality is of clinical or underwriting *significance*, and finally to be able to conclude what is likely *due to*.

What is Normal?

Before one can work with abnormals, one needs to be clear about what is meant by normal. The term "*normal*" gets tossed around rather loosely, and Murphy[15] has suggested that "normal" as used in everyday speech can have one (or more) of seven different meanings (Figure 001K4-2).

You will note on the report page for most blood test results that the term "normal range" is not used much anymore because it may wrongly imply a bell-shaped distribution for the lab results. (Many lab results, in fact, have a skewed, bimodal, or other-than-bell-shaped dis-

FIGURE 001K4-2

Meanings of the Word "Normal"

Preferable Term	Paraphrase
Gaussian normal	Bell-shaped distribution
Mean/median/mode	Average/representative
Habitual	Commonly seen
Desirable/optimal	Fittest for survival
Innocuous	Carrying no penalty
Conventional/approved	Consensus/fashionable
Ideal	Aspired to

(after Murphy[15])

tribution.) Instead they are called "reference ranges" or "usual clinical ranges." This implies that these are consensus norms intended to reflect an "average" or typical reference population with which the sample can be compared.

For example, a reference laboratory may report a usual clinical range for cholesterol as 160-240 mg./dl., whereas "desirable" or "optimal" for a healthy or low-risk 40-year-old might be less than 200. Another fact to be aware of is that being too high or being too low may not be equally significant. The "usual clinical range" tends to be a "center cut." This leaves values on both the high-end and the low-end outside the "normal range," but for some lab tests, there is no clinical significance to the low extreme. It is usually only the high end that is of interest or concern.

And just as underwriters must be prepared to ask whether a result flagged as abnormal (outside the range) is really *significantly* abnormal, another phenomenon to be aware of is that some lab results may be abnormal *for that individual* but hidden in the usual clinical range and, therefore, not advertised by an asterisk(*) or a HI/LO symbol. Because the usual clinical range is often a population-based reference range drawn from large numbers of people, the spread of the range can be quite broad. A creatinine for a 100 lb. woman might "normally" (healthily) be 0.3 mg./dl., but a value of 1.2 mg./dl. (4 times "normal" for her and indicative of perhaps only 1/4 of her "normal" kidney function) would lie *within* most usual clinical ranges and *not* be associated with a telltale asterisk. Where available, a person's own prior test values might provide a more valid reference scale, but in the absence of such data, a population reference range is at least one useful yardstick for comparison.

Reference Ranges

Where do these reference ranges themselves come from? Reference ranges are constructed from groups of presumably healthy people, but such reference ranges may, in fact, include individuals with diseases that are subclinical or presymptomatic. We would like the reference range to represent only healthy people so that we can use it for comparison with our own results, in order to find the *abnormals* and detect *unhealthy* people. But invariably any reference range has *some* unhealthy people in it, which is *one* reason why graphs of the test results of healthy and diseased populations commonly overlap instead of cleanly separating. Another reason for overlap is that the "diseased" population includes a *spectrum* of disease, with mild and early cases often toward the low end and more severe cases at the upper end.

Even though the whole reference group is regarded as the "presumably healthy" group, not even all of *its* members are defined as "normal." Rather, the "normal" part of the reference range is defined as the central 95% of the reference population. This gives rise to another phenomenon of testing, namely the possibility that someone who is *healthy* may yet have an *abnormal* test result due to "chance" alone, and not due to any significant condition. In other words, if you did a single "routine" (not for a medical indication) lab test on an individual, and "normal" was defined as the middle 95% of "usual" test results, then you would have a 95% chance of the result coming back normal and a 5% chance of it coming back abnormal, due to just chance alone. What would happen if you ran a battery of tests? If you did a chemistry *profile* (say a Chem-15) and if each of these tests were mutually *independent*, then the chance of being *normal* on *all* 15 is only 0.95 to the 15th power (0.95^{15}) or only 46%! Turn it around, and the chance of being abnormal on *at least one* test is 100% minus 46% or 54%! (Fifty-four percent represents the sum of those individuals who are abnormal on at least one of those fifteen tests — they may be abnormal on only one test, or on various combinations of more than one.)

Abnormal results due to "chance" effects of multiple simultaneous testing tend to be borderline abnormalities that hover near the margins of the "normal" range. (Such results tend to "normalize" (regress toward the mean) on repeat testing, but they can cause considerable head-scratching when first seen.)

Is it Hopeless, Then?

Given all of the caveats and pitfalls to the interpretation of test results mentioned above, you may rightly wonder how it is ever possible to make a meaningful interpretation of a test result. But **interpretation relies upon the totality of the information available and not just the *one* fact of an isolated abnormality.** Doctors and underwriters ask themselves these questions: "How extreme is the abnormality? Is it solitary or not? Is it new or

previously known? If previously known, is there any trend to it?" And most importantly of all, "what is the clinical context?" Do the history, physical exam, medications and previous diagnoses allow for a meaningful interpretation?

Validity

Understanding a bit about reference ranges and meaningful abnormals, the next thing to ask oneself is "how good is the test that is being performed?" A good test is one that has been standardized for the purpose in question, obtained for a worthwhile reason, and one which is a good discriminator for the condition in question. This raises the subject of *validity*. A *valid* test is one which is **appropriate for the intended purpose**. Gamma Glutamyl Transpeptidase (GGTP) as a test for *diabetes* performs poorly; this is because it is not valid for that purpose. *Glucose* measurements as tests for diabetes, however, have validity for that purpose.

It is worth noting here that *few* tests are *unique* discriminators of one condition. While GGTP is most often used for assessing liver function, it is present in other tissues and can occasionally be elevated due to renal disease, for instance. If the GGTP *were* elevated due to renal disease, it would then be a "false positive" test for *liver* disease. This is not because there is anything "false" about the GGTP having been elevated, but rather because it is giving false and misleading information about the condition under consideration — liver abnormality. Or to take a slightly different example, while an elevated GGTP level commonly arouses suspicion for alcohol-related impairment, taken alone it is not *unique to* or even highly *predictive of* alcohol-related disease because elevations can and do occur for other reasons. This does not make it a bad test for underwriting purposes, because most of the *other* causes of significant elevations of GGTP also have important morbidity or mortality concerns to the underwriter; but for *establishing alcoholism* alone, the GGT by itself is of limited value.

There certainly are test results so extreme that you can say, "It's immaterial *what* the exact cause is; this is an unacceptable risk." But to do so, you must understand the test. Where possible, a medical director or underwriter would like to be able to name not only those underlying conditions that *could* cause an abnormal result, but what condition *is* causing it, and then "rate for cause."

Sensitivity and Specificity

There are two more terms which it is important to clearly understand. Just as the word "normal" can mean several different things, the terms "sensitivity" (SN) and "specificity" (SP) have exact technical definitions that are slightly different from their common everyday usage.

Sensitive can sometimes mean touchy, responsive or compassionate. But when the term **sensitive** is applied to a *test*, the exact definition to have in mind is "*positive in disease* (PID)." A highly sensitive test is one which, with high frequency, gives a positive result when the disease is known to be present.

Likewise, the term **specific** in everyday usage might mean precise, definite or particular. However, when we say that a test is specific, we mean that it is "*negative in health* (NIH)": that in healthy people (those without the disease or condition in question) the test is usually negative. One thing to note here is that in loose usage when someone says a test was "specific" for diabetes, it sounds as if he means that it is diagnostic of the disease being present (but note that this is more closely what the term *sensitive* — strongly associated with the presence of disease — technically means). Remember, a sensitive test, by definition is appropriately positive (i.e., *positive when disease is present*) and a specific test is appropriately negative (i.e., *negative when the disease in question is absent*).

True Positives, False Positives, etc.

If we were to graph the test results of a group of disease-free people against the range of values they could have for that test, we would get a curved distribution of results. This would be the reference population or the population that is presumed to not have the disease in question.

A second group of people, the "diseased population," will also have a certain distribution, and the *two curves* will typically *overlap* (Figure 001K4-3). If we now define a particular value of the lab test as the "cut-off point" *above which* we will classify the result as *abnormal*, we can see that we now get *four groups of people*. The cut-off

FIGURE 001K4-3

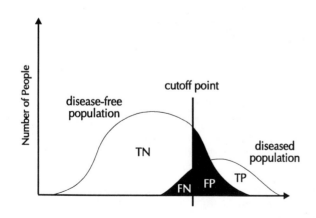

line divides the non-diseased population into two parts, those below the cut-off who are the *true negatives* (TN = the lab result is negative, and the people are truly non-diseased) and *false positives* (FP = those *non*-diseased people who would falsely be called abnormal because their results are above the cut-off). Likewise, the diseased population is divided by the cut-off line into two parts, the *true positives* (TP = those *with* the disease who are testing positive or abnormal, above the cut-off point) and

FIGURE 001K4-4

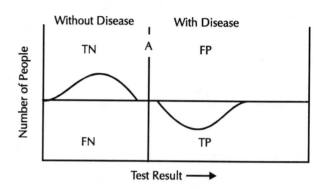

B. Partial overlap = 4 subgroups

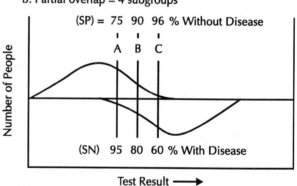

C. Full overlap = "one" population (nested)

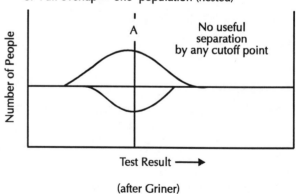

(after Griner)

the *false negatives* (FN = those members of the diseased population who are being missed because they fall below the cut-off point and are being classified as negative for the disease.) As you can see, the relative sizes of these four groups of people will depend upon: the sizes of the two populations, the degree of overlap of the two populations, and *where* the cut-off line is placed.

If you move the cut-off point (Figure 001K4-4B) to the right, you will progressively eliminate the false positives, but at a price. That price is that you necessarily increase the number of false *negatives*. (You might want to try drawing similar graphs for yourself and move the cut-off level around.) Likewise, you could eliminate the false negatives by moving the cut-off level farther and farther to the left, but the price you would pay is increasing the number of false *positives*.

You will note that if the two curves did *not* overlap (Figure 001K4-4A), you could place the cut-off point *between* the two curves and now you would end up with just two groups — true positives and true negatives. But few diseases segregate so cleanly that a test can discriminate this well. Likewise, if the diseased population nestled *completely within* the hump of the non-diseased population (Figure 001K4-4C), it would be impossible to select a useful cut-off point since the degree of overlap of the two populations would be 100%.

Look at Figure 001K4-4 again.

The upper graph shows two populations with no overlap such that decision point A clearly separates the two populations. There are no false positives or false negatives. *Everyone* is properly and "truly" classified. This would be a "perfect test" for distinguishing the disease in question.

The bottom graph has the diseased population as a complete subset of the larger non-diseased population. No value of the test — not A, not anywhere — helpfully separates the groups. This would be a "worthless test." It would have no value for distinguishing between these two populations and would not be valid for that purpose.

But in the middle graph, there is significant overlap, and decision points could be placed at A, B, or C. This is a "typical test." Decision point C would result in high specificity but low sensitivity. Decision point A would have high sensitivity but at the price of low specificity. This is the *inevitable trade-off* when dealing with tests used to discriminate conditions in populations which have overlap: there is no free lunch, and it is hard to get both high specificity and high sensitivity out of a given cut-off level for a particular test.

This, then, is how sensitivity and specificity behave. But where do the numbers come from that tell you *how* sensitive or specific a test is for a particular disease?

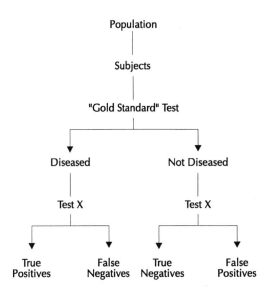

FIGURE 001K4-5

Relationship Test Results and Disease

Typically, someone conducts a study and reports these findings (Figure 001K4-5).

Out of a population, a group of subjects is chosen (according to some criteria) and subjected to a "gold standard" test which allows for them to be divided into two groups — those *with* the disease in question and those *without* the disease. For the condition "coronary artery disease," the gold standard might be coronary angiography.

Having established those "with" and those "without" disease, *another* test — more generally suitable, less invasive — (one, that could ultimately be used on a more general population as a surrogate for the gold standard) is applied. For coronary artery disease, this could be the treadmill test. The results of the treadmill, when applied to the "diseased" and "not diseased" populations, will then be either positive or negative. In the population with *already known* disease, the results will either be *true positives* or *false negatives*. In the population *known not to have* the disease, the results will be *false positives* and *true negatives*.

Let's paint in some numbers (Figure 001K4-6).

Suppose 1,000 subjects are chosen and subjected to coronary angiography. Suppose the decision point for angiography (i.e., the point at which we say "yes, they've got the disease") is >70% obstruction of at least one coronary artery. Let's assume we assemble a study group of 1,000 subjects, 500 *with* coronary disease and 500 *without* coronary disease, according to this definition. Now we apply the treadmill test, and we use a decision

FIGURE 001K4-6

Example

1000 Subjects

Heart Catheterization
(>70% 1VD)

500 CAD   500 No CAD

Stress Test   (1mm ST↓)   Stress Test
⊕   ⊖   ⊖   ⊕

300 TP   200 FN   455 TN   45 FP

$$SN = \frac{300}{500} = 0.60 \qquad SP = \frac{455}{500} = 0.91$$

(Prevalence 50%)

FIGURE 001K4-7

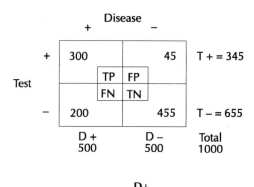

$$Prevalence = \frac{D+}{Total} = 50\%$$

$$SN = \frac{TP}{D-} = \frac{TP}{TP + FN} = 60\%$$

$$SP = \frac{TN}{D-} = \frac{TN}{TN + FP} = 91\%$$

$$PVP = \frac{TP}{T+} = \frac{TP}{TP + FP} = 87\%$$

$$PVN = \frac{TN}{T-} = \frac{TN}{TN + FN} = 69\%$$

point for positive and negative outcomes of "1 mm. horizontal ST-segment depression." The results could look as follows: out of 500 patients with coronary disease, 300 have true positives and 200 have false negatives, according to the stress test; likewise, 455 have true negatives and 45, false positives.

Now recall that *sensitivity* (SN) means "positivity in disease." This is the ratio of true positives to the total number with disease. (This latter number, the total with disease, is the sum of the true positives and the false negatives.) Thus, the sensitivity of this test in this situation is 300/500 or 0.60. Likewise, the *specificity* (SP) of the disease is its "negativity in health" (or negativity in absence-of-disease, according to how the "disease" may be defined). The specificity here is the true negatives over the total number without-disease. Thus, the specificity is 91%. These results aren't bad and are fairly typical of treadmill testing in such circumstances.

We can display the same data in a 2x2 table (Figure 001K4-7).

The usual **convention** for doing so is to have "disease" at the *top* and "test" outcome at the *left* side, and to have the left upper box be the "positive-positive" box. Therefore, according to this convention, sensitivity and specificity are "vertically" arranged.

Sensitivity falls out of the first column, TP/D+ (D+ = disease-positive), and specificity falls out of the second column, TN/D−. Now just replace the abbreviations TP, FN, FP, and TN with the numbers from Figure 001K4-6,

and presto! You have converted the representation of the data from a flow diagram to a 2x2 table. Each is a perfectly good representation of the same data, but the latter form may be more useful to those who think algebraically. Note that in addition to being "positivity in disease," sensitivity could also be called "few false negatives," because the fewer the FN, the higher the sensitivity. Likewise, specificity relies on "few false positives" in order to be as high as it can be.

So, sensitivity and specificity are determined for a *particular disease* (itself defined according to a gold standard) and for a *specific decision point* (such as 1 mm. ST depression) defined according to clinical appropriateness as a discriminator. Are the sensitivity and specificity permanent attributes of the test? The answer is "no." Recall from Figure 001K4-3 that *where* the cutoff point or decision level is placed determines the proportion of results that are true positive and false positive, true negative and false negative, and since the sensitivity and specificity reflect these proportions (Figure 001K4-4B), they necessarily vary according to the cut-off point chosen. For example, a *2 mm.* ST segment depression is more "significant" than 1 mm. depression. Experience teaches that it is more likely to define a "surer" positive (someone with coronary disease) than someone whose level of positivity on a treadmill may only be manifested at the 1 mm. mark. This is the same as saying that in moving to a *stricter* cut-off point (2 mm.), one increases the specificity but reduces the sensitivity of the treadmill test. Or to put it another way, one has reduced the number of false positives by allowing more false negatives.

One final thing to note is that this "standardization" study which gives us the sensitivity and specificity values was conducted on a population in which, quite artificially, there were equal numbers of people "with" and "without" the disease. It is quite common to do it this way, with equal numbers of cases and controls. However, this gives you an inflated "prevalence" of disease of 50% for the subject population (D+/total number of subjects). The significance of this factor will become evident when we next discuss the "**P**redictive **V**alue of a **P**ositive test (PVP)." The baseline prevalences of diseases in the general population almost never run this high, but more commonly run between 0.1% and 10%, and may often be <0.1%.

Predictive Value

The *predictive value* of a test is how well it predicts the presence of the disease when the test is positive, or how well it predicts the absence of the disease when the test is negative. This is what one really wants to know, after all. All those other things are well and good, but predictive value is the bottom line.

Looking again at Figure 001K4-7, the "predictive value of the positive test result (PVP)" is determined "horizontally" on the 2x2 table, i.e., TP/(TP + FP) (or TP/T+). What this says is "what is the likelihood of the disease being present, if the test result is positive?" Likewise, the predictive value of a negative test result is ascertained from the lower pair of boxes going across, i.e., TN/(TN + FN) (or TN/T−) and this expresses the likelihood of the disease being absent when the test outcome is negative. (Remember, "positive" and "negative" test results refer to exceeding or being below whatever your cut-off point is — e.g., 1 mm. or whatever, if you're talking about a treadmill.)

In our last example, where the sensitivity was 60% and the specificity 91%, the PVP = 300/345 = 87%. Notice that it's not 100% — that it doesn't predict the presence of disease with *certainty* but only with probability. (You would need 0 false positives for the equation to give you *that* result.) But 87% is quite good and makes coronary disease "highly probable."

Let's suppose that instead of starting with a population prevalence of 50% CAD, we instead are performing our treadmill test on a population with a pretest probability of disease of 8%. This would correspond to the baseline prevalence of CAD in a group of asymptomatic 50 year-old, American males. Let's start with a group of 1,000 such people and create Figure 001K4-8.

FIGURE 001K4-8

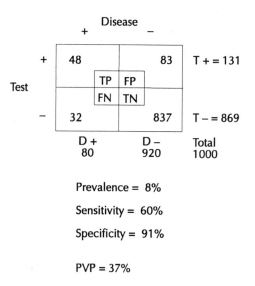

Prevalence = 8%

Sensitivity = 60%

Specificity = 91%

PVP = 37%

Of the 1,000, 8% of them will have the disease (D+ = 80). The remaining 92% will be disease-free (D− = 920). The test sensitivity and specificity remain the same, assuming that we are using the same decision point of 1 mm. ST segment depression, so sensitivity is still 60% and the specificity 91%. So, to finish filling the boxes, TP = 60% x 80 = 48; and FN = the remainder of the 80, or 32. TN = 91% x 920, or 837; and FP = the remainder of the disease-free, or 83. That means T+ = 48 + 83 = 131, and T− = 837 + 32 = 869. The predictive value of the positive test, given this sensitivity and this specificity, and given a population prevalence of 8%, calculates out to be 48/131, or only 37%. Now, this is not a sufficient likelihood for a doctor to make an unequivocal diagnosis of coronary artery disease, but 1/3 chance of having ischemic heart disease might still be more uncertainty than an underwriter might care to live with. This is the problem inherent in screening tests — doing treadmills, etc. on asymptomatic individuals — as opposed to doing it for a medical indication such as substernal chest pain: low initial prevalence (low "pre-test probability") invites high false positive rate (low PVP) and requires further investigation to differentiate true positives from false positives. However, when a test is done after *risk factor* assessment, in light of *complaints*, and after *exam findings* have **raised** the index of suspicion higher, then it is being applied in a situation of much higher pre-test likelihood of disease than the mere population prevalence would suggest (recall Figure 001K4-1). You can begin to see then that a test of a given sensitivity and specificity can give you different probabilities of disease depending on what the pretest prevalence or likelihood was in the first place.

FIGURE 001K4-9

Probability of CAD After ETT
(effects of different kinds of pre-test pain)

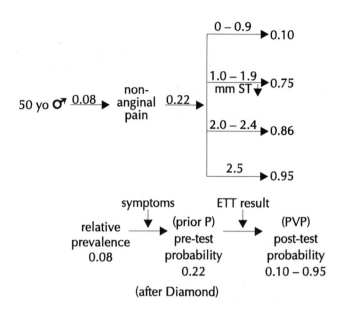

pre-test probability

post-test probability

(after Diamond)

FIGURE 001K4-10

Probability of CAD After ETT
(effects of extreme-ness of abnormality)

You remember we started this whole discussion with a hypothetical applicant. He was a 50 year-old, American male with an abnormal ("positive") ETT (exercise tolerance test).

Figure 001K4-9 shows what the pre-test probability of disease would have been depending on the presence and type of chest pain prior to the positive treadmill. (Please note that the pre- and post-test likelihoods in Figures 001K4-9 and 001K4-10 are adapted from tables developed by Diamond, which is one place such estimates can be obtained. They are based on somewhat different sensitivity and specificity assumptions than some of our other examples, like Figures 001K4-8 and 001K4-11, so this must be kept in mind.) As you can see, our hypothetical applicant has a baseline prevalence of 8% for having coronary artery disease just by virtue of being 50, male and American. If he were having no chest pain prior to this treadmill, this remains his "pre-test probability." If he were having nonanginal chest pain, his pre-test probability becomes 22%; if atypical angina, 59%; and if typical angina, 92%. Following a treadmill test, positive for 1 mm. ST depression, the post-test likelihood of disease ranges from 19% to 96%.

Now we see why the PVP of his abnormal treadmill could be anywhere from 20% to 90%! The Attending Physician wasn't just being noncommittal, he was being Bayesian! He was telling us that the likelihood of the disease was a function of its conditional probability: that

the probability of disease reflected both the *fact* that the test was abnormal *and* the *pre-test likelihood* of disease.

Suppose that rather than screening an asymptomatic patient, the Attending Physician is using the treadmill to help evaluate a chest-pain complaint. Let's suppose the applicant was having non-anginal chest pain. What would we have considered the likelihood of CAD after treadmill if the treadmill abnormalities were something *other* than 1 mm. Figure 001K4-10 shows what different cut-off points for positivity on the treadmill might give you. As you can see, a treadmill result of less than 1 mm. basically revises the applicant's pre-test likelihood from 22% for his nonanginal chest pain to 10%, which was close to his original "population probability" of having CAD just by virtue of being 50 and male. On the other hand, a treadmill result of 2.5 mm. or greater would give him a 95% likelihood of coronary artery disease.

Suppose again that our hypothetical applicant winds up with a 48% post-test likelihood of having coronary artery disease (Figure 001K4-10). Is this the closest one can get to a final risk assessment, or is there a way of trying to further resolve this question? You know the answer to this: look to results of further (sequential) testing using some independent means (that is, a method of investigating for ischemia that uses an end-point other than electrical repolarization abnormality). Typically, thallium perfusion scans are used in this fashion as a means of further evaluating a treadmill abnormality. (An alternative

FIGURE 001K4-11

Probability of CAD After ETT and Thallium Test
(effect of multiple independent tests)

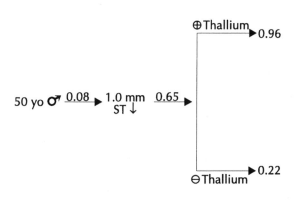

(Assume Thallium SN = 71% SP = 94%)

FIGURE 001K4-12

Variability of SN and SP

Test	Endpoint	For	SN%	SP%	Gold Std.
Treadmill	1.0 mm	CAD	75	85	>50% 1VD
	1.0 mm	CAD	60	91	>70% 1VD
	>2.5 mm	CAD	20	99.5	>70% 1VD
Thallium	reperfusing defect	CAD	71	94	>70% 1VD
GGTP	3xULN	ETOH(L)	88	85	liver BX(H)
	3xULN	ETOH(L)	52	(85)	liver BX(A)
ELISA	OD ⊕	HIV	98.8	99.6	HIV
WB	3 lanes ⊕	HIV	99.6	99.8	HIV
{ Treadmill + Thallium }	1.0 mm + reperfusing defect	CAD	42	98	>70% 1VD
{ ELISA (2) + WB }	O.D. ⊕ + 3 lanes ⊕	HIV	99.995	99.9	HIV

(other studies have yielded other results)

to a Thallium scan might be an RVG — radionuclide ventriculogram — also known as a MUGA or **mul**ti**ga**ted blood pool scan — to investigate wall motion abnormality.) Let's suppose the hypothetical applicant undergoes thallium testing next (Figure 001K4-11).

If his thallium test is positive for a reperfusing abnormality, he goes from a 48% likelihood of disease to a 96% likelihood; and if his thallium scan is negative, his chance of having CAD reverts to about 22%, (which you will recall was the pre-test likelihood of CAD in a 50 year-old male with nonanginal pain before the treadmill was positive). I think you begin to see the pattern here. (Note that a negative thallium scan does not tell you that there is a *zero* percent chance of CAD, but instead, it essentially cancels the effect that the abnormal treadmill had on the likelihood of CAD, i.e., takes the applicant back near his pre-test 20% likelihood.)

Figure 001K4-12 is a table compiled from different articles from the medical literature that gives you some overall sense of variability of sensitivity and specificity according to the disease being assayed for the population being studied, the particular gold standard used, and the cut-off point used to call the test positive. Thus, you can see that when coronary artery disease is defined as "greater than a 50% narrowing of at least one vessel," it has a higher sensitivity and lower specificity than when a stricter gold standard (70% one vessel disease, or more) is used, even with the same 1 mm. ST depression endpoint on the treadmill. (Does this imply that some goldstandards in use are really "gold-plated"? The reader can decide!)

Likewise, when the gold standard for CAD is a 70% -or-more narrowing of at least one vessel, the sensitivity and specificity for coronary artery disease depends on whether an endpoint of 1 mm. or 2.5 mm. is chosen. The sensitivity decreases as the endpoint becomes stricter, but the specificity increases. The thallium scan has a better sensitivity and specificity for coronary artery disease against a gold standard of "70% obstruction" than a 1 mm. treadmill abnormality does. (But it is a much more expensive test to conduct and is generally reserved for sequential testing in those cases where the treadmill is first abnormal, and its success depends on being able to achieve an exertional pulse rate sufficient to produce a reperfusing abnormality [i.e., *resting* Thallium scans are not going to have much information about ischemia].)

Because liver test abnormalities and HIV testing arouse similar concerns about false positives and real PVPs, some representative numbers from the literature are displayed for these as well. For GGT an end point of 3 times the upper limit of normal (ULN) was studied for alcoholic liver disease (not alcoholism, and not just any liver disease, but alcoholic disease of the liver). The gold standard in the first case was liver biopsy in hospitalized patients (H) and in the second instance liver biopsy in ambulatory patients (A). Liver biopsy is not a gold standard that many people willingly volunteer for, so it is appropriate to try to have a noninvasive substitute for such an invasive gold standard. The sensitivities and specificities for GGTP *for this narrow purpose* do not generate impressive PVPs (if you work through the arithmetic as on the treadmill example). But for underwriting purposes, when GGTP is used to assay for "all conditions of substandard implication" instead of merely for detection of alcoholic liver disease, and when a high cut-off point like 3 times (3x) the upper limit is used, the overall sensitivity and specificity are better, and so is the predictive value.

And now we come to "Bayes' Theorem" — summarized in this famous equation arrived at by a country cleric in 1763:

$$PVP = \frac{(P)\,(SN)}{(P)\,(SN) + (1-P)\,(1-SP)}$$

Now, it should no longer be frightening or intimidating. It can be expressed using a variety of symbols or algebraic forms, but the one shown here is one of the more useful ways of rendering it. P is the pre-test probability of the disease being present. (1–P) is 1 minus this probability. SN and SP are the sensitivity and specificity, respectively, for the condition in question. Quite simply,

Bayes' Theorem tells you the predictive value of a positive test — the likelihood that the disease or condition in question is present, given the fact that the test result is positive.

As you can now see, there is *much* more to it than meets the eye. For the test to have been positive means many things — how was it done? what cut-off point was used?, etc. The sensitivity and specificity, likewise, require you to know a little bit about what gold standard was used to define the presence of the condition in question. But now, within those few constraints, all you have to do is fill in the blanks, crank out an answer, and you can do estimations of the likelihood of disease *all on your own.* Rather a powerful little tool!

With just a little experimentation with different numbers and scenarios, you can discover a multitude of uses and ways in which these concepts can help you understand and interpret test results.

Appreciation is hereby expressed to the Home Office Life Underwriter's Association (HOLUA), on whose behalf some of this material was presented as workshops, and to Robert J. Pokorski, M.D., for his ideas and encouragement.

APPENDIX

The discussion of treadmill testing was necessarily simplified for the purposes under discussion. It is important to remember that the information content of a treadmill extends well beyond that of an arbitrarily chosen index like "1 mm. flat or downsloping ST depression." Questions to consider in *fully* evaluating treadmill reports would include such things as: "why was it done and why was it stopped?" Was the context "chest pain" and a high index of suspicion for coronary disease (in which case PVCs, ST segment depression more than 80 msec. past the J point, and other findings may represent ischemic equivalents)? Was it *stopped* because of chest pain and if so, at what exercise level? Was the subject able to achieve 85% of his maximal pulse or not? Was the resting cardiogram abnormal, and if so, in what way? (Repolarization abnormalities with exercise are difficult to interpret meaningfully in the presence of left bundle branch block[LBBB] at rest.) Is there a normal heart exam? How

was the exercise test done: 3 leads or 12 leads? According to Bruce protocol or some other protocol? If ST changes do occur with exercise, do they occur in one lead or more than one lead?

A treadmill test contains much valuable information and generally should be "milked" for *all* of the underwriting information that can be extracted from it.

In the hypothetical case above, in order to conclude that the result was a *false* positive, there was presumably either negative sequential testing, allowing revision of his CAD-likelihood back toward baseline prevalence, or the total universe of information available about his CAD risk, including the specifics of his treadmill "positivity," allowed for such an inference. Underwriting, of course, is the science of applying methods *other than* wishful thinking to the task of risk-assessment!

SOME USEFUL REFERENCES

BASIC

*1. A. W. DeTore, "The Evaluation of Abnormal Laboratory Results," *J. Insur. Med.*, 20 , no. 2 (1988): 5-9.

2. G. A. Diamond, J. S. Forrester, "Analysis of Probabilty as An Aid in The Clinical Diagnosis of Coronary Artery Disease," *N. Engl. J. Med.*, 300 (1979): 1350-58.

3. R. S. Galen, S. R. Gambino, *Beyond Normality* (New York, Wiley, 1975).

*4. H. George, "Analyzing and Underwriting The Blood Chemistry Profile," *Lincoln National Management Services.*

*5. R. J. Pokorski, "Overview of Test Theory," BIM Triennial Course, The Wigwam, Litchfield Park, Arizona, 1988.

*6. R. K. Riegelman, *Studying a Study and Testing a Test* (Boston, Little Brown, 1981).

*7. D. L. Sackett, R. B. Haynes, P. Tugwell, "How to Read a Clinical Journal," *Clinical Epidemiology: A Basic Science for Clinical Medicine* (Boston, Little Brown and Company, 1985), pp. 285-319.

8. G. Siest, et al., *Interpretation of Clinical Laboratory Tests* (Foster City, CA, Biomedical Publications, 1985).

9. C. E. Speicher, J. W. Smith, *Choosing Effective Laboratory Tests* (Philadelphia, Saunders, 1983).

10. J. Wallach, *Interpretation of Diagnostic Tests* (Boston, Little Brown, 1986).

INTERMEDIATE

11. A. K. Bahn, *Basic Medical Statistics* (New York, Grume and Stratton, 1972).

*12. T. Colton, *Statistics in Medicine* (Boston, Little Brown, 1974).

*13. P. F. Griner, et al., "Selection and Interpretation of Diagnostic Tests and Procedures," *Ann. Intern. Med.*, 94 (1981) (4, Part 2): 453-600.

*14. B. J. McNeil, H. Sherman, "Primer on Certain Elements of Medical Decision Making," *N. Engl. J. Med.*, 293 (1975): 211-15.

15. E. A. Murphy, *The Logic of Medicine* (Baltimore, Johns Hopkins Press, 1976).

MORE ADVANCED

16. A. R. Feinstein, *Clinical Biostatistics* (St. Louis, Mosby, 1977).

*17. J. A. Ingelfinger, et al., *Biostatistics in Clinical Medicine* (New York, Macmillan, 1987).

18. M. C. Weinstein, H. V. Fineberg, *Clinical Decision Analysis* (Philadelphia, Saunders, 1980).

(Asterisked references are especially helpful with some of the concepts).

THE CONVERSION OF MORTALITY RATIOS TO A NUMERICAL RATING CLASSIFICATION FOR LIFE INSURANCE UNDERWRITING

Richard B. Singer, M.D.

A question often asked by medical directors attending a mortality seminar is this: "Are mortality ratios the same as table ratings? If not, what is the relation?" The answer is: "No, they are not the same." The relation is complex, and was not explicitly covered in the methodology chapter of *Medical Risks*.[1]* The subject was discussed, but rather briefly, in the panel discussion on *Medical Risks* presented at the 1976 annual meeting of ALIMDA.[2] At the mortality seminars I conducted there was never sufficient time to devote to a satisfactory answer to this question. The topic certainly merits adequate discussion, because a primary purpose of preparing mortality abstracts for the two *Medical Risks* monographs and for the *Journal of Insurance Medicine* is to make available results of follow-up studies for better underwriting. In this review I will attempt to describe a method of conversion as clearly as I can, with the help of detailed results from an excellent follow-up study of post-MI survivors reported from Auckland, New Zealand.

The illustrative data I have chosen provide annualized mortality rates by sex, age and duration, and also by severity, all ages and both sexes combined. They have been developed from a series of reports by Norris and his colleagues[3-6] on a cohort of 757 patients admitted with acute myocardial infarction (MI) to the three general hospitals in Auckland, New Zealand, representing an unselected group of all patients with this diagnosis in this metropolitan area, reaching the hospital alive in a 12-month period, 1966-67. Of 549 survivors discharged alive a mean of three weeks after hospitalization, 530 were successfully traced for 15 years. Distribution data by age and sex were published for the 549 entrants to long-term follow-up[3] and for the 132 survivors at 15 years.[6] Results have been presented in Abstract #614 for the new *Medical Risks* monograph,[7] but I have reworked these to separate the male and female experience in each

age group. At some durations, the results are approximations rather than precise data, but the approximations are close enough to utilize for illustration of the conversion method presented here. Expected mortality has been derived from graduated 1970-72 New Zealand life tables to utilize in this clinical follow-up study. For the conversion of mortality to an insurance standard, expected mortality has been derived from the 1975-80 Basic Select Tables.

The basic method proposed here is to obtain EDR, the excess death rate, in extra deaths per 1000 per year. *Annualized* mortality rates have been calculated for each triennial interval as a geometric mean, $\breve{q}$, for the observed, and $\breve{q}'$ for the population expected mortality, in deaths per 1000 per year. For each interval EDR=$\breve{q}$–$\breve{q}'$, and the mortality ratio, MR=100 $\breve{q}/\breve{q}'$.

The well-known difference between insurance select mortality and population may be seen in Table 3-1, page 27, in *Medical Risks*.[1] In adults, the first-year select rate is about 25% to 35% of the population rate (1965-70 Select Tables vs. U.S. 1969-71 Life Tables). The differential decreases with policy duration, but even the ultimate insurance rates, more than 15 years after policy issue, remain lower than corresponding population rates at the same attained age, the insurance rates being about 78% to 85% of the population. Additional examples of the effect of selection and antiselection on mortality are given in Table 3-2, page 28 of *Medical Risks*.[1] Some degree of selection may be exercised in the formation of clinical series of patients, but the cohort of post-MI patients of Norris et al represents the acute survivors of *all* cases of MI hospitalized during the entry period. Population life tables are, therefore, the proper ones to use for the estimation of $\breve{q}'$ in this clinical series.

To illustrate the variation of the indexes of comparative mortality with duration follow-up, I have chosen the men who survived their acute MI at age 50-59 years (Table 003K1-1). The entire follow-up of 15 years has been divided into five equal intervals of three years each. Number of patients at risk at the start and deaths during each interval are shown first in the Table, then the annualized mortality rates per 1000 (as geometric means), observed $\breve{q}$ and population expected $\breve{q}'$, then EDR as ($\breve{q}$–$\breve{q}'$), and the mortality ratio, MR, as 100 $\breve{q}/\breve{q}'$. Note the

---

* An additional Chapter 17 on "Applications" was originally projected for this volume, but the draft available at the completion of the rest of the manuscript in 1976 was not considered satisfactory, so the chapter was omitted.

Source: R. B. Singer, "The Conversion of Mortality Ratios to a Numerical Rating Classification for Life Insurance Underwriting," *J. Ins. Med.*, 20, no. 2 (1988): 54-61. Reproduced with permission of author and publisher.

independent variation of observed and expected mortality with duration, and the consequent effect on EDR and MR. The mortality ratio decreases steadily with increasing duration, but the pattern for EDR is different: a high initial rate of 90 extra deaths per 1000 per year, then a relatively stable EDR, 56-64, in the intervals from 3 to 12 years, followed by a lower rate of 39 per 1000 at 12-15 years.

In the right-hand portion of Table 003K1-1 are given the data to convert mortality ratio to an expected rate, q'_s, based on the 1975-80 Basic Select Tables. The basic assumption is that the excess mortality, measured as EDR, would be the same, regardless of the expected mortality used as a standard. Therefore, the smaller select q'_s is added to EDR to obtain an "estimated observed" rate, q_s: $q_s = EDR + q'_s$. The assumption is that this is the annual mortality rate that would have been observed in the MI patients if those cases had been excluded that did not meet insurance select standards in all other respects. The new mortality ratio calculated as 100 q_s/q'_s is seen to be substantially higher than the MR as 100 $\breve{q}/\breve{q}'$. The ratio of the mortality ratios, shown as a decimal to avoid confusion with the percentage values, is given in the right-hand column. This ratio decreases from a maximum of 3.4 in the first interval as duration advances, to a minimum of 1.3 in the last interval.

Shown in Table 003K1-2, for duration 0-3 years, are the mortality data by age, separately for male and female patients. EDR shows little difference by sex, but increases from about 50 per 1000 for patients under age 50 to 210 per 1000 in male patients and 170 per 1000 in female patients in the oldest group, age 70-89. Exclusion of older patients in many clinical trials of post-MI patients clearly results in a lower excess mortality for the remaining group. Note the marked difference in age distribution in the two sexes, and the higher expected mortality for the males in each age group. However, for all ages combined, the female $\breve{q}'$ of 26 per 1000 is almost identical to the $\breve{q}'$ of 27 in the male patients. Mean values of $\breve{q}$ and EDR are also very similar in the two sexes, all ages combined. The trend in mortality ratio is opposite to that of EDR: MR decreases with advancing age, and is higher in female than in male patients in each age group, although MR values are very similar, all ages combined.

In the conversion process to Select expected mortality rate, q'_s is invariably much smaller than $\breve{q}'$ for the same age and sex, and MR values are correspondingly higher. It is of interest that the highest mortality ratios are seen in the age group 50-59, not in the youngest age group. The ratio of mortality ratios tends to increase with advancing age to age 60-69, then decreases. This ratio is therefore quite variable with respect to both age and duration of follow-up. Such variability would make it extremely difficult to use as a factor with which to multiply the

population expected mortality ratio. The variability also explains why I have chosen to approach the conversion through use of EDR, which can reasonably be assumed to be nearly constant if the expected mortality table used is appropriate for the series of persons followed. Errors inherent in this assumption are relatively small when there is substantial excess mortality, as there is, of course, in post-MI patients.

Because this series of post-MI patients consisted of the early survivors of all patients hospitalized for confirmed acute MI in a defined area and time period, it includes the entire spectrum of severity of attack, excluding only patients who died before reaching the hospital. One original intent of Norris et al was to develop a quantitative measure of severity, which they called the "Coronary Prognostic Index."[3] This consisted of a weighted numerical score based on clinical ECG and X-ray findings obtained soon after admission. The index is described in Abstract #614; it was found to predict acute in-hospital mortality with great accuracy. Acute mortality was only 3% in patients with the best prognostic index (C.P.I. score under 4) and increased progressively with increasing index score to 78% in those with the worst prognostic index (C.P.I. score 12 or more). All of the factors used in formulating the C.P.I. for acute mortality were re-tested against mortality of hospital survivors during the first three years after discharge. The modified C.P.I., still based on data available in the very early stages of hospitalization, was also found to be highly predictive of long-term mortality at 3 years[4] and at 6 and 15 years, respectively.[5,6] The C.P.I. scores have been divided into five groups, with ascending severity, and comparative mortality has been shown in Table 003K1-3, for the total series, 0-3 years, with mortality rates again annualized as a geometric mean. As a further comparison, similar mortality data have been added in Table 003K1-3 on the 3-year experience for all male and female patients in the total series, regardless of severity. In the total series, EDR is 123 per 1000 per year, and the mortality ratio is 455%. After its conversion to select mortality, MR is seen to be 1,700%, and the ratio of ratios is 3.7. This ratio of ratios, incidentally, is higher for female than for male patients (Table 003K1-2).

The variation in observed annualized $\breve{q}$ in Table 003K1-3 is more than tenfold: $\breve{q}$ is only 37 per 1000 with C.P.I. score of less than 3, but is 457 per 1000 in the group with the worst C.P.I. score of 12 or more. Corresponding extremes are 10 and 430 per 1000 for EDR and 137% and 1,690% for MR. With conversion of MR to Select Basic Tables, the extremes of MR become 160% and 7,300%, respectively. The ratio of ratios is only 1.2 for the group with C.P.I. score less than 3, but increases from 3.5 to 4.3 as the score and mortality increase. Again, it is evident that the ratio of ratios is also influenced by differences in mortality dependent on differences in severity. These data also demonstrate the extent to which overall mortality in a series of post-MI patients can be influenced by the bias of exclusion of more severe or less severe cases. The EDR of 23 per 1000 in Group J1 of the *1983 Medical Impairment Study*, substandard male policyholders with history of MI, is much lower than the 91 per 1000 for males in the series of Norris *et al*, partly because underwriting selection has excluded many of the severe cases, and partly because of the very small proportion of policyholders age 60 and over.

No age distribution data were available by severity score, so I have been forced to use a constant rate of 27 per 1000 for $\check{q}'$ and 6 per 1000 for q'_s in Table 003K1-3. However, the increase in mortality with advancing age seen in Table 003K1-2 also enters into the C.P.I. score. It can reasonably be assumed that the proportion of older patients, the mean age, and the mean annual $\check{q}'$, all increase with the C.P.I. score. Excess mortality has therefore been somewhat underestimated at low C.P.I. scores and overestimated at high C.P.I. scores. I believe that the magnitude of this bias is not large enough to affect the interpretation of the general trends in EDR, MR and the ratio of ratios in Table 003K1-3.

Mortality ratios in this series have generally exceeded 1,000% after conversion, and such high excess mortality is often handled in insurance rating schedules by a combination of flat extra and table ratings, such as $25 per year and a table equivalent to 300% mortality ratio (+200 debits over standard). To achieve a lesser excess mortality, let us assume a group of post-MI patients with a C.P.I. score of 4 or less, a $\check{q}$ of 30 per 1000, a $\check{q}'$ of 15 per 1000, and restrict the age to 50-59 years and duration to 5 years. The EDR would be 15 per 1000 and the MR 200%. If q'_s is 5 per 1000, the converted mortality ratio is then (100) (15+5)/5 or 400%. Would this correspond to +300 debits in the rating schedule? It would, for the given age group, duration and severity characteristics, *provided* the individual company mortality experience is close to that of the 1975-80 Basic Select Tables. If it is only 80% of intercompany mortality, the MR_s of 400% must be adjusted by dividing by 0.8, and this gives a company-adjusted MR_s of 500%, or +400 debits in that company's rating schedule. If the company mortality is higher, say 125% of that in the Basic Select Tables, the adjusted MR_s would be (400/1.25) or 320%, corresponding to +220 debits. Such adjustments may affect the appropriate rating class. If the rating class limits for an average +300 debits are +250 to +349 debits, such adjustment might make the appropriate rating class one table above or one table below the rating class for an MR_s of 400% based on the Intercompany Select Tables. Adjustment is there-

fore essential, based on the level of individual company mortality in relation to the Intercompany mortality rates used, as they are in the *1983 Medical Impairment Study*, for example. Of course, the appropriate individual company mortality rate can be substituted for that used in Tables 003K1-1 to 003K1-3, and then no further adjustment of MR_s would be needed.

I will now revert to one further set of results from the reports of Norris *et al*. A survival curve has been published as Figure 1 in the 1984 report,[6] with annual values of the cumulative survival rate to 15 years. From this and other data, I have reconstructed annual exposure data for the total series, and comparative mortality has been recalculated with observed mortality rates calculated as d/E instead of as a geometric mean. These results are shown in Table 003K1-4, with subdivision of follow-up into more conventional intervals for post-MI patients: 0-1, 1-5, 5-10 and 10-15 years. The purpose of this exercise is to show the very large excess mortality in the first year, and the steady decrease in EDR and MR after the first year. Excess mortality calculated with the use of *aggregate mean* mortality rates is somewhat higher than it is from *geometric mean* rates because of the different weighting used to obtain the average annual rates.[1] Use of a triennial interval has somewhat inflated expected deaths, as shown in the comparison of the two methods for the total series, duration 0-15 years at the bottom of the table. Conversion of mortality ratios to Basic Select expected rates has not been carried out in Table 003K1-4. The trend is similar to that for the male patients age 50-59 in Table 003K1-1; the highest ratio of mortality ratios is 4.1 for the first year of follow-up.

A final comment on patterns and magnitudes of excess mortality. Just as "man cannot live by bread alone," I used to admonish those attending the mortality seminars, "the medical director (and the underwriter) should not live by mortality ratio alone." I hope these illustrative tables and text will reinforce the thesis that excess mortality should always be evaluated in terms of excess death rate, EDR, as well as the traditional mortality ratio. Both of these indexes are functions of two independent variables, observed mortality, q, and expected mortality, q'. Both of these mortality rates should be used as *annual* rather than cumulative or interval rates, if possible, although averaging is often necessary to yield a sufficient number of deaths. In this article, I have had to assume that the reader already has some acquaintance with the rudiments of life table methodology. The methodology is described in *Medical Risks*,[1] in the 1976 panel discussion,[2] and in material distributed to those taking the past courses offered by the Board of Insurance Medicine and the numerous mortality seminars given since 1977.

To assist readers who may wish to review the methodology, I am reproducing two illustrations used in the panel discussion.[2] Figure 003K1-1 shows a bar graph representation of a set of observed mortality rates per 1000 of different orders of magnitude, approximate average Select mortality over the first 5 policy years for issue ages 30, 40, 50 and 60, and the corresponding indexes, EDR=q–q', and MR= 100(q/q'). These data are intended to force the reader to consider age in relation to q', and the impact on EDR and MR. I have also reintroduced the question as to what are appropriate qualifying terms for a wide range of magnitudes of excess mortality. No one at the 1976 meeting ever wrote to me as to the appropriateness of the schema shown (based on EDR rather than MR) or the qualifying adjectives to describe the excess mortality. What do readers of this article think?

The final item reproduced from the 1976 panel is labeled Table 003K1-5. It consists of average annual Select rates per 1000 for combinations of quinquennial entry ages 5 to 75, and follow-up years 0-5, 5-10 and 10-15. The rates are derived from the 1965-70 Basic Select Tables. The diagonal lines connect rates for the same average *attained age*, as described in the explanatory text, which is also reproduced below the table. This can be used as a reference table for values of Select q', averaged over 5-year intervals of follow-up, as part of the conversion method for MR described herein. The more detailed 1975-80 Basic Select Tables, or appropriate company Select tables, may also be used, if desired. If Figure 003K1-1 and Table 003K1-5 are studied in conjunction with the printed Panel Discussion[2] they will provide a useful background to the proposed conversion method for Mortality Ratio described in this article.

REFERENCES

1. R. B. Singer, L. Levinson, eds., *Medical Risks: Patterns of Mortality and Survival* (Lexington, MA, Lexington Books, 1976).

2. H. F. Starr, Jr., Moderator, "Panel Discussion: The Mortality Monograph, a Medico-Actuarial Milestone," *Trans. Assoc. Life Insur. Med. Dir. Am.*, 60 (1976): 142-70.

3. R. M. Norris, P. W. T. Brandt, D. E. Caughey, et al., "A New Coronary Prognostic Index," *Lancet*, 1 (1969): 174-78.

4. R. M. Norris, D. E. Caughey, C. J. Mercer, et al., "Coronary Prognostic Index for Predicting Survival After Recovery from Acute Myocardial Infarction," *Lancet*, 2 (1970): 485-88.

5. R. M. Norris, D. E. Caughey, C. J. Mercer, et al., "Prognosis After Myocardial Infarction. Six-year Follow-up," *Brit. Heart J.*, 36 (1974): 786-90.

6. M. A. Merrilees, P. J. Scott, R. M. Norris, "Prognosis After Myocardial Infarction: Results of 15 Year Follow-up," *Brit. Med. J.*, 288 (1984): 356-59.

7. E. A. Lew, J. Gajewski, eds., *Medical Risks: Trends in Mortality by Age and Time Elapsed* (New York, Praeger, 1990).

CONVERSION OF MORTALITY RATIOS FROM POPULATION EXPECTED TO SELECT EXPECTED RATES

(See Norris *et al.*, Auckland, N.Z., All Acute MI Survivors 1966-67 Followed to 1983, Abstract #614, *Medical Risks: Trends in Mortality by Age and Time Elapsed,* 1990)

TABLE 003K1-1

MALE PATIENTS AGE 50-59 BY TRIENNIAL DURATION INTERVALS

Duration (Hosp. Disch.)	N. Z. Population Rates (1970-72)						1975-80 Basic Select Tables			
	No. at Risk at Start	Deaths in Int.	Mean Ann. Mort. Rate/1000			Mortality Ratio	Mean Ann. Mort. Rate/1000		Mortality Ratio	Ratio of Ratios
			Obs.*	Exp.†	Excess		Exp.**	Est. Obs.		
t to t+Δt	ℓ	d	$\breve{q}$	$\breve{q}'$	$(\breve{q}-\breve{q}')$	$MR=100(\breve{q}/\breve{q}')$	q'_s	$q_s=EDR+q'_s$	$MR_s=100(q_s/q'_s)$	MR_s/MR
0-3 yrs.	127	35	102	12	90	850%	3.2	93	2,900%	3.4
3-6	90	18	72	16	56	450	5.0	61	1,220	2.7
6-9	70	17	86	22	64	390	9.2	73	795	2.0
9-12	53	14	93	29	64	320	15	79	525	1.6
12-15	39	8	74	35	39	210	22	61	275	1.3

* Geometric mean annual rate: $\breve{q}=1-\breve{p}=1-\sqrt[3]{P_3}$. $P_3=1-Q_3=1-(d/\ell)$.

† Basis of expected $\breve{q}'$: 1970-72 New Zealand Life Tables Rates (graduated).

** Basis of expected q'_s: 1975-80 Basic Select Tables.

TABLE 003K1-2

POST-MI PATIENTS BY AGE AND SEX, DURATION 0-3 YEARS

Age Group	N. Z. Population Rates (1970-72)						1975-80 Basic Select Tables			
	No. at Risk at Start	Deaths in Int.	Mean Ann. Mort. Rate/1000			Mortality Ratio	Mean Ann. Mort. Rate/1000		Mortality Ratio	Ratio of Ratios
			Obs.*	Exp.†	Excess		Exp.**	Est. Obs.		
Yrs.	ℓ	d	$\breve{q}$	$\breve{q}'$	$(\breve{q}-\breve{q}')$	$MR=100(\breve{q}/\breve{q}')$	q'_s	$q_s=EDR+q'_s$	$MR_s=100(q_s/q_s')$	MR_s/MR
MALE PATIENTS										
Under 50	67	10	52	4.4	48	1,180%	2.0	50	2,500%	2.1
50-59	127	35	102	12	90	850	3.2	93	2,900	3.4
60-69	108	42	151	30	121	505	7.0	128	1,830	3.6
70-89	61	31	210	86	124	245	20	144	720	2.9
All Ages	363	118	123	27	96	455	6.9	103	1,490	3.3
FEMALE PATIENTS										
Under 50	16	2	43	3.4	40	1,260%	1.3	41	3,200%	2.5
50-59	40	9	81	6.4	75	1,270	1.9	77	4,100	3.2
60-69	55	20	140	15	125	935	3.8	129	3,400	3.6
70-89	56	24	170	58	112	295	11.9	124	1,040	3.5
All Ages	167	55	124	26	98	475	5.8	104	1,790	3.8

* Geometric mean annual rate: $\breve{q}=1-\breve{p}=1-\sqrt[3]{P_3}$. $P_3=1-Q_3=1-(d/\ell)$.

† Basis of expected $\breve{q}'$: 1970-72 New Zealand Life Table Rates (graduated).

** Basis of expected q'_s: 1975-80 Basic Select Tables.

CONVERSION OF MORTALITY RATIOS FROM POPULATION EXPECTED TO SELECT EXPECTED RATES

(See Norris *et al.*, Auckland, N.Z., All Acute MI Survivors 1966-67 Followed to 1983,
Abstract #614, *Medical Risks: Trends in Mortality by Age and Time Elapsed,* 1990)

TABLE 003K1-3

All POST-MI PATIENTS, 0-3 YEARS, BY SEVERITY (CORONARY PROGNOSTIC INDEX)

C.P.I. Score	No. a Risk at Start		Deaths in Int.	Mean Ann. Mort. Rate/1000			Mortality Ratio	Mean Ann. Mort. Rate/1000		Mortality Ratio	Ratio of Ratios
								1975-80 Basic Select Tables			
				Obs.*	Exp.†	Excess		Exp.**	Est. Obs.		
	ℓ (%)		d	$\check{q}$	$\check{q}'$	$(\check{q}-\check{q}')$	MR=100($\check{q}/\check{q}'$)	q'_s	q_s=EDR+q'_s	MR$_s$=100(q_s/q'_s)	MR$_s$/MR
1-2.9	170	(32%)	—	37	(27)	10	137%	(6)	16	160%	1.2
3-5.9	139	(27%)	—	91	(27)	64	335	(6)	70	1,170	3.5
6-8.9	114	(22%)	—	157	(27)	130	580	(6)	136	2,300	4.0
9-11.9	71	(14%)	—	288	(27)	261	1,070	(6)	267	4,400	4.1
12 Up	25	(5%)	—	457	(27)	430	1,690	(6)	436	7,300	4.3
All Pts.	530	(100%)	173	123	27	96	455	6	102	1,700	3.7

* Geometric mean annual rate: $\check{q}=1-\check{p}=1-\sqrt[3]{P_3}$. $P_3=1-Q_3=1-(d/\ell)$.

† Basis of expected $\check{q}'$: 1970-72 New Zealand Life Table Rates (graduated).

** Basis of expected q'_s: 1975-80 Basic Select Tables.

Note: No information on age distribution by C. P. I. score. Probably mean age and $\check{q}'$ and $\check{q}'_s$ increase with C. P. I. score. If so excess mortality is somewhat underestimated at low scores and overestimated at high score.

TABLE 003K1-4

EXPOSURE AND LIFE TABLE DATA, All POST-MI PATIENTS, RECONSTRUCTED FROM ANNUAL SURVIVAL RATES (GRAPH) AND TABULAR DATA

Interval Start-End	No. Alive at Start	Estimated Exposure	No. of Deaths		Mean Ann. Mort. Rate/1000			Mortality Ratio	Obs. Cum. Surv. Rate
			Observed	Expected*	Observed	Expected*	Excess		
t to t+Δt	ℓ	E	d	d'	$\bar{q}$=d/E	$\bar{q}'$	$(\bar{q}-\bar{q}')$	100(d/d')	P
0-1 yr.	530	530	90	13.6	170	26	144	655%	0.830
1-5 yrs.	440	1,512	138	42.4	91	28	63	325	0.557
5-10	294	1,306	102	41.5	78	32	46	245	0.346
10-15	191	832	57	33.0	69	40	29	173	0.258
1-15	440	3,650	297	116.9	81	32	49	255	0.258
0-15	530	4,180	387	130.5	93	31	62	300	0.258
0-15†	530	—	387	140.9†	86**	34††	52	275	0.258

* Basis of expected deaths: annual exposure and 1970-72 New Zealand Life Table Rates.

† Expected deaths = Σ[triennial (ℓ) (Q'$_3$) all age groups, separate M and F]

** Geometric mean q=1–p=1–$\sqrt[15]{P_{15}}$.

†† Geometric mean q'=1–p'=1–$\sqrt[15]{P_{15}}$ =1–$\sqrt[15]{0.5954}$.
   MR=100($\check{q}/\check{q}'$)=100(86/34)=255%.

DEGREES OF EXCESS MORTALITY

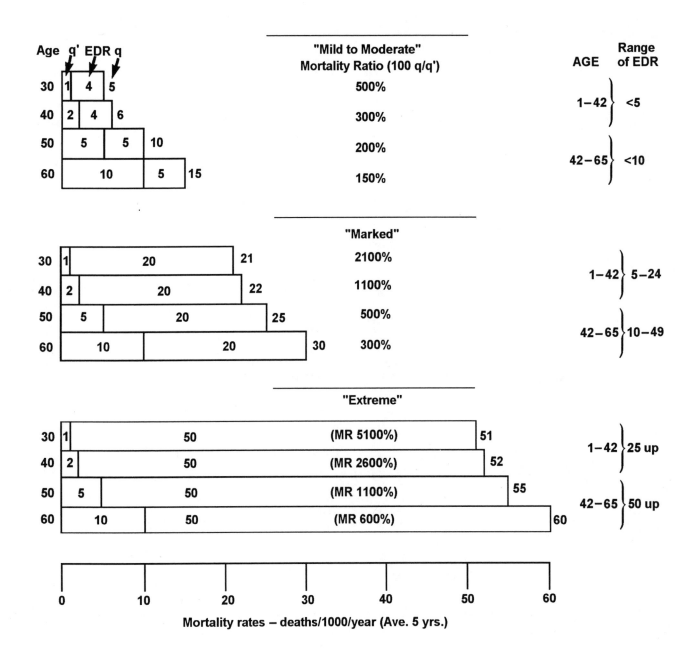

Mortality rates – deaths/1000/year (Ave. 5 yrs.)

TABLE 003K1-5

Average Annual Mortality Rates per 1000 (q′)

| | Male Years of Follow-up | | | | Female Years of Follow-up | | |
| | 0-5 | 5-10 | 10-15 | | 0-5 | 5-10 | 10-15 |
Entry Age	Average Attained Age above Entry Age +2	+7	+12		Average Attained Age above Entry Age +2	+7	+12
5	0.39	0.46	1.01		0.28	0.26	0.37
10	0.42	0.98	1.41		0.24	0.33	0.48
15	0.86	1.24	1.17		0.26	0.41	0.68
20	0.97	1.01	1.18		0.30	0.57	0.90
25	0.74	0.96	1.55		0.42	0.68	1.11
30	0.78	1.4	2.7		0.63	1.1	1.7
35	1.2	2.4	4.9		0.84	1.6	2.9
40	2.1	4.1	7.8		1.3	2.6	4.2
45	3.2	6.4	12.3		1.9	3.8	6.2
50	4.9	10.0	19.2		2.5	5.2	9.3
55	7.3	15.1	29.3		3.5	7.0	15.2
60	10.6	20.9	43.4		5.7	11.7	26.7
65	15.6	28.7	65.0		8.9	19.6	41.8
70	22.2	43.3	98.3		13.9	32.2	65.7
75	35.3	67.1	155.4		25.1	53.9	114.7

(Diagonal lines link Average Attained Age values: 22, 32, 42, 52, 62, 72, 82.)

The diagonal lines slanting upward lead to the average *attained age* common to the combinations of entry age and follow-up duration for which the mortality rates are thus linked. For example, men with entry age 40 have an average q′ of 2.1 per 1000 per year for years 0-5 of follow-up, corresponding to attained ages 40 through 44 or an average attained age of 42. Proceeding horizontally in the table q′ is 4.1 at durations 5-10 (average attained age 47) and 7.8 at durations 10-15 years (average attained age 52). However, attained age 42 is also produced by a combination of entry age 35 and follow-up 5-10 years (q′ of 2.4), and a combination of entry age 30 and follow-up 10-15 years (q′ of 2.7). Such values of q′, linked by the diagonal lines, reflect an increase in q′ with increasing duration of follow-up at the same attained age, due to gradual loss of the effect of selection on entry (issue of standard insurance). However, the effect of life insurance selection never disappears completely, as ultimate mortality rates, more than 15 years after policy issue, are still considerably lower than mortality rates in the general population for the same sex and attained age (ultimate insurance and population rates are not shown in the table).

MORTALITY RATIOS TO
NUMERICAL RATING CLASSIFICATION

Orrin S. Tovson, F.S.A.

Dear Editor:

Underwriters are indebted to Dr. Richard Singer for his excellent article "The Conversion of Mortality Ratios to a Numerical Rating Classification for Life Insurance Underwriting." The approach he illustrated is especially useful in the instance of impairments with extra mortality which is substantial in the early durations at all ages and which decreases sharply among the survivors in later years.

In mortality studies for which advance preparation is possible, significant characteristics of individual lives can be recognized. Impaired lives and lives set up as a standard for comparison can be selected carefully. In analyzing studies of previous years this careful selection of lives may not be possible. Frequently the number of lives is so small that the desired breakdown into homogenous groups is impractical.

To measure the mortality significance of an impairment, the absence of other impairments is desirable, but probably not vital for useful results. However, comparison with a group of lives reasonably similar in all respects, but for the impairment, is essential for reliable indication of its effect on mortality.

Selecting an appropriate group of lives for comparison is difficult especially when information about the impaired group is limited. Mortality is affected by many measurable physical characteristics of the body and its impairments; sex; habits such as tobacco, drug, and alcoholic beverage usage, rest, physical activity, and diet; occupation; consistency of diagnosis; and many other facets of an individual. Some of these characteristics vary by geographical area and ethnic background, and some tend to change as the years pass.

Unfortunately, medical reports do not include the details on individual lives which are available for insurance impairment studies; so, a problem exists in selecting a suitable standard for comparison. A frequent choice is population mortality of the same period covering the same geographical area. Population groups contain impaired lives, the percent impaired tending to increase with age. Since these impaired lives experience higher mortality rates, the population group as a whole experiences higher than standard mortality; so, the rate of extra mortality is understated.

Dr. Singer stated that first year select rates are about 25% to 35% of the population rates with the differential decreasing with increasing policy duration. Insurance pricing recognizes this and allows for it. Hence, when extra mortality is based on only the excess over population life mortality, excess mortality in the early durations will be understated.

On the other hand, the presence of any other impairments in the impaired life group being studied tends to increase the mortality of that group and thus overstate the extent of extra mortality.

The study Dr. Singer selected for his illustration, 530 lives with 387 deaths, summarized the problem an analyst faces. This study covered 2 sexes, 4 broad age groups, 5 duration groups, and 5 Coronary Prognostic Index ranges —200 groups of impaired lives, averaging 2.65 lives and 1.94 deaths per group. Dr. Singer further demonstrated that variations in each of the four characteristics affected mortality significantly. By itself each of the 200 possible groups was too small for the results of its experience to be significant.

While the underwriter is helped considerably by Dr. Singer's illustration of how to use the abstracts in the *Medical Risks* book, its sequel, and similar mortality studies, he must include his own informed judgement regarding approximations and assumptions included in mortality studies when incorporating this information in his composite underwriting decision.

One last word must be added. All medical reports and studies thereon are in the past. Medical science, its technology, and methods of treatment, are being improved constantly. Many individuals are responding to these advances, and persons insured today might enjoy lower mortality rates than those on whom the studies were made.

Sincerely,

Orrin S. Tovson, F.S.A.

Source: O. S. Tovson, "Correspondence — Mortality Ratios to Numerical Rating Classification," *J. Ins. Med.*, 20, no. 4 (1988): 76. Reproduced with permission of author and publisher.

FEINSTEIN'S REPORT OF THE "WILL ROGERS" PHENOMENON: ADVANCES IN DIAGNOSIS, RESULTING STAGE MIGRATION, AND THEIR IMPACT ON 6-MONTH LUNG CANCER MORTALITY BY STAGE

Richard B. Singer, M.D.

"When the Okies left Oklahoma and moved to California they raised the average intelligence level in both states."

Attributed to Will Rogers

References:

1. A. R. Feinstein, D. M. Sosin, C. K. Wells, "The Will Rogers Phenomenon — Stage Migration and New Diagnostic Techniques as a Source of Misleading Statistics for Survival in Cancer," *N. Engl. J. Med.*, 312 (1985): 1604-8.

2. M. E. Charlson, A. R. Feinstein, "A New Clinical Index of Growth Rate in the Staging of Breast Cancer," *Am. J. Med.*, 69 (1980): 527-36.

3. A. R. Feinstein, "An Additional Basic Science for Clinical Medicine: IV. The Development of Clinimetrics," *Ann. Int. Med.*, 99 (1983): 843-48.

4. A. R. Feinstein, J. A. Pritchett, C. R. Schimpff, "The Epidemiology of Cancer Therapy. IV. The Extraction of Data from Clinical Records," *Arch. Int. Med.*, 123 (1969): 571-90.

Background: In the course of two decades of the study of cancer epidemiology, Dr. Alvan R. Feinstein has made important observations and presented innovative concepts that are fundamental to the methodology and analysis of all types of follow-up studies. To cite only three examples, he has used the term "auxometric" in a report on a new clinical index of growth rate in the staging of breast cancer,[2] he has stressed the importance of accurately defined descriptors as a science of "clinimetrics," and he has added much to basic aspects of the carrying out of follow-up studies by attention to accuracy of recording clinical data.[4] Other references my be found in Feinstein's report on the "Will Rogers Phenomenon,"[1] which is the source for this mortality abstract. An objective of this 1985 report[1] was to compare 6-month survival in a 1977 cohort of patients treated for lung cancer with survival in an earlier cohort, according to stage and other characteristics, including newer diagnostic techniques used in the 1977 staging, but not available for use in the earlier cohort. Six-month survival by TNM stage appeared to have improved in the 1977 cohort, but on analysis by staging procedures used in the earlier cohort it was found that this change was due to migration of cases from a less advanced stage in accordance with the earlier criteria, to a more advanced stage according to the 1977 criteria, which employed new diagnostic imaging techniques. These effects have been discussed in detail, and Feinstein has also demonstrated that no change in survival between cohorts has occurred according to symptom stages, an alternate method of classification of stage of the cancer that is unaffected by the new imaging techniques.

Subjects Studied: In the 1977 cohort there were 131 patients treated for lung cancer and in the 1953-64 cohort, 1,266 patients, both cohorts treated and observed at the Yale-New Haven and the West Haven V.A. Hospitals in Connecticut. Mean age was 63 years in both cohorts; the 1977 cohort contained 27% female and 9% black patients, in contrast to only 12% female and 4% black patients in the 1953-64 cohort. "Old-stage" data used for TNM staging in both cohorts included examination findings, bronchoscopy, biopsy and cytology, and conventional and contrast X-rays. "New-stage" data used in the 1977 cohort only, included radio-nuclide imaging of liver and spleen, brain, and bone, as well as other procedures, such as CT scan, ultrasound, etc. These were used in the initial TNM staging of the 1977 patients, then this was redone with only the old-stage criteria. An independent set of symptomatic criteria for lung cancer was defined and used in both cohorts. Four categories were used: *Asymptomatic; Primary* (symptoms such as hemoptysis, change in cough pattern, wheezing, dyspnea or chest pain); *Systemic* (symptoms such as anorexia, weight loss, fatigue or existence of a paraneoplastic syndrome); *Metastatic* (symptomatic evidence of a metastatic lesion, excluding asymptomatic patients with morphologic evidence of metastasis).

Follow-up: Deaths and survival data at 6 months were available in all patients in both cohorts. "Zero-time" for

Source: R. B. Singer, "Feinstein's Report of the 'Will Rogers' Phenomenon: Advances in Diagnosis, Resulting Stage Migration, and Their Impact on 6-Month Lung Cancer Mortality by Stage," *J. Ins. Med.*, 22 (1990): 141-44. Reproduced with permission of author and publisher.

start of follow-up was defined as the date of the first antineoplastic treatment for lung cancer, or the date of a decision not to undertake any antineoplastic treatment. Staging was based only on data available at zero-time.

Results: The distribution, survival, and comparative mortality of the two cohorts by stage are shown in Tables 006K1-1, 006K1-2, and 006K1-4. Observed survivors are given as the observed data in Tables 006K1-2 and 006K1-4 instead of deaths; overall, 715 patients in the 1953-64 cohort and 59 in the 1977 cohort had died at the end of 6 months from zero-time. Results are annualized by obtaining the square of the 6-month survival rate, and deriving an annual mortality rate (based on the experience in the first 6 months) as the complement of the survival rate. This is compared with an approximation of age/sex-matched U.S. 1959-61 population rates for the 1953-64 cohort, the approximation made from the aggregate first-year expected rates for all lung cancer patients by stage in Table 142b of the *1976 Medical Risks* monograph (the experience from End Results Group, Report No. 4). For the 1977 cohort these q' values have been adjusted for the secular decrease in mortality during this period by multiplying by a factor of 0.82. In the absence of age/sex data on the symptom-stage distribution, a constant overall q' has been assumed in both cohorts in Table 006K1-4.

The extremely high mortality characteristic of lung cancer is evident in Tables 006K1-2 through 006K1-4. Both mortality ratio and EDR increase with stage, but even in Stage I EDR is 425 extra deaths per 1000 per year in the 1953-64 cohort, with a mortality ratio of 1,470% despite a mean age of 63 years. Note that in the 1977 cohort in Table 006K1-2 excess mortality is lower (survival is higher) in each stage, as compared with the 1953-64 cohort, although the overall experience is not very different. The TNM classification for the 1977 cohort in Table 006K1-2 employed all data from new-stage diagnostic techniques, including radionuclide imaging and other methods not available in 1953-64.

Table 006K1-3 shows the stage migration and results when the 131 patients of the 1977 cohort are reclassified according to old-stage TNM criteria. The number of Stage I patients would be increased from 24 to 42 by migration of 18 patients, all but one from Stage III. The annual mortality rate of the migrating Grade III patients, 0.720, is much higher than the rate of 0.160 of the 24 patients in the new-stage Grade I. This results in an overall old-stage I EDR of 393 per 1000 and an MR of 1,560%, very close to the level of excess mortality in the Stage I patients of the 1953-64 cohort (Table 006K1-2). The apparent decrease in Stage I excess mortality in Table 006K1-2 is therefore seen to be due to the change in TNM staging criteria. When the old-stage criteria are used for both

cohorts, there is virtually no difference in excess mortality. A similar effect is observed when 8 Grade III patients migrate to the 17 remaining in Grade II: EDR and MR are raised to levels slightly above those in the 1953-64 cohort. The excess mortality in the 64 patients remaining in Grade III in the 1977 cohort is about the same as the respective levels for both cohorts in Table 006K1-2: an EDR over 800 per 1000 per year and an MR about 3,000%.

Comparative mortality for the two cohorts by symptom staging is shown in Table 006K1-4. These criteria are just as effective as the TNM staging in separating the lung cancer patients into a graded series with excess mortality that increases with the severity group. The asymptomatic patients, although smaller in number, have an excess mortality similar to that found in the Grade I patients of the 1953-64 cohort and in the old-stage Grade I patients of the 1977 cohort, with an MR close to 1,500% and EDR under 400 per 1000. The patients in the most severe symptom category, with *clinical* evidence of metastasis, showed extremely high excess mortality, about the same in both cohorts, and similar to the level shown when the morphologic criteria for TNM Grade III were used (Tables 006K1-2 and 006K1-3). For each of the symptom stages in Table 006K1-3 mortality is nearly the same in the two cohorts. Symptom staging is unaffected by the new diagnostic techniques, and Feinstein in his article stresses the similarity of the 6-month survival in each of the symptom stages in the two cohorts (these survival rates are also given in Table 006K1-4).

Comment: To me this is a highly important observation, of potentially great significance in the design and analysis of follow-up studies, with respect to technical advances in diagnostic methods and their application to methods of severity classification. If either survival or mortality is compared in series with a similar severity classification of the same condition, but the entry periods differ by as little as 10 years, the Will Rogers phenomenon must be taken into account. Is any difference observed in supposedly similar groups due to a secular trend, some change in treatment, or is it due to stage migration? The TNM system for grading cancer stage (a measure of severity) is obviously vulnerable to diagnostic technical advances. Earlier detection of metastatic extension of cancer in an otherwise asymptomatic patient results in a "zero-time" shift, with some prolongation of survival as compared with patients who have symptomatic evidence of metastasis. Further discussion of this and other important statistical matters may be found in the original article.[1] In this discussion Feinstein describes how a friend called his attention to a remark attributed to the famous commentator, Will Rogers, made during the Depression of the 1930s, which I quote as given in the article: "When the

Okies left Oklahoma and moved to California they raised the average intelligence level in both states." Although unable to confirm the author, Feinstein clearly felt that the remark was so apt for the taxonomic and statistical effects of the stage migration he has described that it was fitting to use Will Rogers' name as an eponym for the phenomenon. This reviewer agrees completely! Inciden-

tally, the zero-time shift has been featured in a previous abstract on use of Vitamin C in advanced cancer (*J. Ins. Med.*, 21 (1989):127-30). Although I did not use this descriptive phrase in the abstract, the controversy described illustrates how important such statistical bias can be.

THE WILL ROGERS PHENOMENON

TABLE 006K1-1

DISTRIBUTION OF LUNG CANCER PATIENTS BY STAGE

TNM Stage	1953-64 Cohort		1977 Cohort	
	No. Alive at Start	Distribution (Percent)	No. Alive At Start	Distribution (Percent)
I	281	22.2%	24	18.3%
II	172	13.6	18	13.7
III	813	64.2	89	68.0
All	1,266	100.0	131	100.0

TABLE 006K1-2

6-MONTH COMPARATIVE MORTALITY IN LUNG CANCER BY TNM STAGE

TNM Stage	No. Alive at Start	No. 6-Mo Survivors	Survival Rate		Annual Mortality Rate		Excess Death Rate	Mortality Ratio
			at 6 mos.	Proj. 1-yr	Observed	Expected*		
	ℓ	s	s/ℓ	p_1	q	q'	EDR	$100(q/q')$
1953-64 COHORT								
I	281	211	0.751	0.564	0.456	0.031	425	1,470%
II	172	98	0.570	0.325	0.675	0.028	647	2,400
III	813	242	0.298	0.089	0.911	0.029	882	3,100
All	1,266	551	0.435	0.189	0.811	0.029	782	2,800
1977 COHORT								
I	24	22	0.917	0.840	0.160	0.027	133	595%
II	18	13	0.722	0.522	0.478	0.025	453	1,910
III	89	37	0.416	0.173	0.827	0.026	801	3,200
All	131	72	0.550	0.302	0.698	0.026	672	2,700

$P_1=(s/\ell)^2$ EDR=1000(q–q').

* Basis of expected rates: End Results Report No. 4, aggregate age/sex-matched U.S. population rates for 1955-64 cohort. See Table 142b, *1976 Medical Risks* monograph. Rates for 1977 cohort adjusted by factor of 0.82 for secular decrease 1960 to 1977.

TABLE 006K1-3

6-MONTH COMPARATIVE MORTALITY IN 1977 COHORT, SUBDIVIDING BY THE TNM 1953-64 STAGING CRITERIA ALONE AND THE 1977 CRITERIA

TNM Stage New	TNM Stage Old	No. Alive at Start	No. 6-Mo. Survivors	Survival Rate at 6 mos.	Survival Rate Proj. 1-yr	Annual Mortality Rate Observed	Annual Mortality Rate Expected*	Excess Death Rate	Mortality Ratio
		ℓ	s	s/ℓ	p_1	q	q'	EDR	$100(q/q')$
I	I	24	22	0.917	0.840	0.160			
II	I	1	1	1.000	0.000	0.000			
III	I	17	9	0.529	0.280	0.720			
All	I	42	32	0.762	0.580	0.420	0.027	393	1,560%
II	II	17	12	0.706	0.498	0.502			
III	II	8	5	0.625	0.391	0.609			
All	II	25	17	0.680	0.462	0.538	0.025	513	2,200%
III	III	64	23	0.359	0.129	0.871	0.026	845	3,400%

$P_1=(s/\ell)^2$ EDR=1000(q–q').

* Basis of expected rates: End Results Report No. 4, aggregate age/sex-matched U.S. population rates for 1955-64 cohort. See Table142b, *1976 Medical Risks* monograph. Rates for 1977 cohort adjusted by factor of 0.82 for secular decrease 1960 to 1977.

TABLE 006K1-4

6-MONTH COMPARATIVE MORTALITY IN LUNG CANCER BY SYMPTOM STAGING

Symptom Stage	No. Alive at Start	No. 6-Mo. Survivors	Survival Rate at 6 mos.	Survival Rate Proj. 1-yr	Annual Mortality Rate Observed	Annual Mortality Rate Expected*	Excess Death Rate	Mortality Ratio
	ℓ	s	s/ℓ	p_1	q	q'	EDR	$100(q/q')$
1953-64 COHORT								
Asympt.	84	65	0.774	0.599	0.401	(0.029)	372	1,380%
Primary	298	186	0.624	0.390	0.610	(0.029)	581	2,100
System.	305	152	0.498	0.248	0.752	(0.029)	723	2,600
Metast.	579	148	0.256	0.065	0.935	(0.029)	906	3,200
All	1,266	551	0.435	0.189	0.811	0.029	782	2,800
1977 COHORT								
Asympt.	18	14	0.778	0.605	0.395	(0.026)	369	1,520%
Primary	61	41	0.672	0.452	0.548	(0.026)	522	2,100
System.	20	10	0.500	0.250	0.750	(0.026)	724	2,900
Metast.	32	7	0.219	0.048	0.952	(0.026)	926	3,700
All	131	72	0.550	0.302	0.698	0.026	672	2,700

$P_1=(s/\ell)^2$ EDR=1000(q–q').

* Basis of expected rates: End Results Report No. 4, aggregate age/sex-matched U.S. population rates for 1955-64 cohort. See Table 142b, *1976 Medical Risks* monograph. Rates for 1977 cohort adjusted by factor of 0.82 for secular decrease 1960 to 1977. Values of q' by stage assumed to be the same as for total q' in the absence of detailed age/sex data in the source article.[1]

MORBIDITY/MORTALITY ABSTRACTION — FINDING SUITABLE ARTICLES

Michael W. Kita, M.D.

For medical directors, keeping up with the medical literature means not only staying clinically abreast of developments in medicine, but also appraising morbidity and mortality data for their insurance implications. One of the obstacles to morbidity and mortality data analysis, whether formal (mortality abstract preparation) or informal (simply estimating risk or general prognosis), is the absence of tools which facilitate critiquing articles or quickly judging their suitability for such purposes.

Advice to clinicians on how to critically read medical literature and how to distinguish "good" articles (worth spending time and effort on) from less valuable ones (deserving of only casual attention) is available from a variety of sources (see references below). Advice to *medical directors* on how best to judge the quality and suitability of articles for insurance applications is addressed in such places as Dr. Singer's Advanced Mortality Methodology Workshop, but is less readily available to the average medical director.

The Committee on Mortality and Morbidity of ALIMDA, the ALIMDA Research Center, the Center for Medico-Actuarial Statistics of the MIB, the Board of Insurance Medicine, and other bodies within our industry have been interested in promoting quantitative methods as they apply to insurance medicine, and in simplifying the medical director's risk assessment and prognostic activities. This article notes some of the issues involved in assessing the merit of medical articles for medical director use and offers two examples of "checklist" approaches to ascertaining that merit. The checklists are a preliminary attempt to define key information in an organized fashion, and it is hoped that further modifications and revisions will eventually result in a variety of practical tools for the working medical director.

Upon identifying a condition of interest in a medical study, the medical director will judge the pertinence of the information to his or her work by some yardsticks of relevancy and usefulness. We will typically be interested in information on prevalent or significant conditions,

information which either clarifies vague risks or better differentiates classes of severity, or information which contributes to knowledge about prognosis or outcome (e.g., treated vs. untreated; new treatment vs. traditional treatment; etc.). In other words, the initial **relevance** of the information has to do with the degree to which it extends or refines existing knowledge of risk or outcome.

The utility of the findings will also depend on such factors as the **generalizability** and **definitiveness** of the findings. In general, there is value inherent in articles which provide data on the likelihood of condition "X" leading to event or outcome "Z" in "y" years (where X = a risk factor, diagnosis, exam/lab finding, history, or some other variable of interest, and Z = medical expense, complications, morbidity, disability, or death) depending on the work-focus of the medical director. If the sample is representative of populations of insurance interest, and if the selection criteria studied are at all replicable to applicants or insureds, then the findings may be applicable to our day-to-day work. Whether a result is interesting but only preliminary, or conclusive and compelling, will depend on such factors as the effect size or magnitude of differences shown, the carefulness and thoroughness of the study, and the type and quality of the study (prospective or retrospective, randomized clinical trial or case control study, etc.). The medical director also has need of data which document or better support a particular risk position, which permit better risk classification or stratification, or which allow more accurate quantification of risk (i.e., reducible to mortality ratios, excess death rates or other useful measures).

The potential value of an article to a medical director will also depend on the size of the experience reported and whether satisfactory prior data are available. For example, while a medical director who is contemplating doing a mortality abstract might generally look for a study reporting a sizable mortality experience (greater than 100 deaths, say), he might be equally interested in reporting a follow-up study involving fewer deaths (0-25) if existing mortality sources were negligible. Also, if good prior studies *do* exist, but the new information updates the old or renders the observations more current, then the study likely has practical value.

Source: M. W. Kita, "Morbidity/Mortality Abstraction — Finding Suitable Articles," *J. Ins. Med.*, 22 (1990): 287-88. Reproduced with permission of author and publisher.

CHECKLIST A
Morbidity/Mortality Data Reported

	Minimum	Optimal
Demographic Data @ Entry		
at least mean age and % female	☐	
age breakdown (e.g., by decade)		☐
sex proportions (e.g., by ages)		☐
other stratifiers		☐
Exposure & Follow-Up (F/U) Data		
at least mean (or min/max) duration of F/U	☐	
entry period		☐
detailed durations of F/U		☐
at least % lost to F/U	☐	
detail on age/sex/durations, etc. of those lost to F/U		☐
Observed Experience		
at least outcome (deaths) for total series	☐	
at least % (#) surviving for various durations/intervals	☐	
detailed outcome (e.g., by age, sex, diagnostic group, features of Hx, exam, test results, severity, disease stage, etc.)		☐
interval survival data for all intervals of interest		☐
Expected (comparison/control group) Experience		
comparative data available from *some* source	☐	
appropriate "expected" table supplied or referenced		☐
Significance Test		
enough information given to derive or estimate confidence limits		☐
References (prior studies)		☐

CHECKLIST B
Follow-Up (F/U) Article Evaluation Checklist
(If "no" for a major heading, omit the subheadings)

	Yes	No
1. Demographic Data	☐	☐ (None)
• Age groups & distribution	☐	☐
• Mean age and range	☐	☐
• Sex distribution	☐	☐
• Race or other pertinent demographics	☐	☐
2. Severity/Groupings/or Diagnostic Groups	☐	☐
• If so, number and type:		
3. **Observed** Exposure & F/U Data	☐	☐
• Life table data by age & sex	☐	☐
• Life table data, all ages	☐	☐
• Mean duration of F/U with # entrants and # deaths	☐	☐
• Survival rates to 3 decimals, tabular	☐	☐
• Survival curves only, or P to 2 places	☐	☐
• Information given on loss to F/U	☐	☐
4. **Expected** deaths/events given	☐	☐
• Expected survival/mortality rates given	☐	☐
• If not given, are they available?	☐	☐
• Source tables:_____		
5. Randomized Clinical Trial	☐	☐
• Factor studied:_____		
6. Case-Control Study	☐	☐
• Group(s) studied:_____		
7. Significance Test	☐	☐
• Type of test used: _____	☐	☐

After qualitatively judging the suitability of an article or report, based on its pertinence and the adequacy or currency of existing sources, a quick survey of the *quality of the data* is desirable. This entails judging the level of detail of the observed experience, relating this to some yardstick of expected experience for the purpose of deriving mortality ratios or other comparators, and estimating whether the differences are meaningful (e.g., whether the lower confidence limit differs significantly from 1.0 [100% or standard]). This is where a checklist might be handy.

Checklist A attempts to identify some of the key variables (the minimum required for analysis and the optimal level of detail, if available) that an article should contain.

Even for "rough or approximate" estimates of comparative morbidity or mortality, these are the types of variables (especially the **minimum** ones) that would hopefully be present in the article of interest.

A Checklist more specifically geared to identifying those articles suitable for formal mortality abstraction might look more like Checklist B.

These checklists may not be definitive instruments in their present form, but they represent an initial attempt to provide tools for surveying and critiquing relevant medical literature. Input and suggestions from practicing medical directors would be welcome. Ultimately a number of different such instruments geared to the different types of work medical directors engage and consult in could be developed.

Appreciation is expressed to the members of the Committee on Mortality and Morbidity of ALIMDA and to Richard B. Singer, M.D., for their ideas and contributions.

REFERENCES

1. T. Colton, "Critical Reading of the Medical Literature," *Statistics in Medicine* (Boston, Little Brown, 1974), pp. 315-22.

2. R. K. Riegelman, R. P. Hirsch, "Questions to Ask in Studying a Study," *Studying a Study and Testing a Test: How to Read the Medical Literature,* 2nd ed., (Boston, Little Brown, 1989), pp. 75-77.

3. D. L. Sackett, R. B. Haynes, P. Tugwell, "How to Read a Clinical Journal," *Clinical Epidemiology: A Basic Science for Clinical Medicine* (Boston, Little Brown and Company, 1985), pp. 285-319.

MEDICAL RISKS:
TRENDS IN MORTALITY BY AGE AND TIME ELAPSED

Edward A. Lew, A.M., F.S.A.

A reference volume sponsored by the Association of Life
Insurance Medical Directors of America and the Society of Actuaries

Price $195.00
PRAEGER PUBLISHERS
An imprint of Greenwood Publishing Group, Inc.
88 Post Road West, Box 5007, Westport, CT 06881

Introductory Comments by Edward A. Lew

These two volumes on Medical Risks, sponsored by the Association of Life Insurance Medical Directors of America and the Society of Actuaries, constitute the largest compendium of quantitative information on mortality and survival for a wide variety of physical impairments, based on recent medical literature and mortality investigations among insured lives and special groups. They include synopses of the findings for broad classifications of medical risks as well as actuarial analyses of some 400 follow-up studies by sex, age, time elapsed and certain salient characteristics.

In particular, much new information was assembled for

- Coronary Heart Disease
- Coronary Bypass Surgery
- Cancer
- Underweight and Overweight
- Lifestyle Hazards

Analysis of data from diverse sources resulted in a more revealing perspective on the nature of medical risks and especially on the ranges of mortality associated with such risks under different circumstances.

Thus it became apparent that the disparities between findings of different studies reflected in the main the different characteristics of the various study populations, notably the different ways in which the subjects had been

selected, differences in co-existing impairments including smoking habits, and differences in socio-economic status. Studies of insured lives clearly relate to middle-class persons in ostensibly good health, except for the impairment under study. On the other hand clinical studies have rarely excluded persons with several impairments. Patients in some city hospitals have been heavily weighted with subjects from the lower income segments. Patients in tertiary care hospitals have tended to include more of the severe cases.

The *Medical Risks* volumes contain considerable data on variations in mortality by socio-economic status and life styles. A series of abstracts based on the Framingham Study present findings separately for non-smokers, light smokers, heavy smokers, subjects in ostensibly good health and subjects in impaired health.

The actuarial analyses have focused on comparisons of the death rates recorded in a study with contemporaneous death rates among ostensibly healthy persons (such as individuals insured under group life insurance) or when this was not feasible, with contemporaneous death rates in the general population. It has been demonstrated that comparisons with general population death rates may seriously understate the relative mortality experienced in mild or moderate physical impairments.

Actuarial analyses by time elapsed have shown that the length of time covered by a mortality study could markedly affect the overall mortality level. These analyses indicated that mortality ratios decreased with time elapsed for most physical impairments. Accordingly, short term studies — which include a great many clinical studies — tend to overstate the relative mortality in the long run, as illustrated by the mortality experience among

Source: E. A. Lew, "Medical Risks: Trends in Mortality by Age and Time Elapsed," *J. Ins. Med.*, 22 (1990): 289. Reproduced with permission of author and publisher.

underweights. For some impairments, however, notably overweights, rheumatoid arthritis and diabetes, mortality ratios tend to increase with time elapsed. In the case of these impairments mortality in the short run understates the relative mortality in the long run. Mortality investigations of insured lives have been especially valuable in furnishing information on mortality over an extended period of years.

On the basis of data from mortality investigations of insured lives, it was possible to calculate 25-year temporary life expectancies for various degrees of underweight, overweight and numerous medical impairments, and to compare such figures with corresponding 25-year temporary life expectancies for persons in the normal range. Such comparisons provide a measure of the 'years of life lost' attributable to specific conditions.

This publication should be very useful not only to medical directors, actuaries and underwriters but also to all concerned with the evaluation of medical risks, whether in medical research, the health sciences or even legal appraisals, as in structured settlements.

Much of the credit for the debut of these volumes is due to Dick Singer. He pioneered in the field with the production in 1976 of *Medical Risks: Patterns of Mortality and Survival*. He then recommended to the Liaison Committee that additional mortality and morbidity statistics be assembled and published, and was instrumental in getting the recommendations adopted. He gave us invaluable counsel on difficult problems in putting the present volumes together and contributed (with Jerzy Gajewski) the key chapter on Cardiovascular Diseases.

COMPARATIVE MORBIDITY — WHAT ARE THE PROSPECTS?

Richard B. Singer, M.D.

Thanks to the efforts of many illustrious medical directors and actuaries, comparative mortality was developed in the early part of this century as the indispensable tool for life insurance underwriting of individual applicants. The work of Rogers and Hunter culminated in the publication of the numerical rating system. Over the years results of many insurance mortality studies of impaired risks have provided the basis for underwriting manuals that are in use in all companies offering individual life insurance.[1] More recently follow-up studies have been culled from the medical literature and the mortality systematically presented in a comparative format.[2] Thus the risk classification of applicants with all degrees of excess mortality has been steadily refined since the early years of this century.

Health insurance protection has evolved much more recently, from small beginnings prior to World War 2, burgeoning rapidly in the 1950s, and expanding to provide hospital expense and other benefits to a high percentage of the U.S. population. The bulk of this health insurance is provided on a group basis by insurance companies and Blue Cross or Blue Shield associations, but some of the providers continue to offer health insurance to individual applicants. This means underwriting and assessment of a morbidity instead of a mortality risk. Although I have had only peripheral exposure to health insurance underwriting in my career in insurance medicine, what I have seen leads me to picture underwriting as still being in an early stage of development, with manuals that are based much more on opinion than they are on the application of follow-up studies of morbidity. Do you think I am right in this impression? If so, what accounts for this failure to develop a truly scientific basis for health insurance underwriting during the 50 years or so in which it has been practiced?

In my opinion there are two principal reasons for the lack of development of health insurance underwriting: the passive attitude of health insurance companies in not aggressively going ahead with intercompany morbidity follow-up studies tailored to their own needs, and the absence of successful innovation among medical directors and others responsible for such underwriting, innovation displayed to such a remarkable degree by our predecessors in the first two decades of this century. This phenomenon is definitely not due to the lack of a methodology with which to carry out morbidity follow-up studies, nor is it due to lack of such studies reported in the medical literature. It is my objective in this article to demonstrate how easily familiar life table methodology can be applied to morbidity follow-up, and to cite examples of articles of this sort from the abundant supply in current medical literature. Instead of the usual mortality abstract, I have submitted to our willing Editor a Morbidity Abstract on recurrent myocardial infarction (MI), to accompany and illustrate this article (See Abstract #345K1).

Application of Life Table Methodology to Morbidity Follow-up

Although the traditional use of life tables has been in data on human mortality and survival, there is absolutely no mathematical requirement for this. With a human population series one can readily substitute for death a morbid event as the object of study. From the biological point of view, life table methodology can be applied to a follow-up cohort of any living species, not just Homo sapiens. Finally, life table methodology has often been applied to non-living groups, such as failure rates of light bulbs, in quality control of industrial products. This application has been widely used since World War 2. The mathematical principle is to start with a defined cohort and to follow in time the rates of occurrence of a defined event, and the complementary survival rates of members free of this event. This involves counting in each time interval the number of members entering the interval, the number of events during the interval, and the average number of members exposed to risk during the interval. In a mortality study exposure is calculated as ℓ–0.5w, where w is the number of subjects withdrawn alive during the interval, because of loss to or end of follow-up, or other valid reason, such as dropping out of a treatment plan that was a basis for definition of the group being followed. In a morbidity study exposure is calculated in the same way, but now includes deaths during the period, since this removes the member from being a subsequent risk for the defined morbid event. All of this is set forth in the accompanying Table.

Source: R. B. Singer, "Comparative Morbidity — What are the Prospects?" *J. Ins. Med.*, 20, no. 3 (1988): 47-50. Reproduced with permission of author and publisher.

FACTOR DEFINED	MORTALITY	MORBIDITY
Number available for FU at start of interval	ℓ	ℓ
Number of events during interval	d = deaths	n = morbid events
Number of event-free withdrawn from exposure to risk during interval	w = all alive (deaths excluded)	w = both alive and deaths during interval (but n excluded)
Number exposed to risk of event during interval (usually 1 year)	$E = \ell - 0.5w$	$E = \ell - 0.5w$
Interval event rate (observed)	q = d/E = interval mortality rate	r = n/E = interval morbid event rate
Interval event rate (expected)	q′ from age/sex-matched mortality table	r′ from age/sex-matched data
Number of expected events during interval	d′ = (q′)(E) (expected deaths)	n′ = (r′)(E) (expected events)
Interval observed event-free survival rate	p = 1–q = interval survival rate	p = 1–r = interval event-free survival rate
Interval expected event-free survival rate	p′ = 1–q′	p′ = 1–r′
Cumulative event-free survival rate (observed)	$P = (p_1)(p_2)(p_3)...$	$P = (p_1)(p_2)(p_3)...$
Cumulative event-free survival rate (expected)	$P' = (p'_1)(p'_2)(p'_3)...$	$P' = (p'_1)(p'_2)(p'_3)...$
Cumulative event rate (observed)	Q = 1–P	R = 1–P
Cumulative event rate (expected)	Q′ = 1–P′	R′ = 1–P′
Percentage event ratio	Mortality ratio MR = 100(d/d′)= 100(q/q′)	Morbidity ratio MR = 100(n/n′)= 100(r/r′)
Excess event rate	Excess death rate EDR = 1000(q–q′)	Excess event rate EER = 1000(r–r′)
Cumulative survival ratio	SR = 100(P/P′)	SR = 100(P/P′)

When the exposures are all in units of person-years, the total E, and total d or n can be obtained by adding values of any set of consecutive intervals, and the aggregate mean $\bar{q}$ calculated as (total d)/(total E), or the aggregate mean $\bar{r}$ calculated as (total n)/(total E). When the numbers of deaths or events in each interval, such as one year, are very small, it may be desirable to pool the data over 5 years, for example, in order to calculate a mean with a larger number of events and smaller random error. If full life table data are not available but cumulative survival curves are given in the published article, then a geometric mean annual $\check{q}$ or $\check{r}$ can be calculated as the complement of the 5th root, for example, of the 5-year period survival rate. All of this set forth in the Methodol-

ogy Chapter of *Medical Risks*,[2] and in the homework material for the Mortality Seminars, and lecture notes for the Board of Insurance Medicine courses. The above table covers the same ground, with the addition of a few new symbols for the morbidity application of the life table methodology, to replace d, d′, q, and q′.

For clinical investigators this application of life table methodology has been reported in a 1974 paper in the *Journal of Surgical Research*,[3] and in a later 1977 article.[4] The authors were associates, including a biostatistician, of Dr. Albert Starr, developer of the caged ball device widely used in valve replacement surgery. Not only cardiothoracic surgeons but surgeons and investigators in other specialties often refer to these reports as the basis of their life table methodology, not only for mortality and survival, but also for morbid events. The methodology is a time-honored one for actuaries, and many descriptive articles have appeared in the medical literature long before 1974. One reason for the interest in morbid events displayed by Dr. Starr and others involved in valve replacement surgery is the importance of characterizing the mean rate of occurrence of long-term complications of valve replacement: embolic stroke, serious hemorrhage due to anticoagulation, bacterial endocarditis, and valve failure. All of these are serious complications, but not 100% fatal, and they are best measured as morbid events. Tabular data on the incidence of these complications have been given in Abstracts 667-673 of the *1990 Medical Risks* monograph,[5] abstracts which also deal with comparative mortality following valve replacement surgery.

Examples of Morbidity Follow-up Studies

The first study I wish to cite is Section 32 of the series of Framingham Study detailed reports of data, as distinct from the profusion of articles published in the medical literature about this unique long-term follow-up of a defined segment of a Massachusetts town population.[6] This 150-page section contains 51 tables and 13 graphs of follow-up data on cardiovascular (CV) diseases and deaths occurring after first myocardial infarction (MI) or angina pectoris, during the first 20 years' observation of the Framingham cohort, in which 21% of the men and 11% of the women developed their first evidence of CV disease. The morbid events, as distinct from death, sudden death and CV death, were MI, angina pectoris without MI, coronary attack, coronary insufficiency, cerebrovascular accident, and congestive heart failure. Section 32 also contains mortality and morbidity on the Framingham cohort still free of CV disease at the time of the last biennial examination. These data provide the needed expected rates of MI incidence. Please refer to Abstract #345K1 for my chief illustrated application of life table methodology to MI as a morbid event. The table footnotes and text provide some details of the calculations, which I will not discuss further. The reader who makes a careful study of Section 32 and the MI Morbidity Abstract will be rewarded with a better understanding of the wealth of information available from the Framingham Study, and a detailed illustration of how comparative morbidity results can be derived from the observed data.

Two CV morbidity studies will be cited from a plethora of recent articles I have on file. Herlitz et al. have reported on a 5-year morbidity (and mortality) follow-up of patients with suspected MI or chest pain in three hospitals in Goteberg, Sweden.[7] There were four diagnostic categories: possible MI, angina, chest pain of uncertain origin, and nonischemic chest pain. Baseline characteristics and outcomes are reported in great detail, of potential significance for underwriting. Rehospitalization, anginal pain, dyspnea and cessation of working in patients under age 65 were some of the morbid events studied. Hospital mortality was only 0.7% for all patients, but the 5-year cumulative mortality appeared to me to be elevated for all groups except those with chest pain of uncertain origin. Nevertheless, 40% of the 181 latter patients developed anginal pain with an attack frequency at least once a week, and 26% were hospitalized during the 5-year follow-up. The second example is a very detailed report by Flemma et al. on observation for more than 10 years of 785 patients with valve surgery involving the tilting disc (Bjork-Shiley) valve.[8] This group of cardiovascular surgeons in Milwaukee has maintained an excellent computerized file of operated patients, and provided additional data to supplement previous articles at the time of a visit I made in 1982. These data were used in Abstracts 669 and 672 of the *1990 Medical Risks* monograph.[5] Dr. Flemma kindly provided a typescript of this updated study in response to Ed Lew's January 1988 inquiry, and Ed passed on a copy to me. It was too late to revise the abstracts, but mortality and morbidity results in this latest article certainly deserve the preparation of new abstracts. Follow-up results are given for three different age and four valve groups, with tabular data of events, total exposure and mean annual event rates, as well as survival and event-free survival curves. For example, in patients age 50-59 years the exposure, E, was 2,356 patient-years, there were 39 events involving the complication of clotted valve and arterial emboli, 4 involving clotted valve without embolus, and 7 each involving paravalvular leak and endocarditis. The corresponding mean annual morbid event rates for these complications were 17, 1.6, 7.0 and 7.0 per 1000 pt.-yrs., respectively. Such data are additive with respect to both events and rates, as the exposure is the same, so the total for these complications is 57, for a mean event (complication) rate of 24 per 1000 per year.

Four recent morbidity articles can be quickly cited from the Framingham Study, one of which is not concerned with CV disease. One deals with cigarette smoking and cardiovascular morbidity in women over 50, with or without the use of estrogens. Estrogen use was associated with an increase in stroke morbidity rate in smokers and nonsmokers, but the increase in overall CV morbidity was found only in estrogen users who also smoked.[9] A 1988 article has examined in greater detail cigarette smoking as a risk factor for stroke in both men and women.[10] Blood pressure at the biennial examinations was analyzed for 95 subjects who had received drug therapy for hypertension but were normotensive at the first examination after treatment was stopped.[11] The event-free survival curve for these subjects consisted of the cumulative percentage of those remaining free of hypertension (blood pressure under 140/90). Only 32% remained normotensive without medication at 2 years, and only 14% at 4 years, illustrating the importance of continued medication to control blood pressure in most patients with responsive hypertension. (Seminar graduates, can you calculate a geometric mean annual relapse rate, ř, from these lapse-free survival rates?) In another recent paper[12] postmenopausal estrogen usage was found to be associated with a reduced incidence of hip fracture: only 3 fractures in 1,799 person-years with recent use of estrogen, for a rate of 1.7 per 1000, significantly less than the rate of 7.3 per 1000 (135 fractures in 18,326 person-years) among women who never used estrogen. In some of the articles cumulative incidence (R) is used for a period such as 8 years, contrasting the rates when a factor is present versus not present. Often adjustment is made in R for age, sex and other factors. The variety of formats used in presenting results is a challenge to anyone eager to apply them to our formal view of comparative morbidity. Sometimes relative risk as a decimal is used, and this is analogous to a morbidity ratio. All of these articles contain a wealth of morbidity information, much of it of potential value to the health insurance underwriter.

One very recent article[13] provides data on cancer recurrence, a subject I have always been interested in because of its importance for the length of the waiting period before the applicant with a history of complete removal on an internal cancer can be accepted with a rating. The Local Cancer Study Group reported a retrospective (more accurately, an historical prospective) follow-up of 1,532 patients with "complete" surgical removal of non-small-cell lung cancers, in which there were 98 patients with metastatic recurrence in the brain, only after a maximum follow-up of 8 years. Tabular data are given for annual "hazard rate" (recurrence rate) per patient-year, and hazard or morbidity ratios are presented for four other groups against T_1N_0 (smallest tumor size, no lymph node extension) as the "expected" lowest recurrence rate. Life table data (without E) for the combined experience are given up to 8 years; these show 64 recurrences in the first year, 27 in the second, and only 13 in durations 2-8 years. An article based on data from the first National Health and Nutrition Examination Survey and a follow-up study of this NHANES cohort showed that shorter stature in adults was associated with a significantly reduced occurrence of cancer, especially in men.[14] Bone sarcomas occurring after two-year survival from an earlier cancer of any type in children were reported to be related to dose of radiation and to use of chemotherapy for the initial cancer.[15] Table 1 gives comparative morbidity data (except for E values), including n, n', relative risk (n/n'), and "absolute excess risk" (excess events per 10,000 patient-years). Cumulative event curves are also shown up to 25 years. This paper deserves study by the medical director interested in the methodology of morbidity follow-up in children with a history of cancer. An epidemiologic study was carried out in three plants in Sweden in which workers were exposed to ethylene oxide.[16] Eight cases of leukemia were observed in circumstances with only 0.8 cases expected.

Side-effects of antihypertensive drugs were investigated in the Stepped-Care category of patients enrolled in the Hypertension Detection and Follow-up Program.[17] Patients were divided into four age groups, and over a five-year follow-up the number of side-effects and cumulative incidence rate (R) were reported for six antihypertensive drugs, and for a long list of individual side effects. Definite side effects, sufficient to result in discontinuance of the drug, were observed in 9.3% of cases, cumulative overall to five years. Another study reports recurrence of seizures after withdrawal of anticonvulsant drugs in patients with epilepsy.[19] Of the 92 patients who have been seizure-free for two years when medication was withdrawn, 31 relapsed and 61 remained seizure-free in a maximum follow-up of five years. The morbid event of a recurrent seizure is one that can be well defined.

Conclusion

Perhaps I have raised many difficult questions, for which answers are better attempted by medical directors much more experienced in the practical problems of health insurance underwriting than I am. One important question is how to translate the impact of a single excess event rate into overall excess morbidity. Another is to account for the cost of the benefit, which is not fixed as is the benefit in the life insurance contract. Disability income, not discussed at all in this brief review, has its own adverse claim incentives that affect the cost in ways very difficult to predict. However, we do not know that these problems are insoluble; we are certain only that not enough has been done to gather the data for health insurance underwriting. Medical directors, actuaries and underwriters of the health insurance world unite, and devise a cooperative program to accomplish this! Perhaps this small initial step will provide a needed stimulus to get moving.

REFERENCES

1. R. B. Singer, "Mortality Follow-up Studies and Risk Selection: Retrospect and Prospect," *Trans. Assoc. Life Insur. Med. Dir. Amer.*, 62 (1978): 215-38.

2. R. B. Singer, L. Levinson, eds., *Medical Risks: Patterns of Mortality and Survival* (Lexington, MA, Lexington Books, 1976).

3. R. P. Anderson, L. I. Bonchek, G. L. Grunkemeier, et al., "The Analysis and Presentation of Surgical Results by Actuarial Methods," *J. Surg. Res.*, 16 (1974): 224-30.

4. G. L. Grunkemeier, D. R. Thomas, A. Starr, "Statistical Considerations in the Analysis and Reporting of Time-Related Events," *Am. J. Cardiol*, 39 (1977): 257-58.

5. E. A. Lew, J. Gajewski, eds., *Medical Risks: Trends in Mortality by Age and Time Elapsed* (New York, Praeger, 1990).

6. P. Sorlie, *Section 32. Cardiovascular Diseases and Death Following Myocardial Infarction and Angina Pectoris: Framingham Study, 20-year Follow-up* (Bethesda, Md., National Institutes of Health, DHEW Publication No. [NIH] 77-1247, 1977).

7. J. Herlitz, A. Halmarson, B. W. Karlson, et al., "Long-Term Morbidity in Patients Where the Initial Suspicion of Myocardial Infarction Was Not Confirmed," *Clin. Cardiol.*, 11 (1988): 209-14.

8. R. J. Flemma, D. C. Mullen, M. L. Kleinman, et al., "Survival and 'Event-Free' Analysis of 785 Bjork-Shiley Spherical Disc Valves at 10-16 Years," *Ann. Thor. Surg.*, 45 (1988): 258-72.

9. P. W. F. Wilson, R. J. Garrison, W. P. Castelli, "Postmenopausal Estrogen Use, Cigarette Smoking, and Cardiovascular Morbidity in Women Over 50 — The Framingham Study," *N. Engl. J. Med.*, 313 (1985): 1038-43.

10. P. A. Wolf, R. B. D'Agostino, W. B. Kannel, et al., "Cigarette Smoking as a Risk Factor for Stroke — The Framingham Study," *JAMA*, 259 (1988): 1025-29.

11. A. L. Dannenberg, W. B. Kannel, "Remission of Hypertension — The 'Natural History' of Blood Pressure Treatment in the Framingham Study," *JAMA*, 257 (1987): 1477-83.

12. D. P. Kiel, D. T. Felson, J. J. Anderson, et al., "Hip Fracture and the Use of Estrogens in Postmenopausal Women — The Framingham Study," *N. Engl. J. Med.*, 317 (1987): 1169-74.

13. R. A. Figlin, S. Piantadosi, R. Field, Lung Cancer Study Group, "Intracranial Recurrence of Carcinoma after Complete Surgical Resection of Stage I, II, and III Non-Small-Cell Lung Cancer," *N. Engl. J. Med.*, 318 (1988): 1300-5.

14. D. Albanes, D. Y. Jones, A. Schatzkin, et al., "Adult Stature and Risk of Cancer," *Cancer Res.*, 48 (1988): 1658-62.

15. M. A. Tucker, G. A. D'Angio, J. D. Boice, Jr., et al., "Bone Sarcomas Linked to Radiotherapy and Chemotherapy in Children," *N. Engl. J. Med.*, 317 (1987): 588-93.

16. C. Hogstedt, L. Aringer, A. Gustavsson, "Epidemiologic Support for Ethylene Oxide as a Cancer-Causing Agent," *JAMA*, 255 (1986): 1575-78.

17. J. D. Curb, N. O. Borhani, T. P. Blaszkowski, et al., "Long-term Surveillance for Adverse Effects of Antihypertensive Drugs," *JAMA*, 253 (1985): 3263-68.

18. N. Callaghan, A. Garrett, T. Goggin, "Withdrawal of Anticonvulsant Drugs in Patients Free of Seizures for Two Years," *N. Engl. J. Med.*, 318 (1988): 942-46.

CHAPTER 4

GUIDELINES FOR
EVALUATION OF FOLLOW-UP ARTICLES AND
PREPARATION OF MORTALITY ABSTRACTS

Richard B. Singer, M.D. and Michael W. Kita, M.D.

Introduction

Clinical medicine and insurance medicine both grow by accretion — by the gradual augmentation and improvement of what is known and measurable. There is an ongoing need to *extend* the results of previous follow-up (FU) studies, to *update* them, to *collect data on impairments never before studied*, and to *apply* all of these results in more meaningful ways. Articles with useful FU data not previously used in published mortality and morbidity abstracts provide a ready stockpile of sources of potential value to insurance medicine. Criteria by which "*suitability*" of FU studies might be judged were the subject of a recent article in the *Journal of Insurance Medicine*.[1] In Part I of the present article we will develop a more extended discussion of the many factors that contribute to the suitability of non-insurance studies, or their unsuitability. Part II will provide an in-depth critique of methods that have been found to be useful in the transformation of observed FU data into tables of comparative mortality or morbidity and text for an abstract. We will not discuss methods and strategies for searching medical literature through the numerous on-line services that make use of the computerized index of the National Library of Medicine. However retrieved, once a FU article becomes available to a medical director, Part I may be helpful in the evaluation of the applicability of the data to the concepts of comparative mortality. Part II is intended to assist any volunteers interested in the creative process of preparing a formal abstract for submission to this Journal. However, the same methods may also be applied by the medical director who wishes to make a rapid and informal mortality estimate in a particular underwriting or claim case. We urge all medical directors to keep in mind this potential for personal application of life table methodology in their daily work, even if they do

not aspire to prepare a formal mortality or morbidity abstract.

Part I—Evaluation of Articles

Condition Studied. The prevalence of the disease or condition under study in a FU article has an important bearing on the degree of classification needed and the usefulness of the results despite small size of the series. The reviewer should have some familiarity with the inter-company and other insurance studies, and with the mortality abstracts published, and should also have reference data on disease prevalence. Mortality and morbidity FU studies are made not only on chronic (and acute) diseases, but also on examination findings, such as blood pressure and weight in relation to height, test findings such as ECG or serum cholesterol, and nonspecific history such as chest pain or a single episode of febrile convulsion in childhood. To these we apply the term "conditions," as opposed to diseases. The term "impairment" has been used in underwriting literature.

Classification. A mortality study of coronary heart disease (CHD) patients should be classified in much greater detail for subsequent use than a study of patients with amyloidosis. Those interested in comparative FU data in CHD patients will probably focus their attention on a particular aspect, such as myocardial infarction (MI), or bypass surgery, or the prognosis of acute MI patients with complicating ventricular arrhythmia. On the other hand, it is unlikely that anyone would wish to classify in great detail abstracts on a rare disease such as amyloidosis. The topic of disease classification will be dealt with in a *JIM* article now in preparation.[2]

Size of Series. A frequent question asked by reviewers of FU articles is, "what is the minimum size of a series (or minimum number of deaths), for the data to be worth the effort of preparing a mortality abstract?" Although there is no simple answer to this question, some criteria can be outlined. For example, a huge volume of cases, exposures and deaths is available in the 1979 and earlier Blood Pressure Studies. A clinical series of 2,000 hypertension

Source: R. B. Singer, M. W. Kita, "Guidelines for Evaluation of Follow-up Articles and Preparation of Mortality Abstracts," *J. Ins. Med.*, 23 (1991): 21-29. Reproduced with permission of authors and publisher.

patients with over 100 deaths would add little to the results of these studies, unless the report included special aspects not found in the Blood Pressure Studies, aspects such as malignant hypertension, now a relatively rare disease. For any rare disease, with no known previous study, a series with fewer than 50 patients and only 0-5 deaths might be of value for a mortality abstract. If minimum size standards can be developed in the future, it will have to be in relation to the prevalence of the disease, ranging from common to very rare, and to the existence of previous comparative mortality studies. With respect to comparative morbidity, such abstracts are extremely rare, although morbidity FU observations are being reported with increasing frequency in the medical literature.

Type of Follow-up Study. There are several different methods of designing and carrying out FU studies, some of which provide for "controls," but more often than not a suitable "expected" mortality is not given in the article. Features of these types are given briefly below; details are more important to the analyst who prepares the tables than they are to the reviewer.

- Prospective Study, planned in advance, to define a group with a common disease or condition, to determine all needed characteristics of each entrant, and to follow the entire group at stated intervals. Examples are the Framingham Study (entry at nearly the same starting date), and most Cancer Registries (entry over a period of years). The duration of entry period is important because many entrants will be withdrawn as survivors at the cutoff date, with differing durations of FU, because they have come to the end of follow-up. If all entrants have the same starting and ending dates and none are lost to FU, the only attrition is death, an important factor in rate calculations.

- Historical Prospective Study, planned and carried out after the beginning of the entry period. Intercompany and individual company mortality studies are of this type, also studies utilizing the very complete record systems of the Mayo Clinic and the related Rochester (Minnesota) Epidemiological Project. Studies of this type outnumber purely prospective studies.

- Randomized Clinical Trials are prospective studies in which patients from a large pool are assigned in randomized fashion to two or more groups, at least one of which serves as a placebo control, while a particular method of treatment is used for the other group(s). Randomization is often done on a double-blind basis, and such studies are often sponsored by one of the National Institutes of Health in the U.S. or public health agencies in other countries. Epidemiologists tend to consider these the "gold standard" for the efficacy of a drug or other treatment method, perhaps

a term made more appropriate by their great expense. However, clinical trials share many of the problems of other FU studies, and some students of mortality studies believe that a good observational study, of the historical prospective type, may provide information as useful and as statistically conclusive as that derived from a clinical trial.

- Case Control Studies involve identification of patients having a certain characteristic to be studied (such as adverse effect of a drug) from a large set of records, then identification from the same record pool of another series of patients lacking the study characteristic, but matched as closely as possible with respect to age, sex and other factors that are felt to be important to the outcome, either death or some morbid event.

- Retrospective Studies involve investigation of the *preceding* course of a disease in a series of patients identified at some endpoint of the course, such as death and autopsy, or hospitalization. Rare exceptions are possible, but generally autopsy series cannot be utilized to prepare data for a mortality abstract. Almost all articles of this type would be rejected as unsuitable for abstract preparation.

Formation of the Series is a matter of direct concern for the representativeness of the experience. All kinds of bias may enter into the way in which the subjects or patients are selected for the study. A study of life insurance policyholders is biased to lesser degrees of severity in persons from a higher than average socioeconomic group. A study of a series of hospitalized patients is usually biased to higher degrees of severity of the disease studied. A proper sample of the population is needed to obtain all degrees of severity; this is the advantage of a registry such as the Rochester Epidemiological Project, which provides unusually complete case detection and follow-up of the residents of Olmsted County, Minnesota.

Demographic Data at Entry are important, because accurate expected mortality is dependent on accurate matching of the study group(s) followed by age and sex. Race, socioeconomic status and selection characteristics are also important. Race data are often omitted, but usually mean age and percentage of females are given as a minimum. The problems generated in deriving expected mortality when more complete age/sex distribution is not provided are difficult for the abstract preparer to handle, but will not be detailed here.

Follow-up Notes. Salient characteristics are important in describing the FU achieved in the study, and usually these must be deduced from the data given in the *Material and Methods* section of the article. These include the entry period, the cutoff date, minimum, maximum and mean durations of FU, adequacy of methods used in FU, and percentage of patients lost to FU. If the authors rely on questionnaires for FU without supplementing data on non-respondents by other means, it will generally be evident that a large fraction of the entrants has been lost, and follow-up is so incomplete as to be unsatisfactory. One reason for non-response, of course, is death of the entrant, and the proportion of deaths in the lost patients or subjects may be higher than in those successfully followed. This part of the study should be evaluated with a critical eye. These and other aspects of FU and death ascertainment are very important for the analyst who prepares the abstract.

Classification of Patients or Subjects. In most FU articles the experience is given not only for the total series but also for subdivisions thereof. The total may be broken down by sex, by age, by diagnostic group, by features of the history, examination or test results at entry, or by a severity classification, such as the New York Heart Association functional class, or cancer stage, or some other method, including a scoring system. Division may be one factor at a time (univariate), combination of factors (cross-classification), or one of the statistical methods of multivariate analysis. Such classification information is important in describing results of the FU article.

Derivation and Presentation of Results appear in almost infinite variety in FU articles. Graphs of cumulative survival curves (P) are the most common method of presentation, sometimes with additional data, such as the numbers of survivors at various durations after entry. Actuarial or other life table methods are used to derive the curves, but observed life table data are given in only a minority of articles, and then in a variety of tabular formats, some omitting essential data. Expected mortality and survival are given in less than 20% of articles, although control rates of cumulative mortality or morbidity may be used for comparison with observed rates in clinical trials and case control studies. Terms such as risk ratio and relative risk are generally used instead of the more familiar term, mortality ratio. These are problems the abstract preparer must cope with, but the responsibility of the reviewer is to note with care the presentation of results. If expected rates are given, the source table should also be noted.

Significance Tests. Such tests are available in great profusion, and the methods used in any article are generally cited by name and reference. This information is of importance to the analyst who prepares the abstract.

Article References. These are an extremely important part of the article review, because they often point to other articles with good FU data, which may assist the task of abstract preparation. The authors often have done a good job of reviewing the literature, and references to this are apt to appear in the introduction or the discussion section of the article. The text and references of the article

should therefore be read carefully with this point in mind. References that appear to be of potential value should be listed, with the page number of the text in which the citation appears, for future use.

Potential Value of a FU Article. With many factors to be weighed it is extremely difficult to devise a satisfactory method of grading the value of an article as a source for a mortality abstract. The method proposed here is a provisional one, little tested and subject to change with accumulation of experience in its use. A formal evaluation sheet of this sort is designed primarily for a cooperative review effort. If such an effort should be developed in the future it would probably be organized and supervised by the Mortality and Morbidity Committee and would involve a descriptive sheet for the article, of which this proposed evaluation system could be the final part. The guidelines in Part I can be used either independently or as part of an organized article review process. Five evaluation grades are defined:

A – highest value (top priority)

B – intermediate value

C – relatively low value by itself

Q – questionable value, article to be referred to other reviewer

U – unsuitable for abstract

At present it is impractical to define a numerical grading score. The two chief factors to evaluate are the number of existing sources of comparative mortality or morbidity, and the size of the experience (number of observed deaths) reported. Total deaths are sometimes not reported if the data are in the form of survival curves; in this case estimate mean duration from maximum and minimum FU in years, estimate exposure as product of number of entrants and mean FU in years, and then expected deaths as product of E and q', using q' of 0.002 for a predominantly young series, 0.01 for a mean age in the 50s, and 0.02 for a mean age over 60. The reviewer will have to rely on his own knowledge of the literature of mortality abstracts and insurance mortality studies to decide whether existing studies are abundant, limited, or virtually non-existent, but a bibliographic summary is in preparation to aid in classification of this factor. Unsuitable articles include those with case reports only, most autopsy series and retrospective studies, those with an approximate exposure yielding less than 1 expected death, and those with a serious defect in design, methods used, or the reporting of the FU data. If the reviewer cannot classify properly or is doubtful about the methodology, the article should be given a Q grading and referred to the most experienced reviewer for evaluation. If methodology appears to be satisfactory, most articles not considered unsuitable can be given a grading of A, B, or C in accordance with the following table:

Size of Mortality Experience Reported

Existing Mortality Sources	Deaths >100	Deaths 26-100	Obs. deaths 0-25 & exp. deaths >1*
Almost nil	A	A	A
Limited	A	B	C[†]
Abundant	B (>1000)	Q	U
	C (101-1000)		

*See text above for estimating d' in absence of report of total deaths.

[†]If there are several new articles in this class for a given condition, their value will be enhanced by combining them in a "composite" abstract.

Part II—Abstract Preparation

The preparer of an abstract may utilize an article that he has personally reviewed or one from a stockpile, with a descriptive sheet. In either case, the preparation of an abstract is a creative process, one that requires a thorough knowledge of the standard format used, and an equally thorough knowledge of life table methodology (see Pokorski's full seminar text[3]). The following guidelines are intended to be of further assistance in the preparation.

Duration Questions. Are results given by duration, or only for all durations combined? Is the maximum duration of follow-up short (e.g., 1-2 months), or long-term (about 4 years or more), or in between? This assumes a prospective or historical prospective study: a case-control, period, or retrospective study does not ordinarily involve duration as a factor. In some conditions, such as acute myocardial infarction (MI) or stroke, the early or short-term mortality may be extremely high, in which case the rate usually decreases quite rapidly over a period of days, weeks or months until it becomes more stable, a duration pattern that can be properly described on a yearly basis, or even by longer intervals. When early mortality is much higher than it is subsequently, the early experience should be excluded from the long-term experience and presented in a separate table. It may not be necessary to put the early mortality in comparative terms. For example, in acute MI of hospitalized patients only three variables need be shown for each age, sex, severity or other category: the number of MI patients hospitalized, the number of deaths to the end of the early duration, such as 30 days after admission, and the early mortality rate, often given as a percentage, unlike the decimal units or deaths per 1000 exposed to risk, used for long-term intervals. When this separation is made, long-term mortality and survival have, as a starting-point, the end of the early observation period. If annual duration intervals are used, the first interval is truncated and is labeled in the duration column as "30d-1yr," or "1-12mo," or "HD-1yr," where HD stands for hospital discharge, when this is designated as the end of the early period. The first long-term interval is therefore shorter than the subsequent intervals of one full year, and one must be careful to make sure that exposure in *person-years* and *annual* mortality and survival rates are adjusted for the duration of less than 1 full year in the first interval. However, if annual rates are shown, the first-year cumulative survival rate, P_1, must be derived from the *interval* survival rate, p_i, *not* the first-year annual survival rate, $1-q$. Thereafter the interval and the annual survival rates are identical. If graphs of cumulative survival rates are the primary source of data in the article, the curve and the caption of the graph should be examined carefully to determine whether the early deaths have been excluded or not. If early MI deaths have not been excluded, the P curve should show a steep initial dip reflecting the high mortality in the first month, and then should have much less of a slope in the remaining portion of the first year. The time scale or the caption should make it clear that 0 time is hospital admission. However, if early deaths *have* been excluded, there will be no initial steep dip, and P=1.00 will correspond to 0 time of 1 month, or whatever the end of the early period is. Such a starting point for the rest of the time scale means that the first year is a full 12 months, not the truncated year that results from using hospital admission as the starting point for long-term as well as the early follow-up. Alternatively, the graph may show P=1.00 at t=1 month or 1/12 year, in which case duration and the time scale are not based on hospital admission as the starting-point, and the first year of long-term follow-up is a truncated period. These details are important because, if they are not recognized, errors may result in calculation of the first-year mortality rate and in all values of P.

Another important aspect of duration is the statement in the article regarding the calendar years of entry, in relation to the calendar year(s) of cutting off follow-up. In most published studies patients have been entered in the study over a period of years, such as 1970-79, and followed to a year close to the last year of entry, such as a cutoff at the end of 1980. In this case the minimum duration of follow-up is 1+ year, and the maximum is 10+ years. A follow-up range of 1-10 years implies that patients must have been withdrawn alive due to end of follow-up in each year of observation after the first. Such a follow-up may be called a "double-decrement" study because patients are withdrawn either because of death (one decrement), or because of end of follow-up or becoming untraced while still alive at last observation (the second decrement). In contrast is the less common situation in which the study is designed so that all patients in effect have the same entry point and the same end point of observation w=0 and E =ℓ. It is no longer mandatory to calculate Q as 1– P from annual values of q and p. If there are 1,000 entrants and 100 deaths over a uniform follow-up of 5 years, and no annual data are given, Q can be calculated by the "ad hoc" method as Q=100/1000=0.1, and P=1–Q=0.900. Geometric mean annual rates of survival and mortality may then be derived. It can be shown mathematically that this value of P, the cumulative survival rate, will be derived regardless of the distribution of the 100 deaths over each of the five observation years. This uniform follow-up duration for all entrants presents a very different situation from the usual one of a wide range of follow-up durations and many patients withdrawn because of end of follow-up, even when there are very few or no patients lost to follow-up.

When the authors do not present annual life table data, including w, E, and d, it may still be possible to approximate the total E and the mean annual mortality rate, *if* the mean follow-up duration, Δt, is given with the total number of deaths. Suppose there are 200 entrants with a Δt of 5.0 years; then E=(200)(5.0)=1,000 person-years. If 50 deaths were observed, then the mean annual mortality rate, q=50/1000=0.050, or 50 deaths per 1000 per year. If a valid matching q' can be derived, so can d', the MR and EDR. This approximation is accurate, because the only way to calculate mean q is by the quotient, d/E: the authors must have calculated total E even if they do not report it as such in the article.

It should be evident that analysis of these duration aspects is most important in the development of life table calculations for comparative mortality and in the design of the abstract tables. Without separation of the high early mortality experience, if it is present, first-year and average 5-year observed mortality rates will not be representative of the greater part of the long-term experience. There is no high excess acute mortality, of course, in the follow-up of chronic conditions which lack an initial period of high risk, or in which the entrants have survived this period (post-MI survivors, for example). On the other hand, a common type of follow-up reported is for patients treated with major surgery, and the early perioperative experience *should* be separated from the long-term experience. All too frequently this is not done in the cumulative survival curves reported. P values based on P=1 at operation can be adjusted easily by dividing by p_o=1–q_o, where q_o is the early, perioperative mortality rate.

Age/Sex and Other Patient Groupings. The Methods and Results section, the tables and figures, and the other text of the article should be carefully examined to ascertain the scope of the age/sex groups, and the diagnostic, severity and other patient groupings. The calculation of expected deaths, mortality and survival rates will depend on the extent of detail in the age/sex entry data, and whether results by duration are given by age and sex. With several age/sex groups at entry, it is possible to derive accurate values of d' and q' for the first year

(calculate d' in each age/sex group as the product of first-year E and q' taken from the table of expected rates, with the central age of the age group, then add the d' values, and divide this by the total E to get the first-year q', all ages and both sexes combined). But if there is no follow-up by separate age/sex groups, the *progression* of q' by duration becomes a difficult problem (see section on expected mortality below). Bear in mind that mean age and age distribution will probably differ from one patient group to another, and q' will vary accordingly. If age/sex distribution data are requested from the authors, they should be requested for all patient groups for which mortality or survival results are given. The diagnostic and severity groups will determine many features of table format and size. Subdivision of the total series should not be attempted if numbers of deaths are too small in the individual data cells.

Need for Additional Data. It is important to decide on the need for additional data as early as possible in the evaluation of the article. Is an initial age/sex distribution given, and if not, how essential is it to have this information from the authors? In patient series with myocardial infarction, coronary heart disease with angiogram, coronary bypass surgery, aortic and mitral valvular heart disease, and some types of cancer, it is possible to use a mean age and obtain a good approximation of first-year mean q' (see section on expected mortality). A less accurate approximation from the mean age is possible in other diagnoses if the age distribution is similar to the age distribution of one of the above. Age distributions reported in the *Medical Risks* monographs or in other reference sources should be consulted. Furthermore, it is of the utmost importance to obtain any earlier papers of the authors which may describe the age/sex distribution or other essential data pertaining to the series being reported in the current article. If the study is of special value, with large exposure and numbers of deaths, it is usually desirable to write to the authors requesting the age/sex distribution, if available, not only for the total series but for the diagnostic and severity groups also. A similar need may arise for exposure data, or for life table data supporting cumulative survival curves in graphs, or tabular P values given only to two decimal places. Occasionally there is no reply, but often the requested data are made available. It should always be made clear that the data are desired for a mortality abstract that will be published, but with full credit to the original paper(s), and to the author(s) for the additional data received. Many mortality abstracts made in the past have been greatly enhanced by such additional data.

Expected Mortality. The choice of the "best" (most appropriate) mortality table to be used as a comparative standard for expected mortality is a most important one.

Contemporaneous select and ultimate tables are the best for most studies of individual life insurance applicants and policyholders. Population life tables are appropriate for studies of patients or subjects that can reasonably be considered to be a random population sample. This assumption may be true for some clinically generated series, but a careful reading of the description of how the series was formed will *frequently* reveal that a considerable degree of selection has been used: age has been restricted, patients with certain severity or other characteristics have been excluded, patients with other high-risk conditions have been excluded, etc. If selection has been used it may be better to utilize a Group Life Insurance table or similar table, giving a lower expected mortality than would be derived from a population table. Race information is important, but often not available in the article; it will be necessary to decide first on use of a total population or white population table from U.S. Tables. Because of the large sex difference in mortality at most ages it is better to separate the male and female age groups, even when the sex distribution is given only for the total series, not for the various age groups. Data are available that show the age variation and the male/female percentages in CHD and some other conditions (see the *Medical Risks* monographs). If early deaths are excluded, the age distribution should be that for the early survivors, not the initial entrants (early mortality is usually higher at the older ages). All of this involves careful review of the article, good judgment in selecting the expected tables for use, and in the derivation of the first-year rates matched by age/sex group to obtain an overall mean expected mortality, q'. Except for the age/sex distribution these derivation calculations seldom appear in the abstract. The work-sheets should always be made available to the reviewer of the abstract, and both text and all tables should define the expected tables used.

It is well known that, regardless of the table of expected mortality used, the rate increases geometrically by a nearly constant factor of 1.1 per year between the ages of 40 and 80 years. From age 2 to age 36 years annual mortality rates in the U.S. white population are very low, under 1 per 1000 in females, and under 2 per 1000 in males. Starting under age 80 in males and over age 80 in females, the geometric factor commences a gradual decrease, and is less than 1.02 at age 110. In chronic diseases, such as coronary heart disease (CHD), the patient sample usually has a wide age range, even if older patients are excluded, as they often are in clinical trials. The mean age ($\bar{x}$) is often of the order of 50 to 65 years, with a 95% range about ±20 years around the mean. Given the geometric increase in q' in the life table and such a mean age and age distribution about the mean, it can be easily shown that q' values at ages older

than $\bar{x}$ will contribute more to the mean q' than q' values at the younger ages. In other words, the mean q' in a male or female cohort will *always* exceed the tabular q' corresponding to the mean age, $\bar{x}$ (i.e., *mean q' exceeds the q' of the mean age*). If only the mean age is given in an article, with a range or S.D., one can approximate the mean q' by entering the male or female table with an adjusted age, e.g. ($\bar{x}+3$). For example, a group of men surviving a coronary bypass operation (CBPS) might have a typical age distribution that yielded a mean age, $\bar{x}$, of 51 years, and a mean q' of 0.0106. The tabular q' for white men age 51 is only 0.0078, but the q' for age (51+3) or 54 years is 0.0103, a much better approximation of the mean q'. Such an approximation has been confirmed empirically in a large number of cohorts of patients or subjects when the mean age is of the order of 50 to 65 years and the range is of the order of ±20 years. If the range is only 10 years, as in a group of patients 40-50 years old, the mean age, such as 45 years, can be used to enter the table to obtain a accurate mean q', unless the age distribution is extremely skewed. Both mean age and range of age are therefore of importance in any use of the empirical factor of +3 years to add to the mean age. When age/sex distribution is not given in the article, authors usually report the percentages or numbers of men and women. An overall mean q' for this sex distribution may be approximated by obtaining the adjusted q' values separately from the male and female expected tables and weighting them according to the respective male and female percentages. Data on the derivation of an accurate mean q' from mean age and range of age are given in Table 642D,[5] for post-CBPS patients. Unpublished data also exist (RBS files) for patients surviving an acute myocardial infarction (MI), patients with aortic or mitral valve disease, treated surgically, and patients with cancer of the colon or thyroid.

Unfortunately, an accurate first-year mean q', all ages combined, does not solve another problem in the *progression* of mean q' with duration, so that accurate values of q' will be available to match annual or mean annual values of observed q. Despite the fact that each annual *survivor* in the cohort is, indeed, one year older than he or she was in the preceding year, the *mean age of the cohort* very often advances at a variable fraction of a year with each year of duration, and may even *decrease* temporarily after the first year. This is due primarily to the effect of a higher observed mortality at the older ages, which results in a significant shift in age distribution to a younger mean age, despite the fact that all survivors are a year older in the next successive year of follow-up observation. This observed mortality effect is abetted by a wide initial age range and a high rate of withdrawal due to end of follow-up. It is difficult to make any valid recommendation as to decreasing the geometric increase factor of 1.1 by a given amount. Only about one-half of the series of CBPS patients tested from follow-up of individual age groups showed a factor much below 1.1, averaged over at least 5 years (there may be considerable random variation from year to year). The annual factor in the CBPS cohorts varied from 1.05 to 1.08 when it was less than 1.09. In the series of patients surviving an acute MI, with higher mean ages and wide ranges of age, the increase factor ranged from 1.03 to 1.08. In cancer of the colon, the annual increase factor may range from 0.93 to 1.08 in localized and regional extension stages, with a mean of about 1.02 at 1-5 years, and 1.04+ at 5-10 years. The decrease in mean q' at 1-2 years was even more striking in metastatic cancer of the colon, with a factor of 1.00 averaged over 1-5 years and about 1.05 over 5-10 years. In thyroid cancer, which is characterized by an unusually wide range of age, the early decrease in mean age and mean q' is very prominent and persistent, giving a mean factor of only 0.68 in duration years 1-5! There is a need for similar testing of other patient cohorts, not only in cancer, but in a wide range of other diseases, to establish some sort of pattern of progression of q' in annual survivors of such cohorts. It is important to remember that editors or reviewers of any formal mortality abstract will be desirous of seeing all calculations of expected mortality, and they should be provided with any worksheets (legible and labeled!) that will permit them to follow your derivations. For many abstracts, a new section, **Expected Mortality**, would be proper to add to the standard abstract format, as illustrated in Table 338K1-1 of the Mortality Abstract on the Aspirin Component of the Physicians' Health Study (See Abstract #338K1).

Tables Based on Life Table Data

1. *Early Mortality Results.* Generally the observed mortality rate is given as $q_o = d_o/\ell_o$, this subscript indicating the early mortality period of 4 weeks, hospital admission to discharge, or however it is defined. These three variables are apt to be the only ones displayed (expected deaths or rates and comparative indices are seldom used), and the acute mortality rate is often given as a percentage rather than a decimal or rate per 1000. The table design may vary widely according to the type of data displayed. Many examples can be found in the first *Medical Risks* monograph,[4] and additional ones in the tables of Abstract 609, or Tables 613A-B, 618A-B, and 620 A in the new monograph.[5]

2. *Extensive Life Table Data.* The essential observed data are ℓ, E, and d, from which are derived the mortality and survival rates; E itself is derived from ℓ and w, but it has become the practice in mortality abstracts of the past 10 years to omit the column of w data to save space. If ℓ

values are available they probably should be included, even though it was not the custom to report them in the tables of the 1983 Impairment Study. Life table data in an article are considered extensive when they include results by age and duration, or a combination of age and duration. Prototypes of detailed life table results of this sort may be found in Tables 625A and 650C-D.[5] Subheadings within the table may be used to distinguish different severity, diagnostic or other categories of the data. As shown in Table 625A, 9 columns are needed to present what are generally considered to be the minimum essential results for observed and expected data, and comparative mortality: duration, ℓ, E, d, d' MR, q, q', and EDR. With omission of all survival data, survival ratio and cumulative mortality ratio, this compresses into one table what used to be shown in two companion tables in the *1976 Medical Risks*.[4] In the new monograph[5] a strenuous effort was made to reduce the number of data columns and thus "simplify" the tables. One of us (RBS) had to fight to retain data considered essential in some of the important abstract drafts, and longer tables did not always prevail. Even with 9 columns the detailed tables still omit all survival results, and they do not contain confidence limits, which the reader has to take out of a reference table of Poisson limits. Formerly q and q' were given as 3-place decimals, but the tendency now is to give them as deaths per 1000 per year, to match EDR. When the life table data are given by a combination of age and annual duration it is generally necessary to save vertical space by combining individual years into longer intervals, such as 2-5, 5-10, etc. If the results are for all ages combined, separate annual data may be presented up to 5 or even 10 years. The pattern of mortality with duration determines at what follow-up year it is possible to combine results without sacrificing a trend that may be important for the reader. Age groupings are most commonly decennial, but there may be even fewer groups, such as <55 and 55 up. Detailed life tables of this sort are the easiest ones in which to develop q' and d', and hence the indices of comparative mortality. Unfortunately, such detailed results are not often available in the published article. If the authors are cooperative, the data they supply sometimes include quite detailed life table results.

3. *Abridged Life Table Results.* This term is applied to a variety of life table formats that are less detailed than those containing data by age and duration. The results are based on E, d, and d', with derived q, q', MR and EDR, but not infrequently one or more of these variables may be lacking. If both E and EDR are missing, the life table is incomplete as well as abridged. An example of a fairly complete life table is Table 324A,[5] in which mortality ratios are given for widowed and married persons by sex and age in the same table. The two groups are matched

for age and sex, so that ℓ and E values are identical for them. Two sets of data are given for d, d' and MR. EDRs can be derived from the E, d, and d' data, but have been omitted because the table already contains 10 columns of data. Table 623A[5] contains only d, d' and MR data for the CHD experience of the Prudential Insurance Company of London; with E data omitted it is impossible to calculate EDR. It is a disservice to the potential users of the tabular results to omit essential exposure data, so that EDR cannot be derived when all ages are combined. EDR is a more reliable estimate of excess mortality than MR, because it is less sensitive to age differences between groups. In the *1976 Medical Risks* monograph,[4] tables at the end of each major disease section present combined limited results from various sources. These do contain E, d, d', MR and EDR data, generally for all ages and durations combined from one source; such tables may be regarded as collections of abridged life table data.

Occasionally "oddball" presentations of data are encountered. An abridged life table containing P by duration may give the P value for the *start* of the interval, instead of the *end*, as is the usual custom. In a follow-up study of asymptomatic carotid bruit, Thompson et al.[6] reported, not life table data, but follow-up data by annual duration consisting of three columns: "No. of Long-term Survivors," "No. of Long-term Deaths," and "Total No. of Patients." In one table the grand total at the bottom of the third column was 132 patients, with 89 total survivors and 43 total deaths in 16 years of follow-up. Since the authors state that no patient was lost to follow-up, the distribution of survivors in the first column represents annual values of w, patients withdrawn alive due to end of follow-up. The annual distribution of deaths in the second column is clear enough, but it may not be easy to recognize the significance of the data in the first column as actual values of w. They are not so labeled — the mortality abstract preparer must figure this out for himself, and how to take the data and construct the actual observed life table data, with columns of ℓ, w, E, d, q, and, if desired, p, P, and Q. Both the reviewer of articles and the preparer of tables must be prepared to cope with such special situations.

4. *Ad Hoc Life Table Data.* When follow-up is complete to the end of the period of observation, w=0 for each year of observation, ℓ=E, and Q may be calculated directly as $\Sigma d/\ell_1$. Or, if ℓ is given annually, mean annual q=$\Sigma d/\Sigma\ell$. An average value of q over several years may be annualized as an aggregate or a geometric mean, depending on the available data. Examples of these may be found in two different post-MI series,[5] Table 613C and 614E.

5. *Life Table Data by Cause of Death.* In all tables of this sort there is a common value of E for each cause of

death and for the total. An example is Table 624I,[5] the experience by cause of death in the Japanese Declined Lives Study of applicants with CHD. E is given in the total row at the bottom of a separate E column, but it could have been given in the Table heading. In addition to the cause of death column, other data in this table were d, d', MR, aggregate mean annual q, and EDR. Mathematically, the EDR values for each cause of death are additive to the total EDR. There is, however, no simple relationship between the MRs for individual causes of death and the total MR.

Tables Based on Cumulative Survival Curve Data

1. *Tabular P Data.* These are more accurate than measurements from a survival curve graph provided the results are given to three places (72.5% or 0.725, rather than 72% or 0.72). Interval survival rates are calculated with the needed accuracy as the quotient of the P values at the end and the beginning of the desired interval. The mean annual $\breve{q}$ is then derived as $1-\breve{p}$, where $\breve{p}$ is the geometric mean of the interval survival rate. If the P data are reported faithfully, values to only 2 decimal places produce less accurate values of mean annual $\breve{q}$ than if they are given to 3 decimal places. Three-place P data are given in Table 628A at 5, 10 and 15 years in various groups of post-MI men followed in Dublin, Ireland. The data in this table include P, P', the survival ratio, and mean annual $\breve{q}$, $\breve{q}'$, EDR and MR as $100\breve{q}/\breve{q}'$. More often the data for survival ratio may be omitted, and a column of interval p_i data is provided, giving the intermediate step in the derivation of geometric mean annual $\breve{q}$. Remember, if early deaths have not been excluded, although they should have been, it is necessary to adjust each P value by dividing by the p_o value, and to adjust the first interval to start at the end of the early period.

2. *Graphic Survival Curve Data.* The estimation of P from measurement of points on the curve of a graph is beset with error because of (1) the generally small scale of the graph, (2) inaccuracy in plotting the curve, and (3) optical distortion in photographic reproduction of the graph. The survival scale may be truncated, e.g., 100% down to below 50%, interruption in scale, then 10% to 0%. In this case measurements must be made of Q rather than P, downward from a horizontal line at P=100%, parallel to the time scale at the bottom. The length of such a vertical scale must be derived from the measurement of the portion that is not truncated, in this case twice the measurement from P=50% to 100%. With a millimeter rule and a magnifying glass our experience has been that the best one can do is measure to the nearest 0.2 millimeter, and we recommend that you measure the scale and each point several times and use the average for each point. As a decimal, P is then calculated as the ratio

y(point)/y(scale), where y is the vertical measurement in mm. Occasionally the graph gives a curve for Q, not P. The measurement process is the same, and then $P=1-Q$. You must observe the same precaution in adjusting the P values from the graph to exclude the early mortality experience, if this is indicated and has not been done in construction of the graph. For the duration intervals chosen, such as 5 years, interval survival rates, p_i, may be derived as the quotient of the appropriate P values, and then the geometric mean *annual* survival rate calculated as follows: $\check{q}=1-\check{p}_i^{0.2}$, if the interval is 5 years ($1/5=0.2$). Finally, $\check{q}=1-\check{p}$. The mean annual mortality rates are preferred to interval mortality rates, because they are more closely related to the aggregate means that are always used when ΣE and Σd are available. Mortality ratios based on cumulative or interval mortality rates are always lower than annualized mortality ratios. Furthermore, interval mortality rates cannot be used for the direct calculation of EDR.

Derived rates are given in the table to 3 decimal places, for example the final geometric mean annual $\check{q}$ might be 0.026 or 26 per 1000. However, it should be recognized that the error of this derived rate could be ±0.003, or more than 10%, because of the error of measurement of P. Another example of a table based on survival rates is Table 671B,[5] giving results on mitral valve replacement by duration and type of prosthetic valve, all ages combined. After the duration column the variables are P, p_i, $\check{q}$, $\check{q}'$, EDR as ($\check{q}-\check{q}'$), and MR. Readers unfamiliar with this type of table may be baffled by the derivation of $\check{q}$; the relationship can be given in a footnote, for the sake of completeness. It is always desirable to have tables (and figures) self-explanatory, without forcing the reader to go to the text.

3. *Graphic Survival Curve with Values of ℓ by Duration.* In this situation you should remember that $\ell_1-\ell_2=d_1+w_1$. It may sometimes be possible to reconstruct a life table by a method of successive approximations, given the various relations, $E=\ell-0.5w$, $q_1=1-(P_2/P_1)$, $q_i=d_1/E_1$, and the fact that the sum of the individual d values must equal the total deaths as given in the article. If the total is not stated, a valuable check of the allocation of d by duration is lost. The calculation of an *annual* q from successive annual P values is generally inaccurate. If annual deaths tend to be relatively small and w values large, this approximation method would be impractical, and it would be necessary to rely on the usual development of the survival rates, without any use of the ℓ values. Despite the uncertainties, a successful life table approximation by this method will probably yield EDR and MR results that are more accurate than those derived from the survival curve alone. However, in the text or in a table

footnote or both it should be emphasized that E and d are not exact observed data, but approximations.

Other Tables

1. *Clinical Trials.* A randomized double-blind clinical trial is generally considered to be the acme of statistical testing of the effectiveness of a type of therapy by comparing the test group mortality or morbidity against an age/sex-matched control group, with similar characteristics. Despite the matching process, both groups should have expected rates of deaths calculated from the appropriate standard tables, just as in observational studies. Failure to do so may obscure features of the selection process that are important: for example, in the clinical trial conducted under the auspices of the University Group Diabetes Program, controversy arose about the validity of the finding of no reduction in mortality with use of an oral drug. The clinical investigators and those on both sides of the argument never tested the mortality of the control group, which one of us (RBS) found to be almost the same as that of the general population, indicating selection of a very mild set of diabetics for both control and test groups. Comparative mortality should therefore be shown for both the placebo and the treatment groups. An example of a table based on a clinical trial is 639A,[5] giving mortality by age and sex in a randomized trial of propranolol in early survivors of acute MI. The first two columns contain the age group and proportion of females. Subsequent columns give the data for ℓ, d, d', MR, $\bar{q}$, $\bar{q}'$, and EDR. These results were derived from one of the reports of the "BHAT" Study, a large multicenter study sponsored by the National Institutes of Health. In this study, as in many clinical trials, older MI patients were excluded (age 70 and up in this instance). The significant reduction in mortality from that in the placebo group is reflected in the lower EDR and MR values found in the group treated with the chosen beta-blocker. Numbers of deaths were very small under age 40, but were substantial at older ages, and excess mortality increased with advancing age in a pattern typical of post-MI patients.

2. *Intra-Series Comparison.* In some large-scale prospective studies such as the Framingham Study or that of the Pooling Project, the total cohort or a large fraction thereof is used to provide the "expected" mortality experience. The total series is subdivided into parts, for example quintiles, according to levels of systolic or diastolic blood pressure, and comparative mortality is derived. In Table 601B[5] this has been done for results of the Pooling Project in this manner. The table shows the rank of the quintile in the left-hand column, and comparative mortality in two sets of columns, systolic pressure on the left and diastolic pressure on the right. The data reported are

d, d', MR and EDR. In this table format E has been omitted to conserve space, but the presence of positive EDR values indicates that E was observed. With this type of expected mortality, in the Pooling Project, all subjects without ECG abnormalities, some of the group divisions will have lower mortality and some higher than the average for the total. As a consequence some MRs will be under 100% and some EDRs will be negative (Ed Lew chose to omit the negative EDR values from the tabular results of the *1990 Medical Risks* monograph[5]).

3. *Abridged Risk Ratio Data.* The authors of some follow-up studies have chosen to present only the final comparative result in terms of what they call a "risk ratio," given as a decimal to one place, or sometimes an "odds ratio," if a morbid event is under consideration. These are age/sex-adjusted, and are equivalent to a mortality ratio or a morbidity ratio, but they are not expressed as a percentage. If an abstract is prepared from such an article, only the MR results can be given. EDR cannot be calculated, and the authors generally do not give the observed data from which the risk ratio has been calculated. This form of data presentation is often used in occupational risk studies. Special significance may be given by the statistician to terms such as odds ratio , if a case control study is involved (see below). "Relative risk" is another term that is sometimes used.

4. *Case Control Studies.* Usually regarded as retrospective studies rather than prospective, the design involves identification of a group of patients or subjects from past records with a particular type of treatment modality, and from current follow-up the mortality or occurrence of a morbid event, such as development of a type of cancer. The database must be such as to permit identification of a control group, matched by age, sex and perhaps confounding risk factors, who did *not* have the treatment under study. A large database of nurses has been used to produce various case control studies on questions such as the possible relation of progesterone to breast cancer. Such studies have generally not been used for the preparation of mortality or morbidity abstracts, but they might be used if their limitations are recognized. See Feinstein and Horwitz's excellent review.[7]

5. *Attained Age Cohort.* In chronic diseases that are severe or conspicuous enough to result in most cases in the population coming to medical attention, it may be justified to create a cohort of a series of such patients and analyze comparative mortality by attained age from an early age as a starting point. An example of this is shown in Table 633A,[5] results of 257 patients with Marfan's syndrome, diagnosed and followed at a Johns Hopkins Clinic over a period of many years. Survival curves from age 10 to age 60 were used to construct comparative mortality results by decade of attained age. After the age

column the data shown in order are P, interval p_i, q_i, q'_i, MR (interval q), annualized $\breve{q}$, $\breve{q}'$, EDR, and MR from the annual mortality rates. Another example[5] is based on data from a Danish registry of patients with Tetralogy of Fallot alive on January 1, 1950. Incidence rates of this severe congenital heart disorder and numbers of live births back to 1890 were used to estimate cases and deaths by attained age. Such reconstructed life tables from observations of this sort constitute a real challenge to the student of life table methodology. Very careful consideration must be given to the circumstances of series of this sort. Generally it is not permissible to use retrospective exposure from date of first contact with a patient back to date of onset, because deaths prior to first contact have been automatically eliminated. Congenital conditions present a special situation.

6. *Organizing Data from Several Articles into a "Composite Abstract."* This task arises either from the need to increase the aggregate number of deaths by giving results from several small series of patients, or from the desirability of showing together the results of several series of patients with a particular feature of their generic diagnosis, for example results of several series of patients with single-vessel disease after coronary bypass surgery (CBPS). Quite a few examples of this sort may be found in the new reference monograph.[5] One example is Abstract 648, in which post-CBPS patients are analyzed with respect to age and sex. In the long-term results the usual detailed life table format is used: age, reference to series, ℓ (at 30 days after operation), E, d, d', MR, $\bar{q}$, $\bar{q}'$, and EDR. Results in this case are sufficient to fill 6 pages, even though the basic information on the various series had been given previously. It is very difficult to attempt general instructions for preparing composite abstracts; everything depends on the nature of the data and the desired objectives. In the new reference monograph[5] several composite abstracts were prepared for acute MI and for CBPS patients. Miscellaneous limited data were also combined in the *1976 Medical Risks* monograph[4] at the end of each major disease section. These may be studied as examples of what may be achieved with such a presentation.

Conclusion

There appears to be a strong consensus within ALIMDA membership, including the Executive Council and the Mortality and Morbidity Committee, that mortality abstracts are a useful supplement to the intercompany Impairment Studies, which provide the data essential to medical underwriting and risk classification. The Board of Insurance Medicine now sponsors the Mortality Methodology Courses as one requirement for Board certification. Some members of ALIMDA worked hard with members of the Society of Actuaries in the formidable task of preparing the two *Medical Risks* reference monographs.[4,5] Our *Journal of Insurance Medicine,* under the editorial leadership of John Elder, now offers high-quality mortality abstracts in each issue. The ALIMDA Research Center was started two years age, partly with the idea of facilitating systematic search for and retrieval of FU articles from the medical literature. Despite all of this support in principle, the production of mortality abstracts for publication in the *JIM* has remained modest. Efforts to organize greater production and encourage a wider network of contributors have not met with much success, but there has been a stirring of professional interest.

In May 1990, in Portsmouth, NH, a two-day workshop sponsored by the Board of Insurance Medicine provided a lively "hands-on" opportunity for ALIMDA members to intensively study methods of Life Table analysis and to formally abstract an article from a medical journal for themselves. This present article is, in part, an outgrowth of that workshop. Another such workshop is scheduled for May 1991, in Portland, ME. It is our sincere hope that the practical suggestions, hints, and empirical rules offered in this article and in these workshops will encourage more than just a few medical directors to try their hand at the rewarding task of transforming the results of a medical FU study into a high-quality abstract.

Among the things that distinguish insurance medicine as a discipline are its quantitative approach to matters of prognosis and outcome and its application of actuarial methods to risk classification and assessment. Formal mortality abstraction is only one part of the universe of quantitative reasoning that medical directors engage in, but it is still an important part. Not merely a relic of our history and heritage, it clearly involves skills and perspectives that are also part of our future as a profession. Making these methods more generally accessible, identifying and overcoming obstacles to their use, and supporting a spectrum of approaches from the soundly reasoned, curbside estimate to the detailed, published abstract are goals worthy of pursuit!

This article is by no means exhaustive in its description of topics. Nothing has been said about articles involving survival models, meta-analysis, life expectancy, the intricacies of statistical analysis and the like, but there is much that each of us can do by simply applying basic methodologies to the abundantly available medical literature and generating valuable mortality abstracts. Let's do it!

REFERENCES

1. M. W. Kita, "Morbidity and Mortality Abstraction — Finding Suitable Articles," *J. Ins. Med.,* 22 (1990): 287-88.

2. R. B. Singer, J. R. Avery, M. W. Kita, "A Classification System for Mortality and Morbidity Abstracts and Related Data," *J. Ins. Med.,* 23 (1991): 94-96.

3. R. J. Pokorski, "Mortality Methodology and Analysis Seminar," *J. Ins. Med.,* 20, no. 4 (1988): 20-45.

4. R. B. Singer, L. Levinson, eds., *Medical Risks: Patterns of Mortality and Survival* (Lexington, MA, Lexington Books, 1976).

5. E. A. Lew, J. Gajewski, eds., *Medical Risks: Trends in Mortality by Age and Time Elapsed* (New York, Praeger, 1990).

6. J. E. Thompson, R. D. Patman, C. M. Talkington, "Asymptomatic Carotid Bruit," *Ann. Surg.,* 188 (1978): 308-16.

7. A. R. Feinstein, R. I. Horwitz, "Double Standards, Scientific Methods, and Epidemiologic Research," *N. Engl. J. Med.,* 307 (1982): 1611-17.

CHAPTER 5

A CLASSIFICATION SYSTEM FOR
MORTALITY AND MORBIDITY ABSTRACTS
AND RELATED DATA

Richard B. Singer, M.D., John R. Avery, and Michael W. Kita, M.D.

Introduction

Readers of the *1976* and *1990 Medical Risks* reference monographs[1,2] are aware that all mortality abstracts have been numbered according to a disease or impairment classification system, although the system differs somewhat in the two books. Tables in each abstract have been assigned a letter following the abstract number code. A reverse order has been used in the 1951 and the 1983 Impairment Studies:[3,4] a letter has been used for the impairment category (these differ in the two studies), and a number has been used for the tables and results for each impairment within the letter category. No classification code at all has been used for the separate mortality abstracts, the morbidity abstracts, or other articles that report mortality data, when they have appeared in the *Journal of Insurance Medicine (JIM)* in the past few years (such results as were not included in the *1990 Medical Risks* monograph[2]).

As a subcommittee of the ALIMDA Mortality and Morbidity Committee, we have recognized the need for a uniform classification system to provide a unique identifier for these miscellaneous abstracts and articles, and for future abstracts, articles and mortality results, in the *JIM* or other sources. It is possible that all of these may be collected periodically for publication in a smaller but much more timely volume than the massive *Medical Risks* monographs, which took so many years to produce. The feasibility of such volumes is being considered by our subcommittee, together with the possibility of a looseleaf volume for early distribution of abstracts and updating. Our subcommittee has agreed that it would also be desirable to prepare a general index of the abstracts and mortality results already published in the books referred to,[1-4] in various intercompany insurance reports,[5-9] and in other follow-up studies, whether in abstract format or not. The period of publication covered by this index will be 1951-90; prior studies are now chiefly of historical interest. The index will require a source code, to be described later, in order to accommodate the different methods used to identify the abstracts or the mortality results. The classification system will also be used for future abstracts and articles published in the *JIM*, and in other ALIMDA publications.

The Disease Classification System and Numerical Code*

The proposed classification system consists of a 3-digit numerical code covering neoplasms, seven major disease categories by system in an order commonly seen in textbooks of medicine, and a diagnostic test category. The third digit will be used only when additional subdivision is needed and will not be included in the outline shown below. An initial category of "General Factors" encompasses such factors or causes external to the human body as environmental, socioeconomic and occupational ones; injuries; poisons; and in addition, family history and infectious diseases. The final category is a new major group for diagnostic test results.

Nosology is a highly intricate subject, with no existing classification accepted as a standard for general medical use. The subcommittee felt that our design should not be modeled after complex systems such as the ICD, MEDLARS, and others, but should be easy for the medical director, actuary, underwriter, epidemiologist and any interested physician to learn and use. The basic classification outline is as follows:

Source: R. B. Singer, J. R. Avery, M. W. Kita, "A Classification System for Mortality and Morbidity Abstracts and Related Data," *J. Ins. Med.*, 23 (1991): 94-96. Reproduced with permission of authors and publisher.

---

* Editor's Note: Since publication of the original article, this list has been revised and expanded. The revised list in the Appendix of Chapter 5 should be used in place of the original list reprinted here.

MORTALITY/MORBIDITY DATA CLASSIFICATION
(As originally printed)

GENERAL FACTORS

001	Methodology
010	Environmental (climate, pollution, radiation hazards, etc.)
020	Socioeconomic (income, type of work, education, etc.)
030	Occupational (governmental and insurance classifications)
040	Lifestyle (smoking, hazardous sports, physical activity, etc.)
050	Trauma and other types of injury
060	Toxins, poisons, side effects of drugs and any treatment method
070	Family history, excluding specific genetic factors (see 870)
080	Viral diseases
090	Bacterial, fungus and parasitic diseases

NEOPLASMS

100	Benign tumors
110	Cancers and precancerous lesions
120	Cancers of brain and nervous system
130	Leukemias, polycythemia vera, multiple myeloma
140	Cancers of lung and respiratory system
150	Cancers of digestive system
160	Cancers of genito-urinary system
170	Cancers of endocrine system
180	Cancers of bone, cartilage and soft tissues
190	Other cancers not included above

DISORDERS OF THE NERVOUS SYSTEM

200	Cerebrovascular disorders
210	Other brain disorders, extrapyramidal disorders
220	Spinal cord disorders
230	Peripheral nerve disorders
240	Disorders of the eye and ear
250	Psychoses
260	Neuroses
270	Character disorders
280	Addictions and substance abuse, alcoholism
290	Other neurological and psychiatric disorders, demyelinating disorders

DISORDERS OF THE CARDIOVASCULAR SYSTEM

300	Arrhythmias, pulse rate
310	ECG abnormalities
320	Hypertension, blood pressure
330	Latent coronary heart disease (CHD), risk factors
340	Acute CHD, MI and other acute coronary events
350	Chronic CHD, angina pectoris, chest pain, asymptomatic disease
360	Valvular heart disease
370	Ventricular failure, congestive heart failure, heart enlargement
380	Other heart disorders
390	Congenital cardiovascular disorders
400	Disorders of the aorta and arteries
410	Disorders of the veins
420	Other CV disorders, pulmonary vascular disorders

DISORDERS OF THE RESPIRATORY SYSTEM

430	Disorders of the nose, throat, sinuses; hay fever
440	Disorders of the larynx and trachea
450	Bronchial disorders, except asthma
460	Asthma
470	Lung infections, TB, pneumonia, pleural infections, etc.
480	Other lung disorders, emphysema, fibrosis, COPD, etc.
490	Other respiratory disorders not included above

(Pulmonary function evaluation - see 940)

DISORDERS OF THE DIGESTIVE SYSTEM

500	Mouth, tongue, and pharynx
510	Esophagus
520	Stomach, peptic ulcer
530	Small intestine
540	Colon, appendix, rectum
550	Liver and gallbladder
560	Pancreas
570	Peritoneum, abdominal cavity
580	Spleen
590	Other digestive system disorders not included above

DISORDERS OF THE GENITO-URINARY SYSTEM

600	Urinary abnormalities except glycosuria
610	Disorders of the bladder
620	Disorders of the ureters
630	Disorders of the kidneys
640	Disorders of the prostate
650	Male genital disorders
660	Vaginal disorders
670	Disorders of the uterus and adnexa

680   Breast disorders

690   Pregnancy and other GU disorders not included above

DISORDERS OF THE ENDOCRINE AND IMMUNE SYSTEMS

700   Diabetes mellitus, including glycosuria and blood glucose tests

710   Other adrenal disorders

720   Thyroid and parathyroid disorders

730   Male gonadal endocrine disorders

740   Female gonadal endocrine disorders

750   Pituitary, thymus and other endocrine disorders

760   Immune system disorders except asthma (460) and hay fever (430)

770   Metabolic disorders other than diabetes

780   Nutritional disorders

790   Other general disorders

MUSCULOSKELETAL SYSTEM AND OTHER DISORDERS

800   Disorders of the skin and connective tissues

810   Joint and back disorders

820   Other bone and cartilage disorders

830   Muscle disorders

840   Overweight, obesity, underweight, weight loss

850   Other musculoskeletal and integumentary disorders

860   Congenital disorders

870   Genetic disorders

880   Disorders of the blood and lymphatic systems

890   Miscellaneous disorders not classified elsewhere

DIAGNOSTIC TESTS

900   Chest X-ray and other X-rays

910   Other imaging techniques (CT, MRI, etc.)

920   Endoscopy; angiography

930   Exercise and other cardiac testing (resting ECG, see 310)

940   Pulmonary function tests

950   Liver and GI function tests

960   Renal function and bladder function tests

970   Cytological, genetic, and related tests

980   Blood chemistry and related tests (glucose, see 700)

990   Other tests not included above

(Urinary abnormalities - see 700 for glycosuria, 600 for all others)

Source Classification

The individual abstract or results identifier varies according to the book in which it is published. As a consequence, it becomes necessary to provide for a source code. The number of sources in the period 1951-90 is limited, and it suffices to use a single letter code appended to the numerical disease code. The list of source codes is as follows:

SOURCE OF ABSTRACT/MORTALITY STUDIES

A   *1951 Impairment Study*[3]

B   *1959 Build and Blood Pressure Study, Volume 1*[5]

C   *1959 Build and Blood Pressure Study, Volume 2*[6]

D   *1967 Occupation Study*[7]

E   *Medical Risks: Patterns of Mortality and Survival, 1976*[1]

F   *1979 Build Study*[8]

G   *1979 Blood Pressure Study*[9]

H   *1983 Medical Impairment Study, Volume 1*[4]

I   *1983 Medical Impairment Study, Volume 2* (in preparation, 1993)

J   *Medical Risks: Trends in Mortality by Age and Time Elapsed, 1990*[2]

K   Other abstracts/mortality studies published 1951-90

L   Reserved for any special mortality studies published prior to 1960

M   Abstracts/mortality studies published 1991-99

The Unique Identifier

We intend to retain the identifying number (or combination of letter and number) used in each of the books that contain large numbers of mortality abstracts or impairments studied. A 3-digit number was used in the first *Medical Risks* monograph,[1] but the numbers in the second *Medical Risks* monograph[2] extend to 4 digits because they are based on the numbers of the chapters, from Chapter 3 to Chapter 14, in which the abstracts are distributed. In the *1951 Impairment Study*,[3] the impairments are allocated into 9 lettered classes and given a number; an entirely different classification system with 25 letters, and a number for each impairment, is used in the *1983 Medical Impairment Study*.[4]

Coding Examples (Codes have been changed)

The new classification and source codes will be used anteriorly, followed by a hyphen and the identifier exactly as given in the source. Thus coding for the recent intercompany mortality experience on insured lives with diabetes mellitus would be 700H-U1. The 700 code is for the diabetes, the H code is for the *1983 Medical Impairment Study,* and the U1 code is the unique identifier in that source. The mortality experience in a group of diabetic patients followed in Edinburgh would be coded as 700J-1114. The same disease code is used (700 for diabetes), with source code J for the *1990 Medical Risks* monograph, and 1114 for the abstract number in Chapter 11, which covers Endocrine and Metabolic System Diseases.[2]

Mortality abstracts published separately, often in the *Journal of Insurance Medicine*, would have to be assigned a unique identifier, chronologically by date of publication at the date of assignment. For example, a mortality abstract on a group of Harvard College alumni classified by habits of physical exercise would be coded as 040K1. Habitual physical exercise is a "Lifestyle" descriptor, for which the 040 code is used, and the letter K for an individual abstract published in 1987. Since this is the first such abstract with this classification and source code,

it is currently assigned the unique identifier, number "1." This abstract was published in the *Journal of Insurance Medicine* in 1987, volume 19, issue number 4.

Conclusion

Our subcommittee of the Mortality and Morbidity Committee has prepared this classification system for coding mortality/morbidity abstracts and studies. This is for use in the future construction of a general index of such studies published during the period 1951-90, and for current and future use in coding new abstracts and related studies as they appear in publication in the *Journal of Insurance Medicine* or in other ALIMDA-sponsored publications. The disease classification system may be expanded by defining the third digit of the code. In addition, the system may be subject to future revision if experience in its use indicates the need for such revision.

REFERENCES

1. R. B. Singer, L. Levinson, eds., *Medical Risks: Patterns of Mortality and Survival* (Lexington, MA, Lexington Books, 1976).

2. E. A. Lew, J. Gajewski, eds., *Medical Risks: Trends in Mortality by Age and Time Elapsed* (New York, Praeger, 1990).

3. 1951 Impairment Study (Compiled and published by the Society of Actuaries, 1954).

4. Medical Impairment Study 1983, Volume I (Boston, Soc. Actuaries and Assoc. Life Ins. Med. Dir. Amer., 1986).

5. 1959 Build and Blood Pressure Study, Vol. 1(Compiled and published by the Society of Actuaries, 1959).

6. 1959 Build and Blood Pressure Study, Vol. 2 (Compiled and published by the Society of Actuaries, 1960).

7. 1967 Occupation Study (Compiled and published by the Society of Actuaries, 1967).

8. Build Study 1979 (Boston, Soc. Actuaries and Assoc. Life Ins. Med. Dir. Amer., 1980).

9. Blood Pressure Study 1979 (Boston, Soc. Actuaries and Assoc. Life Ins. Med. Dir. Amer., 1980).

APPENDIX

REVISED 2-DIGIT CODE LIST AND
3-DIGIT CODES USED FOR THIS VOLUME

GENERAL FACTORS 001-099

001-009	Methodology
001	Statistics, significance testing, computer applications
002	Vital statistics; prevalence, incidence; classification of diseases
003	Life table methodology (actuarial, Kaplan-Meier, etc.)
006	Mortality/Survival, follow-up studies, clinical trials, selection and bias, sampling
008	Morbidity studies (non-fatal event, disability, etc.)
010	Environmental Risk Factors
020	Socioeconomic Risk Factors
030	Occupational Risk Factors
038	Armed services personnel and veterans
040	Good Health and Personal Lifestyle Risk Factors
041	Habitual physical activity
050	Physical Injury, Trauma
060	Toxicology and Therapeutic Accidents
070	Family
080	Viral Diseases
086	AIDS and HIV infection; lymphogranuloma venereum, herpes genitalis
090	Bacterial, Mycotic and Parasitic Diseases

NEOPLASMS 100-199

100	Benign Tumors
110	Malignant Tumors
120	Malignant Tumors of the Nervous System
130	Cardiovascular, Blood, RE and Lymphatic Systems
140	Respiratory System
149	Other respiratory system malignant tumors
150	Digestive Tract
160	Genito-urinary Malignant Tumors
169	Other male and other female
170	Breast
180	Bone and Soft Tissue
190	Other Cancer Aspects - Epidemiology

DISEASES OF THE NERVOUS SYSTEM 200-299

200	Nervous System Disorders
210	Brain Disorders
220	Spinal Cord Disorders
230	Peripheral Nerves and Muscles
240	Degenerative and Demyelinating Nervous System Disorders
250	Psychoses
260	Neuroses (Psychoneuroses)
270	Character Disorders

280	Addictions
290	Other Neuropsychiatric Disorders

CARDIOVASCULAR DISEASES 300-429

300	Cardiovascular diseases, in general or in combination
301	Rate and rhythm, pulse rate
305	Ventricular fibrillation, cardiac arrest, cardioversion
310	ECG (electrocardiographic) abnormalities
319	Exercise test ECG, Holter monitor, other ECG tests *(see also 930)*
320	Blood pressure, in general or in combination
330	Latent CHD (coronary heart disease), incidence and prevalence
338	Prevention of CHD
340	Acute CHD, acute coronary event (ACE) and sequelae
345	Post-MI mortality and morbidity, recurrence
350	Chronic CHD
354	Angiography and ventriculography
355	Thallium imaging and related tests
358	Coronary bypass surgery, other surgery in chronic CHD
360	Valvular heart disease, heart murmurs in general
369	Valve repair and valve replacement, open-heart surgery
370	Congestive heart failure, general aspects
380	Other cardiac disorders, general aspects
390	Congenital CV disorders, general and in combination
400	Diseases of the Aorta and Arteries, Atherosclerosis
410	Diseases of the veins
419	Other diseases of the veins
420	Other cardiovascular diseases

DISEASES OF THE RESPIRATORY SYSTEM 430-499

430	Diseases of the Respiratory System
431	Diseases of the Nose, Sinuses, Throat and Middle Ear
440	Diseases of the Larynx and Trachea
450	Bronchial Disorders, Emphysema and Asthma
460	Noninfectious Pulmonary Diseases
466	Chronic obstructive pulmonary disease
470	Infectious Diseases of the Lungs
480	Diseases of the Pleura, Diaphragm and Mediastinum
490	Other Respiratory Disorders

DISEASES OF THE DIGESTIVE SYSTEM 500-599

500	Diseases of the Digestive System
501	Diseases of the Oropharynx
510	Diseases of the Esophagus
520	Diseases of the Stomach
530	Diseases of the Small Intestine
540	Diseases of the Colon and Rectum
550	Diseases of the Liver and Gall Bladder
560	Diseases of the Pancreas *(Diabetes mellitus - see 701)*

563	Cystic fibrosis (mucoviscidosis)
570	Diseases of the Peritoneum and Abdominal Cavity
580	Diseases of the Spleen and Hemorrhagic Disorders
590	Other Gastro-intestinal Diseases

DISEASES OF THE GENITO-URINARY SYSTEM 600-699

600	Diseases of the Genito-urinary System
601	Urinary Abnormalities
609	Other urine tests
610	Diseases of the Bladder and Ureters, Obstruction
611	Malformations of the bladder
620	Renal Diseases (Kidneys)
621	Congenital cystic disease
630	Acute glomerulonephritis, streptococcal
640	Diseases of the Prostate
650	Male Genital Diseases
660	Diseases of the Female Genital Tract
670	Disorders of the Uterus and Adnexa
680	Diseases of the Female Breast
690	Other Genito-urinary Disorders

DISEASES OF THE ENDOCRINE AND OTHER SYSTEMS 700-799

700	Diseases of the Endocrine and Other Systems
701	Diabetes mellitus
710	Endocrine Diseases of the Adrenal Cortex
720	Diseases of the Thyroid and Parathyroid Glands
730	Endocrine Disorders of the Male Gonads
740	Endocrine Disorders of the Female Gonads (Ovaries)
750	Disorders of the Pituitary and Other Endocrine Glands
760	Immune System Disorders, Excluding Hay Fever (433) and Asthma (458)
770	Metabolic Disorders
780	Nutritional Disorders; Diet
790	Other General Disorders

DISEASES OF THE MUSCULOSKELETAL SYSTEM AND OTHER DISEASE CATEGORIES 800-899

800	Diseases of the Musculoskeletal System and Other Diseases
801	Diseases of the Skin
810	Joint and Back Disorders
820	Diseases of Bone and Cartilage
830	Muscle Disorders
840	Body Build, Somatotype; Disorders of Body Weight and Body Fat
850	Collagen-vascular and Connective Tissue Diseases
860	Congenital Disorders (see also Genetic Disorders, 870)
870	Genetic Disorders
876	Hemochromatosis (iron storage disease)
880	Disorders of the Blood and Blood-forming Organs
890	Diseases of the Lymphatic System

LABORATORY AND OTHER DIAGNOSTIC TESTS 900-999

900	Laboratory and Other Diagnostic Tests
901	X-rays (excluding other imaging techniques)
903	X-rays of heart and great vessels
904	Chest X-ray
910	Other Imaging techniques
920	Endoscopy
930	Exercise and Other Cardiac Testing with ECG *(see also 319)*
940	Pulmonary Function Tests
950	Liver and Digestive Tract Function Tests
960	Tests of Genito-urinary Functions *(urine examination - see 601-609)*
970	Cytological and Genetic Testing
980	Blood Chemistry, Blood Tests and Histochemistry
981	Total base, osmolality, ionic constituents (sodium, chloride, etc.), iron, trace elements
983	Serum proteins (albumin, globulins, fibrinogen, blood coagulation)
984	Enzymes, hormones, antigens, antibodies, vitamins
990	Other Diagnostic Tests

CHAPTER 6

COMMENTARY ON ABSTRACTS AND ARTICLES

Richard B. Singer, M.D. and Michael W. Kita, M.D.

INTRODUCTION

This *Compend* has been modeled after the two *Medical Risks* monographs of 1976[1] and 1990.[2] However, because of the *Compend's* much smaller size, Chapter 6 is a single chapter that takes the place of the introductory overview text in each of the predecessor books. Because of the much smaller number of abstracts or articles in each disease area in this *Compend*, it has been impractical to follow the previous system of providing an epidemiological overview in each disease area, with national cause of death and related statistics. Attention has been focused on discussion of the abstracts or articles in the order in which they appear with the present coding system used (Appendix of Chapter 5). In each disease area, however, an effort has been made to refer to other sources of mortality data, such as the *Medical Risks* monographs[1,2] and the *1983 Medical Impairment Study*.[3] The reader should understand that the numbering system in each of these references differs from the coding used in this *Compend*, not only for individual abstracts, but also for the Chapters and the order in which disease groups are considered.

METHODOLOGY 001-009

Articles on this subject are not mortality abstracts. They have been added to the coding system for abstracts because of the obvious interest in the topic among contributors to and readers of the *Journal of Insurance Medicine* over the recent years during which the source material for this *Compend* has been collected. The inclusion of this subject matter adds to the heterogeneity of the major index group of GENERAL FACTORS 001-099. We have decided to comment very briefly on the methodology articles in Chapters 2-5, before starting the commentary on the other mortality abstracts or articles which follow Chapter 6.

Chapter 2 is a revised version of the text prepared by Pokorski for his basic course on "Mortality Methodology" and the triennial course sponsored by the Board of Insurance Medicine. It was originally published in the *Journal of Insurance Medicine* in 1988, and provides a logical, stepwise development of the key variables in the life table, including the use of worksheets. Most of the revisions have been made to clarify the proper usage of

exposure, E, in person-years, and number-exposed-to-risk, NER, in follow-up intervals generally shorter than 1 year.

Chapter 3 contains 10 further contributions covering a range of additional methodological topics. DeTore begins with a general discussion of "Medical Informatics," and in a second article he describes a decision-tree method for the cost-benefit analysis of abnormal laboratory test results in life underwriting. Iacovino and Kita discuss the predictive value of laboratory test results, using conditional probability by Bayes' theorem to draw appropriate statistical inferences. Singer provides a method for adjusting mortality ratios based on population mortality rates to mortality ratios based on insurance select rates, which can be used to approximate numerical ratings; a letter of actuarial comment by Tovson is appended. (Figure 003K1-1 in this article is a helpful aid for the visualizing of excess mortality in terms of both mortality ratio and excess death rate at different ages.) Singer also describes the effects of ascertainment bias on stage migration in lung cancer (the "Will Rogers phenomenon"). To assist those interested in identifying articles suitable for mortality or morbidity abstract preparation, Kita provides two checklists — one for rapid screening, and the other for a more detailed analysis. Lew presents a descriptive review of the *1990 Medical Risks* monograph.[2] Finally, Singer applies life table methodology to the calculation of morbid event rates and the preparation of morbidity abstracts, as distinct from mortality abstracts.

Chapter 4 is a fairly lengthy article that describes many of the aspects and problems of converting data in follow-up articles to tables of comparative mortality. This is done in greater detail than in the Methodology chapters in the two *Medical Risks* monographs.[1,2] The reader is referred to these chapters for additional information on basic methodology, and also to new Chapters 3-6 in the third edition of the text of Brackenridge and Elder,[4] published just prior to the completion of this text. Chapter 5 provides an outline of the coding system which has been adopted for use in this *Compend*. The reader should use the modified list of index codes in the Appendix of Chapter 5, because changes have been made in some of the codes since publication of the original article, and the coding has been expanded to three digits. This list is restricted to the basic codes of the original list, and the more detailed three-digit codes for the abstracts and articles contained in this volume. Publication of the complete, expanded three-digit list will be made in a forthcoming volume to be entitled, *A Descriptive Index of Selected Sources for Mortality Studies, 1951-90.* Work has already commenced on the preparation of this volume.

GENERAL FACTORS 010-099

The term GENERAL FACTORS has not been used in the previous *Medical Risks* monographs. It is used in this *Compend* to include infectious diseases and various risk factors for potential excess mortality or morbidity that are usually not classified as "diseases." The nine subgroups included are, in order:

010-019	Environmental Risk Factors
020-029	Socioeconomic Risk Factors
030-039	Occupational Risks Factors
040-049	Good Health and Personal Lifestyle Risk Factors
050-059	Physical Injury, Trauma
060-069	Toxicology and Therapeutic Accidents
070-079	Family (including family history, growth and development, and aging)
080-089	Viral Diseases
090-099	Bacterial, Mycotic and Parasitic Diseases

Only a few of these subgroups are represented by abstracts or articles in this volume. At the end of the commentary on these abstracts, reference will be made to other sources.

Abstract #038K1 is based on an article in which 9,324 male Army veterans who had served in Vietnam were compared with 8,989 matched male veterans who had had contemporaneous service in the U.S. or theaters other than Vietnam. All veterans had a minimum of 16 weeks of service, 1965-71, and were discharged with pay grade E1 to E5. Servicemen who died while on active duty were excluded. Nearly 250,000 man-years of exposure were accumulated in the two cohorts, and their mortality experience was compared with that for U.S. males matched by age, race and year of follow-up. Mortality rates were lower than expected (mortality ratios under 100%) in both cohorts in all duration periods, except for 0-5 years in the Vietnam cohort, for which a mortality ratio (MR) of 114% was observed. When total deaths were broken down into those due to natural and those due to external causes (violent deaths), the MR for natural causes for the Vietnam veterans was 54%, but for death by external causes the MR was 127%. Virtually all of the rather modest excess mortality was due to external causes in the first five years after discharge. The low mortality in both cohorts of veterans is due to the selection process prior to enlistment, the so-called "healthy worker" effect. The abstract contains some discussion of the choice of the most appropriate life table to use when selection has been involved in formation of the cohort under study. A group life table might have been more appropriate than the U.S. population tables in this case. For comprehensive mortality results in a variety of occupations the reader is referred to the latest insurance *Occupational Study.*[5]

Abstract #041K1 contains outcome data in relation to self-recorded physical activity of 16,936 Harvard College alumni age 35 to 74 at entry (questionnaires were mailed in 1962 and 1966). Maximum follow-up to 1978 was 12 or 16 years, and follow-up was 99 percent complete. Alumni with a history of coronary heart disease were excluded. Data on the habitual level of physical activity were converted into weekly rates of energy expenditure. Mortality rates adjusted for age and four risk factors were found to increase with decreasing physical activity. Mortality ratios against mortality in the total group as the "expected" rate ranged from a minimum of 65% to a maximum of 142% for the 15.4 percent of exposure in the most sedentary men with an energy expenditure under 500 kilocalories per week. Comparative mortality results were also derived for a combination of age and physical activity, and for the associated risk factors of blood pressure level in college or subsequent history of hypertension, weight index, smoking history, and history of parental death under age 65. There were 1,413 deaths recorded in an exposure of 213,716 person-years, a rate of 6.6 per 1,000 per year, all ages combined. Rates by attained age were lower than those in tables for the U.S. white male population, as would be expected on the basis of level of education.

In Morbidity Article #050K1 Butz analyzes his company's experience with 6,461 severely injured litigants seeking a structured settlement between 1982 and 1986. Reduced survival was estimated in terms of the reduction of projected age-at-death (life expectancy plus current age) below age 70 as an approximate life expectancy at birth in the U.S. white population. This reduction has been designated as "potential years of life lost to age 70" (P.Y.L.L. –70), a quantity that can be used by the actuary to calculate annuity benefits needed to support the injured person over his or her estimated remaining lifetime. Numerous tables are used to show the distribution of cases by age, sex, setting of the accident, type of accident, type of injury and P.Y.L.L.–70. The male-female ratio was highest for work-related injuries. The predominant type of severe injury was craniocerebral (39.0%), and the next highest prevalence was for spinal cord injury (21.2%). Severe injuries in children and young adults can shorten life drastically (very high values for P.Y.L.L.–70 of 10 or more years). Butz calls attention to unexpected findings, such as the large number of injuries due to iatrogenic causes, and the high proportion of birth injuries with anoxic brain damage. Valuable prevalence data are given in this article, together with the estimates of reduced life expectancy and 34 references to the medical literature. For additional information on structured settlements the reader should consult Chapter 6 of the new edition of the Brackenridge and Elder text.[4]

Although there is only one Mortality Abstract, #086K1, on AIDS (Acquired Immune Deficiency Syndrome), Braun and Singer have included results from seven different studies in 12 tables, thus presenting a comprehensive and detailed review of recent experience in this lethal disease epidemic. The data assembled consist of follow-up information on 12,016 AIDS patients from four community-based and three hospital-based series, five in the U.S. and one each in Australia and the United Kingdom. The multiple tables permit comparison of AIDS mortality by age, sex, follow-up duration, secular trend, and type of AIDS manifestation. One study of perinatally acquired HIV infection also provides data on the rate of development of clinical AIDS in these infants, as well as their survival. Most of the study articles contain additional information on AIDS that could not possibly be included in the abstract tables; for this the reader is referred to the original articles. In Table 086K1-1 and the initial text of the abstract the authors provide full details of the nature of each series, follow-up methods and derivation of expected mortality. Excess mortality is extremely high in AIDS patients; in the first year after entry, EDR (the annual excess death rate per 1000) is of the order of 500 per 1000 (or 50%) in the three largest U.S. series (Tables 086K1-2 to 086K1-4). In San Francisco and Maryland there was little or no improvement in the second year of duration, but there were no data after two years. In New York City EDR did decrease with duration, but was still 110 to 223 per 1000 per year at durations 2-5 years. EDR was somewhat higher in the minority of female patients (Table 086K1-5). Although there does appear to be a downward secular trend in first-year mortality with the introduction of treatment such as zidovudine, mortality is still very high (Tables 086K1-6 and 086K1-7). Because AIDS is such a new disease with a low survival, there is very little information available on excess mortality at long-term durations beyond 5 years. Other aspects of AIDS mortality are covered in Tables 086K1-8 to 086K1-12. As the authors point out the AIDS epidemic has had a tremendous economic impact, in addition to the personal tragedy it has brought to patients and their families.

They quote an estimate of one million persons infected with HIV in the U.S., and another estimate of 165,000 to 250,000 U.S. deaths from AIDS in the period 1991-93.

The medical literature on AIDS and HIV infection continues to expand at a high rate. There is one 1987 report by Cowell and Hoskins[6] that deserves careful study because of its methodology. The authors have used a Markov chain model to describe then existing data on the stage progression of HIV infection and clinical AIDS to ultimate death, thus presenting a more detailed description of the natural history of the infection. Chart 3 shows virtually no deaths at 2 years after infection, but over 70% of patients have developed lymphadenopathy syndrome or AIDS-related complex, precursor states for clinical AIDS. Less than 5% of infected persons have developed AIDS at 2 years, but this has increased to a cumulative rate of about 30% at 5 years at which time the cumulative mortality was 19%. The modeled progression and cumulative mortality curves of Cowell and Hoskins have a good fit with observed data as of 1987. Such a model should be updated periodically as additional observations are reported.

Volume I of the *1983 Medical Impairment Study*[3] contains only two sets of tables on GENERAL FACTORS, one on family history of cardiovascular disease, and the other on alcohol misuse, both of which showed substantial excess mortality, including policyholders issued a standard policy. Chapter 3 of the *1990 Medical Risks* monograph[2] contains 33 mortality abstracts on social class, smoking, drug addiction, and other lifestyle risk factors, an abundance of data on risk factors not covered here. In addition, Chapter 4 of the same monograph provides 12 abstracts with comparative mortality by occupational classes and exposure to workplace hazards such as petrochemicals, anesthetic gases and asbestos fibers. It should also be pointed out that Article #050K1 contains morbidity and limited mortality data on various types of accidents and injuries, as well as iatrogenic accidents, which are classified as "complications of therapy" (066-069 in the three-digit code). Cross-classification would be needed to specify the contents of such articles in more detailed fashion. Finally, the *1976 Medical Risks* monograph[1] has 12 mortality abstracts on alcoholism, smoking, family history and occupational exposure of anesthesiologists to halothane. There is one additional abstract which summarizes some of the results of the *1967 Occupation Study*,[5] previously referred to.

NEOPLASMS 100-199

There are five mortality articles dealing with six types of malignant disease in this section of the *Compend*, but Abstract #006K1, classified under Methodology in Chapter 3, actually provides mortality data in lung cancer, a site additional to the six mentioned above. The *1990 Medical Risks* monograph[2] contains 51 mortality abstracts from SEER and other source data on at least 33 different sites, including leukemias as a form of cancer. Earlier SEER results from what was formerly called the End Results Study of the National Cancer Institute may be found in the *1976 Medical Risks* monograph.[1] Some mortality data are also in the *1983 Medical Impairment Study*,[3] but insurance records generally supply results that are limited in numbers and in detail as to the cancer site. Other sources are to be preferred for mortality in cancer.

The interesting Article #110K1 by Butz describes in some detail a registry known as the Centralized Cancer Patient Data Systems (CCPDS), to which 21 Comprehensive Cancer Centers began contributing patient data in July, 1977. The data processing was done in a special section of the Fred Hutchinson Cancer Research Center in Seattle. From a 1987 report of 5-year follow-up[7] Butz has extracted aggregate experience for testicular cancers and for Hodgkin's Disease, subdivided by histological type and by stage. Overall EDR for the cancers of the testis was 37 per 1000 per year, all stages combined, but only 7.4 per 1000 for cancers classified as localized. This excess mortality is much smaller than reported in the SEER (cancer Surveillance, Epidemiology, and End Results program) data in Abstract 515[2]: EDRs of 33 and 90 per 1000, respectively for localized and all stages, 0-5 years duration. In Hodgkin's Disease (Table 110K1-4) EDR ranged from about 40 per 1000 per year for stages I and II to 86 per 1000 for Stage IV. Again, these EDRs appear to be much lower than the EDRs for men and women under 65 in Abstract 521,[2] durations 0-5 years, all stages combined. The reasons for these differences are not evident, unless the later period of observation and superior treatment in the CCPDS data are part of the explanation.

In Mortality Article #149K1 Iacovino has reviewed in detail the diagnosis and classification of bronchial carcinoids as the predominant one of four histological types of bronchial adenoma (truly benign bronchial adenomas are uncommon). Tables of comparative mortality were developed from two different source articles for typical and atypical bronchial carcinoids. The estimated EDR for atypical bronchial carcinoids was 61 per 1000 per year at 0-5 years, and 40 per 1000 at 5-10 years. In typical bronchial carcinoids excess mortality was either not evident or at a low level (6 per 1000 per year) within 10 years in both studies. In the long-duration study, up to 25 years, estimated mortality ratios were under 100% after 10 years. Iacovino emphasizes the need to examine the detailed pathologist's report before any attempt is made to underwrite an insurance applicant with a history of surgically removed bronchial carcinoid.

A clinical trial of Vitamin C in advanced colorectal cancer was reported from the Mayo Clinic in an effort to confirm or refute the claim of Linus Pauling and Cameron that large doses prolong the survival of patients with various types of advanced cancer. In Mortality Abstract #150K1 Singer has made a detailed analysis of the mortality in the 100 patients in the trial over two years, by Vitamin C or placebo, and the first-year mortality in the combined groups by age, sex, site of metastasis, Broder's grade of malignancy, and interval from diagnosis to entry into the study. Vitamin C had no effect on survival — the 6 survivors at two years duration were all in the placebo group. The important observation was that first-year EDR decreased sharply as the interval from diagnosis to entry into the study increased: 898 per 1000 with an interval <3 weeks, 482 per 1000 at 3-8 weeks, and 296 per 1000 with the interval >8 weeks. With the extremely high but decreasing weekly or monthly mortality in the first year after diagnosis of advanced cancer, it is evident that one-year mortality and survival are extremely sensitive to the timing of entry into any follow-up study. It is hypothesized that this is the explanation for the observation of Cameron and Pauling that survival was longer in their patients treated with Vitamin C than it was in their historical controls not so treated. In an additional table annual comparative mortality has been developed from a much larger number of patients with advanced cancer (End Results Group), all ages combined, to demonstrate the duration pattern of annual q, q', EDR and mortality ratio. Because mortality is higher in the older patients, q' *decreases* from the first to the second year of follow-up, and is still below the first-year level in the fifth year of follow-up. These methodological problems are of obvious importance in any study of a disease with very high and changing mortality early in follow-up, especially when the cohort has a wide age range.

Although classified as a "Mortality Article," #169K1 actually contains survival curves that have not been converted into comparative mortality. The article deals with nephroblastoma (Wilms' Tumor), diagnosed in young children and very rarely over age 7 years. A National Wilms' Tumor Study project (NWTS) has standardized staging and histological classification and maintained a registry for the follow-up of patients. Survival curves to a maximum of 10 years or less are shown for patient cohorts treated 1968-74, 1974-80, and 1980-85. Wilms' Tumor has shown remarkable sensitivity to chemotherapeutic agents since the 1970s, and 10-year survival for the 1974-80 patients with metastasis but favorable histology (89% of cases) was about 0.70, with most of the deaths occurring in the first five years. This corresponds to a mean annual mortality rate of about 35 per 1000, but the rate would be much lower at 5-10 years.

Because the mortality rate in children is so small (under 1 per 1000 per year from age 1 to age 14 years), EDR would nearly equal the annual observed rate.

For grade I patients (tumor confined within the capsule of the kidney) with favorable histology the 10-year survival is about 0.90, giving an estimated EDR slightly under 10 per 1000 per year. Clinically this is a favorable result, but from the standpoint of life insurance the corresponding mortality ratio would be well in excess of 1,000%. It would be necessary to examine the life table data from which the survival curves were constructed to determine the trend in EDR with duration, in order to project residual excess mortality after 10 years. The author states that tumor recurrence after 2 years is uncommon, but second malignant tumors occur in about 1% of patients by 10 years after removal of the Wilms' Tumor.

Cancer of the breast in Swedish women is the object of study in Mortality Abstract #170K1. This is an unusually large study, with patients entered in the Swedish National Cancer Registry 1960-78 and followed a minimum of 1 year. Additional life table and other data were supplied by Adami, the senior author of the 1986 published report. The size of the cohort and inclusion of all stages permitted a breakdown by quinquennial age distribution from 20-24 years to 75-79 years, with the oldest group age 80 years and up. In almost all age groups comparative mortality is given annually to 5 years, then in aggregate for 0-5, 5-10, 10-15 and 15-20 years, in the total cohort. In addition, cumulative survival rates and survival ratios are given for the total cohort, and all of the foregoing data for the 1975-78 patients are given at 0-5 years. The 30,216 deaths permit an exceptionally detailed analysis of patterns of mortality in total breast cancer, as shown in three very large tables and described in the abstract. All mortality ratios decrease with increasing age at any given duration period, because of the predominant increase in population mortality. Patterns of excess mortality are better judged from EDR values. In the first year the EDR curve is U-shaped: EDR 78 per 1000 per year at age 25-29, a minimum of 45 per 1000 at age 45-49, and 134 per 1000 at age 80 and up. In the older age groups, 70 and up, EDR decreases with advancing duration, although there is some irregularity at durations over 10 years, perhaps due to random variation in the small numbers of survivors at 15 years. However, in all age groups under 70-74 years the EDR *increases* in the second or third follow-up year before it starts to decrease with advancing duration and attained age. In all age groups EDR persists at durations over 10 years, generally at a level in excess of 20 per 1000 per year. This is one of the important findings of this very large cancer study. Further discussion may be found in the Comment section of the abstract.

NEUROLOGICAL DISEASES 200-299

Only a single abstract, #222K1, in this *Compend* falls in the group of Neurological Diseases. However, a previous article by the same author is coded under the General Factor of Trauma (050), as justified by its title and content, despite the fact that 60 percent of the injuries involved the brain or spinal cord. The reader is referred to Article #050K1 for an extensive and detailed discussion of the epidemiology of damage to the brain or spinal cord, with some limited discussion of survival.

In Abstract #222K1 Butz has described results of a 7-year multicenter study of paraplegia or quadriplegia due to spinal cord injury. Severity has been further classified as incomplete or complete paralysis involving only the legs or the body below the neck, for cervical lesions of the spinal cord. Excess mortality is given in Table 222K1-1 by duration to 7 years for all age and severity groups combined. EDR was found to be 40 per 1000 per year in the first year, 21 per 1000 in the second year, after which it appeared to stabilize at about 11 per 1000 at durations 2-7 years. The corresponding range in mortality ratio, based on U.S. Population rates, was from 1,290% to about 350%. In Table 222K1-3 Butz has made an approximate estimate of the mortality ratio by a combination of age and severity for the period of follow-up after the first 2 years. Table 222K1-2 provides accurate data by the same combination of age and severity for all durations, 0-7 years, combined. EDR increased with age in each severity group, but the highest mortality ratios were in the middle age group, 25-49 years. By severity, excess mortality was almost the same in complete as in incomplete paraplegia, and similar levels were observed under age 50 for incomplete quadriplegia. Excess mortality was higher in patients age 50 up in incomplete quadriplegia, and much higher in all age groups for complete quadriplegia (EDR 291 per 1000 in patients age 50 up, an extremely high level). These results may be compared with comparative mortality in Abstracts 1210-1215 in the *1990 Medical Risks* monograph.[2]

CARDIOVASCULAR DISEASES 300-429

As in previous collections of mortality abstracts, cardiovascular (CV) disorders constitute the major disease area, with the largest number, 14 of 38 articles or abstracts in the *Compend*. In the *1976 Medical Risks* monograph,[1] 39 of 190 abstracts or 20 percent dealt with CV disorders, and the proportion in the 1990 monograph[2] was even higher, 118 out of a total of 377 abstracts. Journals of general medicine, internal medicine, surgery and other specialties continue to publish their highest proportion of follow-up (FU) studies in the CV disease area. As noted previously, this *Compend* also differs from the previous monographs in featuring articles on methodology, with 13 such articles in Chapters 2-5.

Epidemiological data on CV diseases will not be recapitulated here. The reader is referred to the summaries in Chapters 6 and 7 of the *1990 Medical Risks* monograph[2] and to the current publications of the National Center for Health Statistics. (It should be noted that annual volumes of U.S. Mortality Statistics are published about three years after the year reported, and the decennial volumes, about five years after.) For comparative mortality, in CV series with no age distribution given in the article, the reviewer may find the age/sex data useful in Abstract 607,[2] for CHD (coronary heart disease) patients after acute MI, and Abstract 642,[2] for CHD patients who have had coronary angiography or bypass surgery.

Arrhythmias and ECG Abnormalities, 300-319. The first article in this group of CV disorders is #305K1, which presents data from a population-based survey of successful cardiopulmonary resuscitation (CPR) in King County, Washington, with FU of survivors to 4 years, and similar results of two smaller series. Sudden collapse and death are most often cardiac in origin, due to ventricular fibrillation or ventricular arrest. Most of these patients have CHD, and early mortality is very high: about 64 percent of the 1,567 cardiac arrest cases in the King County series died in or prior to being brought to the emergency room of the reporting hospital, despite the attempted CPR. Of those who survived long enough for hospital admission about one-half died in the hospital, and only one-half were discharged alive. Both risk of recurrent cardiac arrest and risk of death continued to be very high in those who were discharged alive, not only in the first year of FU (EDR 200 per 1000 per year or more), but also in long-term FU, duration 1 to 4 years (EDR of 84, based on 31 deaths in 228.5 patient-years of exposure). Mean ages in the three patient series were 65±12.7, 63 and 63 years, respectively; only 23 percent of the King County series were women, and their mean age was 70 years. The 4-year survival rate of the discharged patients was only 45 percent. More recent reports of patients resuscitated from cardiac arrest do not indicate significant improvement in immediate or long-term survival.[8] The subject of sudden cardiac death has been intensively reviewed in a symposium sponsored by the New York Academy of Sciences.[9]

Follow-up studies on some types of ECG abnormalities are reported in abstracts in both *Medical Risks* monographs.[1,2] Abstract #702[2] also provides data on relative frequency of ECG abnormalities, as well as comparative mortality, in a study of 21,415 British civil servants age 40-64 years. This series was divided into symptomatic and asymptomatic groups, thus providing comparative mortality in clinically healthy men, as well as those with symptoms at the time the tracing was made.

Abstract #319K1 is based on the results of Bruce's FU study of three cohorts of men with a maximal exercise test, entered in the Seattle Heart Watch Registry 1971-81. The first cohort consisted of 4,105 healthy men with a normal resting ECG; the second, 1,396 men with a history of hypertension but no CHD; and the third, 2,371 men with chronic CHD. Mean ages for the three cohorts were 44.6, 50.0, and 53.6 years, respectively. Each cohort was subdivided into a low-risk, moderate-risk, or high-risk group according to a defined combination of exercise test results, and four non-ECG risk factors: (1) family history of premature CHD event or death; (2) cholesterol of 250 or higher; (3) borderline systolic pressure; and (4) history of smoking cigarettes. A quinquennial age distribution permitted accurate calculation of expected deaths in each of the nine combinations of cohort and risk group. Because of the favorably low mortality in the 99 percent of the healthy men in the low- and moderate-risk group, insurance select mortality rates were used to calculate expected deaths.

Results of this well-designed study demonstrate the value of the maximal exercise test (Bruce protocol) and other risk factors in separating men into groups with widely different mortality observed over a 9-year FU period. The healthy men with normal resting ECG, except for the 1 percent in the high-risk group, experienced a mortality lower than that found in male policyholders issued standard life insurance. But the 44 "healthy" men in the high-risk group were found to have an EDR of 22 extra deaths per 1000 per year, and a mortality ratio of 550%. This was a significant excess in mortality despite the small numbers (5 deaths and 186 person-years of exposure). A moderate degree of excess mortality was observed in the hypertension cohort: mortality ratio of 200% and EDR of 4.8 per 1000 per year. Excess mortality was considerably higher in the men with chronic CHD: EDR 18 per 1000 per year in the low-risk group, 29 in the moderate-risk, and 97 in the high-risk group. These rates are for all ages combined. Distinctive patterns of excess mortality with age were observed in the different combinations of cohort, risk group and age group. The results of this Seattle Heart Watch experience are more comprehensive and more detailed than those in previous abstracts[1,2] on results of exercise test ECGs.

Blood Pressure 320-329. The single article on hypertension in this Compend (Article #320K1) provides an extensive summary of the results on men in the *1979 Blood Pressure Study*.[10] This article supplements the results in the published volume, because data for policyholders issued life insurance rated for elevated blood pressure as the sole reason for rating are given separately from data for men issued standard policies. Furthermore, the exposure data and excess death rates (EDRs) shown in the tables of this article were not given in the published volume. These results are therefore of importance to any reader interested in the mortality in insured men classified according to a wide range of blood pressure classes (systolic/diastolic combinations), age, and duration.

The enormous size of the *1979 Blood Pressure Study* is evident in the nearly 3.8 million standard and 591,000 rated policy records that were entered in the database. These were divided into 9 systolic and 11 diastolic blood pressure categories, as shown in Table 320K1-1 and the blood pressure grid for distribution of deaths. A smaller number of blood pressure combinations has been shown for men in two age groups in the tables of this article: eight blood pressure classes, designated A through H, as defined in the grid and in Tables 320K1-1 to 320K1-4.

Salient features of the standard experience are as follows:

1. A relatively large increase in mortality from the lower normotensive Class A (BP <128/<83) to the upper normotensive Class B (BP 128-137/ 78-87). The mortality ratio increased from 87% to 116% in men age 15-39 years at policy issue, and from 82% to 109% in men age 40-69 years.

2. Lower excess mortality in borderline hypertension Class C (BP 138-147/88-92) in men with standard than in men with rated insurance: in men age 15-39, a standard MR of 166% versus a substandard MR of 224%, and in men age 40-69, a standard MR of 134% versus 179% substandard. The mortality differences were undoubtedly due to more careful underwriting selection in the approximately 75 percent of the men with Class C blood pressure who were issued standard policies. Yet their increased mortality did not justify the standard policies issued, on the basis of a mortality ratio of 130% as an upper limit for issue of policies on a standard basis.

Salient features of the experience in the men rated for BP elevation were as follows:

1. A relatively small number of men were rated despite current BP readings in the normotensive range, Classes A and B. The reason for rating was a history of past hypertension. Overall mortality ratios were about 200% in men age 15-39, and about 180% in men age 40-69.

2. Excess mortality in terms of EDR increased with BP level progressively from Class C (BP 137-148/88-92) through Class F (BP >167/>97) and was higher in the older age group, the maximum being an EDR of 42

per 1000 per year in Class F at durations 15-22 years (based on 17 deaths). Hypertension is a potent mortality risk factor, based on casual blood pressure readings alone, without regard to other findings and tests used to establish the diagnosis.

3. In all rated BP classes B through H, EDRs increased with policy duration, from minimum levels of about 1-3 extra deaths per 1000 per year at durations 0-2 years to maximum levels of 40 or more per 1000 at durations 15-22 years.

4. Men with predominantly systolic hypertension (Class G, BP 148-167/78-87) had a higher overall excess mortality than that observed in men with predominantly diastolic hypertension (Class H, BP 128-147/93-102). By a considerable margin men in these Classes G and H outnumbered men with both systolic and diastolic BP elevation (Classes E and F, BP >157/>92).

For further information on BP elevation as a mortality risk factor the reader should consult the *1979 Blood Pressure Study*[10] itself, and Chapter 7 of the *1990 Medical Risks* monograph.[2] Chapter 7 also contains results on arrhythmias and ECG abnormalities.

Coronary Heart Disease 330-359. The value of a small dose of aspirin in reducing the incidence of acute MI was demonstrated in a large clinical trial as part of the Physicians' Health Study (see Abstract #338K1). The 22,071 male physicians were selected for volunteer enrollment in this study only if there was no prior history of CHD, cancer, liver and renal disease. Because of this selection, the overall mortality was found to be close to that in select insurance tables, and far below mortality in the U.S. population. We are indebted to Dr. Charles Hennekens, Director of this study, for supplying the additional data needed for the complete observed data in Table 338K1-1, data needed for the accurate calculation of expected deaths from insurance select rates. There was almost no difference in total number of deaths between the two matched groups: 217 in the men given aspirin, and 227 deaths in those given placebo. Age distribution was virtually identical, and exposure was just under 55,000 person-years in both groups. Table 338K1-3 shows that a reduction in deaths due to MI in the aspirin group was counterbalanced by an increase in sudden deaths, with almost no difference in other CV and non-CV deaths between the two groups. However, the morbidity results did show a highly significant reduction in non-fatal MIs: 213 in the placebo, to 129 in the aspirin group (Table 338K1-4).

Physicians are sometimes confronted with the problems of how to manage patients with a clinical history strongly suggestive of acute MI, yet without confirmation by abnormal Q waves in the ECG or elevation of serum enzyme levels. Evidence from several sources is presented in Article #340K1, with this pattern described, together with FU observation of the patients. Among such patients there is a high incidence of in-hospital MI and deaths within one year of the acute episode. Out of a total of 648 patients from five series, 77 deaths were recorded within one year (Table 340K1-1). In the absence of age data, this rate of 119 per 1000 per year has been compared with pooled mortality for patients during the first year after an acute MI. First-year mortality rates after acute MI may be found in Abstracts 608-618 and in the text of Chapter 6 in the *1990 Medical Risks* monograph.[2] These provide a basis for additional comparison. It is reasonable to suspect that the normal ECGs and serum enzyme levels in these series represented a false negative test result.

Excellent data are available from the very long-term Framingham Heart Study on the recurrence of MI following an initial MI, and these have been presented in a formal Morbidity Abstract, #345K1. (The methodology has been described in Article #008K1 at the end of Chapter 3 in this *Compend.*) Published rates of *initial MI* by age and sex in the members of the Framingham series provide the needed "expected" incidence rates for MI. The annual MI recurrence rate was higher in Framingham men than in Framingham women, and the rate increased with age in both sexes (Table 345K1-1). There were 29 recurrent MIs in an exposure of 965 person-years for men who survived at least one MI, with an excess event rate (EER) of 21 per 1000 per year. In women recurrence rates were even higher, with an EER of 67 per 1000 per year, based on 13 MIs in only 183 person-years. These numbers are not large, and any EER trend by age or duration is therefore unreliable. This abstract is a good example of the application of life table methodology to comparative morbidity, with recurrent MI as an easily defined morbid event.

The illustrative follow-up study detailed in the Methodology Article #003K1, Chapter 3, gives the 15-year experience of a cohort of MI patients in Auckland, New Zealand. These results may be reviewed apart from the methodology aspects as supplementing the other MI series referred to in Chapter 6.

A useful addition to the extensive body of FU studies of post-MI patients[1,2] is Fessel's analysis of 426 policy records of European men reinsured 1956-85 by a large international reinsurance company (Abstract #345K2). Overall mortality was high, with 78 deaths observed in an exposure of 2,250 policy-years, a mortality ratio of 575% and an EDR of 29 per 1000 per year. Mortality ratios exceeded the rating classes used (Table 345K2-1). Excess mortality expressed as EDR tended to increase with increasing age and policy duration (Tables 345K2-2 and 345K2-3). When excess mortality was analyzed by interval from MI to the year of application, the highest EDR, 43 per 1000, was found in a small group of applicants for whom this interval was unknown (Table 345K2-4); it is possible that other risk factors were also not known to the underwriter in these cases. Excess mortality was higher in association with elevated BP (Table 345K2-5). The overall EDR of 29 per 1000 was higher than the overall EDR of 22 per 1000 found in a larger series of men insured by U.S. and Canadian companies, in which there were 330 death claims.[3] Results of many clinical series of post-MI patients[1,2] indicate a somewhat higher overall excess mortality, but with a wide range, depending on severity factors. The underwriting selection process undoubtedly eliminates many applicants whose MI history was associated with complications or sequelae that are recognized as increasing the mortality risk.

A different area of CHD is marked off by the diagnostic tools of coronary angiography and ventriculography in the evaluation of chronic CHD. These tests have made possible selection of whole armies of CHD patients for coronary bypass surgery (CBPS) by use of grafts to bypass one or more obstructions in any of the three major coronary arteries. In Abstract #354K1 Palmer has reported a FU study of 5,306 patients who had a cardiac catheterization at the Cardiac Laboratory of the Hartford Hospital from 1971 through 1981. The patients were characterized in detail as to their age/sex distribution and other medical characteristics. The FU experience included 26,989 person-years of exposure and 631 deaths; 46 percent of the patients were treated medically, and 54 percent were treated with CBPS. In his printed report Palmer presented comparative mortality results based on both select insurance rates and on U.S. population rates. The insurance select rates were chosen for the tables in this abstract for reasons described in the text. When excess mortality was analyzed by a severity score, 0-9, for the degree of coronary obstruction (single or multiple), both the mortality ratio and EDR were found to rise progressively from 0 score (no significant obstruction) to score 9, the maximum degree of 3-vessel disease (Table 354K1-4). Excess mortality was somewhat higher in male patients and in older patients, both medical and surgical treatment combined (Table 354K1-6). However, as found in many other series when severity of the coronary obstruction and age are comparable,[2] mortality was higher in the medically treated patients than in those treated by CBPS (Table 354K1-5). This differential was greater in the patients with more severe disease, score 5-9, the EDR being 50 per 1000 per year in the medically treated, and 14 per 1000 per year in those treated surgically. The mortality pattern of CBPS patients by duration is consistent with the trend clearly demonstrated in the many abstracts of the *1990 Medical Risks* monograph:[2] a minimum EDR at durations 1-4 years, followed by a progressive increase with increasing duration, especially after 5 years. This is due to atherosclerotic narrowing that continues in the non-bypassed portions of the major coronary arteries, and appearance of the disease in the bypass grafts themselves. The principal benefit of bypass surgery occurs in the first five years after surgery, and is much greater in older patients.[2] Tables 354K1-7 through 354K1-10 detail the increase in mortality with decreasing ejection fraction, increasing left ventricular end-diastolic pressure, or the presence of other risk factors.

Table 354K1-10 provides a cross-comparison of the medically and surgically treated cases, in terms of a decimal ratio of the respective mortality ratios, and the difference in the respective EDR values. The largest difference was found in the existence of overt congestive heart failure, with an EDR difference of 152 per 1000 per year.

Abstract #354K2 is based on a FU study of medically treated CHD patients also classified by angiography and ventriculography at Erlangen University Polyclinic, Germany, 1969-76. Three severity grades for coronary stenosis were used, based on the American Heart Association scoring system, and three severity grades for impairment of left ventricular function, based on the ejection fraction. Only the least severe classes had an excess mortality comparable to that observed as an *average* for the medically treated patients in the Hartford Hospital series described above. Mortality was calculated as an average from 5-year survival rates, and EDR exceeded 100 per 1000 per year in the most severe stenosis group, and in both groups with abnormal ejection fraction (under 60 percent). As evident in Tables 354K2-2 and 354K2-3 excess mortality was very high in the categories of more severe disease, and 71 percent of the patients were placed in the more severe stenosis groups. The source article on which this abstract is based was part of a published European symposium with the title "Prognosis of Coronary Heart Disease. Progression of Coronary Atherosclerosis" (see reference in the abstract).

Another study of 2,842 patients evaluated by angiography and treadmill exercise test at the Duke University Medical Center has been analyzed by Reardon in Abstract #354K3. A severity score was developed from the duration of exercise, the ST segment depression, and an index of angina experienced by the patient during the test. Although all patients had definite or suspected anginal symptoms, 39 percent were found to have no significant coronary obstruction in their angiogram. It is not surprising, therefore, that no excess mortality in comparison with Group Life Insurance rates was observed in the 968 patients (one-third of the total) who had a low-risk test score (Table 354K3-1). During the first five years of FU, patients with a moderate-risk score had an EDR of 12 per 1000 per year and those with a high-risk score had a much higher EDR of 57 per 1000. The test score was equally effective in differentiating excess mortality in the patients with 3-vessel disease, as shown in Table 354K3-2: the mean annual EDR over five years' duration increased from 6 per 1000 in the low-risk group, to 26 per 1000 in the moderate-risk, to 69 per 1000 in the high-risk patients. Only 16 percent of the patients with 3-vessel disease were in the low-risk group; mortality would have been higher in these patients if those with obstruction of the left main coronary artery had not been excluded.

The role of thallium imaging has been evaluated by Mackenzie in Article #355K1, with respect to estimating probability of the existence of coronary artery obstructive disease from clinical history and exercise test results, including ST segment depression in the ECG. The analysis is based on noninvasive test results, prior to any coronary angiography. A table of pre-test probability of CHD is given, based on age and sex, and on increasingly suspicious chest pain history. Post-test probability of CHD may then be read off curves of ST segment depression in the exercise test ECG, against pre-test CHD probability in one graph, and from positive and negative thallium test result curves in the other graph. In one example given, the probability of CHD is rendered very low by the negative thallium test, but in another, a rather high probability of CHD is only slightly reduced. The emphasis of this article is therefore on analysis of probability as a diagnostic aid in risk classification. However, the author does cite a follow-up study in which mean annual death rates were in the range of 2 to 5 per 1000 in patients with suspected CHD but a negative thallium stress test. The extent to which these rates might exceed average select rates in the first five years of policy duration would depend on the age and sex of any insurance applicant.

Two mortality abstracts on patients with CBPS appear in this *Compend* in the form of supplements to results published in the *1990 Medical Risks* monograph. The first, #358K1, gives data on coronary bypass reoperations from the very extensive experience with CBPS at the Cleveland Clinic. It is based on 1,500 consecutive patients who required such reoperation following an initial coronary bypass procedure. Overall perioperative mortality of 3.4% was higher than the 1.5% experienced in the many thousands of first CBPS operations performed at the Clinic from 1967 to 1980.[2] Long-term EDR over a FU of 6 years averaged 7 per 1000 per year, but with a range from 0 to 46 per 1000, depending on degree of abnormality of left ventricular function. The authors felt that overall results were nearly as good as those following initial CBPS. Results from the Cleveland Clinic appear in several abstracts of their experience with medically and surgically treated patients, but without the reoperation data in this abstract.

The second CBPS abstract, #358K2, provides age and sex distribution data that were lacking in a different article used as a source for the experience of the St. Luke's Hospital in Kansas City, previously published as Abstract #655.[2] The latter was the only abstract lacking even a mean age and proportion of females, and average values from a dozen other series of CBPS patients were used to derive the expected mortality. The recently discovered age/sex distribution is given in Table 358K2-1. During the first 4 FU years, excess mortality was found to be higher in the female than in the male patients. The accurate EDR values derived from this age/sex distribution average about 8 to 10 percent higher than those estimated in Abstract #655, which have now been superseded by the new results of Abstract #358K1.

Other Cardiovascular Diseases 360-429. Only one FU article was retrieved that involved a CV disease outside the area previously discussed. This was a study of 210 patients who had mitral valve repair for mitral insufficiency without mitral stenosis (Abstract #369K1). The report is from the Medical Center of the University of Alabama at Birmingham. Only 86 of the patients had isolated mitral valve repair without other cardiac surgery; of the remainder 63 also had CBPS, 31 had aortic valve replacement, 27 had repair of a congenital defect, and 3 had other cardiac procedures. Perioperative mortality was only 3.5% in isolated mitral valve repair, but was 8.9% when other cardiac procedures accompanied the valve repair. The same findings prevailed with long-term mortality after hospital discharge: EDR estimated from 5-year survival rates was 14 per 1000 per year from the patients with mitral valve repair; EDRs were higher in the other groups with associated cardiac surgery, the highest value, 82 per 1000 per year, in the patients who also had an aortic valve replacement. Detailed results are in Table 369K1-3. Comparative mortality by duration is reliable only for the total series (Table 369K1-2). This shows a high excess mortality in the first year after hospital discharge and a lower but substantial EDR averaging 23 per 1000 per year at durations 1-10 years. Such results are difficult to interpret because of the heterogeneous nature of the operative procedures in the total series. Mitral valve repair, when it can be done without the need for other cardiac operations, offers advantages over mitral valve replacement. Both perioperative and long-term mortality are lower (see Abstracts 667 and 671-673 in the 1990 Medical Risks monograph[2]), there is a lower incidence of complications, and there is no need for the continuous use of anticoagulants, with their attendant complications.

The reader interested in other CV diseases will find in the 1990 Medical Risks monograph[2] six abstracts on congenital heart disorders, eleven on valvular heart disease, six on cardiac disorders, such as heart enlargement, congestive heart failure and cardiac myopathy, and seven on vascular diseases. Additional mortality data on CV diseases are given in the 1983 Medical Impairment Study,[3] and abstracts of earlier studies in the 1976 Medical Risks monograph.[1]

RESPIRATORY DISEASES 430-499

In Abstract #466K1 Butz has developed comparative mortality results from an interesting FU study of subjects with a forced expiratory volume at one second (FEV1) less than 65 percent of that predicted for age and height. Such a reduced FEV1 test is indicative of chronic obstructive pulmonary disease or asthma with reversible broncho-constriction. The series was drawn from a random population sample tested by spirometry in Tucson, Arizona, and subjects were excluded if they had evidence of restrictive pulmonary disease. There was no excess mortality in the 27 subjects of Group I, all of whom had confirmed asthma, and 56 percent of whom had never smoked. In contrast, subjects in Group III all had a smoking history, a negative skin test for allergy, and a negative history for asthma. The 45 subjects in this group experienced 24 deaths in 10 years, a high excess mortality, with EDR of 46 per 1000 per year and mortality ratio of 280% (average age was 65 years). Group II subjects consisted of those who could not be classified in either Group I or Group III. At durations 0-5 years their EDR was only 9 per 1000 per year, but EDR increased sharply at 5-10 years to 70 per 1000 per year, approximately the same as the rate in the Group III patients at the same duration range. A distinctive feature of this study is the clear separation of asthmatic patients, most of whom were not current smokers, from the smokers without asthma or positive skin test for allergy. Mortality was very different in the two groups. This feature should be kept in mind when these results are compared with results of nine abstracts on abnormal pulmonary function tests or chronic obstructive pulmonary disease in the 1990 Medical Risks monograph.[2]

Abstract #466K1 is the only one culled from the Journal of Insurance Medicine that deals with a respiratory disease. Comparative mortality results on other types of respiratory diseases may be found in the recent reference volumes previously cited.[2,3]

DIGESTIVE TRACT DISEASES 500-599

Again, the next disease system, digestive tract disorders, is represented in this Compend by only a single article, #563K1, in which Butz has summarized mortality and survival data collected by the Cystic Fibrosis Foundation. It is true that cystic fibrosis, or mucoviscidosis, is a disease that involves the pancreas, and textbooks of medicine generally classify it with other pancreatic disorders. In actual fact, cystic fibrosis is an autosomal, recessive, genetic disease that involves multiple body systems: the pancreas; exocrine glands, including sweat glands and mucous glands of the intestinal and respiratory tracts; a fundamental disorder of the composition of sweat and mucus; and important secondary problems of malabsorption in the intestinal tract and bronchial obstruction and infection in the lungs. The lung complications are probably the most important cause of disability and excess mortality. Cystic fibrosis, as a consequence, is a good example of the nosological difficulties encountered in the construction of any system of disease classification. For practical reasons we have decided to retain the usage of medical texts, so that this disease can be the sole occupant of a 3-digit code, because it is such a common genetic disease.

The tables and figures of the article demonstrate that excess mortality increases with attained age and is higher in females than in males. In male patients the EDR increases from 5 extra deaths per 1000 per year at ages 1 through 4 years to 58 at ages 25 through 29; in female patients the corresponding increase is from 8 to 72 per 1000 per year. Such high excess mortality in children and young adults entails a sharply reduced survival to age 30. The 1976-85 experience (Figure 563K1-2) shows a cumulative survival rate of 31.8% for male patients and 23.2% for females. When male and female experience is combined, the recent mortality experience for 1985 reflects a potential cumulative survival rate of 38.1% at 30 years, a substantial improvement over the 27.6% survival rate computed for the 1976-85 experience (Figure 563K1-4 in the article).

GENITO-URINARY DISEASES 600-699

In Morbidity Article #609K1 Stout has reported 140 confirmed positive tests for HIV in 103,000 urine specimens submitted on life insurance applicants whose urine was routinely tested, a prevalence of 1.36 per 1000. This was higher than the rate of 0.85 per 1000 found for routinely tested serum specimens. These results were based on a nationwide distribution of applicants. Higher rates for HIV positive urine specimens were found in California (1.83 per 1000) and New York (3.12 per 1000). This was a screening survey, and no follow-up was attempted.

Mortality Abstract #611K1 gives results of a small series of children with the congenital malformation of exstrophy of the bladder. There were only 6 deaths observed, against 3.0 expected from an estimated expo-

sure of 2,246 patient-years. Certain assumptions had to be made in these calculations, because the authors of the report utilized retrospective exposure prior to the attained age of the patient at the time first seen at the Babies Hospital, New York City. Mortality may be underestimated in the first decade of life, because prior deaths of potential entrants are automatically eliminated from retrospective exposure. Overall excess mortality (EDR 1.3 per 1000 per year) was significant at the 91 percent, but not the 95 percent confidence level, by the Poisson distribution. The authors cite two earlier Mayo Clinic follow-up studies on children with exstrophy of the bladder. Survival rates in these studies yield much higher EDR values, mostly in excess of 30 per 1000 per year, suggesting a marked improvement in survival with newer techniques of medical management. This abstract shows the potential value of small numbers of cases and deaths in evaluating prognosis in uncommon chronic conditions.

Another genetic disorder, polycystic kidney disease, is reported by Dalgaard in Article #621K1. This autosomal dominant disease of the kidneys is estimated to occur in about 1 per 1000 live births, and the follow-up was done on Dalgaard's original 1957 series of cases sought for and identified in Denmark. The disease is latent in the early decades of life and has seldom been diagnosed prior to age 40. The lowest attained age range given in Table 621K1-4 of the article is 20-29 years. Excess mortality is virtually the same to age 60 for male and female patients in terms of EDR, which increases with attained age from a minimum under 1 per 1000 per year in the youngest patients to 61 per 1000 in men age 70 up, and 111 per 1000 in women age 70 up. Overall EDR values are identical for male and female patients at 20 per 1000. Polycystic kidney disease is a good example of a chronic disorder in which EDR increases steadily with attained age, while the mortality ratio increases to age 40-49 years, then starts to decrease because of the characteristics of the natural rise in the population mortality rate.

ENDOCRINE AND OTHER DISEASES 700-899

The mortality experience of a large European reinsurance company is given by Fessel in Abstract #701K1 for men with diabetes mellitus. It should be recognized that the underwriting selection process would have eliminated most of the very severe cases, including those with complications. Overall excess mortality, with an EDR of 7.4 per 1000 per year, was somewhat higher than the EDR in the larger experience of men rated for diabetes alone in the *1983 Medical Impairment Study*.[3] EDRs increased with age and policy duration, and with the severity of the rating imposed, as they did in the *Impairment Study* experience. Fessel in his abstract calls attention to some differences between these two insurance studies of mortality in insured diabetics. Despite these differences, the patterns of excess mortality are similar. The detailed tables in the abstract provide a clear picture of mortality among insured men with diabetes mellitus.

In Article #876K1 Iacovino has reviewed some clinical, mortality, and underwriting aspects of idiopathic hemochromatosis. This is an autosomal recessive genetic disease characterized by excessive storage of iron in the liver, with complications of serious liver disorders. Mean survival times and survival rates quoted by Iacovino from follow-up studies indicate a very high mortality in idiopathic hemochromatosis, even when treated by the standard method of regular phlebotomy. The 5-year survival of 0.66 and 10-year rate of 0.32 reported by Bomford in 1976 permit the calculation of geometric mean annual mortality rates. During the interval from 0 to 5 years after diagnosis the mean annual mortality rate so calculated was 80 per 1000, but this increased to 135 per 1000 at 5 to 10 years after diagnosis. These rates were for patients, "about 55 years," who were under treatment, and they imply a correspondingly high degree of *excess* mortality for idiopathic hemochromatosis. As Iacovino points out, the varying degrees of severity of the liver damage and any complications must be taken into account in the interpretation of the excess mortality.

DIAGNOSTIC TESTS 900-999

Ferrer has reported a survey of 6,000 chest X-rays made on life insurance applicants at the Equitable Life Assurance Society, and read by the author (Article #904K1). Additional insurance and medical data were available in 4,209 or 70 percent of these cases, of which 463 were found to have 470 abnormalities in their chest X-rays. Table 904K1-1 lists the 312 pulmonary abnormal findings, which outnumbered the 158 abnormal findings in the heart and aorta by a ratio of 2/1. It should be understood that chest X-rays are often obtained by life insurance companies, along with an ECG, as a screening procedure when the amount applied for is large, especially for applicants at the older ages. Others are obtained for review because of the medical history or other evidence of pulmonary or cardiovascular disease, some of these on loan, others newly taken at the request of the medical underwriter. The predominant abnormality, found in 225 or 5.3 percent of the detailed cases, was evidence of old pulmonary tuberculosis, either calcified nodes or parenchymal lung changes. Cardiac enlargement, defined as a cardiothoracic (CT) ratio of 50% or more, was found in 78 X-rays, and aortic calcification in 65 X-rays. Ferrer found that only 15% of the abnormal chest films resulted in an insurance rating or declination. This translates into a proportion of only 1.2% of the 4,209 detailed cases. This low yield of abnormality with under-

writing significance was partly due to the fact that the reason for obtaining the chest X-ray was generally a routine large-amount requirement rather than a medical reason.

Two additional articles, #903K1 and #903K2, also concern chest X-ray findings in insurance applicants, but the chief emphasis is on relative heart diameter (RHD) by the Clark-Ungerleider tables.[11,12] These tables of transverse heart diameter were based on measurements of transverse heart diameter correlated with height and weight of ostensibly normal subjects, with a P-A chest film taken at a distance of 6 feet. They have been used in insurance medical departments since about 1940 as a more accurate measure of increased heart diameter than the more widely used CT ratio. Relatively few cardiologists and radiologists in clinical medicine have utilized the Clark-Ungerleider tables or other methods of making a more accurate estimate of increased heart size than that derived from the CT ratio; the most intensive use of these tables has been in insurance medicine.

The source for the data in both articles was a computerized file of applicants to the New England Mutual Life Insurance Company, with ECGs interpreted 1954-66 who were also coded as having had a chest X-ray reviewed at the same application as the ECG. Out of this file 4,962 applicants age 20 to 74 years, with a chest X-ray, were analyzed with respect to the distribution of relative heart diameter in Article #903K1, and 4,143 of these with a minimum follow-up of one year were evaluated in a mortality study in Article #903K2. Almost all of the chest X-rays had been preserved; these were reinterpreted by a single observer, a board-certified radiologist, the senior author of the first article, with the detailed record of the current interpretation used in a small percentage of cases for which the X-ray was no longer available. Data observed on the X-ray reinterpretation were coded with other information for data processing. The most important information was cardiovascular, the relative heart diameter, the ratio of the observed transverse heart diameter to that predicted from the Clark-Ungerleider table, derived from the individual's height and weight. The table in Article #903K1 gives the quinquennial age distribution for the 4,962 applicants in the total series, for the 4,713 men and 249 women, and for three other groups. These groups were defined as applicants who were issued standard insurance (65.7 percent), those rated for any cardiovascular risk (23.8 percent), and those rated for non-cardiovascular reasons (10.5 percent). Normal (bell-shaped) distribution curves of RHD for various of these groups are shown in Figures 903K1-1 to 903K1-6 in the article, in terms of relative frequency. These were analyzed for mean values of RHD (97.2% in the groups issued standard insurance or insurance rated for non-cardiovascular reasons), standard deviation (±7.1%) in the largest group, men issued standard insurance), and coefficients of skewness and kurtosis, which were small, indicating minimal departure from the shape of the normal curve. The mean RHD of 97.2% was significantly less than the mean of 100.0% predicted from the Clark-Ungerleider table. This difference was interpreted as being due to improvement in chest X-ray technique over a period of about 30 years, with better definition of the location of the cardiac apex in those individuals with an obscuring periapical fat pad. This mean RHD of 97.2% was also significantly smaller than the mean of 99.3% for the group of applicants rated for any cardiovascular risk. Despite the statistical significance of the difference in the means, the overlap of the distributions curves makes it difficult to set an upper confidence limit for a normal value of RHD. The article includes a detailed discussion of the statistical results and their interpretation.

Expected rates were derived from the 1965-70 Select and Ultimate Intercompany tables, which were about 15 percent higher than the rates prevailing in the New England Mutual Life Insurance Company (Article #903K2). This accounts in part for the favorable mortality ratio of 73% in all standard cases. The rest of this favorable selection was doubtless due to the screening out of applicants with abnormalities in their ECG or chest X-ray, abnormalities considered to be of enough significance to warrant a rating. However, in the group rated for cardiovascular reasons the mortality ratios were under 125% when the RHD was less than 90%, but excess mortality was observed at a maximum when the RHD was 105% and higher (see Table 903K2-5). The EDR was close to 11 per 1000 in males age 50-74 for both RHD levels of 97-104% and 105% and up. These were RHD values unadjusted for the standard mean of 97% being 3% below the predicted mean of 100%. Cases rated for increased RHD alone were too few to permit a meaningful analysis, but it is apparent that applicants rated for cardiovascular reasons experience a lower comparative mortality when the RHD is below the mean of 97%, and a higher mortality when the RHD is above the mean, in both younger and older applicants. The article should be consulted for further results on mortality in relation to RHD and other factors, including the Sheridan Index for aortic width.

"Normal" standards in blood chemistry — the concentrations of constituents of blood, plasma or serum — are an ever-present problem for the physician, whether engaged in clinical medicine or insurance medicine. The problem is well illustrated by an interesting report from the Mayo Clinic, which was the basis for the Test Article #981K1. Heath et al. investigated the annual incidence of hyperparathyroidism diagnosed in Rochester, Minnesota, during the period 1965 to 1976, and found an apparent jump from a rate of 7.8 per 100,000 prior to July 1, 1974, to 37.1 per 100,000 after that date. This date was critical because serum calcium levels were obtained only at the request of the Mayo Clinic physician through June, 1974. Starting in July the Mayo Clinic Laboratory began to report routine serum calcium concentration as part of a 12-channel chemistry combination utilized for most Mayo Clinic and hospitalized patients as part of their diagnostic workup. It was found from the medical records that the diagnosis was based on a serum calcium over 10.1 mg. per dl., *without* clinical manifestations in only 18 percent of the diagnoses prior to July 1, 1974, but this rose to 51 percent of the diagnoses made after the autoanalyzer came into routine use. Of the 84 cases with serum calcium recorded nearly half were 10.5 mg. per 100 dl. or lower; that is, any elevation above the accepted upper limit of normal of 10.1 was a relatively small elevation. The apparent increase in the incidence rates was very probably due to false positive diagnoses made on the basis of the "elevated" serum calcium, without corroboration by clinical or other evidence. Additional details and other data are discussed in the article.

Another article, a mortality abstract dealing with serum chemistry, #983K1, describes an unanticipated inverse association of mortality with serum albumin concentration within the normal range. The blood chemistry data were drawn from a regional population sample (the practice of a single physician in each of 24 towns in England, Scotland and Wales in 1978-80). A total of 7,690 men age 40-59 years had serum albumin and other data collected as part of the British Regional Heart Study. Adjustments were made for the significant cross-correlations of serum albumin with age, serum cholesterol, systolic blood pressure and forced expiratory volume at 1 second (FEV1), as shown in Table 983K1-1. Over an average follow-up of 9.2 years, when adjusted mortality rates were used, the EDR was 11 per 1000 per year and the mortality ratio, 220%, in the group with the lowest serum albumin, under 40 g./L. (Table 983K1-2). Mortality decreased as the serum albumin increased, regardless of whether adjusted or crude mortality rates were used. Phillips et al., authors of the report, offer no hypothesis that might explain this inverse association between mortality and serum albumin; they caution that the association might be coincidental. Nevertheless, this is a most interesting observation that deserves further study.

The final article, #984K1, is a cost-benefit analysis of screening older male life insurance applicants with a test for PSA (prostate-specific antigen), a test that has recently received much attention in pre-clinical or clinically evident prostate cancer. Variables considered by Bergstrom, the actuary-author of this article, included excess mortality data for prostate cancer derived from SEER data published in 1989,[13] preliminary incidence rates for a positive test in two age groups of insurance applicants, average policy lapse rates, the present value of projected death claims per $1,000 of insurance applied for, the potential mortality savings, and return on investment of the cost of screening for various application amounts. The preliminary incidence data were obtained in a large reference laboratory used by insurance companies for various types of screening tests. Although only a few companies have utilized PSA testing for larger amount applications, the incidence rates were low, 0.3% for men age 50-59, and 0.7% for men age 60-69 years. Bergstrom estimated the "return on investment" (the investment being the cost of the testing, with over 99% negative tests) on a $50,000 policy to be 60% for men age 50-59, and 193% for men age 60-69. Returns were higher for larger policy amounts.

A dissenting view was expressed by Alexander on the desirability of routine PSA testing for older male insurance applicants (letter to Editor, #984K2).

There are many factors for insurance management to consider before adopting new screening tests of this nature. "Tumor markers" are a new subject of great interest to physicians involved in epidemiology and clinical practice, as well as those involved in life insurance medicine. Appended to the above is a letter to the Editor of the *Journal of Insurance Medicine*, in which the writer, an insurance company medical director, expresses reasons for *not* subjecting life insurance applicants who are older males to routine PSA screening, despite the apparent attraction of a favorable cost-benefit analysis. The editors of this volume maintain a discreet silence on the merits and drawbacks of PSA testing as one example of detecting tumor markers in the selection process for individual life or health insurance. The topic is too extensive for review here.

REFERENCES

1. R. B. Singer, L. Levinson, eds., *Medical Risks: Patterns of Mortality and Survival* (Lexington, MA, Lexington Books, 1976).

2. E. A. Lew, J. Gajewski, eds., *Medical Risks: Trends in Mortality by Age and Time Elapsed* (New York, Praeger, 1990).

3. *Medical Impairment Study 1983*, Volume I (Boston, Soc. Actuaries and Assoc. Life Ins. Med. Dir. Amer., 1986).

4. R. D. C. Brackenridge, W. J. Elder, eds., *Medical Selection of Life Risks, 3rd Edit.* (New York, Stockton Press, 1992).

5. *1967 Occupation Study* (Chicago, compiled and published by the Soc. Actuaries, 1967).

6. M. W. Cowell, W. H. Hoskins, *AIDS, HIV Mortality and Life Insurance, a Joint Special Report of the Society of Actuaries* (Itasca, IL, Soc. Actuaries, 1987).

7. K. A. Kealey, ed., *Survival Rates for U.S. Comprehensive Cancer Center Patients, Admissions 1977-82* (Seattle, Centralized Cancer System Statistical Analysis and Quality Control Center, 1985).

8. J. W. Bachman, G. S. McDonald, P. C. O'Brien, "A Study of Out-of-Hospital Cardiac Arrests in Northeastern Minnesota," *JAMA*, 266 (1986): 477-83.

9. H. M. Greenberg, E. M. Dwyer, Jr., eds., *Sudden Cardiac Death* (New York, vol. 382 of Ann. N.Y. Acad. Sci., 1982).

10. *Blood Pressure Study 1979* (Boston, Soc. Actuaries and Assoc. Life Ins. Med. Dir. Amer., 1980).

11. H. E. Ungerleider, C. P. Clark, "A Study of the Transverse Diameter of the Heart Silhouette and Prediction Table Based on the Teleoroentgenogram," *Trans. Assoc. Life Insur. Med. Dir. Amer.*, 25 (1938): 84-103.

12. H. E. Ungerleider, C. P. Clark, "A Study of the Transverse Diameter of the Heart Silhouette and Prediction Table Based on the Teleoroentgenogram," *Am. Heart J.*, 17 (1939): 92-102.

13. M. H. Myers, L. A. G. Ries, "Cancer Patient Survival Rates: SEER Program Results for 10 Years of Follow-up," *CA-A Cancer Journal for Clinicians*, 39 (1989): 21-32.

PART II

ABSTRACTS AND ARTICLES

POSTSERVICE MORTALITY IN ARMY VIETNAM VETERANS

Richard B. Singer, M.D.

References:

1. C. A. Boyle, et al., "Postservice Mortality Among Vietnam Veterans," U.S.P.H.S. Centers for Disease Control, Atlanta, GA 30337 (1987).

2. The Centers for Disease Control Vietnam Experience Study, "Postservice Mortality Among Vietnam Veterans," *JAMA*, 257 (1987): 790-95.

Object of the Study: To identify the possible adverse health effects in Army Veterans who served in Vietnam.

Subjects Studied: 9,324 male Army Veterans who served in Vietnam (VS) and 8,989 male Army Veterans of the same era, who served in the U.S., Germany, or Korea, but not in Vietnam (NVS). The cohorts were selected from a random sample of 48,513 Army personnel on the basis of these criteria: males with first enlistment between January 1, 1965 and December 31, 1971, with single term of enlistment, at least 16 weeks of service, and with pay grade from E-1 to E-5 at the time of discharge. Excluded from the cohorts were 234 men in the VS group who died while on active duty (181 deaths were hostility-related), and 34 in the NVS group who also died before the end of their enlistment. All but 8.3% of the men in the VS cohort were in an age range of 18-24 years, all but 11.3% in the NVS cohort; the mean ages were estimated at 22.3 and 22.2 years, respectively, at the time of discharge. The two groups were compared with respect to age, race, region of birth, percent volunteers, health status, aptitude test scores, type of Army unit, and other characteristics. Most of the group differences were small, but VS Veterans had a higher prevalence of honorable discharge (97.3% vs. 91.1%), a higher prevalence of pay grade E-4 to E-5 after an average of 26 months of service, and a higher prevalence of assignment to the infantry (26.6% vs. 14.6%). All men had passed the selection criteria for Army enlistment.

Follow-up: Was carried out to December 31, 1983, with 446 deaths determined through records of the Veterans

Source: R. B. Singer, "Postservice Mortality in Army Vietnam Veterans," *J. Ins. Med.*, 21 (1989): 47-48. Reproduced with permission of author and publisher.

Administration, Social Security Administration, Internal Revenue Service, or the National death Index. Death certificates were obtained in all but nine of these reports. Cause of death was determined by a medical review panel. Veterans not identified as deceased were traced and interviewed in all except 590 (6.3%) of the VS group, and 722 (8.0%) of the NVS group. The men whose status was not confirmed were "considered to be alive at the end of follow-up for analytic purposes."[1] In various categories observed deaths were compared to expected, based on person-years of exposure and rates among U.S. males standarized for calendar year, race and age.

Results: As shown in Table 038K1-1, the expected mortality rate for this very young series of adults males was about 2.1 per 1000 per year, and increase with duration was minimal (U.S. Life Tables actually show an increase in q' from age 18 to 24, then a slight decrease from age 25 to 32). Except for the first 5 years after discharge in the VS group, the observed mortality rates were consistently lower in all of the other categories shown. Mortality ratios ranged between 76% and 85%, with negative EDR values, –0.3 or –0.5 per 1000 per year. With the low mortality rate prevailing in young men, these differences are small, but they are significant in the two duration periods within 10 years, as evaluated by 95% confidence limits from the Poisson distribution for observed deaths. The slight excess mortality observed at 0-5 years duration in the veterans who served in Vietman was not significant: mortality ratio of 114%, with 95% CL of 89%-131%, and EDR of +0.3 per 1000 per year.

In Table 038K1-2 deaths have been divided into those due to natural causes (disease) and those due to external causes (accident, homicide, suicide and poisoning). The mortality ratios for deaths from natural causes are seen to be even lower, only 54% to 68%, regardless of duration or service in Vietnam. Such deaths were greatly outnumbered by the deaths due to external causes, as is true for cause of death in the U.S. population of young men in their 20s. Excess mortality was found only at 0-5 years in the veterans who had served in Vietnam, with a mortality ratio of 127%, and EDR of +0.8 per 1000 per year (not shown in the table).

In both the monograph and the *JAMA* article most of the voluminous mortality results compare rates in the VS cohort with corresponding rates in the NVS cohort, in terms of a decimal "rate ratio" (RR), with emphasis on cause of death RR values. There are five tables presenting such results in the article, and only one comparing observed deaths with expected deaths from U.S. population tables — the source of results in Table 038K1-2. Results in Table 038K1-1 were derived from the monograph.[1] Within 5 years of discharge the RR was 1.45 for total deaths, and 1.61 for deaths due to external causes. The mortality excess, VS over NVS, was highly significant. A curious finding was a significantly lower rate in the VS group as compared with the NVS group for deaths due to circulatory diseases and for deaths due to all natural causes. RR values were reported for seven of the covariates recorded, but all differences were small and not statistically significant. When RRs were adjusted by the Cox proportional hazard model, the adjustment tended to make the crude ratios more rather than less significant. For more detail on these results the reader should consult the sources. [1,2]

Comment: These results clearly demonstrate the "healthy veteran" effect: as a well-defined group, originally selected to meet the physical and mental requirements of the armed forces, veterans have a significantly lower mortality than that found in the U.S. population. To epidemiologists such results are analogous to the "healthy worker effect." In insurance medicine the phenomenon is well known in the mortality pattern of select vs. ultimate mortality tables. Because of the exclusion of disabled persons and the effects of pre-employment screening, mortality in group life insurance tables is also lower than in population tables. The healthy veteran effect has been documented by Seltzer and Jablon ("Effects of Selection on Mortality," *Am. J. Epidemiol.*, 100 [1974]: 367-72). Further evidence is provided in another article from the Medical Follow-up Agency (Robinette and Fraumeni, "Asthma and Subsequent Mortality in World War II Veterans," *J. Chronic Dis.*, 31 [1978]:

619-24). A control group for the veterans with asthma was obtained by matching them with an otherwise equivalent group of veterans who had been hospitalized for the medically inconsequential diagnosis of acute naso-pharyngitis. Follow-up continued from 1946 to 1974, a total of 29 years. Mortality ratios matched against U.S. men by calendar year, race and age, were all less than 100%, but showed a steady increase from 71% in the first interval, 1946-49, to 96% in the final interval, 1970-74, 24-29 years after the 1946 entry year. In cross-section the socioeconomic status of veterans of World War II was apparently similar to that in the U.S. male population, but the selection effect endured for nearly 30 years.

Those preparing mortality abstracts from studies reported in the medical literature should take note of the importance of choosing expected life tables that are most appropriate to the group being reported. For example, it would have been wiser, in retrospect, to have used "normal veteran" life tables to calculate expected deaths in the post-MI patients described in Abstracts 303, 310 and 311 in the *1976 Medical Risks* monograph. These series consisted of Army men admitted to service hospitals in World War II and male veterans admitted to VA hospitals after 1945. U.S. Life Tables were used, because the healthy veteran effect had not been well documented at that time. Ed Lew and I have been careful to use mortality from the total Framingham experience as the basis for comparison of mortality in any Framingham Study group, because the overall mortality is significantly lower than in the U.S. Life Tables. Group life rather than population tables have been used in the many series of coronary bypass patients reported in the *1990 Medical Risks* monograph, because most patients with advanced cancer and other serious diseases or complications would not be referred for surgery. For bypass surgery one must postulate a selection bias of this sort, even when the surgeon is willing to operate on all patients who are referred.

COMPARATIVE MORTALITY BY VIETNAM SERVICE AND DURATION

Duration Post-Dis.	Exposure Man-yrs.	Observed Deaths	Expected Deaths*	Mortality Ratio	Mean Annual Mortality Rate per 1000		
					Observed	Expected	Excess
Years	E	d	d'	100(d/d')	q	q'	(q–q')

8,989 VETERANS, NO SERVICE IN VIETNAM

0-5	44,747	73	92.8	79%	1.63	2.07	−0.44
5-10	44,233	74	92.0	80	1.67	2.08	−0.41
10 up	32,350	53	67.9	78	1.64	2.10	−0.46
All	121,330	200	252.7	79	1.65	2.08	−0.43

9,324 VETERANS WITH SERVICE IN VIETNAM

0-5	46,350	110	95.9	114%	2.37	2.07	+0.30
5-10	45,855	72	95.4	76	1.57	2.08	−0.51
10 up	35,692	64	75.0	85	1.79	2.10	−0.31
All	127,897	246	266.3	92	1.92	2.08	−0.16

* Basis of expected deaths: U.S. Male Rates by Calendar Year, Race and Attained Age.

COMPARATIVE MORTALITY BY VIETNAM SERVICE, TYPE OF DEATH AND DURATION

Type of Death	Vietnam Service	Exposure Person-yrs.	Observed Deaths	Expected Deaths*	Mortality Ratio
		E	d	d'	100(d/d')

0-5 YEARS AFTER DISCHARGE

Type of Death	Vietnam Service	Exposure Person-yrs.	Observed Deaths	Expected Deaths*	Mortality Ratio
Natural	No	44,747	16	23.4	68%
	Yes	46,350	13	24.2	54
External	No	44,747	55	69.4	79
	Yes	46,350	92	72.5	127

MORE THAN 5 YEARS AFTER DISCHARGE

Type of Death	Vietnam Service	Exposure Person-yrs.	Observed Deaths	Expected Deaths*	Mortality Ratio
Natural	No	76,583	39	63.4	62%
	Yes	81,547	38	65.8	58
External	No	76,583	88	96.8	91
	Yes	81,547	96	102.7	93

* Basis of expected deaths: U.S. Male Rates by Calendar Year, Race and Attained Age.

LONG-TERM MORTALITY OF HARVARD COLLEGE ALUMNI 1962-78, CLASSIFIED BY LEVEL OF PHYSICAL ACTIVITY

Richard B. Singer, M.D.

Reference:

R. S. Paffenbarger, Jr., R. T. Hyde, A. L. Wing, C. H. Hsieh, "Physical Activity, All-Cause Mortality, and Longevity of College Alumni," *N. Engl. J. Med.,* 314 (1986): 605-13.

Subjects Studied: Health and life-style questionnaires were returned from 16,936 Harvard Alumni who entered college 1916 to 1950. This total includes only men who were age 35 to 74 in the year of entry (questionnaires mailed in 1962 and 1966), and excludes 732 men (4.1%) who gave a history of physician-diagnosed coronary heart disease (CHD) on their questionnaire. The series was thus selected to exclude known CHD, but not to exclude a history of cancer, stroke or other high-risk disease (less than 4% of the total). Habitual physical activity was estimated from the number of blocks walked and the number of stairs climbed daily, and the average weekly hours engaged in various sports since college. Physical activity levels were estimated in kCal/week, in 8 classes ranging from less than 500 to 3,500 or more kCal/week. Alumni were also classified in this study according to systolic blood pressure under 130 mm. or 130 mm. and higher in their college examination records, or any physician diagnosis of hypertension, type of sports participation in college, family history of number of parental deaths prior to age 65, history of cigarette smoking, and current height and weight. All mean annual mortality rates (all durations combined) were calculated as number of deaths divided by the exposure in person-years in each category studied. The rates were adjusted for all age differences in all physical activity and other risk categories.

Follow-up: Was extended to 1978, for a duration of 12 or 16 years from the entry years 1966 and 1962. More than 75% of alumni surviving in the entry years responded to the mailed questionnaires. From weekly updating of death notices by the Harvard Alumni Office death certificates were obtained. The authors report that

Source: R. B. Singer, "Long-Term Mortality of Harvard College Alumni 1962-78, Classified by Level of Physical Activity," *J. Ins. Med.,* 19, no. 4 (1987): 15-18. Reproduced with permission of author and publisher.

fewer than 1% of alumni were lost to follow-up without death notification.

Results: With 1,413 deaths observed in 213,716 person-years of exposure the mean annual mortality rate was 6.61 per 1000. Age-adjusted mortality rates, prevalence of exposure, and deaths have been given in the article for a variety of physical activity classes (walking, stair-climbing, light sports, vigorous sports, and physical activity level by estimated caloric expenditure per week), and for the previously mentioned risk factor classes. In all of the classes except family history the death total was less than the 1,413 deaths reported for the entire series. The mean annual mortality rate of 6.61 per 1000 for the entire series has been used to estimate exposure in the physical activity classes, for which 1,349 total deaths were reported: $E=d/\bar{q}=1,349/0.00661$, or approximately 204,100 person-years. Exposure for each physical activity class shown in Table 041K1-1 was calculated from this total E of 204,100 and the prevalence distribution for E. Crude mortality rates (d/E) are shown in Table 041K1-1, as well as the reported age-adjusted rates rounded off to the nearest 0.1 per 1000 per year. As a uniform expected rate I have used 6.6 per 1000 per year. Comparative mortality in the abstract tables has been derived as the excess death rate, $EDR=(\bar{q}-6.6)$, and as a mortality ratio, $MR=100(\bar{q}/6.6)$. With the average used as the expected rate, some of the classes show excess mortality, and some show negative values of EDR and MRs under 100%. In the article tables, "relative risks of death" have been reported in terms of the group with the highest mortality: all of these decimal indices are therefore less than 1.00.

From the results in Table 041K1-1 it is apparent that excess mortality was highest in the group with the lowest physical activity level, less than 500 kCal/week. Mortality rates decreased steadily with increasing level of physical activity to 3,499 kCal/week, but then increased by 9% at the highest activity level of 3,500 kCal/week and up. This general trend of mortality downward with increasing physical activity was highly significant, with $p<0.0001$. A similar downward trend was observed in miles walked and hours per week of light sports activity. In the other measures of physical activity, stairs climbed and vigorous sports, the class with the highest level of physical activity also exhibited a higher mortality than in the proximate class, but lower than that of the class with the least physical activity. It is probable that most alumni who engaged in vigorous sports were also in the class with the highest level of energy expenditure, 3,500 kCal/week or more. One can only speculate whether a high exposure to vigorous sports may result in some increase in mortality relative to that associated with equivalent energy expenditure in less stressful sports.

As shown in Table 041K1-2, mortality decreased with increasing activity level in each of the four age groups analyzed. Three activity levels were used: under 500, 500-1,999, and 2,000 or more kCal/week. The mortality was almost twice as high in the most sedentary as compared with the most active groups at age 60 and up. Differentials were less marked in men under age 60, but consistent in their trend. "Expected" rates in each age group had to be approximated from the rates in the three physical activity classes as their average weighted according to the exposure prevalence, all ages combined. The rates in Table 041K1-2 were estimated from Figure 1 of the article, with the use of the logarithmic q scale. The authors reported no exposure or death data by age.

Table 041K1-3 contains results for age-adjusted mortality, exposure prevalence, and deaths in other associated risk factors, regardless of the level of physical activity. The same uniform average annual mortality rate of 6.6 per 1000 was used as the expected rate in each class; all observed rates were age-adjusted. As would be expected from previous studies the highest mortality was observed in alumni with hypertension, in those who smoked a pack or more of cigarettes per day, and in those with both parents dead before the age of 65. Levels of excess mortality are somewhat reduced in comparison with excess mortality in insurance studies, since the high-risk subjects have not been excluded from the expected mortality rate. All of the trends were highly significant ($p < 0.0001$) for these risk factors. However, anomalous results were obtained for body mass index, with no significant trend at intermediate levels, and the highest mortality observed at both the lowest index, under 32, and the highest, 38 or more. The body mass index is calculated as the function, $1000(wt./ht^2)$, where weight is in pounds and height in inches. The conversion of actual height-weight combinations to this body mass index makes it virtually impossible to compare results with those of the 1979 Build Study. I cannot identify reasons for the mortality relation seen in Table 041K1-3, except that higher mortality at the extremes of the body mass index classes is not inconsistent with the higher mortality observed in overweights and in subjects who are under "ideal" weight.

Additional results not shown here include three dimensional bar graphs of combinations of physical activity class with the associated risk factors, a multivariate analysis of "attributable risks of death" for the associated risk factors, a table of added life expectancy associated with an active life style by quinquennial age group, and a table of proportions of active and sedentary men surviving to age 80. The original article should be studied by readers interested in these results.

Comment: The evidence is convincing that a sedentary life style is associated with a relatively high level of mortality at any age in this rather large group of college alumni. Mortality decreased with increasing physical activity level, but turned upward in the class with the highest activity level, which probably included a large proportion of men who engaged regularly in vigorous sports. There appears to be an upper limit to the favorable association of physical activity with decreased mortality. It should be noted that the average mortality rates in these Harvard alumni are much lower than the 1969-71 U.S. rates for white males at corresponding approximate attained ages. Part of this is attributable to the selection process, excluding men with a CHD history. However, I would attribute a major part of this favorable mortality differential to educational and socioeconomic factors. This study is an example of the need to use an internal expected mortality for the calculation of comparative results. Use of population mortality rates would have resulted in all mortality ratios being well under 100%. The authors of the study chose to use the class with the highest instead of the lowest mortality as the standard for comparison in each category studied, whereas I have used the average mortality in the entire series.

TABLE 041K1-1

COMPARATIVE MORTALITY TO 16 YEARS, BY PHYSICAL ACTIVITY LEVEL, ALL AGES COMBINED

Physical Activity Level	Exposure		No. of Deaths	Ann. Mort. Rate per 1000		EDR-Excess Death Rate	Mortality Ratio
	Prevalence	Person-yrs.		Crude	Adjusted[†]		
KCal/Week	%	E(est)*	d	d/E	$\bar{q}$	$(\bar{q}-6.6)$	$100(\bar{q}/6.6)$
<500	15.4%	31,400	308	9.8	9.4	+2.8	142%
500-999	20.9	42,700	322	7.5	7.4	+0.8	112
1000-1499	15.2	31,000	202	6.5	6.8	+0.2	103
1500-1999	10.4	21,200	121	5.7	5.9	–0.7	89
500-1999	46.5	94,900	645	6.8	6.9	+0.3	105
2000-2499	8.1	16,500	89	5.4	5.8	–0.8	89
2500-2999	6.9	14,100	62	4.4	4.8	–1.8	73
3000-3499	5.0	10,200	42	4.1	4.3	–2.3	65
2000-3499	20.0	40,800	193	4.7	5.1	–1.5	77
3500 up	18.1	36,900	203	5.5	5.8	–0.8	88
2000 up	38.1	77,700	396	5.1	5.4	–1.2	82
All Levels	100.0*	204,100*	1,349	6.61	6.61	—	—
Total Series	(>100)	213,716	1,413	6.61	6.61	—	—

* E for all activity levels estimated from d and $\bar{q}$ for total series (total d/total E). E for each activity level estimated from prevalence of E and E ≅204,100, all levels. The overall $\bar{q}$ of 6.6 per 1000 is used as the expected annual mortality rate, $\bar{q}$.

[†] Adjusted for differences in age, blood pressure, weight class, smoking class, and family history.

TABLE 041K1-2

COMPARATIVE MORTALITY TO 16 YEARS BY AGE AND PHYSICAL ACTIVITY GROUP

Physical Activity Level	Prevalence* Exposure (Assumed)	Mean Annual Mortality Rate per 1000			Mortality Ratio
		Observed	Expected[†]	Excess	
KCal/Week	%	$\bar{q}$	$\bar{q}'$	$(\bar{q}-\bar{q}')$	$100(\bar{q}/\bar{q}')$
MEN AGE 35-49					
<500	(15.4%)	2.7	2.4	+0.3	112%
500-1999	(46.5)	2.6	2.4	+0.2	108
2000 up	(38.1)	2.1	2.4	–0.3	88
MEN AGE 50-59					
<500	(15.4)	6.2	4.9	+1.3	127%
500-1999	(46.5)	5.3	4.9	+0.4	108
2000 up	(38.1)	4.0	4.9	–0.9	82
MEN AGE 60-69					
<500	(15.4)	21	15	+6	140%
500-1999	(46.5)	14.5	15	+0.5	97
2000 up	(38.1)	11.5	15	–3.5	77
MEN AGE 70-84					
<500	(15.4)	36	25	+11	144%
500-1999	(46.5)	26	25	+1	104
2000 up	(38.1)	18.5	25	–6.5	74

* Based on distribution, all ages combined.

[†] Weighted mean, based on prevalence distribution for all ages combined (Table 041K1-1), applied to each age group.

LONG-TERM MORTALITY OF HARVARD COLLEGE ALUMNI

TABLE 041K1-3

COMPARATIVE MORTALITY TO 16 YEARS BY ASSOCIATED RISK FACTOR, ALL AGES COMBINED

Category	Exposure Prevalence	No. of Deaths	Ann. Mort. Rate per 1000		Mortality Ratio	Significance of Trend
			Observed*	Excess		
	%	d	$\bar{q}$	$(\bar{q}-6.6)$	$100(\bar{q}/6.6)$	p Value
BLOOD PRESSURE STATUS†						
Hypertension History	9.4%	283	11.7	+5.1	177%	
Normal, College S ≥130	21.4	275	6.8	+0.2	103	<0.0001
Normal, College S <130	69.2	714	5.9	−0.7	89	
SMOKING HISTORY — CIGARETTE PACKS PER DAY						
1+ pack/day	27.2	480	11.0	+4.4	167%	
<1 pack/day	11.0	129	6.4	−0.2	97	<0.0001
None	61.8	648	5.5	−1.1	83	
WEIGHT INDEX**						
38 and up	18.2	286	7.6	+1.0	115%	
36-37	19.0	236	6.1	−0.5	92	
34-35	25.3	331	6.5	−0.1	98	0.63
32-33	21.0	259	6.3	−0.3	95	
≤31	16.5	259	8.0	+1.4	121	
PARENT DEAD BEFORE AGE 65						
Both	4.1	87	8.1	+1.5	123%	
One	29.2	491	7.7	+1.1	117	<0.0001
Neither	66.7	835	6.3	−0.3	95	

* Age-adjusted mortality rate. Uniform age-adjusted expected rate of 6.6 per 1000 per year (See Table 041K1-1).

† Hypertension on basis of physician diagnosis. In absence of hypertension history alumni were classified according to systolic pressure of less than 130 at college examination, or 130 up.

** Weight in pounds divided by height in inches squared, multiplied by 1000.

THE EPIDEMIOLOGY OF SEVERE INJURIES
IN STRUCTURED SETTLEMENT APPLICANTS

Roger H. Butz, M.D.

Abstract

This study describes the epidemiologic characteristics of 6,461 severely injured individuals. These attributes include age, sex, race/ethnic group, injury settings, and mechanisms, types and severity of injury. The injuries were 28.4% work-related, 23.3% iatrogenic, and 48.1% from personal injuries. The overall male: female ratio of persons injured was 2.2:1. Craniocerebral injuries accounted for 39.1% of the total, and spinal cord injuries 21.2%. These two injury types are described in considerable detail. It is concluded that the group described, which consisted entirely of individuals applying for structured settlements in satisfaction of claims for recovery of injury, probably do not differ significantly from population-based groups of injured persons of similar severity.

Introduction

Unintentional physical injuries are a major public health problem worldwide. In the United States, injuries from any cause are the fourth leading cause of death, following heart disease, cancer and stroke, and the treatment of nonfatal injuries is a major contributor to the cost of health care (Nahum and Melvin, 1985).

There are a number of ways to measure the impact of various health problems. The one most often reported is comparison of number of deaths or death rates attributable to a particular disease or health problem. In 1980 injuries caused 71 deaths per 100,000 of U.S. population, compared to 336 for diseases of the heart, 184 for cancer, and 75 for stroke. The total of 160,551 deaths from injury in the U.S. were about equally represented by deaths from motor vehicle crashes (53,172), deaths from all other unintentional injuries (52,246), and deaths from intentional acts (26,869 suicides and 24,726 homicides). Another 3,686 were unclassified (Nahum and Melvin, 1985).

Mortality comparisons, ubiquitous though they are, tend to minimize the real impact of injuries. Unlike the other leading causes of death, injuries tend to predominate among the young. For ages 1 through 44 injuries are the leading cause of death, and for most ages in that group injuries kill more people than all other causes combined.

A method for better illustrating the significance of injuries is to compare the various causes of death after weighting the effect of each death by the factor of the number of years of potential remaining life that are lost as a result of that death. For example, if one assumed a probable life span of 70 years as an average, then death from heart attack at age 55 would cost 15 Potential Years of Life Lost prior to 70 (P.Y.L.L.-70), while a motor vehicle crash death at age 25 would cost 45 P.Y.L.L.-70, a "significance" three-fold that of the heart attack. Expressed in terms of P.Y.L.L.-70, death from injury has the leading impact among causes of premature death in the United States. (Romeder and McWhinnie, 1977; Budnick and Chaiken, 1985).

Fatal and non-fatal injuries have an economic impact on society through direct costs of medical resources and indirect costs of lost productivity. Measured in this fashion, injuries from motor vehicle crashes are found to be second only to the costs of cancer, with direct costs from motor vehicle injuries totalling twice that from coronary heart disease (Nahum and Melvin, 1985). Munoz (1984) estimates that 1977 costs of nonfatal injuries in the U.S. included $18.9 billion of direct treatment-related costs and $9.7 billion of foregone earnings. Some injuries are spectacularly expensive, such as paralytic spinal injuries. Expressed in 1982 dollars, Munoz (1984) indicates that the *direct* costs of an incomplete paraplegia are $161,867, complete paraplegia $211,543, incomplete quadriplegia $355,438 and complete quadriplegia $439,995.

Sources for the recovery of the costs incurred as a result of traumatic injury included individual medical and disability income insurance plans, group employer-sponsored insurance coverages, workers' compensation programs, and others including tort liability actions. In this latter setting a successful personal injury claimant has traditionally received a lump sum of money from the responsible defendant in exchange for a release from liability. The lump sum settlement is then the injured

Source: R. H. Butz, "The Epidemiology of Severe Injuries in Structured Settlement Applicants," *J. Ins. Med.*, 18, no. 3 (1986): 2-16. Reproduced with permission of author and publisher.

claimant's to use for attendant expenses, to invest for future needs, or to squander.

In recent years the concept of periodic payments in lieu of single lump sums has been developed for settlements, and in a growing number of states there is legislation authorizing courts to enter judgments which require periodic payments in appropriate circumstances (Hindert et al., 1986). Periodic payments received as recovery of the costs of injury are most commonly presented as part of a structured settlement whereby the injured claimant receives an immediate cash payment for past and current expenses, along with an annuity contract promising payments at regular intervals, usually monthly, over the claimant's lifetime, intended to cover any future costs attributable to the injury. These structured settlement annuity contracts are purchased from a life insurance company by the responsible defendant or sponsor. They are structured or tailored to meet the anticipated needs of the injured claimant and commonly include some or all of: payments which inflate annually at a modest rate, usually 3-5% throughout the lifetime; additional lump sums at specified future dates, e.g. when a dependent child reaches college age; payment schedules with "step" increases or decreases at various times; a lump sum for beneficiaries upon death of the annuitant; payments at regular intervals for a fixed period of years regardless of the annuitant's survival ("period certain"); and, variations of these and others (Hindert et al., 1986).

The use of structured settlements for recovery of the costs of injury is increasing rapidly. This mechanism was first applied significantly in the U.S. in 1976, and has grown since to about 200,000 cases of placed annuities, by our best estimate. This alternative to the traditional settlement is generally accepted as being in the best interest of all parties concerned, especially the injured annuitant. This dramatic growth has been encouraged by the current tax advantage of postponing "constructive receipt" of the award coming from a recovery action.

Purpose

The purpose of this study is to describe the epidemiologic characteristics of unintentional injuries to individuals seeking recovery of costs of severe injury by structured settlement techniques. The description includes physical characteristics of sex, age, race/ethnic group, and the settings, mechanisms, types and severity of injuries. The results will add to the knowledge of the epidemiology of injury, especially for craniocerebral and spinal cord injury which will be considered in additional detail. The study also will describe similarities and differences between this study group and other reported injury groups who are not engaged in this new, unique claim activity.

Method

This study reviews data concerning a group of 6,461 injured applicants whose medical reports were consecutively submitted to the Medical Department of Safeco Life Insurance Company, Seattle, Washington, from October 1982 to May 1986. The purpose was assessment of the probable impact upon life expectancy of severe injuries leading to a settlement in recovery of attendant costs. The author applied generally accepted actuariomedical considerations to these cases, translating the anticipated increase in mortality rate or reduction in life expectancy into the assignment of an "adjusted age," i.e., the age at which the corresponding population mortality rate and overall average life expectancy most closely approximated the reduced life expectancy of the injured claimant. (See Appendix for detail concerning this underwriting process.) Subtracting the chronological age from the assigned adjusted age gives an estimated P.Y.L.L. The medical records upon which this underwriting judgment was based varied in extent and timeliness, but usually included hospital records from the initial care for injury, subsequent medical and/or rehabilitation records reflecting the results of follow-up care, and sometimes extensive expert examinations or depositions intended to describe the injury in great detail. (The largest of these was delivered in a box and was five inches thick!) Each of the 6,461 cases was entered into a Database II file on an IBM PC. Each record included name, age, sex, type of injury, the adjusted age, and business data.

For the 2,908 cases entered after July, 1985, an added notation of the injury setting was also made, recording whether the injury arose out of a work-related (workers' compensation) injury, an iatrogenic (medical liability) injury, or a personal setting. Work-related injuries included all of those arising out of gainful employment and included claims for medical conditions which were attributed to adverse effects of the working environment (such as myocardial infarction on the job which was judged to be due to the stress of the workplace). Iatrogenic injuries included all actions against physicians, dentists, nurses, hospitals, pharmaceutical suppliers, nursing homes, ambulance attendants (only one), etc. Personal injuries included all home, recreational, and motor vehicle injuries arising out of activities of individuals not in a setting of gainful employment or under medical management at the time. This subset will be identified as the N=2,908 group.

An additional subset from those cases was specifically searched for mechanisms of injury and for race/ethnic group of the claimant. For 1,188 cases submitted during November and December 1985, January, March and April 1986, mechanism of injury appeared in 1,140 of the medical records, but could not determined in 48 instances. A clear statement of race/ethnic group was present in 921 (77.5%) of the medical records, permitting assignment of those individuals to one of the following groups: white, black, Asian/Pacific Islander, Native American, Hispanic, or other. This subset of the N=2,908 group will be identified as the N=1,188 group.

Findings: Age and Sex

The distribution of the study group injuries by age decade and sex is shown in Table 050K1-1. As shown, the male:female ratio was 2.2:1 overall, with a maximum difference of 3:1 occurring in the sixth decade. The excess of these severe injuries among men was significant at each age group through the seventh decade ($p<0.01$).

TABLE 050K1-1

TOTAL INJURIES, BY DECADE OF AGE AND SEX

(The assumption is made that the population male: female ratio approximates 1:1)(χ^2=107.5, df=8, $p<0.0001$)

Ages	Male	Female	Total	(%)	[M:F]
0-9 yrs	626	421	1,047	(16.2)	[1.5:1]*
10-19	432	254	677	(10.5)	[1.7:1]*
20-29	1,020	382	1,042	(21.7)	[2.7:1]*
30-39	807	320	1,127	(17.4)	[2.5:1]*
40-49	623	245	868	(13.4)	[2.5:1]*
50-59	564	191	755	(11.7)	[3.0:1]*
60-69	334	132	466	(7.2)	[2.5:1]*
70-79	61	42	103	(1.6)	[1.5:1]*
80+	3	13	16	(0.2)	[0.2:1]*
Total	4,641	2,000	6,461	(100.0)	[2.2:1]*

* M:F difference, $p<0.01$

At age 80 and beyond, the ratio actually reversed, but when compared to the proportion of octogenarians in the U.S. population who are female, the ratio is not significantly different.

One purpose of this study is to attempt to define the extent to which non-injury factors influencing this study group of claimants to seek structured settlement recovery might cause the group to differ from the overall population of injured persons in the U.S. For this purpose the study group must be compared only to severely injured populations, because the study group represents only persons whose injuries were sufficiently severe that an adverse impact on life expectancy is anticipated, truly a severely injured group. The mean estimated P.Y.L.L. among the 2,000 injured women was 11.7 years (median of 8.5 years) and for the 4,461 men it was 10.9 years (median of 8.4 years).

For comparison of the male:female ratio by age group, Table 050K1-2 shows the ratios for all unintentional injury deaths in the U.S. in 1982 (Hoskin et al., 1985). The overall male:female ratio is similar to the study

group, and the age groups show the same trends, although the age groups are divided differently making exact comparison impossible. The difference between overall male:female ratio and that of the study group, and the difference in peak ratios, are probably due to the effect of iatrogenic injuries in the study group. In fact, as shown in Table 050K1-3, 23.2% of the study group were claimants following iatrogenic injuries, and for this group there was no significant male:female difference. If the iatrogenic injuries are factored out from the study group, in the fourth decade for example, then the male:female ratio becomes 676:189, or 3.6:1, which is comparable to the injury fatality ratio for the population in that age range. The iatrogenic injuries might also explain the high proportion of injuries in the youngest decade of ages in the study group, since birth injuries were the largest group of iatrogenic injuries. Aside from this definable difference in composition of the study group of injured persons, the age and sex distributions appear similar to the fatally injured in the population of the United States.

TABLE 050K1-2

ACCIDENTAL DEATHS IN THE UNITED STATES DURING 1982, BY AGE GROUP, BY SEX[1]

Ages	Male	Female	Total	[M:F]
0-4 yrs	2,452	1,654	4,108	[1.5:1]
5-14	3,045	1,459	4,504	[2.1:1]
15-24	16,856	4,450	21,306	[3.8:1]
25-44	19,932	5,203	25,135	[3.8:1]
45-64	11,487	4,420	15,907	[2.6:1]
65-74	5,055	3,169	8,224	[1.6:1]
75+	6,925	7,973	14,898	[0.9:1]
Total	65,754	28,328	94,082	[2.3:1]

[1] From Hoskin et al., *Accident Facts*, 1985.

TABLE 050K1-3

NUMBER OF INJURIES BY SETTING OF INJURY AND SEX
(χ^2=261.9, df=2, $p<0.0001$)

Injury Setting	Male	Female	Total	(%)	[M:F]
Work-related	743	82	825	(28.4)	[9.1:1]*
Iatrogenic	360	316	676	(23.2)	[1.1:1]
Personal Activity	913	494	1,407	(48.4)	[1.8:1]*
Total	2,016	892	2,908	(100.0)	[2.3:1]*

* M:F difference, $p<0.01$

Findings: Race/Ethnic Group

It was possible to determine the race/ethnic group from 77.5% of the medical record sets searched for this information. The distribution of injury setting by racial/ethnic group is shown in Table 050K1-4, along with a comparison of the total injuries by racial/ethnic group

TABLE 050K1-4

NUMBER OF INJURIES BY INJURY SETTING AND RACE/ETHNIC GROUP
Compared To Expected From Racial/Ethnic Distribution In The U.S. Population*,
Not Adjusted For Age Or Sex

Race/Ethnic Group	Injury Setting					
	Work Related	Iatrogenic	Personal Activity	Total	(%)	Expected (95% C.I.)
White	187	159	336	682	(74.1)	706.4 (681.3-731.5)
Black	49	30	38	117	(12.7)	107.8 (88.6-126.9)
Asian	5	5	8	18	(2.0)	12.9 (5.9-19.9)
Hispanic	19	17	40	76	(8.3)	59.9 (45.2-74.5)
Native American	1	1	0	2	(0.2)	5.5 (0.9-10.1)
Other	4	10	12	26	(2.8)	28.6 (18.2-38.9)
Total	265 (28.8%)	222 (24.1%)	434 (47.1%)	921	(100.0)	

* From *Statistical Abstract of the United States*, 1986.

to the expected distribution if the U.S. population proportions of racial/ethnic groups were similarly represented in the study group (Statistical Abstract of the United States, 1986). In fact, black, Asian and Hispanic groups appear to be over-represented, although only the Hispanic group fell beyond the 95% confidence limits of expected representation. It has been reported that injury mortality in minority groups does differ from the white U.S. population by the relative ratios shown in Table 050K1-5 (Report of the Secretary's Task Force on Black and Minority Health, 1986). These figures are consistent with data relating the mortality from fires/explosions by ethnicity (Leads from the MMWR, 1985), and reports of spinal cord injuries and severe traumatic head injuries by race (Bracken et al., 1981; Young et al., 1982; Whitman et al., 1984; Jagger et al., 1984). If the expected racial/ethnic representations for the study group in Table 050K1-4 are adjusted by the applicable relative ratio (Table 050K1-5), then significant differences in representation, falling above and below 95% confidence intervals respectively, are Asians and Native Americans. Significant differences from expected proportions of racial/ethnic groups in the study group probably reflect non-injury factors, such as relative access to legal counsel and understanding of the systems for making claims, or propensity to exploit the structured settlement means of recovering the costs of injury between the various minority groups. The distribution described by this study group is an interesting and unexpected finding. Also apparent from Table 050K1-4 is the different distribution of injury

TABLE 050K1-5

RATE RATIOS OF MORTALITY FROM INJURY BY RACE/ETHNIC GROUP
United States 1978-81[**]

Race/Ethnic Group	Relative Ratio	
	Male	Female
White	1.0	1.0
Black	1.2	1.1
Asian	0.5	0.6
Hispanic	1.7	1.0
Native American	2.1	2.3

** Report of the Secretary's Task Force on Black and Minority Health, Morbidity and Mortality Weekly Report, 1986.

setting among blacks, with work-related injuries more common than for the overall group, and personal injuries less common ($p < 0.01$).

Relating severity of injury to the racial/ethnic groups was limited by the small group sizes for minorities, and the analysis was only done for white/nonwhite differences. Table 050K1-6 shows the results when injuries are differentiated for severity by those which result in a predicted P.Y.L.L. of less than 10, and the group with 10 or more P.Y.L.L. Severity of injury is significantly greater for nonwhites in the study group, but only for work-related and iatrogenic injuries, and not for personal injuries.

135

This severity for nonwhites is consistent with the earlier report that mortality is generally higher among injured nonwhites, and perhaps indicates that both the increased frequency and the extra severity account for the reported additional mortality among minority groups (except for the Asian subgroup).

Findings: Types of Injuries

The types of injuries incurred among the study group are detailed in Table 050K1-7, by sex. The male:female preponderance was significant for each type of injury and for the study group overall ($p<0.01$). When comparing each type of injury to the proportions of male:female for the overall group, males had excess spinal cord injuries and cardiovascular injuries relative to females, while females had excessive craniocerebral injuries and medical injuries.

Comparable data are available for craniocerebral and spinal cord injuries and show similar ratios (Tator and Edmonds, 1979; Young et al., 1982).

The types of injury seen by injury setting where incurred are shown in Table 050K1-8 for women and Table 050K1-9 for men for the 2,908 cases where the injury setting was recorded. When personal injuries are considered separately, the male:female differences in numbers of burns and medical conditions arising out of injury no longer are significant, but craniocerebral and spinal cord injuries continue to afflict males predominantly ($p<0.01$).

TABLE 050K1-6

NUMBER OF INJURIES BY SEVERITY OF INJURY, WHITE/NONWHITE AND INJURY SETTING, NOT ADJUSTED FOR AGE OR SEX
(χ^2=14.77, df=5, *p*=0.01)

Setting of Injury	White	Nonwhite	Odds Ratio
Work-Related			
<10 P.Y.L.L.	155	55	2.0*
10+ P.Y.L.L.	32	23	
Iatrogenic			
<10 P.Y.L.L.	71	19	1.9*
10+ P.Y.L.L.	88	44	
Personal Activity			
<10 P.Y.L.L.	210	59	1.1
10+ P.Y.L.L.	126	39	
Total			
<10 P.Y.L.L.	436	133	1.4*
10+ P.Y.L.L.	246	106	
	682	239	

* *p*<0.01 for this O.R.

TABLE 050K1-7

NUMBER OF INJURIES BY TYPE OF INJURY AND SEX
(χ^2=167.27, df=5, *p*<0 .0001)

Type of Injury	Males		Females		Total	[M:F]
Craniocerebral	1,610		916		2,526	[1.8:1]
Traumatic		886		413		
Anoxic		433		336		
Other		291		167		
Spinal Cord	1,098		274		1,372	[4:1]
Paraplegia		467		128		
Quadriplegia		631		146		
Burns	153		59		212	[2.6:1]
Injuries, Other	709		302		1,011	[2.3:1]
Cardiovascular	194		30		224	[6.5:1]
Medical, Other	697		419		1,116	[1.7:1]
Total	4,461		2,000		6,461	[2.2:1]

TABLE 050K1-8

NUMBER OF INJURIES BY TYPE OF INJURY AND INJURY SETTING FEMALES ONLY, FROM N = 2,908 GROUP

Type of Injury	Work-Related		Iatrogenic		Personal Activity		Total (%)	
Craniocerebral	12		192		189		393	(44.1)
Traumatic		10		4		173		
Anoxic		0		141		0		
Other		2		47		16		
Spinal Cord	2		21		86		109	(12.2)
Paraplegia		1		12		39		
Quadriplegia		1		9		47		
Burns	0		0		22		22	(2.5)
Injuries, Other	26		7		115		148	(16.6)
Cardiovascular	5		3		8		16	(1.8)
Medical, Other	37		93		74		204	(22.9)
Total	82	(9.2%)	316	(35.4)	494	(55.4)	892	(100.0)

**NUMBER OF INJURIES BY TYPE OF INJURY AND INJURY SETTING
MALES ONLY, FROM N = 2,908 GROUP**

Type of Injury	Work-Related		Iatrogenic		Personal Activity		Total(%)	
Craniocerebral	112		240		338		690	(34.2)
Traumatic		91		8		290		
Anoxic		0		180		2		
Other		21		52		46		
Spinal Cord	126		21		281		428	(21.2)
Paraplegia		75		10		97		
Quadriplegia		51		11		184		
Burns	29		1		36	66		(3.5)
Injuries, Other	181		11		163		355	(17.6)
Cardiovascular	71		17		21		109	(5.4)
Medical, Other	224		70		74		368	(18.3)
Total	743	(36.9%)	360	(17.9)	913	(45.3)	2,016	(100.0)

Findings: Work-Related Injuries

The mechanisms of injury are displayed by injury setting in Tables 050K1-10, 050K1-11 and 050K1-12. First, the 28.4% of injuries which were work-related were 92% in males (Table 050K1-10). This probably results in part from the predominantly male work force, and perhaps that jobs with greater injury risk probably are more likely to be filled by men. When adjusted for the overall ratio of males:females, the differences by mechanism of injury were not significant. It is notable that all 48 cases of toxic inhalation occurred in men. This probably reflects the working environment of jobs more likely to be filled by men. Eleven of these cases were of asbestosis.

The two cases of injury to women from interpersonal violence were both attacks upon women working as security guards and consisted of physical assaults. The four men suffering the same mechanism in the course of employment were victims of gunshot wounds in three of the instances. One of the more remarkable occupational back injuries was an acute herniated vertebral nucleus pulposus occurring in an orthopedic surgeon as he worked in the operating room. He completed the operation, according to the medical history, and then became a patient himself with cord compression, resulting in permanent disability due to incomplete paraplegia.

Findings: Iatrogenic Injuries

Iatrogenic injuries (Table 050K1-11) made up 23.2% of the study group, and were not significantly more common for men or women in any category of mechanism of injury ($p>0.05$). The proportion of iatrogenic injuries in the study group was a surprise. Perhaps claimants with iatrogenic injuries are especially prone to seek economic recovery, and thus appear to such a large extent. Birth injuries were the leading source of iatrogenic injury, accounting for 43.5% of the total. These were almost entirely anoxic cerebral injuries, although other injuries included spinal cord injury and high cervical quadriplegia with permanent respiratory dependence. The cases of missed diagnosis injury were notable for several cases of infantile meningitis which were not recognized upon initial medical intervention, and for several cases of breast cancer which were not recognized as such in timely fashion. The patient or physical injuries were mostly falls by elderly or infirm patients, but one was a claim against a psychiatric inpatient facility on

TABLE 050K1-10

**NUMBER OF CASES OF WORK RELATED INJURIES
BY MECHANISMS OF INJURY AND SEX**
($\chi^2=11.7$, df=11, $p>0.05$)

Mechanism of Injury	Men	Women	Total	(%)
Motor Vehicle	20	0	20	(6.4)
Occupant	5	0	5	(1.6)
Pedestrian	52	6	58	(18.5)
Fall	37	1	38	(12.1)
Falling Object	20	1	21	(6.7)
Explosion/Fire	10	0	10	(3.2)
Electrical	13	2	15	(4.8)
Toxic Inhalation*	48	0	48	(15.3)
Back Strain	35	6	41	(13.1)
Stress from Job	30	6	36	(11.5)
Interpersonal Violence	4	2	6	(1.9)
Misc./Unknown	15	1	16	(5.1)
Total	289	25	314	(100.0)
	(92%)	(8%)		

* Includes 11 cases asbestosis.

TABLE 050K1-11

NUMBER OF IATROGENIC INJURIES BY MECHANISMS OF INJURY AND SEX
($\chi^2=8.813$, df=6, $p=0.18$)

Mechanism of Injury	Men	Women	Total	(%)
Birth Injury	79	58	137	(43.5)
Surgical Complication	31	28	59	(18.7)
Missed Diagnosis	20	31	51	(16.2)
Adverse Treatment Effect	13	15	28	(8.9)
Anesthetic Complication	12	14	26	(8.3)
Physical Injury of Patient	3	6	9	(2.9)
Unknown	1	4	5	(1.6)
Total	159	156	315	(100.0)
	(50.5%)	(49.5%)		

behalf of a patient who was rendered quadriplegic from cervical spine fracture dislocation upon her third unsuccessful attempt to commit suicide by diving from her bed to the concrete floor of her room.

There are very little published data with which to compare this distribution of mechanisms of iatrogenic injuries. One brief report recently suggested that among the ten most frequent errors by physicians, surgical mishaps account for 17.7% of "malpractice" suits, 9.9% from failure to diagnose, 7.2% from adverse treatment effect, and only 5.3% due to "improper treatment while giving birth" (HEF News, 1984). An older article shows that in Federal medical facilities a failure to diagnose was responsible for 21.3% of claims for alleged negligence (Rudov et al., 1973). Information from a large professionals liability insurance carrier indicates that in 1983, among the ten leading allegations in claims some 27.7% related to unsatisfactory surgical outcomes, 25.1% patient injuries due to falling, 17.3% adverse treatment effects, and 8.2% due to missed diagnosis (AMA Special Task Force Report, 1984). A review of anesthetic complications in King County, Washington, revealed 192 cases from 1971 to 1982 resulting in 62 deaths but only 27 "brain damage" injuries. Thus individuals surviving with anesthetic injury total fewer than three per year for that period in an area with nearly one million in total population, making this an uncommon injury (Solazzi and Ward, 1984).

The literature is too sparse to conjecture if the large number of birth injuries in the study group represents a secular trend or an unusual concentration among structured settlement applicants. Structured settlements do provide a particular economic advantage for individuals facing a long life of need during which they may be incompetent to handle their own financial planning.

Findings: Personal Injury

Traffic, home and recreational injuries (Table 050K1-12) were attributable to motor vehicles 64.4% of the time. Traffic injuries alone, shown in Table 050K1-13, appear to be distributed for the study group similar to population data for fatalities in 1983 in the U.S. (Statistical Abstract of the United States, 1986). A total of 107 injuries in the study group could be classified as home injuries, if one assumes that personal injuries unrelated to highway traffic or sports activities are home injuries. The mechanisms of these injures are compared to published data in Table 050K1-14 (Insurance Facts, 1985). Unfortunately, data for home injuries of severity comparable to the study group cases could not be located in literature, so these data for home injury fatalities must suffice.

The study group has significantly more injuries due to falls than the proportion of fatal home injuries shown ($p<0.01$). Perhaps falls at home have a lower mortality rate than the other injuries shown, so the study group of surviving injured persons would not be comparable though similar in incidence of falls. Another explanation might be a difference in ages of the groups, since falls are known to be much more common among elders (Oreskovich et al., 1984). Significant age differences did not

TABLE 050K1-12

NUMBER OF PERSONAL ACTIVITY INJURIES BY MECHANISMS OF INJURY AND SEX FROM N = 1,188 GROUP
($\chi^2=54.83$, df=14, $p<0.00001$)

Mechanism of Injury	Men	Women	Total	(%)
Motor Vehicle				
Automobile-Driver*	118	65	183	(32.7)
Automobile-Passenger	40	59	99	(17.7)
Pedestrian	20	16	36	(6.4)
Motorcycle*	27	2	29	(5.2)
Other	9	4	13	(2.3)
Bicycle**	11	3	14	(2.5)
Fall	22	25	47	(8.4)
Falling Object	7	3	10	(1.8)
Explosion/Fire/Burn	8	4	12	(2.1)
Electrical	5	0	5	(0.9)
Toxic Inhalation/Poisoning	6	1	7	(1.3)
Interpersonal Violence	14	2	16	(2.9)
Asphyxia/Near-Drowning	5	5	10	(1.8)
Recreation Sports**	36	10	46	(8.2)
Misc./ Unknown	21	11	32	(5.7)
Total*	349	210	559	(100.0)
	(62.4%)	(37.6%)		

* M:F difference, $p<0.01$

** M:F difference, $p>0.01$, <0.05

appear in our earlier analyses; specific ages are not available for this subgroup. The differences in injuries from toxic ingestions/inhalations is also significant ($p<0.01$). Possibly a personal injury of this mechanism is less likely to result in a claim for recovery from a responsible payor because responsibility might more commonly rest solely with the injured party, in which case the study group would not include such injuries to a proportional extent.

Significant male:female differences among personal injury mechanisms of injury are limited to automobile driver and motorcycle (at $p<0.01$) and possibly bicycle and sports injuries ($p>0.01$, but <0.05), when compared to the male:female ratio overall among personal injuries (Table 050K1-12).

In Table 050K1-15 the motorcycle injuries are compared with reported specific injuries among a group including some of minor severity (Zettas et al., 1979). One report indicates that 98% of motorcycle crashes result in injury and that 45% are "major" injuries (Bray et al., 1985). If one adjusts the proportion of injuries reported by Zettas et al. (1985) (Table 050K1-15) upward

by that factor, then comparability to the study group is true for skull fractures and paraplegias.

The bicycle injuries listed in Table 050K1-12 consisted of nine craniocerebral injuries and five spinal cord injuries. The interpersonal violence included nine gunshot wounds, comprising both of the injuries to women and half of those to men.

The recreational injuries are further described in Table 050K1-16. The injuries associated with diving, football and gymnastics were quadriplegic spinal cord injuries, with the exception of one paraplegia among the gymnasts. The diving injuries, which made up 63% of the recreational injuries, were particularly severe with 23 complete quadriplegias, three at a high cervical level resulting in permanent respirator dependence. A report

TABLE 050K1-13
PERCENT TRAFFIC INJURIES BY MECHANISMS OF INJURY, COMPARED TO TRAFFIC DEATHS OCCURRING IN THE U.S. DURING 1983

Mechanism of Injury	Study Group	Statistical Abstracts[*]
Motor Vehicles/	86.2%	87.5%
Motorcycles	7.3	7.6
Pedestrian	10.3	12.1
Bicycle	3.5	1.4
Total	100.0%	100.0%

[*] Statistical Abstract of the United States, 1984

TABLE 050K1-14
PERCENT HOME INJURIES BY MECHANISM OF INJURY, COMPARED TO ALL DEATHS FROM "HOME ACCIDENTS" OCCURRING IN THE U.S. DURING 1984[**]

Mechanism of Injury	Study Group	"Insurance Facts"[**]
Falls	43.9%	30.5%
Fire/Explosion/Electrical	15.9	19.5
Toxic Ingestion/Inhalation	6.5	19.9
Asphyxia	9.3	12.5
Gunshot Wound	8.4	4.5
Other/Unknown	16.0	13.5
	100.0%	100.0%

[**] Insurance Facts, 1985

TABLE 050K1-15
NUMBER OF MOTORCYCLE INJURIES BY TYPE OF INJURY, COMPARED TO REPORT OF ZETTAS ET AL. FROM N = 1,188 GROUP

Type of Injury	Study Group	Zettas et al.
Craniocerebral		
Fracture	6 (20.7%)	29 (11.2%)
No Fracture	10 (34.5)	84 (32.3)
Spinal Cord Injury		
Paraplegia	4 (13.8)	12 (4.6)
Quadriplegia	2 (6.9)	1 (0.4)
Other	7 (24.1)	134 (51.5)
	29 (100.0%)	260 (100.0%)
Male	27 (93.1)	236 (90.8)
Female	2 (6.9)	24 (9.2)
	29 (100.0%)	260 (100.0%)

TABLE 050K1-16
NUMBER OF RECREATION AND SPORTS INJURIES BY MECHANISM OF INJURY AND SEX, FROM N = 1,188 GROUP

Mechanism of Injury	Male	Female	Total	(%)
Diving	23	6	29	(63.0)
Football	3	0	3	(6.5)
Gymnastics	2	1	3	(6.5)
Horseback Riding	0	2	2	(4.3)
Wrestling	1	0	1	(2.2)
Track and Field	1	0	1	(2.2)
Ice Hockey	1	0	1	(2.2)
Auto Racing	1	0	1	(2.2)
Rodeo	1	0	1	(2.2)
Skiing	1	0	1	(2.2)
Snowmobile	1	0	1	(2.2)
All-Terrain Vehicle (A.T.V.)	1	0	1	(2.2)
Cheerleading	1	0	1	(2.2)
Total	36	10	46	(100.0)
	(78.3%)	(21.7%)		

of spinal cord injuries from the Toronto area shows 38 of 55 sports and recreational injuries to be diving-related, with 32 in males and six in females, with 25 complete quadriplegias and 13 incomplete quadriplegias (Tator et al., 1981). The horseback riding, track and field, ice hockey and A.T.V. all resulted in craniocerebral injury, with skull fracture in each except for one horseback fall. In this small group there were no football head injuries, even though this is now reported to be a more common serious football injury than quadriplegia (Torg et al., 1985).

Findings: Craniocerebral Injuries

Craniocerebral injuries are the most common injury seen in this study group, making up nearly 40% of the total. The male:female ratio is 1.8:1, as shown in Table 050K1-7. This compares with 2.1:1 reported in the National Head and Spinal Cord Injury Survey, but when we limit comparison to traumatic head injuries, then the ratio is 886:413, exactly duplicating the published figure (Kalsbeek et al., 1980). Of the total, 52.7% were traumatic head injuries, and 43.2% of the traumatic injuries included a fracture of the skull, as shown in Table 050K1-17. Surprisingly, surgical ventricular shunt was performed in 10.9% of the traumatic head injuries, with 11.9% of those with skull fracture having a shunt procedure. The mechanisms of injury for craniocerebral injury are shown in Table 050K1-18. Iatrogenic injuries account for 47.1% and traffic injuries for another 37.1%.

TABLE 050K1-17

NO. OF CRANIOCEREBRAL INJURIES BY TYPE OF INJURY AND PRESENCE/ABSENCE OF SURGICAL VENTRICULAR SHUNT FROM N = 6,461 STUDY GROUP
Surgical Ventricular Shunt Procedure

Type of Injury	No		Yes		Total	
Traumatic	1,157		142		1,299	(52.7%)
No Fracture		663		75		
Fracture		494		67		
Anoxic	723		46		769	(31.2%)
Birth Injury		613		40		
Anesthetic		110		6		
Cerebral Injury Other	351		46		397	(16.1%)
Total	2,231	(90.5%)	234	(9.5%)	2,465	(100.0%)

TABLE 050K1-18

NO. OF CRANIOCEREBRAL INJURIES BY MECHANISM OF INJURY FROM N = 1,188 GROUP

Mechanism of Injury	N	% of Total
Motor Vehicle		
Automobile-Driver	87	16.3%
Automobile-Passenger	50	9.4
Motorcycle	16	3.0
Other Vehicle	8	1.5
Pedestrian	28	5.3
Bicycle	9	1.7
Fall	36	6.8
Falling Object	16	3.0
Asphyxia/Near-Drown	8	1.5
Work-Related, Other	18	3.4
Recreation/Sports	13	2.4
Interpersonal Violence	12	2.3
Iatrogenic—Birth Injury	141	26.5
—Anesthetic Complication	25	5.3
—Other Iatrogenic	53	9.9
Other/Unknown	10	1.9
Total	533	100.0%

TABLE 050K1-19

PERCENT TRAUMATIC HEAD INJURIES BY MECHANISM OF INJURY, STUDY GROUP COMPARED TO OLMSTED COUNTY POPULATION

Mechanism of Injury	Study Group	Annegers et al.
Automobile	50.7%	42.2%
Motorcycle	5.9	8.3
Bicycle	3.3	5.0
Fall	13.3	19.3
Occupational	14.8	7.3
Recreation	5.2	4.6
Assault	2.2	4.6
Gunshot Wound	2.2	2.3
Other/Unknown	2.4	7.4
Total	100.0%	100.0%

TABLE 050K1-20

CRANIOCEREBRAL INJURIES, MEAN ESTIMATED P.Y.L.L. (MEDIAN IN PARENTHESES) BY TYPE OF INJURY FROM N = 4,661 STUDY GROUP (χ^2=1.89, df=9, p=0.99)
Potential Years of Life Lost

	Men		Women		No. Cases
TRAUMATIC					
No Fracture					
No Shunt	8.8	(6.7)	8.9	(6.9)	663
Shunt	14.6	(13.1)	13.8	(11.3)	75
Fracture					
No Shunt	7.8	(6.3)	8.4	(6.7)	494
Shunt	14.0	(12.2)	18.3	(14.3)	67
ANOXIC					
Birth Injury					
No Shunt	17.5	(14.2)	17.9	(14.5)	613
Shunt	20.2	(17.9)	26.6	(19.2)	40
Anesthetic					
No Shunt	18.1	(15.0)	16.3	(14.8)	110
Shunt	22.5	(25.0)	20.0	(20.0)	6
Cerebral Injury, Other					
No Shunt	17.6	(12.8)	19.1	(15.6)	351
Shunt	21.1	(17.3)	24.3	(21.7)	36
					2,465

Limiting comparison to traumatic head injuries only, the mechanisms of injury for the study group are similar to those reported from Olmsted County, Minnesota, for "severe" injuries in 1935-74, as shown in Table 050K1-19 (Annegers et al., 1980). Craniocerebral injuries are particularly severe in terms of P.Y.L.L. They tend to occur in the young and have a high case-fatality rate for those mechanisms of injury peculiar to the young, including bicycle injuries, motorcycle crashes and pedestrian traffic injuries in the very young (0-9 years), where one study showed the highest case-fatality rate (Klauber et al., 1981). Table 050K1-20 displays the mean estimated P.Y.L.L. for the various types of craniocerebral injuries in the study group. Published data concerning reduced long-term health after severe head injury are difficult to compare but they are certainly not inconsistent with these figures (Roberts, 1979). The data in Table 050K1-20 can be compared to the overall mean estimated P.Y.L.L. for the 2,000 injured women in the study group of 11.7 years, and the mean of 10.9 years for the 4,461 men, as noted earlier.

Findings: Spinal Cord Injuries

Spinal cord injuries accounted for 21.2% of the total in the study group, or 1,372 cases. The male:female ratio was 4:1 as shown in Table 050K1-7, with 43.4% paraplegic injuries and 56.6% quadriplegia. Twenty-seven cases, 2.0% of the total, were high cervical cord lesions resulting in permanent respirator dependence. Table 050K1-21 displays this distribution of lesions and com-

TABLE 050K1- 21

PERCENT SPINAL CORD INJURIES BY LEVEL OF LESIONS, COMPARISON WITH FOUR PUBLISHED SERIES

Spinal Cord Injury Study Group	Paraplegia			Quadriplegia		
	Incomplete	Complete	Total	Incomplete	Complete	Total
Study Group[1] N=1,372	7.7%	35.6%	43.4%	15.1%	41.5%	56.6%
Young et al.[2] N=5,915	18.7	28.2	46.9	28.4	24.7	53.1
Clifton[3] N=183	20.2	37.7	57.9	29.5	12.6	42.1
Griffin et al.[4] N=154	27.4	21.4	48.8	32.1	19.1	51.2
Fine et al.[5] N=356	17.7	34.8	52.5	25.8	21.6	47.4

[1] N = 6,461 Study Group; [2]Young et al., 1982; [3]Clifton, 1983; [4]Griffin et al., 1985; [5]Fine et al., 1980

TABLE 050K1-22

NO. OF SPINAL CORD INJURIES BY MECHANISM OF INJURY AND LEVEL OF LESION, FROM N = 1,188 GROUP

Mechanism of Injury	Para-plegia	Quadri-plegia	Total	(%)
Motor Vehicle				
Automobile-Driver	22	35	57	(21.8)
Automobile-Passenger	12	19	31	(11.9)
Motorcycle	4	2	6	(2.3)
Other Vehicle	3	2	4	(1.9)
Pedestrian	3	1	4	(1.5)
Bicycle	1	4	5	(1.9)
Recreation*	4	37	41	(15.7)
Fall	21	20	41	(15.7)
Falling Object*	17	6	23	(8.8)
Iatrogenic	9	9	18	(6.9)
Interpersonal Violence	6	4	10	(3.8)
Other/Unknown	12	8	20	(7.7)
Total	114 (43.7%)	147 (56.3%)	261	(100.0)

* Paraplegia:Quadriplegia ratio differs from distribution of overall group, $p <0.01$

TABLE 050K1-23

PERCENT SPINAL CORD INJURIES BY TYPE OF ACCIDENT, COMPARISON OF DISTRIBUTION OF STUDY AND THREE PUBLISHED REPORTS

Type of Accident	Study Group	Young	Griffin	Fine
Automobile, total	33.7%	37.6%	40.9%	30.4%
Motorcycle	2.3	6.6	11.7	9.8
Other Vehicle	1.9	1.5	1.3	—
Pedestrian	1.5	1.7	8.4	2.2
Bicycle	1.9	0.7	4.5	—
Interpersonal Violence	3.8	13.9	3.2	21.2
Diving	11.1	9.5	3.3	7.0
Other Recreation	4.6	4.9	4.5	—
Fall	15.7	15.8	13.0	—
Falling Object	8.8	5.0	—	—
Iatrogenic	6.9	1.3	—	—
Other/Unknown	7.7	1.3	9.1	29.4
	100.0	100.0	100.0	100.0

* From N = 1,188 Study Group, with 261 spinal cord injuries (See Table 050K1-22)

**PERCENT SPINAL CORD INJURIES BY MECHANISM OF INJURY
AND LEVEL OF LESION, COMPARED TO THE REPORT OF YOUNG ET AL.**

	Study Group		Young et al.		Total	
Mechanism of Injury	Paraplegia	Quadriplegia	Paraplegia	Quadriplegia	Study Group	Young et al
Vehicular	41.7%	58.3%	47.1%	52.4%	41.4%	48.4%
Penetrating Wound	66.7	33.3	72.4	27.6	3.4	13.8
Recreation, except diving	33.3	66.7	20.2	79.7	4.6	4.9
Diving	0	100	1.7	98.4	11.1	9.5
Falls	51.2	48.8	51.5	48.6	15.7	15.8
Falling Object	73.9	26.1	72.3	27.7	8.8	5.0
Others	53.8	46.1	49.3	50.6	15.0	2.6
					100.0	100.0

TABLE 050K1-25

**SPINAL CORD INJURIES, MEAN ESTIMATED P.Y.L.L.
(MEDIAN IN PARENTHESES) BY TYPE OF INJURY,
FROM N = 6,461 STUDY GROUP
(χ^2=0.167, df=4, p=0.99)**

	P.Y.L.L.				Cases
	Men		Women		
Paraplegia					
Incomplete	6.2	(5.6)	5.9	(5.5)	106
Complete	11.5	(11.3)	12.6	(13.2)	489
Quadriplegia					
Incomplete	11.5	(11.9)	12.4	(13.0)	207
Complete	17.8	(16.9)	18.0	(17.1)	543
Respirator					
Dependent	31.3	(27.2)	27.5	(27.5)	27
					1,372

pares with four published reports of sizeable series of spinal cord injuries (Fine et al., 1980; Young et al., 1982; Clifton, 1983; Griffin et al., 1985). The proportion of study group paraplegias to quadriplegias is comparable to the largest of the groups, which showed 46.9% and 53.1 respectively (N=5,915).

The mechanisms of injury for spinal cord injuries are shown in Table 050K1-22. Recreational injuries significantly differ from the overall subgroup in terms of paraplegia:quadriplegia ratio (p<0.01). The only other significant difference is the preponderance of paraplegias among those injured by a falling object. Comparison with mechanisms of injury in other reported studies appear in Table 050K1-23, again showing similarity of the study group and other reported series (Fine et al., 1980; Young et al., 1982; Griffin et al., 1985). In addition, Table 050K1-24 compares mechanisms of injury to level of lesion of the spinal cord for the study group and nearly 6,000 cases reported from Regional Spinal Cord Injury Systems (Young et al., 1982). The mean age of spinal cord

injury in the study group was 28.8 years for men and 31.0 for women, with an overall mean age of 29.2 years. This compares with respective mean ages of 31 years and 37 years reported for men and women from Toronto, with a mean age of 32 years (Tator and Edmonds, 1979). Finally, Table 050K1-25 demonstrates the mean estimated P.Y.L.L. due to spinal cord injuries, by level of lesion and sex of the injured person. These figures compare with mortality ratios reported in clinical literature for similar injuries when applied to the mean ages noted (Geisler et al., 1977; Mesard, 1978; Devivo et al., 1980).

Summary

A study group of 6,461 claimants applying for structured settlements in recovery of the cost of severe injury has been described in detail. Male:female ratios of 9.1:1 were found among the 28.4% of injuries which were work-related, 1.1:1 among the 23.2% iatrogenic injuries, and 1.8:1 among the remaining 48.4% of injuries occurring in home, traffic and recreational activities, and personal injuries. The distribution of injuries by racial/ethnic group closely paralleled the proportions of the minority groups reported in the overall U.S. population. Detailed analyses included injury settings, mechanisms of injury, types of injuries and severity of injury in terms of Potential Years of Life Lost (P.Y.L.L.), with particular attention to the two most common injuries seen, craniocerebral injuries (39.1% of the total) and spinal cord injuries (21.2%).

Unexpected findings included the large number of injuries due to iatrogenic causes, and the high proportion of those that were due to birth injury (43.5%). The frequency with which surgical ventricular shunt followed craniocerebral injury (9.5%) was also surprising. Finally, the frequency and severity of spinal cord injuries due to diving into shallow water was remarkable.

The distribution of injuries by age, sex, race/ethnic group, setting of injury, mechanism of injury, type of injury, and severity of injury appeared to be similar to reported data from population-based groups of severely injured persons. Conclusions are limited by the fact that age and sex adjustment was not done when comparing the study group to population-based data. Despite this limitation, the data presented suggest that the application of population-based mortality data, and reference to literature drawn from population-based groups of injured persons, in dealing with this unique structured settlement applicant group, probably carries little risk of major biases influencing the outcome. This has practical signifi-cance, because without this investigation it would have appeared plausible to assume that socioeconomic and other variables might skew this group rather remarkably. Also, with the limitations mentioned, it appears that information from the study group could be generalized to the population, making this rapidly growing group a valuable resource for study of epidemiology and long-term mortality of severe injuries in general, even though this study group has experienced too few deaths during its short existence to allow any opinions about mortality.

APPENDIX

Determining "Adjusted Age"

The underwriting process applied to severely injured applicants for structured settlement annuities involves classifying each applicant by major diagnosis or impairment, and then tailoring the published mortality expectation drawn from clinical or insurance experience to fit the unique features of the individual applicant. For example, there is literature showing that young, complete quadriplegics have experienced an average of 750% of the population mortality rate for individuals of similar age and sex (Mesard, 1978). By applying a 7.5-fold multiplication to the population mortality rate for each year from the chronological age of the injured quadriplegic upward, one can determine the "adjusted age" at which the population age group would experience the mortality rate and average life expectancy predicted for the impaired applicant. For a 20-year old male with a 750% mortality rate expectation, the adjusted age would be 46 years using the 1980 U.S. population life tables, i.e., 26 P.Y.L.L. But in this example, the final adjusted age will include consideration of variables such as presence/absence of decubiti with/without complicating infection with/without underlying osteomyelitis, urinary drainage efficiency with/without complicating infections with/without calculi, pulmonary function, evidence of suicide risk, presence of other disease or risk factors, etc. In addition, since the published mortality experience comes from long-term mortality studies covering the past four decades, prediction of probable changes from the historical experience during the next several decades of anticipated life of the individual applicant must be factored into the final action.

It is the Medical Director's challenge to: 1) Be certain that the medical information submitted with each claim is correctly interpreted so the individual is classified accurately by diagnosis; 2) Be certain that the most reliable and current experiential data are applied in predicting outcome; 3) apply judgment in adjusting for the individual factors that might influence outcomes among those of similar diagnosis; 4) anticipate the probability, magnitude, and nature of trends, treatments or breakthroughs which may influence outcomes during future decades for applicants with significant expectancy for life. It is, of course, impossible to predict the life span of any individual. Nevertheless, the ability of life insurance companies to successfully compete in the current structured settlement annuity marketplace, while assuring their solvency to meet future commitments, depends upon the overall accuracy of this process. The same process has been inherent in the life insurance side of the business since its inception.

REFERENCES

1. Annegers, et al., "The Incidence, Causes and Secular Trends of Head Trauma in Olmsted County, Minnesota, 1935-74," *Neurology,* 30 (1980): 912-19.

2. M. B. Bracken, et al., "Incidence of Acute Traumatic Hospitalized Spinal Cord Injury in the United States, 1970-77," *Am. J. Epidemiol.,* 113 (1981): 615-22.

3. T. Bray, et al., "Cost of Orthopedic Injuries Sustained in Motorcycle Accidents," *JAMA,* 254 (1985): 2452-53.

4. L. D. Budnick, B. P. Chaiken, "The Probability of Dying of Injuries by the Year 2000," *JAMA,* 254 (1985): 3350-52.

5. G. L. Clifton, "Spinal Cord Injury in the Houston-Galveston Area," *Tex. Med.,* 79 (1983) 55-57.

6. M. J. DeVivo, et al.," The Prevalence of S.C.I.: A Re-estimation Based on Life Tables," *S.C.I.: Digest,* 1 (1980): 3-11.

7. P. R. Fine, et al., "Spinal Cord Injuries: An Epidemiologic Perspective," *Paraplegia,* 17 (1980): 237-50.

8. W. O. Geisler, et al., "Survival After Traumatic Transverse Myelitis," *Paraplegia,* 14 (1977): 262-75.

9. M. R. Griffin, et al., "Traumatic Spinal Cord Injury in Olmsted County, Minnesota, 1935-81," *Am. J. Epidemiol.,* 121 (1985): 884-95.

10. D. H. Hindert, et al., *Structured Settlements and Periodic Payment Judgments* (New York, Law Journal Seminars Press, 1984).

11. A. F. Hoskin, et al., *Accident Facts, 1985 Edition* (Chicago, National Safety Council, 1985).

12. Insurance Facts, *1985-86 Property/Casualty Fact Book* (New York, Insurance Information Institute, 1985).

13. J. Jagger, et al., "Epidemiologic Features of Head Injury in a Predominantly Rural Population," *J. of Trauma,* 24 (1984): 40-44.

14. W. D. Kalsbeek, et al., "The National Head and Spinal Injury Survey: Major Findings," *J. of Neurosurg.,* 53 (1980): S19-S31.

15. M. R. Klauber, et al., "The Epidemiology of Head Injury," *Am. J. Epidemiol.,* 113, (1981): 500-9.

16. Leads from the MMWR, "Deaths Associated with Fires, Burns, and Explosions, New Mexico, 1978-83," *JAMA,* 254 (1985): 2538-41.

17. L. Mesard, "Survival after Spinal Cord Trauma: A Life Table Analysis," *Arch. Neurol.,* 35 (1978): 78-83.

18. "Mistakes Doctors Make," *HEF News,* Health Education Foundation, Vol. 7, No. 4, Winter 1984.

19. E. Munoz, "Economic Costs of Trauma, United States, 1982," *J. of Trauma,* 24 (1984): 237-44.

20. A. M. Nahum, J. Melvin, eds., *The Biomechanics of Trauma* (Norwalk, Appleton Century Crofts, 1985).

21. M. R. Oreskovich, et al., "Geriatric Trauma: Injury Patterns and Outcome," *J. of Trauma,* 24 (1984): 565-69.

22. Professional Liability in the '80s: Report I, (AMA Special Task Force on Professional Liability and Insurance, 1984).

23. Report of the Secretary's Task Force on Black and Minority Health, *Morbidity and Mortality Weekly Report,* 35 (1986): 109-12.

24. A. H. Roberts, "Chapter 12. Life Expectancy and Causes of Death." In *Severe Accidental Head Injury* (London, Macmillan Press, 1979), pp. 140-51.

25. J. M. Romeder, J. McWhinnie, "Potential Years of Life Lost Between Ages 1 and 70: An Indicator of Premature Mortality for Health Planning," *Int. J. of Epidemiol.,* 6 (1977): 143-50.

26. M. H. Rudov, et al., "Medical Malpractice Insurance Claim Files Closed in 1970," in Appendix, *Report of the Secretary's Commission on Medical Malpractice* (D.H.E.W. Publication No. [OS] 73-89, 1973).

27. R. W. Solazzi , R. J. Ward, "The Spectrum of Medical Liability Cases," *Inter. Anesthesiol. Clin.,* 22 (1984): 43-59.

28. *Statistical Abstract of the United States,* (Washington, D.C., U.S. Department of Commerce, 1986).

29. C. H. Tator, V. E. Edmonds, "Acute Spinal Cord Injury: Analysis of Epidemiologic Factors," *Can. J. Surg.,* 22 (1979): 575-78.

30. C. H. Tator, et al., "Diving: A Frequent and Potentially Preventable Cause of Spinal Cord Injury," *Can. Med. Assoc. J.,* 124 (1981): 1323-24.

31. J. S. Torg, et al., "The National Football Head and Neck Injury Registry: 14-Year Report on Cervical Quadriplegia, 1971 through 1984," *JAMA,* 254 (1985): 3439-42.

32. S. Whitman, et al., "Comparative Head Trauma Experiences in Two Socioeconomically Different Chicago-Area Communities. A Population Study," *Am. J. Epidemiol.,* 119 (1984): 570-80.

33. J. S. Young, et al., *Spinal Cord Injury Statistics* (Phoenix, Good Samaritan Medical Center, 1982).

34. J. P. Zettas, et al., "Injury Patterns in Motorcycle Accidents," *J. Trauma,* 19 (1979): 833-36.

LIFE TABLE ANALYSIS OF AIDS MORTALITY

Richard E. Braun, M.D. and Richard B. Singer, M.D.

References:

1. R. Rothenburg, M. Woefel, R. Stoneburner, et al., "Survival with the Acquired Immunodeficiency Syndrome," *N. Engl. J. Med.,* 317 (1987): 1297-302.

2. B. M. White, C. E. Swanson, D. A. Cooper, "Survival of Patients with the Acquired Immunodeficiency Snydrome in Australia," *Med. J. Aust.,* 150 (1989): 358-62.

3. G. B. Scott, C. Hutto, R. W. Makuch, et al., "Survival in Children with Prenatally Acquired Human Immunodeficiency Virus Type I Infection," *N. Engl. J. Med.,* 321 (1989): 1791-96.

4. G. F. Lemp, S. F. Payne, D. Neal, et al., "Survival Trends for Patients with AIDS," *JAMA,* 263 (1990): 402-6.

5. B. S. Peters, E. J. Beck, D. G. Coleman, et al., "Changing Disease Patterns in Patients with AIDS in a Referral Centre in the United Kingdom: the Changing Face of AIDS," *Br. Med. J.,* 302 (1991): 203-7.

6. R. D. Moore, J. Hidalgo, B. W. Sugland, et al., "Zidovudine and the Natural History of the Acquired Immunodeficiency Syndrome," *N. Engl. J. Med.,* 324 (1991): 1412-16.

7. Y. F. Friedman, C. Franklin, S. Freels, et al., "Long-term Survival of Patients with AIDS, Pneumocystis Carinii Pneumonia, and Respiratory Failure," *JAMA,* 266 (1991): 89-92.

Objectives of Abstract: To analyze data from 7 series of patients with Acquired Immunodeficiency Syndrome (AIDS) for mortality based on age, sex, presenting disease, and risk factor for HIV infection.

Subjects Studied: Data on 12,016 subjects from 7 series in 3 countries were included in the analysis. Table 086K1-1 contains a breakdown of the entry characteristics of the patients studied. All of the subjects, with the exception of those in Reference 3, were diagnosed with AIDS at entry into the respective series. The series reported in Reference 1, 2, 4, and 6 were community-based with data obtained from mandated reporting and public records. The groups in References 3, 5, and 7 were hospital-based with the subjects

receiving treatment and medical follow-up at the institutions.

Series 1 consisted of 5,833 subjects who were reported to the public health authorities in the city of New York as being diagnosed with AIDS before 1986. The majority of subjects were male, and the largest age group was over 40. The racial mix was 47.4% white, 30.5% black and 22.1% Hispanic.

Series 2 was made up of 554 subjects reported to the Australian National Health and Medical Research Council (NHMRC) Special Unit in AIDS Epidemiology and Clinical Research as having AIDS prior to July 31, 1987. The majority of the subjects were male.

Series 3 included all 172 children given the diagnosis of prenatally acquired HIV at the Children's Hospital Center of Jackson Memorial Hospital, Miami, between January 1, 1981 and December 31, 1987. This is the only series in this review in which the authors did not require the diagnosis of AIDS to be made prior to a subject's entry into the series.

Series 4 consisted of 4,323 subjects reported between July 1981 and December 31, 1987 to the San Francisco Department of Public Health as being diagnosed with AIDS. The study excluded those diagnosed with AIDS at autopsy and those whose initial diagnosis met only the revised (1987) CDC surveillance definition of Aids. The study group was 99.3% male and 84.3% white.

Series 5 contained 347 subjects with AIDS who were followed regularly at the St. Mary's Hospital Medical School in London between October 1982 and December 31, 1989. Males comprised 98.6% of those followed and 95.1% were white.

Series 6 contained 1,028 subjects over age 17 identified as meeting the Center of Disease Control (CDC) definition of AIDS in the Maryland Human Immunodeficiency Virus Information System. This system was established by the Maryland Department of Health and Mental Hygiene in 1987. The system identifies AIDS patients through reports to the Health Department and through active surveillance of clinical laboratories, hospitals, and insurance claims files managed by the state. Suspected AIDS patients are then investigated using standard guidelines for the investigation of infectious disease. New cases thus identified are added to the information system. There were more complete data presented on 714 subjects identified between April 1987 and June 1989, and these subjects were included in this analysis. The survival was reported to be better in this later group of subjects. In the group of 714, 83.5% were male and 32.1% were white.

Series 7 consisted of 73 consecutive patients admitted to the Cook County Hospital with the concurrent diagnoses of AIDS, Pneumocystis Carinii Pneumonia, and acute respiratory failure (excluding those who elected not to be resuscitated). These admissions occurred between January 1, 1987 and December 31, 1989. Some 92% of these subjects were male.

Follow-up: The series differed in the type of surveillance with the community-based series relying on public records and some care-giver contact, and the hospital-based studies relying on ongoing patient contact with some further directed follow-up.

Series 1 follow-up was accomplished through the cross linkage of death records. No attempts were made to confirm the vital status of specific subjects. The authors admit that some under-ascertainment of deaths may have occurred due to subjects dying outside of New York City.

Series 2 subjects were followed-up through surveillance of death certificates and direct contact with the care-giving physician or clinic. The authors believed that the follow-up in Series 2 was complete.

Series 3 consisted of a cohort of children followed at one institution. While not explicitly addressed, it is assumed that follow-up occurred through regular medical care at the institution.

Series 4 followed subjects through review of death certificates and newspaper obituaries and contacting physicians caring for the subjects. Patients who were lost to follow-up (n=438) were treated as if they had lived to the midpoint of the interval during which they were lost.

Series 5 included only the subjects that attended the author's institution regularly. There were subjects excluded from the study (n=66) due to inadequate information, temporary treatment due to distant residence, or those lost to follow-up (only 5 patients).

Series 6 did not specifically address the mechanism for ascertainment of vital status. The authors did survey vital records, health insurance claims, institutional systems, and community-based systems. In addition the National Death Index of the National Center for Health Statistics was used to search for deaths when the date of death was unknown.

Series 7 subjects were followed-up through continued medical care at the institution, telephone contact with the subject or the subject's family and through the Chicago Department of Health. Only one subject was lost to follow-up by these methods.

Expected Mortality: The expected mortality rates were derived from population mortality rates with adjustments for the age, sex, and race of the initial study population.

In Series 1, Series 3, and Series 4 the 1986 Abridged U.S. Life Tables were used to determine expected mortality.

The World Health Organization (WHO) *World Health Statistics Annual 1990* was the source of the expected death rates for Australia and the United Kingdom in Series 2 and Series 5, respectively.

The 1988 Abridged U.S. Life Tables were the source of the expected mortality for Series 6 and Series 7.

Results: Detailed analysis of comparative mortality for Series 1 (New York City) is presented in Tables 086K1-2 and 086K1-3. First-year mortality was extremely high (about 500 per 1000) and even at durations 2-5 years was still approximately 200 per 1000. In terms of EDR excess mortality was relatively constant by age; the decrease in mortality ratio with increasing age was due mostly to the higher expected mortality at the older ages. In this series 11.4% of the patients were diagnosed shortly before death; such patients were included in the first-year mortality.

Comparative mortality by age and duration is shown in Table 086K1-4 for Series 4 (San Francisco) and Series 6 (Maryland). Excess death rates were again very high in all age groups in the first two years of follow-up. In Series 6, the trend was for a slight increase in EDR with advancing age, but in Series 4, the highest EDR values were observed in the few patients under age 20 years as well as in the oldest age groups; EDR was higher in the second than in the first year of follow-up. The decrease in mortality ratio with age was due primarily to the increase in expected mortality.

In general, it appears that females diagnosed with AIDS have a higher EDR than males (above three series in Table 086K1-5). Again, the higher mortality ratios in female patients are due more to the lower expected mortality in women than to their somewhat higher observed mortality.

The secular trend for first-year observed mortality, all ages and both sexes combined, is shown in Table 086K1-6 for four series, and comparative mortality for Series 5 (United Kingdom) is shown in Table 086K1-7. The secular trend shows reduced first-year mortality and improved survival since about 1987. In two of the series (4 and 6), it was reported that patients treated with Zidovudine survived significantly longer than those not so treated. In

146

Series 5, the considerable reduction in calendar-year mortality in 1988-89 followed the election of 79% of patients to receive Zidovudine, starting in April 1987. Somewhat higher first-year mortality ratios in Series 5 than in the corresponding U.S. series are at least partly due to lower expected mortality rates in men under 45 in the United Kingdom (U.K.), as compared with expected male mortality rates in the U.S.

When mode of transmission of the HIV virus was used as a risk factor, it was found that differences in EDR were small and inconsistent between patients with homosexual transmission (Table 086K1-8) and those with transmission due to IV drug use (Table 086K1-9). In several series comparative mortality data are also available by the major clinical manifestation of AIDS, either Pneumocystis Carinii Pneumonia (Table 086K1-10) or Kaposi's Sarcoma alone (Table 086K1-11). In a majority of the first two annual periods of observation, the EDR was higher with pneumonia than with Kaposi's Sarcoma. Those presenting with multiple medical complications were noted as having a very poor survival in Series 2 (Australia) and 4 (San Francisco).

Series 3 (Miami) is the only one in this Abstract providing experience for infants and children with perinatally acquired HIV infection. Symptomatic AIDS tended to develop early, within 2 years of age in 78% of the series. As shown in Table 086K1-12, excess mortality was less than in adult series, but EDR averaged 98 per 1000 per year at attained ages 2-5 years in the total series, and was even higher in the first year of life. Furthermore, when the HIV infection was diagnosed under age 1 year, the annual EDR of 258 per 1000 averaged over 5 years duration was significantly higher than the corresponding EDR of 49 per 1000 observed when the diagnosis was made after the first birthday. The authors emphasized the poor prognosis and need for early diagnosis.

Comment: Through 1990 over 100,000 deaths of AIDS patients have been reported to the CDC. An estimated one million persons in the U.S. are infected with HIV, and an estimated 165,000 to 250,000 will die of AIDS during 1991-93. Insurers paid one billion dollars in AIDS-related claims for life and health insurance in 1989, and 1.2 billion dollars in 1990. This set of studies provides consistent evidence for the very high initial and cumulative mortality after diagnosis of AIDS, although there is also evidence of some improvement in survival since about 1987. Despite this improvement, the AIDS epidemic continues to be a catastrophe of historic proportion in medical, economic, and personal terms.

TABLE 086K1-1

ENTRY CHARACTERISTICS IN 7 SERIES OF AIDS PATIENTS

Characteristic	Series Reference						
	1	2	3	4	5	6	7
No. of Patients	5,833	554	172	4,323	347	714	73
Sex: Male	5,281	533	77	4,292	342	596	69
Female	552	21	95	31	5	118	4
Mean Age	(1)	37.3	Newborn	(1)	37.5	(1)	33 (2)
Race: White	2,753		15	3,643	330	229	14
Black	1,769		157	262	10	472	47
Hispanic	1,281		0	333	4	12	12
Other			0	80	3	1	0
Transmission:							
Homosexual	3,400	482	0	3,663	330	337	46
IV Drug Use	1,660	19	0	576	7	300	11
Heterosexual		7	0		10		13
Transfusion		24	0	40	0		2
Combination	335		0		0		
Other	438	2	172 (3)	43	0	77	1
Presentation (DIS):							
PCP	2,541	402 (4)	14	2,105	176	387	73 (5)
Kaposi's Sarcoma	994	107		1,015	86	52	
Other Single DIS.	814	22	} 80	483	} 85	} 275	
Combination	1,569	53		686			

(1) Series 1, 4, and 6 contained detailed age distribution information (SeeTables 086K1-3 and 086K1-4).
(2) Median age.
(3) All newborn infants of infected mothers.
(4) Opportunistic infections, including Pneumocystis Carinii Pneumonia (PCP).
(5) Patients selected based on PCP with respiratory failure.

COMPARATIVE MORTALITY BY DURATION, 5,833 PATIENTS WITH AIDS, NEW YORK CITY 1981-85 ALL AGES COMBINED[†]

Interval Start-End	No. Alive at Start	Exposure Patient-yrs.	No. of Deaths		Mortality Ratio	Mean Annual Mortality Rate/1000		
			Observed	Expected*		Observed	Expected	Excess
t to $t+\Delta t$	ℓ	E	d	d′	100(d/d′)	q	q′	(q–q′)
0-1 yr.	5,833	5,596.0	2,865	21.38	13,400%	512	3.8	508
1-2 yrs.	2,494	2,058.5	869	8.34	10,400	422	4.1	418
2-3	754	554.5	122	2.38	5,100	220	4.3	216
3-4	233	164.5	19	0.80	2,100	115	4.8	110
4-5	77	52.5	12	0.30	4,000	229	5.6	223

* Basis of expected deaths: 1986 Abridged U.S. Life Tables.

[†] Accurate Life Table reconstruction for w, E, and d based on annual Data for ℓ (caption of Figure 1 in reference) and survival rates, P, to 3 decimal places in Table 2.

COMPARATIVE MORTALITY BY AGE, 5,833 PATIENTS WITH AIDS, NEW YORK CITY 1981-85, DURATION 0-1, 1-2, AND 2-5 YEARS

Age	No. Alive At Start	Survival Rate			Mean Annual Mortality Rate/1000			Mortality Ratio
		Cumulative	Interval	Annual	Observed	Expected*	Excess	
	ℓ	P	p_i	p	$\breve{q}$	$\breve{q}′$	$(\breve{q}-\breve{q}′)$	$100(\breve{q}/\breve{q}′)$
DURATION 0-1 YEARS								
<30 yrs.	1,076	0.510	0.510	0.510	490	2.0	488	24,500%
30-34	1,436	0.530	0.530	0.530	470	2.6	467	18,100
35-39	1,377	0.497	0.497	0.497	503	3.4	500	14,800
40 up	1,994	0.437	0.437	0.437	563	6.3	557	8,900
DURATION 1-2[†] YEARS								
<30 yrs.	(483)	0.268	0.525	0.525	475	2.0	473	23,800%
30-34	(673)	0.321	0.606	0.606	394	2.7	391	14,600
35-39	(602)	0.294	0.592	0.592	408	3.6	404	11,300
40 up	(736)	0.251	0.574	0.574	426	7.0	419	6,100
DURATION 2-5[†] YEARS								
<30 yrs.**	(125)	0.191	0.713	0.844	156	2.0	154	7,800%
30-34	(219)	0.177	0.551	0.820	180	2.8	177	6,400
35-39	(189)	0.118	0.407	0.741	259	4.0	255	6,500
40 up	(221)	0.160	0.637	0.860	140	8.4	132	1,670

* Basis of expected deaths: 1986 Abridged U.S. Life Tables.

[†] Values of ℓ at 1 and 2 years estimated from approximate Life Table reconstruction.

** Maximum duration for age <30 in Table 2 of the article is 4 years, interval 2-4 years instead of 2-5 years as in other age groups.

COMPARATIVE MORTALITY OF AIDS PATIENTS BASED ON AGE — SERIES 4 AND 6
(See also Table 086K1-3)

Series	Site	Age	Interval Start-End	No. Alive at Start	Observed Survival Rate		Annual Mortality Rate/1000			Mortality Ratio
					Cumulative	Interval	Observed	Expected*	Excess	
			t to t+Δt	ℓ	P	pᵢ	q̌	q̌'	(q̌–q̌')	100(q̌/q̌')
4	San Francisco	<20	0-1 yr.	14	0.357	0.357	643	1.5	641	42,900%
			1-2		0.119	0.333	667	1.6	665	41,700
		20-29	0-1	585	0.531	0.531	469	1.8	467	26,000
			1-2		0.222	0.418	582	1.9	580	30,600
		30-39	0-1	3,150	0.543	0.543	457	2.3	455	19,900
			1-2		0.218	0.401	599	2.4	597	25,000
		40-49	0-1	1,144	0.509	0.509	491	4.3	487	11,400
			1-2		0.197	0.387	613	4.7	608	13,000
		50-59	0-1	342	0.406	0.406	594	10.8	583	5,500
			1-2		0.131	0.323	677	12.1	665	5,600
		≥60†	0-1	88	0.289	0.289	711	20.5	690	3,500
6	Maryland	≤30	0-1	213	0.610	0.610	390	2.4	388	16,200%
			1-2		0.370	0.607	393	2.6	390	15,100
		31-44	0-1	398	0.570	0.570	430	4.8	425	9,000
			1-2		0.370	0.649	351	5.2	346	6,800
		≥45	0-1	103	0.470	0.470	530	7.9	522	6,700
			1-2		0.230	0.489	511	8.3	503	6,200

* Basis of expected mortality: matched U.S. Population Life Tables.
† No data for duration 1-2 years.

COMPARATIVE MORTALITY OF AIDS PATIENTS BASED ON SEX — 3 SERIES

Series	Site	Sex	Interval Start-End	No. Alive at Start	Observed Survival Rate		Annual Mortality Rate/1000			Mortality Ratio
					Cumulative	Interval	Observed	Expected*	Excess	
			t to t+Δt	ℓ	P	pᵢ	q̌	q̌'	(q̌–q̌')	100(q̌/q̌')
1	NYC	Male	0-1 yr.	5,281	0.497	0.497	503	4.1	499	12,300%
			1-2		0.289	0.581	419	4.5	414	9,300
			2-5		0.155	0.266	357	5.1	352	7,100
		Female	0-1	552	0.402	0.402	598	2.1	596	28,500
			1-2		0.209	0.520	480	2.3	478	20,900
			2-4†		0.139	0.665	185	2.7	182	6,900
4	San Francisco	Male	0-1	4,292	0.517	0.517	483	3.8	479	12,700%
			1-2		0.202	0.390	610	4.2	606	14,500
		Female	0-1	31	0.355	0.355	645	1.9	643	33,900
			1-2		0.176	0.496	504	2.1	502	24,000
6	Maryland	Male	0-1	596	0.590	0.590	410	5.0	405	8,200%
			1-2		0.350	0.593	407	5.4	402	7,500
		Female	0-1	118	0.460	0.460	540	1.9	538	28,400
			1-2		0.280	0.609	391	2.1	389	18,600

* Basis of expected mortality: matched U.S. Population Life Tables.
† No data for duration 4-5.

TABLE 086K1-6

FIRST YEAR MORTALITY OF AIDS PATIENTS BY YEAR OF OBSERVATION — SECULAR TREND IN 4 SERIES

Series	Site/Group	Annual Mortality Rate								
		1981	1982	1983	1984	1985	1986	1987	1988	1989
1	NYC	0.582	0.521	0.544	0.507	0.496	—	—	—	—
4	San Francisco*	100%*	94%*	87%*	82%*	76%*	72%*	67%*	—	—
5	United Kingdom	—	—	—	0.476	0.587	0.645	0.455	0.316	0.266
6	Maryland	—	—	0.53		0.56	0.45	0.42	0.44	—

* Mortality relative to 1981 Mortality.

TABLE 086K1-7

MORTALITY IN AIDS PATIENTS IN THE UNITED KINGDOM BY CALENDAR YEAR, 1984-90
ALL AGES AND DURATIONS COMBINED — SERIES 5

No.	Interval Calendar Yr.	No. Alive[+] Jan. 1	No. New Patients	Exposure** Patient-yrs.	No. of Deaths Observed	No. of Deaths Expected*	Mortality Ratio	Mean Annual Mortality Rate/1000 Observed	Mean Annual Mortality Rate/1000 Expected	Mean Annual Mortality Rate/1000 Excess
i	(1/1-12/31)	ℓ	ℓn	E	d	d'	100(d/d')	q	q'	(q–q')
1	1984	6	30	21.0	10	0.040	25,000%	476	1.9	474
2	1985	26	23	37.5	22	0.071	31,000	587	1.9	585
3	1986	27	67	60.5	39	0.115	34,000	645	1.9	643
4	1987	55	79	74.5	43	0.142	30,000	455	1.9	453
5	1988	91	65	123.5	39	0.235	16,600	316	1.9	314
6	1989	117	74	154.0	41	0.293	14,000	266	1.9	264
	1990	150								
1-6	1984-90	—	338	471	194	0.895	21,700	412	1.9	410

* Basis of expected mortality: U.K. mortality rate, male 1981+, tabular age 41 (3 years older than mean 38 years, all patients).
[+] $\ell_i = 6 = 9$ new patients – 3 deaths 10/82-12/31/83. All patients followed to death or 12/31/89. $\ell_{i+1} = \ell_i + \ell n_i – d_i$
** $E = \ell_i + 0.5\,\ell n_i$

TABLE 086K1-8

COMPARATIVE MORTALITY OF AIDS PATIENTS WITH HOMOSEXUAL ACTIVITY BEING THE ONLY RISK FACTOR FOR HIV — 4 SERIES

Series	Site	Interval Start-End	No. Alive at Start	Observed Survival Rate Cumulative	Observed Survival Rate Interval	Annual Mortality Rate/1000 Observed	Annual Mortality Rate/1000 Expected*	Annual Mortality Rate/1000 Excess	Mortality Ratio
		t to t+Δt	ℓ	P	p_i	$\breve{q}$	$\breve{q}'$	$(\breve{q}–\breve{q}')$	100($\breve{q}/\breve{q}'$)
1	NYC	0-1 yr.	3,400	0.531	0.531	469	4.1	465	11,400%
		1-2		0.300	0.565	435	4.5	430	9,700
		2-5		0.159	0.530	191	5.9	185	3,200
2	Australia[+]	0-1	482	0.400	0.400	600	2.1	598	28,600%
		1-2		0.210	0.525	475	2.3	473	20,700
4	San Francisco	0-1	3,664	0.523	0.523	477	3.8	473	12,600%
		1-2		0.205	0.392	608	4.2	604	14,500
6	Maryland	0-1	337	0.610	0.610	390	5.0	385	7,800%
		1-2		0.360	0.590	410	5.4	405	7,600

* Basis of expected mortality: matched U.S. Population Life Tables, men only.
[+] Used revised CDC definition of AIDS.

TABLE 086K1-9

COMPARATIVE MORTALITY OF AIDS PATIENTS WITH IV DRUG USE BEING THE ONLY RISK FACTOR FOR HIV — 3 SERIES

Series	Site	Interval Start-End	No. Alive at Start	Observed Survival Rate		Annual Mortality Rate/1000			Mortality Ratio
				Cumulative	Interval	Observed	Expected*	Excess	
		t to $t+\Delta t$	ℓ	P	p_i	$\check{q}$	$\check{q}'$	$(\check{q}-\check{q}')$	$100(\check{q}/\check{q}')$
1	NYC	0-1 yr.	1,600	0.430	0.430	570	3.8	566	15,000%
		1-2		0.252	0.586	414	4.1	410	10,100
		2-5		0.187	0.742	95	4.8	90	2,000
4	San Francisco	0-1	53	0.542	0.542	458	3.8	454	12,100%
		1-2		0.353	0.651	349	4.2	345	8,300
6	Maryland	0-1	300	0.540	0.540	460	4.5	455	10,200%
		1-2		0.360	0.667	334	4.8	329	7,000

* Basis of expected mortality: matched U.S. Population Life Tables.

TABLE 086K1-10

COMPARATIVE MORTALITY OF AIDS PATIENTS WITH PNEUMOCYSTIS CARINII PNEUMONIA (PCP) — 6 SERIES

Series	Site/Obs Per.	Interval Start-End	No. Alive at Start	Observed Survival Rate		Annual Mortality Rate/1000			Mortality Ratio
				Cumulative	Interval	Observed	Expected*	Excess	
		t to $t+\Delta t$	ℓ	P	p_i	$\check{q}$	$\check{q}'$	$(\check{q}-\check{q}')$	$100(\check{q}/\check{q}')$
1	NYC	0-1 yr.	2,541	0.454	0.454	546	3.8	542	14,400%
		1-2		0.250	0.551	449	4.1	445	11,000
		2-5		0.167	0.668	126	4.8	121	2,600
2	Australia[†]	0-1	402	0.37	0.370	630	2.1	628	30,000%
		1-2		0.15	0.405	595	2.3	593	25,900
4	San Francisco	0-1	2,105	0.546	0.546	454	3.8	450	11,900%
		1-2		0.171	0.313	687	4.2	683	16,400
5	U.K. 1987	0-1	41	0.70	0.700	300	1.9	298	15,800%
		1-2		0.42	0.600	400	2.1	398	19,000
6	Maryland	0-1	387	0.60	0.600	400	4.5	395	8,900%
		1-2		0.33	0.550	450	4.8	445	9,400
7	Chicago	0-1	72	0.37	0.370	630	3.9	626	16,200%
		1-2		0.19	0.510	490	4.2	486	11,700

* Basis of expected mortality: matched US. Population Life Tables.
[†] Used revised CDC definition of AIDS, includes all opportunistic infections.

TABLE 086K1-11

COMPARATIVE MORTALITY OF AIDS PATIENTS PRESENTING WITH KAPOSI'S SARCOMA ONLY — 5 SERIES

Series	Site/Obs Per.	Interval Start-End	No. Alive at Start	Observed Survival Rate		Annual Mortality Rate/1000			Mortality Ratio
				Cumulative	Interval	Observed	Expected*	Excess	
		t to t+Δt	ℓ	P	p_i	$\check{q}$	$\check{q}'$	$(\check{q}-\check{q}')$	$100(\check{q}/\check{q}')$
1	NYC	0-1 yr.	994	0.721	0.721	279	3.8	275	7,300%
		1-2		0.507	0.703	297	4.1	293	7,200
		2-5		0.309	0.609	152	4.8	147	3,200
2	Australia[†]	0-1	107	0.480	0.480	520	2.1	518	24,800%
		1-2		0.320	0.666	334	2.3	332	14,500
4	San Francisco	0-1	1,015	0.654	0.654	346	3.8	342	9,100%
		1-2		0.351	0.537	463	4.2	459	11,000
5	U.K. 1987	0-1	22	0.535	0.535	465	1.9	463	24,500%
		1-2		0.375	0.701	299	2.1	297	14,200
6	Maryland	0-1	52	0.610	0.610	390	4.5	385	8,700%
		1-2		0.310	0.508	492	4.8	487	10,300

* Basis of expected mortality: matched U.S. Population Life Tables.
† Used revised CDC definition of AIDS.

TABLE 086K1-12

COMPARATIVE MORTALITY IN INFANTS AND CHILDREN WITH HIV INFECTION ACQUIRED PERINATALLY — SERIES 3

i	Interval Start-End	Observed Survival Rate			Ave. Annual Mortality Rate/1000			Mortality Ratio
		Cumulative	Interval	Annual	Observed	Expected*	Excess	
	t to t+Δt	P	p_i	p	$\check{q}$	$\check{q}'$	$(\check{q}-\check{q}')$	$100(\check{q}/\check{q}')$
	(Birth)	ALL 172 INFANTS AND CHILDREN						
1	0-1 yr.	0.83	0.83	0.83	170	18.1	152	940%
2	1-2	0.75	0.904	0.904	96	1.1	95	8,700
3	2-5	0.51	0.680	0.879	121	0.7	120	17,300
	(Diagnosis)	98 INFANTS WITH HIV DIAGNOSIS UNDER AGE 1 YEAR						
	0-5 yrs.[†]	0.22	0.22	0.739	261	4.0	257	6,500%
	(Diagnosis)	74 INFANTS WITH HIV DIAGNOSIS AFTER FIRST BIRTHDAY						
	0-5 yrs.[†]	0.76	0.76	0.947	53	0.7	52	7,600%

* Basis of expected mortality: 1986 Abridged U.S. Life Table, Black Male and Black Female.
† Interval based on time since diagnosis.

SHORT TERM SURVIVAL WITH TESTICULAR CANCER
AND
HODGKIN'S DISEASE

Report of a Cancer Survival Registration System and Mortality Abstracts for Short Term Survival with Testicular Cancer and Hodgkin's Lymphoma

Roger H. Butz, M.D., M.P.H.

The Centralized Cancer Patient Data Systems (CCPDS) was a registration system for patients with malignant neoplasms defined as reportable by the Comprehensive Cancer Centers in the United States. The System was developed as required by one of the ten characteristics defined by the National Cancer Advisory Board for designation of Comprehensive Cancer Centers. CCPDS data items and code definitions were made largely compatible with those in the World Health Organization *Handbook For Standardized Cancer Registration* published in 1976, and the National Cancer Institute Surveillance, Epidemiology, and End Results (SEER) program. The 21 participating Comprehensive Cancer Centers (see Table 110K1-1) began data collection for CCPDS with patients first admitted after July 1, 1977. CCPDS data were forwarded to the Statistical Analysis and Quality Control (SAQC) Center at the Fred Hutchinson Cancer Research Center, Seattle, Washington under the direction of SAQC Center Project Head, Polly Feigl, PhD, with whose permission I have derived the data to the right (see Table 110K1-1).

The CCPDS has released results from a survival study of cancer patients admitted to their programs between July 1, 1977 and December, 1982.[1] The patients under surveillance included a total of 248,866 of which only the "new" patients are described here, the 155,195 who were admitted to the participating cancer centers within 30 days of their initial diagnosis of cancer and prior to receiving specific treatment elsewhere. These patients came from all of the contiguous 48 United States with representation concentrated from major metropolitan areas, especially where the participating cancer centers were located. The new patient disease categories included 22,495 lung cancer cases, 14.5% of the total;

19,298 breast cancer cases, 12.4%; 9,525 uterine cervical cancer, 6.1%; 9,055 colon, 5.8%; 8,981 prostate, 5.8%; 8,124 buccal cavity and pharynx, 5.2%; 6,728 non-Hodgkin's lymphoma, 4.3%; and fewer cases of the other 30 primary sites listed.

TABLE 110K1-1
LIST OF COMPREHENSIVE CANCER CENTERS

Comprehensive Cancer Center, University of Alabama in Birmingham

Colorado Regional Cancer Center, Inc.

Comprehensive Cancer Center, Duke University Medical Center

Fred Hutchinson Cancer Research Center

Georgetown/Howard Universities Comprehensive Cancer Center

Illinois Cancer Council

Johns Hopkins Oncology Center

Kenneth Norris, Jr. Cancer Research Institute, University of Southern California Comprehensive Cancer Center

Mayo Comprehensive Cancer Center

Comprehensive Cancer Center for the State of Florida

The University of Texas Health System Cancer Center, M.D. Anderson Hospital and Tumor Institute

Ohio State University Comprehensive Cancer Center

Roswell Park Memorial Institute

Dana-Farber Cancer Institute

Memorial Sloan-Kettering Cancer Center

UCLA Jonsson Comprehensive Cancer Center

University of Wisconsin Clinical Cancer Center

Yale University Comprehensive Cancer Center

Comprehensive Cancer Center of Metropolitan Detroit

Columbia University Cancer Research Center

Fox Chase/University of Pennsylvania Comprehensive Cancer Center

Source: R. H. Butz, "Short Term Survival with Testicular Cancer and Hodgkin's Disease," *J. Ins. Med.*, 19, no. 3 (1987): 17-19. Reproduced with permission of author and publisher.

The report of CCPDS survival data is a 590-page volume dated December, 1985 and includes data for follow-up periods of no more than 5 years, and shorter periods for the cases admitted later during the enrollment. These initial survival data for CCPDS are interesting but of limited usefulness for insurance underwriting. In some categories, the numbers of deaths are so small as to reduce significance. Also, although some of the patients were self-referred and many had only Stage I or even in-situ disease, it seems plausible to expect a bias in the direction of worst cases appearing at a cancer treatment center in lieu of local physicians and community hospitals. A positive value of these data pertains to the consistency with which microscopic confirmation was documented, the standardization of data elements for the study records, and the consensus concerning staging criteria. It also seems likely that the treatment rendered was "State of the Art," as these cancer centers are academically associated and tend to pioneer in the application of advanced treatment modalities and surgical interventions. Thus, if technological advances in treatment are improving survivability, one might expect to see it in these results early.

In 1986, oncologist Michael Baker, M.D. reported to the 95th annual meeting of ALIMDA that "one of the most exciting developments in modern oncology" has been the change in prognosis for testicular carcinoma, particularly referring to seminomas as curable in a high proportion of cases.[2] Table 110K1-2 shows the comparative mortality for cancer of the testis by histologic type from the CCPDS report for all ages and all stages of disease. Of the 1,539 cases, 480 were seminoma, affording 1,646 person-years of exposure for this group of men with a median age of 36 years. There were 33 seminoma patient deaths giving an annual average mortality rate of 0.0201, and a mortality ratio of 954% of expected mortality based on 1982 United States population mortality rates.

TABLE 110K1-2

CANCER OF TESTIS, COMPARATIVE MORTALITY — BY HISTOLOGIC TYPE, ALL STAGES, ALL AGES, 0-5 YEARS FROM DIAGNOSIS

	N	E	d	d'	Mort. Ratio	Avg. Ann. Mort. Rate	Est. 5-year Surv. Rate	Surv. Index	EDR
Seminoma (Median age = 36)	480	1,646	33	3.46	954%	0.0201	0.9035	91.3%	18
Embryonal (27)	442	1,516	62	2.58	2,403	0.0411	0.8107	81.8	39
Teratoma (26)	452	1,550	60	2.48	2,419	0.0387	0.8209	82.8	37
Choriocarcinoma (26)	133	456	37	0.73	5,069	0.0811	0.6552	65.6	79
Other (47)	32	110	11	0.58	1,897	0.1000	0.5905	60.6	95

N = Number of cases
E = Exposure, person-years
d = Actual deaths
d' = Expected deaths, based on 1982 U.S. population mortality rate.
EDR = Excess Death Rate

In Table 110K1-3, the cases are limited to stage I (localized disease) all ages. Most of the seminomas, 319 of the 480 cases, were admitted at stage I, giving 1,094 person-years of exposure. In this group, the mortality ratio was 274%, for an estimated 97.28% 5-year survival with a median age of 35 years.

TABLE 110K1-3

CANCER OF TESTIS, COMPARATIVE MORTALITY — BY HISTOLOGIC TYPE, LIMITED TO STAGE 1 (LOCALIZED) DISEASE, ALL AGES, 0-5 YEARS FROM DIAGNOSIS

					Mort. Ratio	Avg. Ann. Mort. Rate	Est. 5-year Surv. Rate	Surv. Index	EDR
	N	E	d	d'					
Seminoma (Median age = 35)	319	1,094	6	2.19	274%	0.0055	0.9728	98.3%	3.5
Embryonal (27)	106	364	4	0.62	645	0.0110	0.9462	95.4	9.3
Teratoma (27)	156	535	6	0.91	659	0.0112	0.9452	95.3	9.5
Choriocarcinoma (26)	28	96	1	0.15	667	0.0104	0.9491	95.7	8.9
Other (51)	15	51	3	0.41	732	0.0588	0.7386	76.9	50.8

N = Number of cases
E = Exposure, person-years
d = Actual deaths
d' = Expected deaths, based on 1982 U.S. population mortality rate.
EDR = Excess Death Rate

Another tumor which has been the target of impressive improvement in clinical treatment, also noted by Dr. Baker in his presentation in 1986, is Hodgkin's lymphoma.[2] Table 110K1-4 shows comparative mortality from CCPDS for Hodgkin's lymphoma by stage, histologic type and all ages. These 1,943 cases afforded 7,096 person-years of exposure and demonstrated mortality ratios in excess of 3,000%. Table 110K1-5 demonstrates the experience with the same group comparing histologic types for all ages, all stages. Although the traditionally cited advantage for lymphoid predominant Hodgkin's is noted, the mortality ratios are very high.[3]

TABLE 110K1-4

HODGKIN'S LYMPHOMA, COMPARATIVE MORTALITY — BY STAGE, ALL TYPES, ALL AGES, 0-5 YEARS FROM DIAGNOSIS

					Mort. Ratio	Avg. Ann. Mort. Rate	Est. 5-year Surv. Rate	Surv. Index	EDR
	N	E	d	d'					
STAGE I (Median age = 33)	325	1,167	50	1.63	3,050%	0.0428	0.8036	80.9%	41
STAGE II (29)	577	2,014	83	2.42	3,450	0.0412	0.8103	81.5	40
STAGE III (32)	564	2,092	129	2.72	4,750	0.0617	0.7273	73.6	60
STAGE IV (36)	326	1,275	112	2.04	5,500	0.0878	0.6316	63.7	86
Other (32)	151	548	27	0.71	3,800	0.0493	0.7766	78.6	48

N = Number of cases
E = Exposure, person-years
d = Actual deaths
d' = Expected deaths, based on 1982 U.S. population mortality rate.
EDR = Excess Death Rate

TABLE 110K1-5

HODGKIN'S, LYMPHOMA, COMPARATIVE MORTALITY — BY HISTOLOGIC TYPE, ALL STAGES, ALL AGES, 0-5 YEARS FROM DIAGNOSIS

	N	E	d	d'	Mort. Ratio	Avg. Ann. Mort. Rate	Est. 5-year Surv. Rate	Est. 5-year Surv. Index	EDR
Nodular Sclerosing (Median age = 28)	1,174	4,262	191	5.11	3,750%	0.0448	0.7952	77.0%	44
Lymphoid Depleted (47)	63	229	36	0.96	3,750	0.1572	0.4252	43.4	153
Mixed Cellular (39)	445	1,615	117	3.07	3,800	0.0724	0.6868	69.3	71
Lymphoid Predominant (36)	113	410	12	0.66	1,800	0.0293	0.8618	86.9	28
Hodgkins Not Specified (34)	148	537	45	0.75	6,000	0.0838	0.6456	65.0	82

N = Number of cases
E = Exposure, person-years
d = Actual deaths
d' = Expected deaths, based on 1982 U.S. population mortality rate.
EDR = Excess Death Rate

The CCPDS is apparently doomed to extinction because the National Cancer Institute (NCI) withdrew funding for the project. Local participants felt that this might have been because of an NCI impression that the data duplicated SEER data to a considerable extent, and that NCI felt there was "little interest in the result"! I have written to Dr. Vincent DeVita, Director of NCI, to be certain he is disavowed of this latter (rumored) impression, if true. As insurance medicine specialists we need just such projects and perhaps our interest in such information needs to be reiterated to such agencies.

REFERENCES

1. K. A. Kealey, ed., *Survival Rates for U.S. Comprehensive Cancer Center Patients, Admissions 1977-82*, (Seattle, Centralized Cancer Patient Data System Statistical Analysis and Quality Control Center, Dec. 1985).

2. M. A. Baker, "Determining Prognosis for Cancer Patients," *Trans. Assoc. Life Insur. Med. Dir. Amer.*, 70 (1986): 19-26.

3. P. H. Wiernink, "Hodgkin's Disease," *Clinical Medicine, Vol. 5*, edited by John O. Spittell, Jr., (Philadelphia, Harper & Row, 1986).

BRONCHIAL CARCINOIDS: AN ASSESSMENT OF MORTALITY

John R. Iacovino, M.D.

"As the tumor (bronchial adenoma) has generally a low-grade of malignancy, the prognosis is generally good, even with regional nodal metastases."[1]

Introduction

The preceding statement typifies both the confusion in nomenclature and erroneous mortality assessment of bronchial tumors that appear in the medical literature. A true bronchial adenoma is pathologically and clinically benign. Other tumors in this heterogenous group (bronchial adenoma) exhibiting lymph node metastasis have a dismal prognosis.

The purpose of this review is to assist the medical director and underwriter in the mortality assessment of bronchial adenomas with an emphasis on bronchial carcinoids (BC). Due to confusion in nomenclature, BC can be inappropriately underwritten as a benign tumor. The key to the successful underwriting of this impairment is correct pathological classification, as well as recognition of the highly malignant, atypical BC. This paper is divided into three parts. The first is an overview of BC, the second is an in-depth review of atypical bronchial carcinoids (ABC), and the third is the mortality assessment of typical and atypical bronchial carcinoids.

Definition

Bronchial carcinoid is one of four distinct histologic tumors classified under bronchial adenoma, a heterogeneous tumor group comprising 5% of all primary pulmonary neoplasms.[1] The remaining three are adenoid cystic carcinoma or cylindroma, mucoepidermoid carcinoma and the truly benign bronchial adenoma. The carcinoids comprise 85-90% of the total group.[2]

History

Laennec initially recognized the BC in 1831;[3] however it remained for Müller to definitively describe the tumor in 1882.[4] Nearly fifty years later, Kramer's work established BC as a distinct clinical and pathological tumor.[5] Finally, in 1972, Arrigoni defined the atypical variety.[6]

Source: J. R. Iacovino, "Bronchial Carcinoids: An Assessment of Mortality," *J. Ins. Med.*, 20, no. 1 (1988): 16-20. Reproduced with permission of author and publisher.

Pathology

BC belong to the APUD (amine precursor uptake decarboxylase) neuroendocrine group of tumors.[7] They appear to share with small cell carcinomas (oat cell) a common stem cell, the Kulchitsky cell.[8,9] This enterochromaffin cell is found in respiratory epithelium and is of neuroectodermal origin.[8] There is a spectrum of increasing malignancy from the typical, benign BC to the highly malignant, rapidly fatal, small cell carcinoma.

Histology

Differentiation between BC and small cell carcinomas of the lung is occasionally quite difficult. Eighty percent of BC have secretory granules seen on light microscopy utilizing argyrophil or argentaffin stains; however electron microscopy is, at times, needed for definitive diagnosis.[9] Several studies of long-term survival in small cell carcinoma have revealed that, in retrospect, these tumors were actually BC that were erroneously classified.[9,10] Recently, measurement of nuclear DNA has been advocated as a reliable method of differentiating between these two tumors.[7] The level has been demonstrated to increase with increasing malignant potential. Also atypical BC have been shown to have higher levels of nuclear DNA than the typical variety.

Clinical

The presentation of BC is dependent upon typical and atypical cell types as well as whether the tumor is centrally or peripherally located. Males and females appear to be equally affected, with the diagnosis usually made in the late fifth decade of life. The atypical variety presents up to five years earlier due to its aggressive, malignant behavior.[6] Central lesions manifest symptoms earlier than those of peripheral origin. Most commonly, the presenting symptoms are hemoptysis, cough and recurrent localized pneumonitis. Several authors emphasize the lapse between the onset of symptoms and diagnosis. The average delay is fourteen months; however, not uncommonly, delays of three to five years are noted.[2,11]

Radiology

The ratio of central to peripheral tumors varies widely with an average of three to one.[2,9,11] BC appear as an asymptomatic coin lesion in 18 to 51% of patients.[8,11] One series revealed a 4% incidence of calcification, a finding usually considered a hallmark of benignity.[10]

Carcinoid Syndrome

The occurrence of this neuroendocrine syndrome is unusual with an overall incidence of 2-7%.[8] The majority of carcinoid syndromes are associated with hepatic metastasis; few can be produced by the primary tumor itself.[8] Other neuroendocrine secretory syndromes associated with BC are Cushing's Syndrome[2,9] and acromegaly.[12]

As previously noted, the key to underwriting BC is the identification of the atypical bronchial carcinoid (ABC) by histology. The excessive mortality of this highly malignant tumor will be discussed in this paper.

Histology

Any *one* of the following features will classify the BC as atypical.[6,9,12]

- increased mitotic activity (average one mitotic figure per one to two high power fields)
- pleomorphism of cells, hyperchromatic nuclei with prominent nucleoli and abnormal cytoplasmic — nuclei ratio
- increased cellularity with disorganization of the architecture
- spindling of cells in association with increased mitotic activity
- tumor necrosis

Another classification utilizes the depth of invasion as a guide for malignant potential.[13]

Deeply Invasive:

- tumor invades halfway thru wall of involved organ
- tumor greater than 2½ centimeters in diameter

The superficially invasive tumors do not meet the preceding criteria. The authors are of the opinion that only depth of invasion distinguishes malignant potential and propensity for metastasis. It should be noted however that their study group included carcinoids of multiple organs and may not be applicable to BC alone.

Incidence

ABC comprise between 4 and 13% of most series.[6,9,10,14] One study did, however, note a 24% occurrence.[8]

Metastasis

The incidence of regional and distant metastases in ABC is as high as 70%[6,12] with up to one third dying at an average of twenty-seven months.[6] Another group showed a 45% occurrence of deaths from metastatic disease with an average survival of thirty-three months.[9] The overall rate of metastasis appears to be between 48 and 66%.[8,14] This contrasts dramatically to the incidence of local metastasis of between 3 and 11%[6,8] and distant metastasis of 2.3%[14] in typical BC. Using the deeply invasive — superficially invasive classification, 85% of the former manifested either local or distant metastatic spread whereas the latter had less than 1%.[13] Okike noted not a single recurrence nor lymphatic permeation if the primary tumor was less than 3 centimeters.[8] Metastasis most commonly involves permeation of the local lymphatics with extension to regional lymph nodes. Distant spread is most commonly noted in vertebrae, ribs, sternum and liver.[13] In contrast to most other osseous metastasis, that from BC is osteoclastic.[15] Carcinoid syndrome is usually associated with hepatic involvement. It is important to note that the lung itself can be the end organ for metastatic spread from primary carcinoids in the stomach, large and small intestine, appendix and ovary.[13]

Mortality

Two papers, one by McCaughan[8] the other by Okike[14], are the basis for this mortality evaluation of BC. The former presented disease-free actuarial survival curves by the method of Kaplan and Meier. In the latter, the method of calculating survival is not known nor is it noted if survival is disease-free.

McCaughan used median age, Okike mean age. The effect of these in calculating expected mortality is important due to the very wide age range in subjects studied, 12-82 and 15-73 respectively. The mean age is an arithmetic mean of all ages, whereas the median represents the middlemost value for age after they have been ranked in numerical order. Half the ages lie above, half below the median. The median is a measure of central tendency, and is unaffected by extremely low or high ages. Therefore, in calculating expected mortality rates in studies with wide age ranges, the median age is more representative of the true expected mortality rate than is the mean age.

The mean mortality rate could not be calculated for either of these studies due to the paucity of detailed age and sex distribution. The inability to calculate a mean mortality rate can lead to underestimation of the true expected mortality rate and an overestimation of mortality ratios and excess deaths, with the median age the lesser offender. For this mortality analysis the expected mortality rate is adjusted for the ratio of males and females in each study.

The United States Population Life Table for 1979-81 was used for both studies. McCaughan's series was published in 1984, Okike in 1976. Using this table, the former mortality ratios and excess deaths are probably slightly underestimated, the latter slightly overestimated. Were the 1975-80 Select and Ultimate table used, the mortality ratios would have been two and one-half to three times higher.

Finally, the differences in lymph node metastases (LNM) needs to be addressed. McCaughan noted a 11% incidence of LNM in his typical BC group. No breakdown of regional versus distant metastasis is given. Okike's typical BC group had a 5.4% incidence of LNM with 3.4% local and 2% distant.

Discussion

Clearly, it behooves the medical director to request the surgical pathology report on any bronchial adenoma or carcinoid to evaluate both the histologic type, looking for the hallmarks of atypia, and the presence of lymphatic permeation and local LNM. Controversy does exist in using the atypical versus the depth of invasion classifications. From an underwriting standpoint, the histologic classification is more appropriate since pathology reports rarely, if ever, describe the depth of invasion in BC.

The tables illustrate the single-year and 5-year interval mortality ratios and excess deaths for two groups of typical BC, a single group of atypical BC and a mixed group with and without LNM. The confounding variables in each group have been noted.

It is abundantly clear that typical BC have superior survival when compared to both the mixed groups and atypicals alone.

In McCaughan's typical group, Table 149K1-1, the excess mortality was exclusively in the second 5-year interval, with no deaths noted through year five. Late mortality was likely due to those typical BC that exhibited LNM. Regrettably, McCaughan did not breakdown his metastasis into local and distant as did Okike. As previously noted, the life table used may have slightly underestimated the study's mortality. Conversely, the lack of a mean mortality rate has the potential of greatly overestimating the mortality.

The study by Okike, Table 149K1-2, is superb in that it gives a 25-year follow-up of typical BC. Unfortunately, only 5-year cumulative survival percentages are given, except for the 10- to 20-year interval. In contrast to McCaughan's typicals, this group's mortality in interval 0-5 was approximately 200%, despite having about one half the number of metastases. The 5-10 year interval mortality ratios for each were quite similar. It is important to note that Okike's mortality may be considerably overestimated due to both the mean age factor as well as the life table used. Clearly beyond year 10 there is no excess mortality in typical BC.

Thus it is appropriate to rate, as a standard risk, those typical BC that have no lymphatic invasion. Typicals with LNM could be either declined until the end of 10 years or be approached with aggressive, up front, flat extras to cover the small, later mortality.

TABLE 149K1-1

TYPICAL BRONCHIAL CARCINOIDS (McCAUGHAN)

Confounding Variables	Interval Start-End	Mortality Ratios			Excess Death Rates	
		Interval	Geo. Ave. Ann.	Cumulative	Interval	Geo. Ave. Ann.
	t to t+Δt	$100(q/q')$	$100(\bar{q}/\bar{q}')$	$100(Q/Q')$	$1000(q-q')$	$1000(\bar{q}-\bar{q}')$
• Metastasis — 11%	0-1	0%	—	0%	0	—
• Age — Median	1-2	0	—	0	0	—
• Study Year — 1984	2-3	0	—	0	0	—
• Disease-free survival	3-4	0	—	0	0	—
	4-5	0	—	0	0	—
	5-6	0	—	0	0	—
	6-7	370	—	70	40	—
	7-8	0	—	59	0	—
	8-9	540	—	133	77	—
	9-10	0	—	115	0	—
	0-5	0	0%	0	—	0
	5-10	170	174	114	—	12

160

TYPICAL BRONCHIAL CARCINOIDS (OKIKE)

Confounding Variables	Interval Start-End	Mortality Ratios			Excess Death Rates	
		Interval	Geo. Ave. Ann.	Cumulative	Interval	Geo. Ave. Ann.
	t to t+Δt	100(q/q')	100(q̄/q̄')	100(Q/Q')	1000(q–q')	1000(q̄–q̄')
• Metastasis	0-5	200%	205%	200%	—	6
3.4% Local	5-10	164	166	176	—	6
					9	
2.0% Distant	10-20	78	80	107	—	0
• Age — Mean	20-25	89	89	100	—	0
• Study Year — 1976						
• Type of survival unknown						

Note: Definition of Variables in Tables 149K1-1 through 149K1-5.

Mortality Ratio — The ratio of the number of deaths observed to the number of deaths expected.

Excess Death Rate — The number of extra deaths that occur per 1000 individuals exposed to the risk of death per year.

t — time in year intervals
q' — Expected interval mortality rate
q — Observed interval mortality rate
q̄' — Expected geometric average annual mortality rate
q̄ — Observed geometric average annual mortality rate
Q' — Expected cumulative mortality rate
Q — Observed cumulative mortality rate

In contrast to the typical BC, the atypicals, Table 149K1-3, exhibited their preponderant mortality in the first five years due to their highly aggressive tumor biology. After the fifth year no further deaths were noted. For underwriting purposes it would be ideal to have further follow-up to ascertain the long-term prognosis of this tumor. Possibly they could be declined for the first five to seven years, then insured with moderate flat extras for the next few years. Those atypicals with LNM that survived into the second 5-year interval also appear insurable since, due to the aggressiveness of the tumor, one would expect all the mortality to be early as in the nonmetastatic atypicals.

For illustration purposes I have included two combined groups — typical and atypical BC with and without LNM, Tables 149K1-4 and 149K1-5. It must be reemphasized that under no circumstances should BC be underwritten without the surgical pathology. The combined BC group without LNM has an erratic mortality somewhere between pure groups of typicals and atypicals. The mixed group with LNM reveals an inferior survival comparable to the atypicals alone.

The true bronchial adenoma is benign. No instance of spread beyond the bronchial wall nor metastasis has been reported.[16]

Mucoepidermoid tumors generally have a low malignant potential although cases of highly malignant lesions with metastases are reported.[2,16] Usually they are centrally located and arise from mucous glands. Pathologically, they can resemble salivary gland mucoepidermoid carcinomas. Their clinical behavior correlates well with the degree of invasiveness at surgery rather than with any specific cytologic feature.[16]

Cylindromas are highly malignant, with 50% being unresectable at surgery due to extensive submucosal and lymphatic involvement and regional lymph node metastases.[2,16] Due to the greater tendency for distant metastasis, only 50 to 60% survive five years.[16] As with the mucoepidermoid tumor they arise from bronchial glands and resemble salivary and lacrimal gland tumors. Occasional reports of the carcinoid syndrome associated with this tumor have been noted.[17]

ATYPICAL BRONCHIAL CARCINOIDS

| Confounding Variables | Interval Start-End | Mortality Ratios | | | Excess Death Rates | |
| | | Interval | Geo. Ave. Ann. | Cumulative | Interval | Geo. Ave. Ann. |
	t to t+Δt	100(q/q′)	100(q̄/q̄′)	100(Q/Q′)	1000(q–q′)	1000(q̄–q̄′)
• Metastasis — 48%	0-1	405%	—	405%	27	—
• Age — Median	1-2	395	—	395	28	—
• Study Year — 1984	2-3	1,890	—	890	187	—
• Disease-free survival	3-4	0	—	640	0	—
	4-5	780	—	630	85	—
	5-6	1,810	—	760	230	—
	6-7	0	—	625	0	—
	7-8	0	—	525	0	—
	8-9	0	—	450	0	—
	9-10	0	—	390	0	—
	0-5	610	690%	610	—	61
	5-10	325	355	420	—	40

COMBINED TYPICAL AND ATYPICAL BRONCHIAL CARCINOIDS WITHOUT LYMPH NODE METASTASIS

| Confounding Variables | Interval Start-End | Mortality Ratios | | | Excess Death Rates | |
| | | Interval | Geo. Ave. Ann. | Cumulative | Interval | Geo. Ave. Ann. |
	t to t+Δt	100(q/q′)	100(q̄/q̄′)	100(Q/Q′)	1000(q–q′)	1000(q̄–q̄′)
• Typical — Atypical	0-1	0%	—	0%	0	—
Ratio 3:1	1-2	0	—	0	0	—
• Age — Median	2-3	0	—	0	0	—
• Study Year — 1984	3-4	500	—	144	46	—
• Disease-free survival	4-5	0	—	111	0	—
	5-6	290	—	146	26	—
	6-7	140	—	144	6	—
	7-8	0	—	121	0	—
	8-9	360	—	156	46	—
	9-10	0	—	135	0	—
	0-5	79	78%	79	—	0
	5-10	157	160	141	—	9

TABLE 149K1-5

COMBINED TYPICAL AND ATYPICAL BRONCHIAL CARCINOIDS WITHOUT LYMPH NODE METASTASIS

| Confounding Variables | Interval Start-End | Mortality Ratios | | | Excess Death Rates | |
| | | Interval | Geo. Ave. Ann. | Cumulative | Interval | Geo. Ave. Ann. |
	t to t+Δt	100(q/q')	100(q̄/q̄')	100(Q/Q')	1000(q–q')	1000(q̄–q̄')
• Typical-Atypical	0-1	0%	—	0%	0	—
Ratio 3:1	1-2	980	—	510	84	—
• Metastasis	2-3	1,010	—	660	95	—
Typical — 11%	3-4	0	—	475	0	—
Atypical — 48%	4-5	790	—	510	80	—
• Age — Median	5-6	1,140	—	585	141	—
• Study Year — 1984	6-7	0	—	480	0	—
• Disease-free survival	7-8	0	—	405	0	—
	8-9	860	—	430	134	—
	9-10	0	—	375	0	—
	0-5	510	560%	510	—	48
	5-10	365	400	410	—	48

REFERENCES

1. J. Rozenman, R. Pausner, Y. Lieberman, G. Gamsu, "Bronchial Adenoma," *Chest,* 92, no. 1 (1987): 145-47.

2. G. A. Tolis, W. A. Fry, L. Head, T. W. Shield, "Bronchial Adenomas," *Surg. Gynecol. Obstet.,* 134 (1972): 605-10.

3. R. T. H. Laennec, *Traité de l'auscultation médiate et des maladies des poumons et du coeur,* Third Edition, Vol. 1: 250 (Paris, Chaude, 1831).

4. H. Müller, *Zur entstehungsgeschichte der bronchialerweiterrungen,* (E. Germany, Ermsleben Halle, 1982).

5. R. Kramer, "Adenoma of Bronchus," *Ann. Otol. Rhinol. Laryngol.,* 39 (1930): 689-92.

6. M. G. Arrigoni, L. B. Wollner, P. E. Bernatz, "Atypical Carcinoid Tumors of the Lung," *J. Thorac. Cardiovasc. Surg.,* 64 (1972): 413-21.

7. L. F. DeCaro, R. Paladugu, J. R. Benfield, L. Lovisatti, H. Pak, R. L. Teplitz, "Typical and Atypical Carcinoids Within the Pulmonary APUD Tumor Spectrum," *J. Thorac. Cardiovasc. Surg.,* 86 (1983): 528-36.

8. B. C. McCaughan, N. Martini, M. S. Bains, "Bronchial Carcinoids," *J. Thorac. Cardiovasc. Surg.,* 89 (1985): 8-17.

9. E. W. Wilkins, H. C. Grillo, A. C. Moncure, J. G. Scannell, "Changing Times in Surgical Management of Bronchopulmonary Carcinoid Tumor," *Ann. Thorac. Surg.,* 38, no. 4 (1984): 339-44.

10. R. M. Lawson, L. Ramanathan, G. Hurley, K. W. Hinson, S. C. Lennox, "Bronchial Adenoma: Review of an 18 Year Experience at the Brompton Hospital," *Thorax,* 31(1976): 245-53.

11. J. N. Baldwin, O. F. Grimes, "Bronchial Adenomas," *Surg. Gynecol. Obstet.,* 124 (1967): 813-18.

12. T. R. Todd, J. D. Cooper, D. Weissberg, N. C. Delarue, F. G. Pearson, "Bronchial Carcinoid Tumors," *J. Thorac. Cardiovasc. Surg.,* 79 (1980): 532-36.

13. S. I. Hajdu, S. J. Winawer, W. P. Myers, "Carcinoid Tumors," *Am. J. Clin. Pathol.,* 61 (1974): 521-28.

14. N. Okike, P. E. Bernatz, L. B. Woolner, "Carcinoid Tumors of the Lung," *Ann. Thorac. Surg.,* 22, no. 3 (1976): 270-77.

15. R. G. Fraser, J. A. P. Pare, *Diagnosis of Diseases of the Chest,* 1st ed. (Philadelphia, W. B. Saunders Company, 1970), pp. 724-30.

16. R. H. Ochs, G. G. Pietra, "Neoplasms of the Lung Other Than Bronchogenic Carcinoma," A. P. Fishman, *Pulmonary Diseases and Disorders* (New York, McGraw-Hill, 1980), pp. 1439-41.

17. G. L. Snider, *Clinical Pulmonary Medicine,* 1st ed. (Boston, Little Brown and Company, 1981), p. 415.

ADVANCED COLORECTAL CANCER AND VITAMIN C

Richard B. Singer, M.D.

References:

1. C. G. Moertel, T. R. Fleming, E. T. Creagan et al., "High-Dose Vitamin C versus Placebo in the Treatment of Patients with Advanced Cancer Who Have Had No Prior Chemotherapy," *New Engl. J. Med.*, 312 (1985): 137-41.

2. R. B. Singer, L. Levinson, eds., *Medical Risks: Patterns of Mortality and Survival* (Lexington, MA, Lexington Books, 1976). See Cancer Mortality Abstracts (100), pp. 1-1 to 1-5, 1-30 and 1-48 to 1-51. Source of data: life table computer output for End Results Group Report No. 4, M.H. Myers, personal communication to the editors.

Purpose of This Abstract: To report comparative mortality results of a randomized double-blind study of 100 patients with advanced colorectal cancer and no prior chemotherapy, the therapeutic agent being 10 grams of Vitamin C daily, and to contrast these results with mortality in a much larger combined series of patients with advanced cancer of the colon from Report No. 4 of the End Results Study Group.

Patients Studied: This recent study at the Mayo Clinic was undertaken to find out if beneficial effects of Vitamin C in prolonging survival of patients with advanced cancer, as previously reported by Linus Pauling, could be confirmed. Patients were selected only if they had advanced cancer with histological proof that the cancer originated in the colon or rectum and was beyond any reasonable hope of curative surgery or radiation. None had received chemotherapy; all were ambulatory and capable of taking oral medication. The ethical justification for not offering chemotherapy was the fact that no drug had been shown to produce substantial palliative effect or increased survival in patients with advanced cancer of the large bowel. Of the 100 patients stratified by age, interval from the date unresectable disease was diagnosed, site of metastasis, and measurable size of malignant disease, 51 were assigned to Vitamin C

Source: R. B. Singer, "Advanced Colorectal Cancer and Vitamin C," *J. Ins. Med.*, 21 (1989): 127-30. Reproduced with permission of author and publisher.

therapy, 10 grams daily, and 49 were assigned to placebo (lactose). Assignment was made on a randomized, double-blind basis. There were 57 men and 43 women; 8 patients were under age 50, 55 were in the age range 50-69 years, and 37 were age 70 or older.

Follow-up: Was carried out through examination and chest X-ray at 4 weeks and then at intervals of 8 weeks until death or to 39 months, at which time there were only 5 survivors, all in the placebo group. No patient was lost to follow-up. Progression of disease was defined by one or more of the following: new areas of metastatic tumor; increase by more than 50% in the product of perpendicular diameters of any area of known malignant disease; loss of body weight by 10% or more; substantial worsening of symptoms or performance status. Cumulative survival was derived through the Kaplan-Meier method.

Results: Table 150K1-1 gives reconstructed life table data for the Vitamin C and placebo groups, based on the distribution data and total 1-year survival rates in Table 1 of the article, and the cumulative survival curves of Figure 2. The latter show the typical "ladder" Kaplan-Meier shape, in which each death in each treatment group should be nearly 0.02 (1/51 or 1/49), since there were no live withdrawals. Figure 2 appears to show P=0 for the Vitamin C group and P=0.12 for the placebo group at 2 years (6 survivors). At 39 months there appear to be 0+5=5 total survivors, which leaves 95 deaths in the total series. The total of "85" deaths given in the text must be a typographical error for the total derived from Figure 2. There are slight inconsistencies in the 1-year survival rates for the total series and its subgroups in Table 1, but I believe the reconstructed data for d are accurate in Tables 150K1-1 and 150K1-2, also the data for ℓ at the beginning of the second year, and all values of q, since w=0 in all duration cells. A quinquennial age/sex distribution has been approximated from the broad age groups and overall sex distribution in Table 1, and d' has been derived from the actual or estimated ℓ and mortality rates (q') matched by age and sex in the 1979-81 U.S. Life Tables for the white population. As a result, both q' and d' should be as accurate as possible in Table 150K1-1 and the upper part of Table 150K1-2. Because there are no data on differences in age/sex distribution in the other subgroups, it has been necessary to assume an approximate, constant value of q' in the lower part of Table 150K1-2.

As would be anticipated for advanced cancer of almost any site, excess mortality was extremely high, with EDR nearly 500 extra deaths per 1000 in both groups in the first year, and even higher in the second year (100% mortality for the 24 1-year survivors in the Vitamin C group). As the authors emphasize, there was no statistically significant difference between the Vitamin C and placebo, either for survival or for survival without evidence of progression (their Figure 1). Mortality in the second year was actually somewhat less in the placebo group, but EDR was still 700 per 1000 and the mortality ratio 1,890%. With q' less than 10% of the magnitude of the very high mortality rate, q, EDR is a more useful index of excess mortality than the mortality ratio, when one compares excess mortality by age or sex, in the upper half of Table 150K1-2. If first year mortality for other factors is analyzed (lower half of Table 150K1-2) it is seen that EDR is lower for metastasis in the lung than in the liver or other sites, and higher in cases with Broder's histological grading of 3-4, indicating a higher degree of malignant growth. EDR also decreases with interval from diagnosis to the start of therapy, an important finding that implies higher short-interval mortality in the early intervals from diagnosis to about 14 months.

The number of patients is much too small in this series to attempt to establish a pattern of mortality by duration. For this I have recalculated data from the End Results Group, Report No. 4 (reference 2). Comparative mortality is shown in Table 150K1-3 for 4,523 patients diagnosed as having advanced cancer of the colon in 1950-64 and followed to 1970. Analysis by age and sex shows only modest differences in EDR, but a marked decrease in mortality ratio with increasing age and from male to female (because of the age/sex pattern for q'). However, as shown in Table 150K1-3, EDR decreases steadily with duration, from a maximum of 712 extra deaths per 1000 per year to 132 per 1000 in the 5th year. Not shown in the table is a continued downward trend to 107 in the 6th year and 66 in the 7th year, after which EDR tends to level off at about 50 per 1000. There were only 60 survivors at the end of 10 years, the 10-year cumulative survival rate being 0.023 and the survival ratio, 3.8%. This consistent trend contrasts with what appears as a somewhat lower EDR in the trial series of 100 patients during the first year of observation, and higher EDR in the second year (Table 150K1-1). In all probability the size of the series is simply too small to permit a valid estimate of trend by annual duration.

It should be noted that the oral drug used had to be discontinued after a median duration of 2.5 months in the Vitamin C group, and a median of 3.6 months in the placebo group. Evidence of disease progression was the most common reason for discontinuance. Chemotherapy was used in about 58% of patients in each group after the Vitamin C or placebo was stopped. The median survival time until there was evidence of progression was shorter in the Vitamin C than in the placebo group, 2.9 and 4.1 months, respectively. In none of the 38 patients with areas of malignancy that were measurable at entry did evidence of regression occur (these patients were randomized in equal numbers to the two groups).

Comment: Extremely high mortality as observed in this type of advanced cancer has little relevance for medical selection for life insurance, except to act as a caution to the underwriter who might be so bold as to make an offer to an applicant with this type of history who may have survived more than 5 or 10 years. Since Linus Pauling is a Nobel laureate his report of the beneficial effects of Vitamin C in advanced cancer attracted much public attention. The results reported here were the second clinical trial of Vitamin C carried out at the Mayo Clinic, in an effort to duplicate more closely the conditions thought by Cameron and Pauling to be most favorable for prolonging survival. The report by Cameron and Pauling may be found in *Proc. Nat. Acad. Sci.*, 75 (1978): 4538-72. Apparently Dr. Cameron supervised the treatment of patients with advanced cancer at the Vale of Leven Hospital in Scotland, and Pauling's location is given as the Linus Pauling Institute of Science and Medicine. Tabular data are given in this 1978 report for the age, sex, cancer site and survival time in days for each of the 100 patients treated with Vitamin C, and mean survival time of 1,000 historical control patients, matched by sex, site, and age within 5 years. Based on date of "untreatability" the mean survival time was calculated at more than 293 days for the 100 patients who received Vitamin C (8 patients were still alive at the end), and only 38 days from the 1,000 historical controls. Mean survival time is a poor index of survival, in my opinion, but cumulative survival is shown in graphs for the 8 different cancer sites, and these confirm a 1-year control survival that appears to be under 1% for all sites except breast. This makes it plain that there must be an extreme antiselection bias in the historical controls, because survival is 0.245 in Table 150K1-3 (the complement of q as a decimal). In their text Cameron and Pauling state that 22 of their 100 patients treated with ascorbate survived 1 year, very close to the p value derived from Table 150K1-3. It is my opinion that the survival reported by Cameron and Pauling for their patients treated with Vitamin C is actually representative of survival as found in patients with advanced cancer in general, and specifically in advanced cancer of the colon, as shown by the results in this abstract. I cannot conjecture why the "date of untreatability" was determined so late in the course of the disease of the patients selected as historical controls at the Vale of Leven Hospital, but this bias, whatever it is due to, is clearly demonstrated in terms of comparative survival and mortality. When short-term mortality is extremely high, the timing of entry into a study becomes of critical importance. This is shown in Table 150K1-2 in the wide range of EDR by interval from diagnosis. Moertel et al. randomized their patients with respect to interval from diagnosis to start of their clinical trial, and thus avoided any bias of this sort. It is remarkable that neither set of authors considered their mortality and survival results in comparative terms in relation to the extensive experience published for advanced cancer of the colon and other sites.

I have another reason for displaying the comparative mortality by duration in Table 150K1-3, all ages and both sexes combined. Cancer of the colon is found in a wide age range of patients, although it is predominantly a disease of older persons, age 60 and up. When the mean q' values are examined in the life tables for each of five age groups (<45, 45-54, 55-64, 65-74, and 75 up), separate male and female, they are seen to increase with duration in a fairly smooth fashion, as one would expect from the annual increase of q' seen in population or other life tables at ages over 35. This increase averages about 10% per year. But the mean q' in Table 150K1-3, all age/sex groups combined, *decreases* from 43 per 1000 in the first year to 34 per 1000 in the second, and in the fifth year q' is still below 43, with an annual increase of only about 4%. Each year of follow-up each survivor is a year older, and his individual q' has increased about 10%. Why is the mean q' *lower* at durations 1-5 years than it

is in the first year? The explanation is that the age distribution of the survivors changes by duration in such a way that there is a shift to a relative increase in younger patients, and a decrease in older patients. Thus, in males, I have calculated a mean age of 66.4 years at duration 0, and an actual *decrease* in mean age of the survivors at duration 1 year to 65.5; at duration 4 years the mean age is still only 66.8 years, although all of these men are 4 years older than they were at entry. Furthermore, the mean q' of 51 per 1000 for the *men,* based on their entry age, corresponds to age 70.6 years in the 1959-61 U.S. Life Tables for the white male population. The tabular q' for the mean age of 66.4 years is just under 38 per 1000. The reader should understand the importance of these facts when q' must be estimated from the mean age at entry and when q' must be estimated by duration, if the cohort being followed has a wide age range, and data are not given for age distribution or for follow-up by age group. I have accumulated examples of empirical relationships for mean q' and mean age, and progression of q' in a variety of diseases, and some of these results have been used in the chapter on cardiovascular diseases in the new *Medical Risks* monograph. However, these empirical relations are dependent on the characteristics of the initial age distribution and the patterns of mortality by duration in the various age groups of the male and female portions of this series. The problem of achieving an accurate estimate of q' in the first year and by duration, all ages combined, is therefore a complex and difficult one. I hope to write an article on this subject that may be of practical help to future makers of mortality abstracts, but I have not yet accumulated sufficient examples to attempt this.

TABLE 150K1-1

COMPARATIVE MORTALITY BY DURATION AND VITAMIN C OR PLACEBO TREATMENT

Interval Start-End	No. Alive at Start	Number of Deaths		Mortality Ratio	Mean Annual Mortality Rate per 1000		
		Observed	Expected*		Observed	Expected	Excess
t to t+Δt	ℓ	d	d'	100(d/d')	q	q'	(q–q')
VITAMIN C (10 g. daily)							
0-1 yr.	51	27	1.78	1,520%	529	35	494
1-2 yrs.	24	24	0.94	2,600	1,000	39	961
PLACEBO							
0-1 yr.	49	26	1.72	1,510%	531	35	496
1-2 yrs.	23	17	0.90	1,890	739	39	700

* Expected deaths based on 1979-81 U.S. Life Tables, white males and white females.

COMPARATIVE FIRST-YEAR MORTALITY, BOTH TRIAL GROUPS COMBINED

Factor	No. Alive at Start	Number of Deaths		Mortality Ratio	Mean Annual Mortality Rate per 1000		
		Observed	Expected*		Observed	Expected	Excess
	ℓ	d	d′	100(d/d′)	q	q′	(q–q′)
Age							
<50	8	6	0.025	24,000%	750	3	747
50-69	55	27	0.93	2,900	491	17	474
70 up	37	20	2.58	775	541	70	471
Sex							
Male	57	28	2.43	1,150	491	44	447
Female	43	25	1.10	2,300	581	26	555
Metastasis							
Lung	17	5	0.60	835	294	(35)	259
Liver	58	36	2.03	1,770	621	(35)	586
Other Site	25	12	0.88	1,370	480	(35)	445
Interval from Diagnosis							
<3 weeks	15	14	0.52	2,700	933	(35)	898
3-8 weeks	58	30	2.03	1,480	517	(35)	482
>8 weeks	27	9	0.94	950	333	(35)	298
Broder's Grade (Histological)							
Grade 1-2	71	31	2.48	1,250	437	(35)	402
Grade 3-4	23	18	0.80	2,200	783	(35)	748

* Expected deaths based on 1979-81 U.S. Life Tables, white males and white females. Rates in parentheses based on total age/sex distribution.

COMPARATIVE MORTALITY BY DURATION, ALL PATIENTS, CANCER OF COLON, DISTANT METASTASIS, FROM END RESULTS STUDY GROUP, REPORT NO. 4 (ref. 2)

Interval Start-End	No. Alive at Start	Exposure Pt.-yrs.	Number of Deaths		Mortality Ratio	Mean Annual Mortality Rate per 1000		
			Observed	Expected*		Observed	Expected	Excess
t to t+Δt	ℓ	E	d	d′	100(d/d′)	q	q′	(q–q′)
0-1 yr.	4,523	4,517.0	3,411	196.0	1,740%	755	43	712
1-2 yrs.	1,100	1,099.0	604	37.9	1,590	550	34	516
2-3	494	493.0	189	17.6	1,070	383	36	347
3-4	303	302.0	80	11.7	685	265	39	226
4-5	221	220.0	38	9.0	420	173	41	132

* Expected deaths based on concurrent U.S. white population rates, 1950-70, matched by age and sex.

SURVIVAL DETERMINANTS IN PATIENTS WITH NEPHROBLASTOMA (WILMS' TUMOR)

Daniel M. Hays, M.D.

Nephroblastoma is the only renal neoplasm seen with frequency in childhood[1] and has an incidence of approximately 7.8/million children/year in the United States; and a relatively similar incidence worldwide. The median patient age at discovery of this tumor is three years. The diagnosis is rarely made after the age of seven.

Chromosomal and biochemical studies suggest that there is an uncommon "heritable" form and a much more common "non-heritable" form of Wilms' tumor.[2,3] In the former, the neoplasm develops at a younger age and is more frequently bilateral and multicentric than in the "non-heritable" form. The chance of offspring developing Wilms' tumor in the heritable group is approximately 30% vs. <2% in the non-heritable form with unilateral disease.[4,5]

A group of congenital anomalies are associated with the occurrence of Wilms' tumor, but are found in a relatively small percentage of these children.[6] Hemihypertrophy (asymmetrical enlargement) occurs in 2.9% and aniridia in 1.1% of these children, neither condition having a known effect on long-range survival. Patients with Wilms' tumor and aniridia frequently have a gene defect, an identifiable 11p13 chromosomal deletion.

Clinical Presentation and Diagnosis

Children with nephroblastoma are usually identified initially because of the discovery of an abdominal, usually subcostal, mass. Gross hematuria, hypertension, recognized weight loss, or significant fever occur in less than 10%.

The major differential diagnostic possibilities in such patients include neuroblastoma and forms of benign renal disease. Ultrasonography will demonstrate that the mass is solid or cystic, excretory urograms establish its connection with the kidney, computerized tomography delineates its extent and MRI elucidates the possible involvement of adjacent structures or nodes. Venography may identify extension into the inferior vena cava through the renal veins, and angiography is used in children with bilateral masses to facilitate attempts to preserve renal tissue on both sides when bilateral tumors are found. The diagnosis is routinely confirmed by nephrectomy without prior biopsy.

Significance of Specific Pathologic Features

By approximately 1976, a perplexing situation had developed in the management of Wilms' tumor in the U.S. At this time, if one accepted the results of the most favorable arm in all of the randomized trials of the National Wilms' Tumor Study (NWTS), the overall survival rate among patients with Wilms' tumor was approximately 90% with the patients on relatively non-intensive chemotherapy regiments. Attempting to improve upon this result with more intensive regimens would place 90% of the patients at risk from increased toxicity, not previously a significant problem in the NWTS. Thus, increasing the intensity of therapy might have deleterious overall effects. This quandary was resolved when Beckwith and Palmer, following analysis of 427 specimens from the NWTS, found that they could "blindly" identify a group consisting of approximately 11% of the total patients in the study whose presence contributed over 52% of the mortality.[7] This observation has been confirmed in subsequent NWTS trials and has resulted in worldwide acceptance of the concept that there are two broad histologic categories, i.e., favorable and unfavorable (as well as several subcategories of the latter), and that these two major categories are of paramount prognostic significance. The 11% with unfavorable histologic features have been divided into three subcategories: anaplastic, clear cell, and rhabdoid tumors. Patients with anaplastic tumors, except when disseminated at diagnosis, have survival rates only slightly lower than those of patients in the favorable category. The clear cell sarcomas of kidney metastasize more commonly than favorable forms, particularly to osseous structures. Rhabdoid tumors have the lowest survival rates. It is debatable whether the latter two tumors should be included under the "umbrella" of the term Wilms' tumor.

The National Wilms' Tumor Study Group: Supported in part by USPHS Grant CA-42326.

Source: D. M. Hays, "Survival Determinants in Patients with Nephroblastoma (Wilms' Tumor)," *J. Ins. Med.*, 21 (1989): 72-77. Reproduced with permission of author and publisher.

Staging

A staging system based both on extent of disease and the initial surgical procedure performed, was developed by the NWTS.[8] The distinction between favorable and unfavorable histology was incorporated into the system for assigning therapy regimens in the third NWTS. Otherwise the classification (Table 169K1-1) has been altered relatively little during the 20-year course of this group's activity. The histologic distinctions recognized by Beckwith and Palmer can be correlated with stage or disease, i.e., in NWTS-2, 2/3 of the patients with favorable histologic patterns had early stage lesions, whereas 50% of those with unfavorable histologic patterns had an advanced stage at diagnosis.

TABLE 169K1-1

DEFINITIONS OF STAGES* IN THE NATIONAL WILMS' TUMOR STUDY

I. Tumor limited to kidney and completely excised.

   The surface of the renal capsule is intact. Tumor was not ruptured before or during removal. There is no residual tumor apparent beyond the margins of resection.

II. Tumor extends beyond the kidney but is completely excised.

   There is regional extension of the tumor, i.e., penetration through the outer surface of the renal capsule into perirenal soft tissues. Vessels outside the kidney substance are infiltrated or contain tumor thrombus. The tumor may have been biopsied or there has been local spillage of tumor confined to the flank. There is no residual tumor apparent at or beyond the margins of excision.

III. Residual non-hematogenous tumor confined to abdomen.

   Any one or more of the following occur:

   a. Lymph nodes on biopsy are found to be involved in the hilus, the peri-aortic chains, or beyond.

   b. There has been diffuse peritoneal contamination by tumor such as by spillage of tumor beyond the flank before or during surgery; or by tumor growth that has penetrated through the peritoneal surface.

   c. Implants are found on the peritoneal surfaces.

   d. The tumor extends beyond the surgical margins either microscopically or grossly.

   e. The tumor is not completely resectable because of local infiltration into vital structures.

IV. Hematogenous metastases.

   Deposits beyond Stage III; e.g., lung, liver, bone, and brain.

V. Bilateral renal involvement at diagnosis.

The major determinants of outcome are: (a) the presence of favorable or unfavorable histologic features; (b) evidence of hematogenous metastasis; and (c) lymph node involvement. Relatively *minor* factors in determining prognosis include extension through the lumen of the renal vein to the *vena cava*, intraoperative tumor "rupture," direct abdominal extension of the tumor to adjacent organs, tumor weight, and patients age.[9] The length of this list of factors which do *not* independently influence outcome, reflects the extreme sensitivity of this tumor to chemotherapeutic agents, even when locally invasive or disseminated.

Therapy

The marked responsiveness of nephroblastoma to chemotherapy is almost unique among adult or childhood tumors. During the early history of its therapy, a five-day course of a single agent (actinomycin-D) made a major difference in outcome. Further, such responses have proved to be remarkably durable. Two-agent therapy with actinomycin-D and vincristine was demonstrated to be most effective by 1976, and subsequently, all therapy regimens included both agents. These two agents have remained the sole therapy, following surgery, for favorable-histology, limited-stage disease.

Therapy is now sharply divided between the two major histology-determined groups. The favorable group have received progressively shorter courses of chemotherapy, and reduced or absent radiotherapy. Survival rates continued to be >90% on these short and non-intensive therapy regimens. Patients in the unfavorable category have been placed on more intensive and longer chemotherapy regimens with continued use of local irradiation. The results in this minority group have been mixed, with decided improvement in some categories and little change in others.

The addition of Adriamycin to the basic regimen has resulted in minor improvement in the therapy of some categories of advanced disease (only) and the addition of cyclophosphamide has apparent usefulness in the management of clear cell and advanced stage anaplastic forms. Neither agent is now used in the management of a large majority of patients with Wilms' tumor.

There has been progressive decrease in the use of radiotherapy and of its dosage when used. At the present time, most patients with favorable histology Stage I or II

---

* Staging, which is on the basis of gross and microscopic tumor distribution, is the same for tumors with favorable or unfavorable histologic features. The patient should be characterized, however, by a statement of both criteria; e.g., Stage II, favorable histology or Stage III, unfavorable histology.

disease receive no radiotherapy and patients with favorable histology in Stage III receive relatively low-dose therapy.

Survival rates in the group with favorable histology (NWTS) have been so high that in NWTS-4, the study now in progress, one of the principal questions posed in the randomized trial is a socioeconomic one. It concerns whether a one-day continuous infusion of actinomycin-D can replace the five-day infusion regimen by which this drug has been traditionally administered, and thus reduce costs, inconvenience, and family stress.

The approach to metastatic or recurrent disease in the case of nephroblastoma is more aggressive than in most other tumors and this has been justified by favorable outcome. Historically, a majority of the patients treated with a single course of actinomycin-D, who had subsequent pulmonary metastasis, were "salvaged" by additional courses of actinomycin-D. With the exception of those patients with osseous metastases, or widespread abdominal involvement, both of which are uncommon, the results of salvage therapy following relapse are relatively good. Approximately 50% of these patients enter the group of long-range survivors. These results are the products of combinations of surgery, radiotherapy, and chemotherapy, with or without the addition of additional chemotherapeutic agents.

Survival

The survival experience in NWTS-1-3 for patients in Stages I-IV with favorable histology is illustrated in Figures 169K1-1 to 169K1-4. The influence of unfavorable histology is shown in Table 169K1-2 which provides survival data on each of the small histologic sub-types of this category when treated by two therapy regimens of NWTS-3.[9]

The European experience with Wilms' tumor is best illustrated by the results of the studies carried out by the International Society of Pediatric Oncology (SIOP) which includes major European centers.[10,11,12] These trials have concentrated on the question of the efficacy of presurgical therapy, i.e., irradiation, chemotherapy, or both, before as well as after operation. During the course of their trials, survival rates have been steadily increasing (Figure 169K1-5). The advantages of presurgical therapy have not been generally appreciated in North America; but it is apparent that the results of both forms of management in major institutions result in almost equally high rates of survival.

Survival rates in most developed countries are progressively increasing to reach levels of approximately 90%,[13] where they "plateau;" whereas in the Third World Countries, the survival rates are significantly lower.[14] Some major cancer centers attract patients in advanced stages or with otherwise complex problems, and this is reflected in lower survival rates.

Tumor recurrence occurring more than two years following the end of therapy is uncommon. The therapy of late pulmonary recurrence is reasonably effective and a survival rate of greater than 50% is expected. Abdominal relapse is less common and survival rates, lower. In addition to the influence of Stage and histology on the relapse rate, a number of local relapses have been associated with failure to follow the details of radiotherapy guidelines.[15,16] Death from Wilms' tumor more than five

FIGURE 169K1-1
STAGE I: SURVIVAL

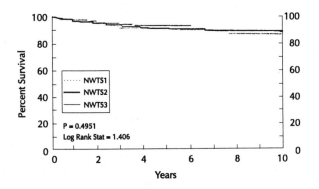

Note: Survival curves of patients in Stage I with favorable histology from NWTS-1, 2, and 3. The total number of patients located for information relative to survival in NWTS-1 (1968-74) (all stages) was 389 at onset, 336 at two years, 312 at four years, 295 at six years, 260 at eight years, and 151 at 10 years. The comparable figures for NWTS-2 (1974-80) were 650 at onset, 564 at two years, 457 at four years, 314 at six years, and 132 at eight years. The comparable figures for NWTS-3 (1980-85) were 972 at onset, 693 at two years, and 267 at four years.

FIGURE 169K1-2
STAGE II: SURVIVAL

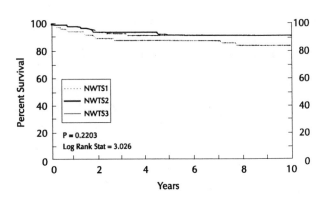

Note: Survival curves of patients in Stage II with favorable histology for NWTS-1, 2, and 3. (See Note for Figure 169K1-1.)

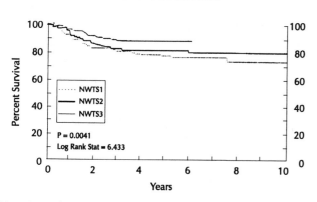

FIGURE 169K1-3
STAGE III: SURVIVAL

Note: Survival curves of patients in Stage III with favorable histology for NWTS-1, 2, and 3. (See Note for Figure 169K1-1.)

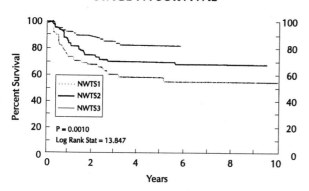

FIGURE 169K1-4
STAGE IV: SURVIVAL

Note: Survival curves of patients in Stage IV with favorable histology for NWTS-1, 2, and 3. (See Note for Figure 169K1-1.)

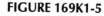

FIGURE 169K1-5

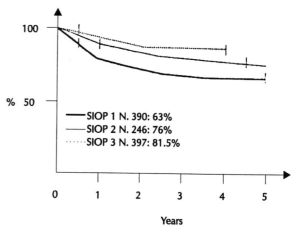

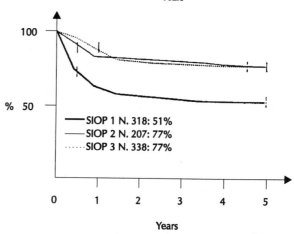

Note: Actuarial survival curves (top) and disease-free survival curves (bottom) in studies carried out by the International Society of Pediatric Oncology (SIOP) with 390 patients entered in the first study (1971-74); 246 in the second study (1974-76); and 397 in the fifth study (1977-80). The survival curves include patients in all stages. The recurrence-free survival curves do not include patients in Stage IV at diagnosis.

years following the end of therapy is a reportable occurrence.

Second Malignant Neoplasms and Other Long-Term Adverse Events

A "follow-up" study of 2,438 patients enrolled in NWTS-1-3 between October, 1969 and December, 1982, identified the occurrence of 15 second malignant neoplasms (SMN).[17] According to U.S. incidence rates for 1973-77, the expected rate of new neoplasms in this group would be 1.77, resulting in a relative risk of 8.5 with a 95% confidence interval (CI) of 4.7-14.0. The

cumulative risk of SMN at 10 years was 1%. Among those patients who received irradiation in their initial treatment, the relative risk compared to standard rates were 12/1.11=10.8 (95% CI=5.6-18.9), and for those who did not receive irradiation, 3/0.60=5.0 (95% CI=1.0-14.6). Among the 15 patients in whom SMN occurred, the original disease process was bilateral in four and multicentric in one. Seven of the 15 patients who developed SMN died from 0.2 to 0.9 years from the time of diagnosis of the SMN. Eight are alive, including four greater than four years and three greater than five years since the appearance of the SMN.

Among the 15 patients with SMN in the NWTS, 12 had received irradiation which was, in almost all instances, of a higher dosage than would have been administered in subsequent NWTS studies. In addition to

(Figures 169K1-1-4 provided by Dr. Nathan Kobrinsky and the NWTS Committee)

WILMS' TUMOR: THE UNFAVORABLE HISTOLOGIC FORMS IN THE NWTS
RELAPSE-FREE SURVIVAL AND SURVIVAL BY HISTOLOGIC SUBTYPE WITH TWO TREATMENT REGIMENS

Histology*	Stage**	Therapy Regimen**	# Patients Evaluated	% Relapse-Free		% Alive	
				2 Yrs.	4 Yrs.	2 Yrs.	4 Yrs.
Anaplastic	I	DD-RT	10	80.0	80.0	77.8	77.8
		J	5	100.0	100.0	100.0	100.0
Anaplastic	II-IV	DD-RT	21	36.7	36.7	43.6	37.4
		J	12	82.5	82.5	81.8	81.8
Clear cell sarcoma	All	DD-RT	25	75.3	70.6	87.8	74.8
		J	25	73.9	60.3	95.7	76.1
Rhabdoid sarcoma	All	DD-RT	13	23.1	23.1	33.8	25.4
		J	18	26.7	26.7	25.9	25.9

* According to Central Pathology (NWTS)

** Final Stage and regimen reported by the institution.

Condensed table from D'Angio, et al, *Cancer* (in press) (Reference #9)

actinomycin-D and vincristine, four of them had received Adriamycin, a drug employed only in advanced disease. Eight of the 15 patients with SMN were in Stage III at diagnosis whereas the incidence of Stage III in the total study population is <25%. In 13 of these 15 patients, the SMN occurred within seven years of the initial registration in the NWTS.

Data regarding SMN for decades after the first 10 years post-diagnosis are less complete. The Late-Effects Study Group, an international body representing large pediatric centers, initially reported a 3.3% incidence of SMN at a point 20 years following diagnosis for *all* childhood cancer survivors.[18] In a more recent report, there was an 8.5% incidence of SMN at the 20 year point among children in this study who survived two years following diagnosis. However, most of the patients in this international study received more irradiation and more intensive chemotherapy than is included in either past or current Wilms' Tumor protocols.[19] Some studies suggest that familial cancer predisposition may be a major factor among patients in which SMN occurs.

Relatively acute toxic effects of therapy—cardiac, hepatic, or renal—occur in a small percent of the larger series of patients treated for Wilms' tumor. As far as can be determined, these are almost always self-limited and identified (and alleviated) during the first decade following therapy. Some musculoskeletal deformity, secondary to irradiation, is seen among Wilms' tumor survivors, particularly those treated with orthovoltage prior to 1975.[20] These have not been associated with lethal complications. Several patients with late recognition of cardiomyopathy secondary to anthrocycline therapy have been reported.[21] This would be of concern only in those patients in advanced stages of nephroblastoma in which Adriamycin was administered.

Several studies have suggested that late renal disease may result from early nephrectomy *per se*,[22] but this has not been seen in the NWTS or other large series.[23]

Summary

The responsiveness of nephroblastoma to chemotherapeutic agents has resulted in a >90% long-range survival in developed countries worldwide. Among groups of patients with localized disease and favorable histologic features, survival rates are significantly higher than this. The incidence of relapse more than five years following the end of therapy is <1%, and after 10 years, almost unknown.

Second malignancy occurs with approximately 8.5 times the frequency of rates in the general population, although only 1% of the total group of survivors are affected. Its occurrence is concentrated among those patient groups with unfavorable histology and advanced-stage disease who have received the most intensive therapy, both irradiation and chemotherapy. It primarily occurs during the initial eight years of surveillance. Other long-range untoward effects of therapy are uncommon and can be recognized in childhood.

REFERENCES

1. J. L. Young, Jr., R. W. Miller, "Incidence of Malignant Tumors in U.S. Children," *J. Pediatr.,* 86 (1975): 254.

2. N. E. Breslow, J. B. Beckwith, "Epidemiological Features of Wilms' Tumor: Results of the National Wilms' Tumor Study," *J. Natl. Cancer Inst.,* 68 (1982): 429.

3. E. Matsunaga, "Genetics of Wilms' Tumor," *Hum. Genet.,* 57 (1981): 231.

4. L. C. Strong, "Genetics of Wilms' Tumor," *Dialogues Pediatr. Urol.,* 6 (1983): 2.

5. F. P. Li, W. R. Williams, K. Gimibrere, F. Flamant, D. M. Green, A. T. Meadows, "Heritable Fraction of Unilatral Wilms' Tumor," *Pediatrics,* 81 (1988): 147-49.

6. T. W. Pendergrass, "Congenital Anomalies in Children with Wilms' Tumor: A New Survey," *Cancer,* 37 (1976): 403.

7. J. B. Beckwith, N. F. Palmer, "Histopathology and Prognosis of Wilms' Tumor," *Cancer,* 41 (1978): 1937-48.

8. G. J. D'Angio, A. E. Evans, N. Breslow, et al., "The Treatment of Wilms' Tumor: Results of the National Wilms' Tumor Study," *Cancer,* 38 (1976): 633-46.

9. G. J. D'Angio, N. Breslow, B. Beckwith, A. Evans, E. Baum, A. deLorimier, D. Fernbach, E. Hrabovsky, B. Jones, P. Kelalis, H. B. Othersen, M. Tefft, P. R. M. Thomas, "The Treatment of Wilms' Tumor: Results of the Third National Wilms' Tumor Study," *Cancer,* (in press).

10. J. Lemerle, P. A. Voute, M. F. Tournade, et al., "Preoperative Versus Postoperative Radiotherapy, Single Versus Multiple Courses of Actinomycin-D, in the Treatment of Wilms' Tumor," *Cancer,* 38 (1976): 647-54.

11. J. Lemerle, P. A. Voute, M. F. Tournade, "Effectiveness of Preoperative Chemotherapy in Wilms' Tumor: Results of an International Society of Pediatric Oncology (SIOP) Clinical Trial," *J. Clin Oncol.,* 1 (1983): 604-9.

12. D. Burger, C. G. Moorman-Voestermans, H. Mildenberger, J. Lemerle, P. A. Voute, M. F. Tournade, C. Rodary, J. F. Delemarre, B. Sandstedt, D. Sarrazin, J. M. V. Burgers, P. Bey, M. Carli, J. deKraker, "The Advantages of Preoperative Therapy in Wilms' Tumor: A Summarized Report on Clinical Trials Conducted by the International Society of Pediatric Oncology (SIOP)," *Z. Kinderchir,* 40 (1985): 170-75.

13. J. W. Clouse, P. R. M. Thomas, R. C. Griffith, C. A. Perez, T. J. Vietti, B. Fineberg, "The Changing Management of Wilms' Tumor Over a 30-Year Period (1949-78)," *Cancer,* 56 (1985): 1484-89.

14. B. de Camargo, M. L. de Andrea, E. L. F. Franco, "Catching up with History: Treatment of Wilms' Tumor in a Developing Country," *Med. Pediatr. Oncol.,* 15 (1987): 270-76.

15. T. H. Kim, G. S. Zaatari, E. S. Baum, N. Jaffe, B. Cushing, R. L. Chard, Jr., G. T. Zwiren, J. B. Beckwith, "Recurrence of Wilms' Tumor After Apparent Cure," *J. Pediatr.,* 107 (1985): 44-49.

16. J. M. V. Burgers, M. F. Tournade, P. Bey, D. Burger, M. Carli, J. F. M. Delemarre, D. Harms, B. Jereb, J. deKraker, J. Lemerle, C. G. M. Moorman-Voestermans, H. Perry, A. Rey, B. Sandstedt, D. Sarrazin, P. A. Voute, J. M. Zucker, "Abdominal Recurrences in Wilms' Tumors: A Report from the SIOP Wilms' Tumor Trials and Studies," *Radiotherapy Oncology,* 5 (1986): 175-82.

17. N. E. Breslow, P. A. Norkool, A. Olshan, A. Evans, G. J. D'Angio, "Second Malignant Neoplasms in Survivors of Wilms' Tumor: A Report From the National Wilms' Tumor Study," *J. Natl. Cancer Inst.,* 80 (1988): 592-95.

18. V. Mike, A. T. Meadows, G. J. D'Angio, "Incidence of Second Malignant Neoplasms in Children: Results of an International Study," *Lancet,* 2 (1982): 1326-31.

19. M. A. Tucker, A. T. Meadows, J. D. Boice, et al., "Cancer Risk Following Treatment of Childhood Cancer," in J. D. Boice, J. F. Fraumeni, Jr., eds., *Radiation Carcinogenesis: Epidemiology and Biological Significance* (New York, Raven Press, 1984), pp. 211-24.

20. A. E. Evans, N. Breslow, P. Norkool, G. J. D'Angio, "Complications in Long-Term Survivors of Wilms' Tumor," *Proceedings of AACR,* 27 (1986): 204, *Abstract #808.*

21. D. Steinhertz, C. Tan, L. Murphy, "Cardiac Toxicity 4-20 Years After Completing Anthrocycline Therapy," *Proceedings of the ASCO,* 8 (1989): 296.

22. T. R. Welch, A. J. McAdams, "Focal Glomerulosclereosis as a Late Sequela of Wilms' Tumor," *J. Pediatr.,* 108 (1986): 105-9.

23. P. Robitaille, J. G. Mongeau, L. Lortie, P. Sinnassamy, "Long-Term Follow-Up of Patients Who Underwent Unilateral Nephrectomy in Childhood," *Lancet,* 2 (1985): 1297-99.

TOTAL BREAST CANCER MORTALITY IN SWEDEN

Richard B. Singer, M.D.

References:

1. H. O. Adami, B. Malker, L. Holmberg, I. Persson, B. Stone, "The Relation Between Survival and Age at Diagnosis in Breast Cancer," *New Engl. J. Med.,* 315 (1986): 559-63.

2. H. O. Adami, Personal communication of life table and other data (April-June, 1987).

Subjects Studied: 59,992 women in Sweden with first diagnosis of breast cancer made 1960 through 1978. Diagnoses of cancer have been submitted to the National Swedish Cancer Registry by hospitals, physicians, pathologists and cytologists since 1958. The proportion of unreported cases subsequent to 1965 has been estimated at less than 2%. From this 98% complete population series 711 patients were excluded because the diagnosis was made only at autopsy, and 1,213 patients (2.1%) were excluded because of lack of follow-up data. The series with follow-up therefore numbered 57,068 patients. In 95% of cases the Registry receives notification from the physician and the pathologist involved. All stages and all types of breast cancer were included in the series. The authors state that total mastectomy and modified radical mastectomy were the dominant surgical procedures used in the surgical treatment of breast cancer, 1960-78. Adjuvant systemic therapy was seldom used.

Follow-up: Was carried out to the end of 1979. The Cancer File was linked annually with the National Causes of Death Registry through national registration numbers which permit identification of every person living in Sweden. A last date of contact with the patient was obtained by linking the name and national registration number of each patient with breast cancer in the Cancer Registry on December 31, 1978 with those in an updated registry of living persons that covers the entire Swedish population. Of the 1,213 patients lost to follow-up, analysis by age at diagnosis showed that the loss was under 2% for patients age 55 and older. The percentage increased progressively at younger ages and reached 12% for the 270 patients under age 30. Most of the loss was attributed

Source: R. B. Singer, "Total Breast Cancer Mortality in Sweden," *J. Ins. Med.,* 19, no. 2 (1987): 13-18. Reproduced with permission of author and publisher.

to incorrect reporting of the registration number, or change in family name, or occasionally to emigration.

Results: In the published article results are given in Table 2 as relative survival rates (survival ratios) for patients under age 30, age 80 and up, and for 10 quinquennial age groups in the range from 30 to 79 years, at 2, 5, 10, and 15 years duration. However, the tables of this abstract show the comparative mortality experience derived from the detailed life table sheets generously provided by Dr. Adami, although the cumulative survival rates and survival ratios are also given in the right-hand columns of the tables. Annual results are shown up to 5 years, then mean annual rates are calculated as d/E and d'/E for durations 0-5, 5-10, 10-15, and 15-20 years, except for intervals in which the exposures and numbers of deaths were too small to give meaningful results. Out of the 57,068 women entering the study the follow-up experience in the tables gives a total of 30,216 observed deaths, nearly three times the number of death claims in women in the 1979 Blood Pressure Study, and a very large number of deaths for analysis by age and duration. Although follow-up was extended to a maximum of 20 years, the high death rates and withdrawals due to end of follow-up combined to produce a large attrition of survivors at 5, 10, and 15 years. The bulk of the experience is found in the first 5 years, and numbers of deaths observed from 15 to 20 years range from none to a maximum of 83 in entrants age 55-59 years (only 504 women out of 6,467 remained for follow-up at 15 years). Nevertheless, this study provides an unusual opportunity for detailed analysis by combination of age and single years of duration to more than 5 years, and for combinations of duration intervals as long as 15-20 years.

For each interval of follow-up the tables provide data for the number alive at the start of the interval, the exposure in patient-years, the numbers of observed and expected deaths, the mortality ratio, the observed, the expected and the excess annual death rates per 1000, and the cumulative observed and expected survival rates and the survival ratio. During the first year after diagnosis the excess death rate (EDR) decreases from 78 or more per 1000 in patients under 30 to a minimum of 45 per 1000 in women age 45-49, then increases with age to a rate greater than 100 per 1000 in the oldest patients, age 75 and up. The pattern of excess mortality during the first 5 years of duration is marked by an increase in EDR to a maximum at 2 or 3 years after diagnosis in patients under age 70, followed by a decrease which tends to persist after 5 years. In older patients, however, EDR is a maximum in the first year of duration and the trend is generally downward thereafter. When mortality rates are averaged over the first 5 years there is an interesting age pattern for EDR: from an initial high level of about 90 per 1000 in the youngest patients, under age 30, EDR falls to its lowest level, 54 per 1000 in women age 45-49, then rises to 86 per 1000 at ages 55-59, dips to 71 per 1000 at ages 65-69, and finally rises again to 98 per 1000 in the oldest patients, age 80 and up. This pattern of three peak levels with two intermediate low levels shows age differences that are statistically of a high order of significance because of the large numbers of deaths in all except the youngest age groups. For example, the 1,350 deaths observed during the first 5 years among patients age 45-49 imply 95% confidence limits of ±5.4%, or limits from 51.1 to 56.9 for the mean EDR of 54 per 1000. The EDR values in the adjacent age groups are both higher than 56.9, that in age group 50-54 substantially higher. With 3,865 deaths during the first 5 years in the oldest age group, the 95% confidence limits about the mean EDR of 98 per 1000 are from 94.8 to 101.2, a relatively very narrow range.

The long-range trend for average EDR is one of decrease with increasing duration interval. In the age groups under 55 EDR tends to be about 35 per 1000 at 5-10 years duration, and under 25 per 1000 at 10-15 years duration. At these durations EDR tends to increase with advancing age and is usually a little above 50 per 1000 over age 65. At durations 15-20 years the numbers of deaths are much smaller, from 13 to 83 in the age groups for which data are shown, and the age trends are irregular, probably because of random fluctuation. The overall level of EDR is below that at durations 10-15 years, except in the age groups 70-74 and 75-79, in which the EDR values are 66 and 140 per 1000, respectively. There were only 6 survivors at 15 years in the age group 80 and up, but 3 deaths occurred. The notable finding at these long durations is the persistence of significant excess mortality in relation to that in the general population more than 10 years after diagnosis and surgery, especially in the patients who were age 65 or older at the time of entry.

With the extremely wide range of age in this series one might anticipate a continuous decrease in mortality ratio with advancing age, and this is indeed shown in the results. For the aggregate exposure in the first 5 years of follow-up the mortality ratio decreased from 18,000% at ages 20-24 to 3,000% in the age group 40-44, to 820% in the age group 60-64, and finally to 173% in the oldest

age group, patients 80 years and older. First-year mortality ratios were higher than these aggregate values, and the ratios tended to decrease with increasing duration beyond 5 years. Because these ratios are so much influenced by the rise in expected mortality with advancing age, the EDR is a much more sensitive and useful index for discerning the patterns of excess mortality in a large series of this kind.

The life tables sent by Dr. Adami included separate 5-year data for patients diagnosed 1975-78. These permit an estimate of secular trend in excess mortality during the first 5 years following diagnosis. EDR values for the 1975-78 patients during this interval were generally about 25% lower than in the total series, which included a preponderance of patients diagnosed from 1960 to 1974. The reduction in mortality ratio was similar in patient groups under age 40-44, but smaller in the 40-44 and older groups. The overall prognosis for the first 5 years after surgery for breast cancer, all stages combined, therefore appears to have improved in Sweden during this observation period that lasted almost 20 years.

In presenting their results in terms of survival ratio the authors concluded that women age 45-49 with breast cancer had the best prognosis, because the survival ratio was highest in this group (75.8% at 5 years). When the age 45-49 group was compared with those 75 and older the differential in cumulative survival ratio between the two groups increased at 10 and 15 years, as is evident from the tabular data in this abstract. There is an inverse mathematical relationship between EDR and the interval survival ratio which has been detailed by Marx in an article entitled "A Life Insurer's Interpretation of Survival Rates," published many years ago in the *Annals of Life Insurance Medicine*, volume 3, pages 1-15. If the cumulative survival ratio is substituted for the interval ratio, the EDR average derived from this relationship is an average for all years up to the duration of the cumulative survival rate.

Comment: The magnitude of the study, a nationwide 98% sample, and the completeness and duration of follow-up make these results peculiarly suited to the analysis of comparative survival and mortality by age, as the authors point out. They have also presented in Figure 2 of their article "annual hazard rates" to 15 years for age groups 30-34, 45-49, 55-59, and 70-74. These are defined as the complement of the annual survival ratio. If the survival ratio is expressed as a decimal, not a percentage, the annual hazard rate is a good approximation of EDR/1000 in Swedish women to about age 75, when the expected mortality rate begins to exceed 0.05, and the annual survival rate falls below 0.95. In their abstract the authors refer to the annual hazard rate as the "long-term mortality rate due to breast cancer," a descriptive term analogous to the excess death rate in this disease. They characterize this rate as approaching "1 to 2 percent at the premenopausal ages but [this] exceeded 5 percent throughout the period of observation in the oldest age group." The above rate of 2% per year approximates an EDR of 20 per 1000 per year. The above description is in good agreement with the EDR values as shown in the tables, and the text of the Results section.

How does breast cancer mortality in Sweden compare with the experience observed in the U.S.? I do not have immediately available the abstracts that have been prepared under Ed Lew's direction for the tables used in End Results Report No. 5, but I have combined the data in age groups 45-49 and 50-54 at durations 0-5 years and compared them with matching results in Table 167a of the *1976 Medical Risks* monograph. These give data at ages 45-54 that can be combined from durations 0-2 and 2-5 years for localized cancer of the breast, and cancer with regional node involvement. There is no age breakdown for cases with distant metastatic involvement, but I have assumed that mortality is the same for age 45-54 as it is for all ages and used 25% of the total metastatic experience for this age group, based on the proportion in the other two stages. Excess mortality is smaller in the Swedish experience than in the U.S., End Results Report No.4, with EDR for total breast cancer in this age/duration category of 65 per 1000 and 98 per 1000, respectively. Partly this may be due to a lower proportion of localized cancer in the End Results experience (45%) than that estimated by Dr. Adami for the Swedish experience.[2] Another factor may be secular difference, as the experi-

ence in Table 167a is based on cases diagnosed in 1955-64, followed to 1972, an earlier period than 1960-78 for the observations in Sweden. Mortality in breast cancer, as in other types, is greatly influenced by the staging classification: EDR was only 34 per 1000 in localized cancer in this age/duration category in Table 167a, but 115 per 1000 in cases with regional involvement, and an estimated 437 per 1000 in the small percentage of cases with metastasis. However, this does not impair the significance of the persisting rather high EDR values beyond 10 years in this Swedish study, because high mortality rates will tend to reduce greatly the proportion of non-localized cases in the total series.

Similar EDR values, of the order of 20 per 1000, were observed in both localized and regional breast cancer cases at 10-20 years of follow-up in the End Results Study, Table 167a. All of these results cast some doubt on the justifiability of the common underwriting practice of employing temporary flat extra premiums for applicants with a history of localized cancer, flat extras that come off automatically 10 years after apparently successful treatment of the cancer. These two large studies clearly show persistence of substantial excess mortality beyond 10 years even when population tables have been used to calculate EDR. The excess mortality would be even higher if select and ultimate tables had been used. It will be important to study such long-term mortality in cancer cases in the tables of the forth-coming mortality reference volume.

TOTAL BREAST CANCER MORTALITY IN SWEDEN, 1960-78
TABLE 170K1-1
COMPARATIVE EXPERIENCE IN WOMEN AGE 20-44

Interval Start-End Yrs	No. Alive at Start ℓ	Exposure Patient-yrs. E	No. of Deaths Observed d	No. of Deaths Expected* d'	Mortality Ratio 100(d/d')	Mean Ann. Mort. Rate/1000 Observed $1000\bar{q}$	Mean Ann. Mort. Rate/1000 Expected $1000\bar{q}'$	Mean Ann. Mort. Rate/1000 Excess $1000(\bar{q}-\bar{q}')$	Cum. Surv. Rate Obs. P	Cum. Surv. Rate Exp. P'	Survival Ratio 100(P/P')
1960-78				**WOMEN AGE 20-24**							
0-5 yrs.	30	113.0	10	0.056	18,000%	88	0.5	87	0.649	0.9976	65.1%
1960-78				**WOMEN AGE 25-29**							
0-1 yr.	203	203.0	16	0.10	16,000%	79	0.5	78	0.921	0.9995	92.2%
1-2	187	181.0	19	0.11	17,000	105	0.6	104	0.824	0.9989	82.5
2-3	156	149.0	19	0.09	21,000	128	0.6	127	0.719	0.9983	72.1
3-4	123	116.0	11	0.07	16,000	95	0.6	94	0.651	0.9977	65.3
4-5	98	93.0	4	0.065	6,200	43	0.7	42	0.623	0.9970	62.5
0-5	203	742.0	69	0.44	15,900	93	0.6	92	0.623	0.9970	62.5
5-10	84	294.0	8	0.24	3,300	27	0.8	26	0.547	0.9929	55.1
1975-78											
0-5	63	172.0	13	0.10	13,000	76	0.6	75	0.750	0.9972	75.2
1960-78				**WOMEN AGE 30-34**							
0-1	643	643.0	38	0.45	8,400%	59	0.7	58	0.941	0.9993	94.2%
1-2	605	577.0	61	0.46	13,200	106	0.8	105	0.841	0.9985	84.3
2-3	488	463.5	46	0.37	12,400	99	0.8	98	0.758	0.9976	76.0
3-4	393	373.5	36	0.34	10,700	96	0.9	95	0.685	0.9967	68.7
4-5	318	302.0	18	0.30	6,000	60	1.0	59	0.644	0.9957	64.7
0-5	643	2,359.0	199	1.92	10,400	84	0.8	83	0.644	0.9957	64.7
5-10	268	974.0	37	1.27	2,900	38	1.3	37	0.536	0.9893	54.2
10-15	131	467.0	16	0.93	1,720	34	2.0	32	0.452	0.9796	46.1
1975-78											
0-5	207	565.0	31	0.45	6,900	55	0.8	54	0.675	0.9960	67.7
1960-78				**WOMEN AGE 35-39**							
0-1	1,574	1,574.0	86	1.73	5,000%	55	1.1	54	0.945	0.9989	94.6%
1-2	1,488	1,443.0	130	1.73	7,500	90	1.2	89	0.860	0.9977	86.2
2-3	1,268	1,222.5	101	1.59	6,400	82	1.3	81	0.789	0.9964	79.2
3-4	1,076	1,038.0	78	1.45	5,400	75	1.4	74	0.730	0.9950	73.4
4-5	922	887.5	38	1.42	2,700	43	1.6	41	0.699	0.9934	70.3
0-5	1,574	6,165,0	433	7.92	5,500	70	1.3	69	0.699	0.9934	70.3
5-10	815	3,096.0	133	6.19	2,100	43	2.0	41	0.562	0.9836	57.2
10-15	426	1,517.5	35	4.40	795	23	2.9	20	0.504	0.9688	52.1
15-20	192	469.5	13	1.97	660	28	4.2	24	0.453	0.9506	47.7
1975-78											
0-5	392	1,092.0	66	1.26	5,200	60	1.2	59	0.738	0.9938	74.3
1960-78				**WOMEN AGE 40-44**							
0-1	3,439	3,439.0	167	5.85	2,900%	49	1.7	47	0.951	0.9983	95.3%
1-2	3,272	3,197.5	227	5.88	3,900	71	1.9	69	0.884	0.9964	88.7
2-3	2,896	2,805.5	196	5.61	3,500	70	2.0	68	0.822	0.9944	82.7
3-4	2,519	2,450.0	140	5.39	2,600	57	2.2	55	0.775	0.9922	78.1
4-5	2,241	2,183.5	110	5.24	2,100	50	2.4	48	0.736	0.9898	74.4
0-5	3,439	14,075.5	840	27.97	3,000	60	2.0	58	0.736	0.9898	74.4
5-10	2,016	7,951.5	269	24.65	1,090	34	3.1	31	0.622	0.9748	63.9
10-15	1,170	4,142.5	101	18.23	555	24	4.4	20	0.552	0.9529	57.9
15-20	500	1,224.5	19	2.69	705	15	6.4	9	0.505	0.9207	54.8
1975-78											
0-5	679	1,892.5	96	3.46	2,800	51	1.8	49	0.756	0.9903	76.3

* Expected mortality compiled from life tables for Swedish female population, 5-year periods, 1960-79.

TOTAL BREAST CANCER MORTALITY IN SWEDEN, 1960-78
TABLE 170K1-2
COMPARATIVE EXPERIENCE IN WOMEN AGE 45-64

| Interval Start-End | No. Alive at Start | Exposure Patient-yrs. | No. of Deaths | | Mortality Ratio | Mean Ann. Mort. Rate/1000 | | | Cum. Surv. Rate | | Survival Ratio |
| | | | Observed | Expected* | | Observed | Expected | Excess | Obs. | Exp. | |
Yrs.	ℓ	E	d	d'	100(d/d')	$1000\bar{q}$	$1000\bar{q}'$	$1000(\bar{q}-\bar{q}')$	P	P'	100(P/P')
1960-78					**WOMEN AGE 45-49**						
0-1 yr.	5,782	5,782.0	280	15.6	1,790%	48	2.7	45	0.952	0.9973	95.4%
1-2 yrs.	5,502	5,357.0	359	15.5	2,300	67	2.9	64	0.888	0.9945	89.3
2-3	4,853	4,709.0	315	14.6	2,200	67	3.1	64	0.828	0.9914	83.6
3-4	4,250	4,116.5	228	14.0	1,630	55	3.4	52	0.782	0.9881	79.2
4-5	3,755	3,629.5	168	13.1	1,280	46	3.6	42	0.746	0.9845	75.8
0-5	5,782	23,594.0	1,350	72.8	1,850	57	3.1	54	0.746	0.9845	75.8
5-10	3,336	12,771.0	458	57.9	780	36	4.5	31	0.625	0.9623	65.0
10-15	1,822	6,259.0	157	41.4	370	25	6.6	18	0.550	0.9301	59.2
15-20	719	1,686.0	54	17.9	300	32	10.6	21	0.463	0.8806	52.5
1975-78											
0-5	1,232	3,525.0	136	8.99	1,510	39	2.6	36	0.832	0.9853	84.4
1960-78					**WOMEN AGE 50-54**						
0-1	6,009	6,009.0	477	24.0	2,500%	79	4.0	75	0.921	0.9960	92.4%
1-2	5,532	5,371.5	499	23.1	2,300	93	4.3	90	0.835	0.9917	84.2
2-3	4,712	4,547.0	381	20.9	1,820	84	4.6	79	0.765	0.9872	77.5
3-4	4,001	3,870.0	291	19.4	1,500	75	5.0	70	0.708	0.9823	72.0
4-5	3,448	3,330.0	204	18.0	1,130	61	5.4	56	0.664	0.9770	68.0
0-5	6,009	23,127.5	1,852	105.4	1,760	80	4.6	75	0.664	0.9770	68.0
5-10	3,008	11,074.0	476	75.3	630	43	6.8	36	0.538	0.9440	57.0
10-15	1,533	5,241.5	125	56.1	230	24	10.7	15	0.470	0.8941	50.5
15-20	601	1,371.0	39	38.4	102	28	28	0	0.394	0.8145	48.3
1975-78											
0-5	1,368	3,788.5	219	16.3	1,340	58	4.3	54	0.721	0.9782	73.7
1960-78					**WOMEN AGE 55-59**						
0-1	6,467	6,467.0	591	39.4	1,500%	91	6.1	85	0.909	0.9939	91.4%
1-2	5,876	5,699.5	584	37.6	1,500	103	6.6	96	0.816	0.9874	82.6
2-3	4,939	4,757.5	489	34.3	1,430	103	7.2	96	0.732	0.9804	74.6
3-4	4,087	3,963.0	352	30.9	1,140	89	7.8	81	0.667	0.9728	68.5
4-5	3,487	3,364.0	244	28.6	855	72	8.5	64	0.618	0.9646	64.1
0-5	6,467	24,251.0	2,260	171.3	1,320	93	7.1	86	0.618	0.9646	64.1
5-10	2,997	10,946.0	619	123.7	500	56	11.3	45	0.464	0.9117	50.9
10-15	1,398	4,634.5	213	88.0	240	46	19.0	27	0.366	0.8291	44.2
15-20	504	1,111.5	83	34.4	240	75	31	44	0.234	0.6983	33.5
1975-78											
0-5	1,504	4,082.0	294	25.3	1,160	72	6.2	66	0.687	0.9921	71.1
1960-78					**WOMEN AGE 60-64**						
0-1	7,155	7,155.0	624	70.1	890%	87	9.8	77	0.913	0.9902	92.2%
1-2	6,531	6,329.5	631	67.7	930	100	10.7	89	0.822	0.9796	83.9
2-3	5,497	5,309.5	511	62.7	815	96	11.8	84	0.743	0.9681	76.7
3-4	4,611	4,407.5	403	57.3	705	91	13.0	78	0.676	0.9555	70.7
4-5	3,927	3,783.0	301	54.1	555	79	14.3	65	0.622	0.9420	66.0
0-5	7,155	26,984.5	2,470	301.9	820	91	11.2	80	0.622	0.9420	66.0
5-10	3,358	11,752.5	777	231.5	335	66	19.7	46	0.444	0.8536	52.0
10-15	1,440	4,538.5	325	154.3	210	72	34	38	0.303	0.7172	42.2
15-20	448	959.0	76	51.8	147	79	54	25	0.219[†]	0.5646[†]	38.8[†]
1975-78											
0-5	1,682	4,577.5	335	44.7	750	73	9.8	63	0.666	0.9471	70.3

* Expected mortality compiled from life tables of the Swedish female population, 5-year periods, 1960-79.

† Survival rates at 19 yrs.

178

TOTAL BREAST CANCER MORTALITY IN SWEDEN, 1960-78
TABLE 170K1-3
COMPARATIVE EXPERIENCE IN WOMEN AGE 65 AND UP

Interval Start-End	No. Alive at Start	Exposure Patient-yrs.	No. of Deaths		Mortality Ratio	Mean Ann. Mort. Rate/1000			Cum. Surv. Rate		Survival Ratio
			Observed	Expected*		Observed	Expected	Excess	Obs.	Exp.	
Yrs.	ℓ	E	d	d'	100(d/d')	$1000\bar{q}$	$1000\bar{q}'$	$1000(\bar{q}-\bar{q}')$	P	P'	100(P/P')
1960-78					**WOMEN AGE 65-69**						
0-1 yr.	7,388	7,388.0	656	123.4	530%	89	16.7	72	0.911	0.9833	92.7%
1-2 yrs.	6,732	6,489.0	619	120.0	515	95	18.5	77	0.824	0.9651	85.4
2-3	5,627	5,437.0	559	112.0	500	103	20.6	82	0.740	0.9453	78.2
3-4	4,688	4,490.5	389	103.3	375	87	23.0	64	0.676	0.9238	73.1
4-5	3,904	3,753.5	299	96.1	310	80	25.6	54	0.622	0.9005	69.0
0-5	7,388	27,588.0	2,522	554.8	455	91	20.1	71	0.622	0.9005	69.0
5-10	3,304	11,207.0	998	381	260	89	34	55	0.391	0.752	52.0
10-15	1,244	3,729.0	381	209	162	102	56	46	0.228	0.546	41.7
15-20	331	698.0	75	66.1	113	107	95	12	0.120	0.313	38.4
1975-78											
0-5	1,951	5,290.0	389	88.4	440	74	16.7	57	0.676	0.9105	74.3
1960-78					**WOMEN AGE 70-74**						
0-1	6,816	6,816.0	838	207.9	405%	123	31	92	0.877	0.9695	90.5%
1-2	5,978	5,775.5	630	194.6	325	109	34	75	0.781	0.9367	83.4
2-3	4,943	4,764.0	507	179.6	280	106	37	69	0.698	0.9014	77.5
3-4	4,078	3,900.5	433	163.8	265	111	42	69	0.621	0.8637	71.9
4-5	3,290	3,162.5	337	148.6	225	107	47	60	0.555	0.8236	67.3
0-5	6,816	24,418.5	2,745	894.5	305	112	37	75	0.555	0.8236	67.3
5-10	2,698	8,863.5	1,019	514.0	198	115	58	57	0.298	0.5915	50.3
10-15	890	2,479.0	392	235.5	166	158	95	63	0.117	0.3377	34.8
15-20	152	268.0	58	40.3	144	216	150	66	0.034	0.1337	25.6
1975-78											
0-5	1,757	4,710.5	384	141.9	270	81	30	51	0.648	0.8419	77.0
1960-78					**WOMEN AGE 75-79**						
0-1	5,667	5,667.0	908	311.7	290%	160	55	105	0.840	0.9450	88.9%
1-2	4,759	4,597.0	677	276.7	245	147	60	87	0.716	0.8879	80.6
2-3	3,758	3,605.0	515	240.8	215	143	67	76	0.614	0.8287	74.1
3-4	2,937	2,810.0	418	207.9	200	149	74	75	0.522	0.7679	68.0
4-5	2,265	2,162.0	304	177.3	171	141	82	59	0.449	0.7060	63.6
0-5	5,667	18,841.0	2,822	1,214.4	230	150	64	86	0.449	0.7060	63.6
5-10	1,755	5,155.0	839	588	143	163	114	49	0.178	0.3990	44.7
10-15	394	980.5	205	151	136	209	154	55	0.050	0.1584	31.6
15-20	40	64.5	25	16.0	156	388	248	140	0.004	0.0347	(10.1)
1975-78											
0-5	1,560	4,010.0	470	220.1	215	117	55	62	0.553	0.7289	75.8
1960-78					**WOMEN AGE 80 AND UP**						
0-1	5,891	5,891.0	1,517	728	210%	258	124	134	0.742	0.8764	84.7%
1-2	4,374	4,189.5	905	542	167	216	130	86	0.582	0.7611	76.5
2-3	3,100	2,964.5	634	411	154	214	139	75	0.458	0.6545	69.9
3-4	2,194	2,105.0	452	316	143	214	150	64	0.359	0.5568	64.5
4-5	1,564	1,494.5	357	239	149	239	160	79	0.274	0.4682	58.4
0-5	5,891	16,644.0	3,865	2,236	173	232	134	98	0.274	0.4682	58.4
5-10	1,068	2,715.0	655	500	131	241	184	57	0.068	0.1586	42.7
10-15	145	306.0	91	80.2	113	297	262	35	0.010	0.0308	31.3

* Expected mortality compiled from life tables for Swedish female population, 5-year periods, 1960-79.

SHORT-TERM SURVIVAL FOLLOWING SPINAL CORD INJURY

Roger H. Butz, M.D.

Reference:

M. J. DeVivo, P. L. Kartus, S. L. Stover, R. D. Rutt, P. R. Fine, "Seven-Year Survival Following Spinal Cord Injury," *Arch. Neurol.*, 44 (1987): 872-75.

Subjects Studied: This study reports on the 5,131 patients who sustained spinal cord injury between 1973 and 1980 and who were admitted to one of seven federally designated Spinal Cord Injury Care Systems during the first year after injury. These facilities and the numbers of patients admitted into each facility were as follows: Spain Rehabilitation Center, University of Alabama at Birmingham (705 patients), University Hospital at Boston University Medical Center (238 patients), Rehabilitation Institute of Chicago at Northwestern Memorial Hospital (1,179 patients), Craig Institute, Englewood, Colorado (1,513 patients), Good Samaritan Medical Center at St. Joseph Hospital, Phoenix (335 patients), Santa Clara Valley Medical Center, San Jose, California (693 patients) and Woodrow Wilson Rehabilitation Center, University of Virginia, Fishersville (468 patients).

Follow-up: These patients were traced until December 31, 1981 when deaths were assessed by a search of the Social Security Administration Master Beneficiary Record and Summary Earnings Record. Deaths occurring within 24 hours of the initial injury were excluded. Losses to follow-up totaled 13.3%. Some misclassification of outcome was shown to be present, based upon known patient status of some who were submitted for Social Security Administration search. It appears that fewer than 1% of live patients were incorrectly reported as deceased, while 2-3% of deceased persons were reported as still living. The maximum period of follow-up was 84 months, but the recruitment of subjects through 1980 resulted in many being followed for fewer years (see Figure 222K1-1).

Results: Mortality was reported for pooled data by year from injury through seven years post-injury (see Table 222K1-1). Mortality was also reported by level of injury by age groups 1-24 years, 25-49 years, and 50 years and over, for the stratified groups, all durations combined. The results, showing comparative mortality by level of injury and age group are shown in Table 222K1-2. The expected mortality was taken from 1977 population mortality with adjustment for age and sex of the patient population in each category. The overall mortality rate during each year after injury is shown in Figure 222K1-2. Despite lack of age, sex and expected mortality data it

FIGURE 222K1-1

DISTRIBUTION BY YEAR OF FOLLOW-UP

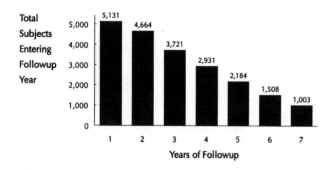

FIGURE 222K1-2

SPINAL CORD INJURY MORTALITY

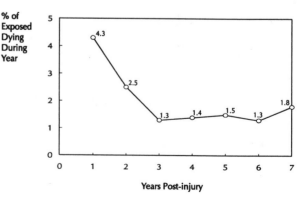

Source: R. H. Butz, "Short-term Survival Following Spinal Cord Injury," *J. Ins. Med.*, 20, no. 3 (1988): 54-56. Reproduced with permission of author and publisher.

can be seen that observed death rates were highest in the first two years and then quite stable through the succeeding five years. If we ignore the effect of increasing ages during follow-up, then 2/7 (29%) of the anticipated deaths might have been expected to occur during years 1 and 2, and 5/7 (71%) during the remaining five years of follow-up. Actually, however, 48% of deaths occurred during the first two years and only 52% in the last five years. Table 222K1-3 shows the attributable extra mortality to duration 2-7 years by reducing the figures in Table 222K1-2 by the proportionate mortality of years 1 and 2. This maneuver, arbitrarily allocating mortality in each age and injury level group by overall distribution of deaths by year for the entire group, may skew results if deaths are maldistributed in age groups or injury levels. However, for purposes of underwriting (structured settlement annuities, especially) it is important to

eliminate the effect of early deaths since most cases are underwritten several years post-injury, and acute mortality is not pertinent.

Comment: These data suggest a stable, significant mortality excess during post-injury years 3 through 7. Noteworthy results of this report include the similarity of age group relative mortality rates for paraplegia and incomplete quadriplegia. Other studies have demonstrated more severe mortality with higher levels of paralysis. This difference in outcome is not easily explained unless it is a temporary phenomenon following the acute injury. Complete quadriplegia was associated with remarkably high mortality ratios, especially at older ages, with 73% cumulative mortality for those over 50 by the end of the seventh year.

TABLE 222K1-1

COMPARATIVE MORTALITY BY INTERVAL FOR COMBINED AGES AND LEVELS OF INJURY

Interval Start-End	No. Alive at Start	Withdrawn or lost	Exposure Person-yrs.	No. of Deaths		Mortality Ratio	Mean Ann. Mort. Rate		
				Observed	Expected*		Observed	Expected	Excess
t to t+Δt	ℓ	w	E	d	d'	100(d/d')	q	q'	1000(q–q')
0-1 yrs.	5,131	252	5,005.0	215	16.62	1,290%	0.0430	0.0033	40
1-2	4,664	838	4,245.0	105	14.99	700	0.0247	0.0035	21
2-3	3,721	746	3,348.0	44	12.50	350	0.0131	0.0037	10
3-4	2,931	710	2,576.0	37	10.16	365	0.0144	0.0039	11
4-5	2,184	648	1,860.0	28	7.67	365	0.0151	0.0041	11
5-6	1,508	489	1,263.5	16	5.47	295	0.0127	0.0043	8
6-7	1,003	437	784.5	14	3.55	395	0.0178	0.0045	13
0-7	5,131	4,120	19,082.0	459	71.04	645	0.0241	0.0037	20

* d' = Number of deaths expected, based on 1977 U.S. Population Mortality.

TABLE 222K1-2

COMPARATIVE MORTALITY FOR SPINAL CORD INJURY DURING 7 YEAR FOLLOW-UP, BY SEVERITY AND AGE GROUP

Injury	Age Group	No. Alive at start	Exposure Person-yrs.	No. of Deaths Observed	No. of Deaths Expected*	Mortality Ratio	Mean Ann. Mort. Rate Observed	Mean Ann. Mort. Rate Expected	Mean Ann. Mort. Rate Excess
		ℓ	E	d	d'	100(d/d')	$\bar{q}$	$\bar{q}'$	1000($\bar{q}$–$\bar{q}'$)
Paraplegia incomplete	1-24 yrs.	417	1,580	12	2.49	480%	0.0076	0.0016	6
	25-49	424	1,508	22	3.34	660	0.0146	0.0022	12
	50+	113	398	23	7.06	325	0.0578	0.0177	40
Paraplegia complete	1-24	688	2,842	23	4.67	495	0.0081	0.0016	6
	25-49	656	2,537	40	5.77	695	0.0158	0.0023	14
	50+	118	456	25	7.67	325	0.0548	0.0168	38
Quadriplegia incomplete	1-24	688	2,561	18	4.27	420	0.0070	0.0017	5
	25-49	506	1,817	30	4.47	670	0.0165	0.0025	14
	50+	247	817	73	18.49	395	0.0894	0.0226	67
Quadriplegia complete	1-24	741	2,861	60	4.84	1,250	0.0210	0.0017	19
	25-49	426	1,489	64	3.08	2,100	0.0430	0.0021	41
	50+	107	220	69	4.89	1,400	0.3136	0.0222	291

* d' = Number of deaths expected, based on 1977 U.S. Population Mortality.

TABLE 222K1-3

CALCULATED COMPARATIVE MORTALITY DURATION 2-7 YEARS FOLLOWING SPINAL CORD INJURY (Rough Estimate, See Text)

Level Injury	Age Group	No. of Deaths Observed*	No. of Deaths Expected†	Mortality Ratio
		d	d	100(d/d')
Paraplegia incomplete	1-24 yrs.	6.24	1.78	350%
	25-49	11.44	2.37	485
	50+	11.96	5.01	240
Paraplegia complete	1-24	11.96	3.32	360
	25-49	20.80	4.10	490
	50+	13.00	5.45	240
Quadriplegia incomplete	1-24	9.36	3.03	310
	25-49	15.60	3.17	490
	50+	37.96	13.13	290
Quadriplegia complete	1-24	31.20	3.44	910
	25-49	33.28	2.19	1,520
	50+	35.88	3.47	1,040

* d = Deaths observed, calculated from year-by-year overall mortality showing 52% of deaths for entire group occurring in duration 2-7 years.

† d'= Deaths expected, calculated as 5/7 of total expected deaths for group.

COMPARATIVE MORTALITY IN SURVIVORS RESUSCITATED FOLLOWING OUT-OF-HOSPITAL CARDIAC ARREST: AN UNDERWRITING NOTE

Richard B. Singer, M.D.

Advances in emergency medicine have included the training of paramedical personnel to utilize advanced cardiac life support measures (defibrillation, parenteral medication, and endotracheal intubation) in the earliest possible treatment of victims of cardiac arrest. In a June 1982 article,[1] Eisenberg and his colleagues report a follow-up study of 276 of 302 patients discharged from hospitals in King County, Washington, following successful cardiopulmonary resuscitation (CPR) by paramedics for cardiac arrest due to heart disease. Since there are more than 300 paramedic programs of this sort in the U.S.,[1] it is not unlikely that survivors of CPR for cardiac arrest may present themselves as life insurance applicants. This underwriting note is intended to present limited comparative mortality data from the King County study and two earlier ones[2,3] and thus aid the medical director who may encounter an applicant with such a history.

CPR is successful in only a minority of victims of cardiac arrest: roughly two-thirds are dead on arrival at the hospital or die in the emergency room, and one-half, more or less, of those admitted die in the hospital.[1,2,3] Successful CPR depends on early arrival of the emergency medical team (or help of a capable bystander), and short time to definitive care, as demonstrated in the King County "Project Restart."[4] The annual incidence rate of cardiac arrest calls was reported as 0.7 per 1000 population, and 81% of the non-trauma cases were due to heart disease, with others caused by cancer, neurologic or respiratory disease, drowning, drug overdose and sudden infant death syndrome.[4] This is not the place to discuss features of the acute phase or the implementation of CPR; details may be found in the articles cited.[1,2,3,4]

Information with regard to early survivors, defined as patients discharged from the hospital, is more complete in the King County study than in the others, but even here the age of the 1,567 cardiac arrest patients is given as a

mean with standard deviation, 65±12.7 years, with only a division at age 60 for those survivors actually followed up. There were 1,202 men and 365 women, with the women considerably older, average 70 vs. 63 years for the men. These cases were gathered in the period from April 1, 1976 to June 1, 1981, in the suburban area around Seattle, Washington, the city itself being excluded because it has a separate program of its own. Of the 557 patients surviving long enough to be admitted to the area hospitals, 255 died and 302 were discharged alive. Since 26 patients were lost to the follow-up, survival curves were calculated on the remaining 276 discharged patients (91%). Only 26 of the 276 patients were discharged to nursing homes or extended care facilities,[1] in contrast to a higher percentage of patients with serious neurological deficit requiring such care in the Hennepin County, Minnesota study[2] and the Miami study.[3] The disturbance associated with cardiac arrest was ventricular fibrillation in two-thirds of the King County cases, and in the patients surviving to hospital discharge, it was 89%.[1] The Miami study was restricted to cases with ventricular fibrillation.[3] Results of the King County study are presented in the form of a series of survival curves. Numbers of cases alive at each year of follow-up to four years, with deaths in the preceding year, are added to Figure 1 in which the curve for all 276 patients combined is compared with curves for age/sex-matched U.S. population rates and recent post-MI rates.[5] There were 99 deaths within four years. In addition, nine graphs are given in Figure 2 for the series divided successively into "with-and-without" groups, with Kaplan-Meier survival curves for each pair. Curves are almost identical in four of the comparisons, including duration of CPR, arrest before or after paramedic arrival, bystander initiated CPR, and single or multiple shocks needed to reinstate cardiac contraction. Survival was significantly higher (p=0.01 to 0.03) in survivors under age 60, in the majority of patients in whom CPR was started less than four minutes after arrest, and in those with similar time to CPR who also had less than ten minutes before receiving definitive care. Survival was also higher in males than females, but not significantly so (p=0.13).

Source: R. B. Singer, "Comparative Mortality in Survivors Resuscitated Following Out-of-Hospital Cardiac Arrest: An Underwriting Note," *J. Ins. Med.,* 14, no. 2 (1983): 29-33. Reproduced with permission of author and publisher.

From the published results just described, I have been able to reconstruct the observed life table constituting the basis of the annual survival curve points in the total series of Figure 1, and I have estimated q' for the first year and q' from one to four years from P' values for the U.S. population. However, inspection of the Kaplan-Meier survival curves in Figure 2 confirms that the survival curve falls most steeply (short interval mortality is highest) in the first three months after hospital discharge. A similar reconstruction has been made of an observed life table at intervals of four months up to 24 months from Table 1 and Figure 4 of the Hennepin County study, in which 34 patients were discharged to chronic care facilities while follow-up was achieved on 47 of the 49 *ambulatory* discharged patients. Exposure data, deaths and observed mortality and survival rates are thus more accurate for these two reports than would be possible to approximate from cumulative survival in the graphs. In the Miami study, exposure can be approximated from mean follow-up duration of 16.8 months for the ultimate survivors and 8.3 months for the deaths; an average annual mortality is thus calculated for comparison with annual mortality in the two other studies. There were 20 deaths among the 42 patients discharged from the hospital. Five patients with severe, and 12 patients with mild neurological residuals were included in the series.

Table 305K1-1 summarizes comparative mortality results developed from the data in these three studies of cardiac arrest early survivors. Maximum follow-up in the Hennepin County[2] and Miami[3] studies was about two years, but the average was slightly over one year, and for this reason, their results have been related to the first-year experience of the King County study.[3] It is evident that excess mortality in all three studies is extremely high, with EDR values ranging from 200 to almost 400 extra deaths per 1000 per year. The expected mortality rate, q', is 0.060 as derived from Figure 1 of the King County article, a high rate reflecting the high proportion of older patients. The average age of 65 years given is a little older than the average of 63 years for the other series. In the absence of age/sex distribution data, I have assumed a q' for the Hennepin County and Miami series of 0.055, a downward adjustment from the rate in the King County series. Because of these high q' values associated with a majority of patients over age 60, the mortality ratios are smaller than might be anticipated from the very high EDRs. After the first year, the King County experience shows a decrease in the level of excess mortality (bottom line of Table 305K1-1), with a mortality ratio of 260%, but an EDR of 84 per 1000 per year, still a very high level and considerably above the excess mortality of the recent series of post-MI patients,[5] shown as one of the survival

curves in Figure 1 of the article on the King County study. Such a decrease in mortality after the first year is typical of conditions that have an extremely high first-year mortality.[6] A peculiar feature of the King County study is that a recurrent episode of cardiac arrest was counted as a "death"; although such recurrences are often fatal, the authors do not state the number of recurrences or the proportion of non-fatal ones. In all of these studies, the incidence of sudden death was very high regardless of the use of anti-arrhythmic drugs in the medical management of these patients.

Table 305K1-2 documents the preponderance of first-year deaths in the first three months of follow-up in the King County series, and Table 305K1-3 is the life table of observed mortality on an annual basis for the four years of this study. Survival rates have been added to the mortality data. These tables support the summary results[1] in Table 305K1-1. Those who have attended one of the mortality seminars sponsored by ALIMDA over the past several years may find it of interest to reconstruct the life tables from Figure 1 of the article and verify the accuracy of my own reconstruction in Tables 305K1-2 and 305K1-3.

Note that q̆' of 0.052 on the bottom line of Table 305K1-1 for duration 1-4 years is *lower* than q' for the first year (0.060, top line). This is due to higher excess mortality in older patients in the first year, with a subsequent decrease in attained average age and average expected mortality rate, a point stressed in the mortality seminars.

What about the age comparison and the sex comparison already mentioned as being in Figure 2 of the article on the King County study? In a somewhat over-elaborate tabular reconstruction, I have confirmed extremely high excess mortality in the first three months for all age/sex categories, with EDR on the order of 500 on an annualized basis. From three months to four years, overall EDR is slightly higher than from one to four years, using the same q̆' as in Table 305K1-1 with 96 vs. 84 extra deaths per 1000 per year. However, the aggregate q' I obtained after reasonable assumptions of average age in separate male and female groups, under 60 and age 60 up, was 0.031, considerably lower than the 0.052 derived from the published U.S. population survival curve, a discrepancy for which I have no explanation. EDR for the younger patients was about 80 from three months to four years, with little difference between male and female, by this rough approximation. For those age 60 up excess mortality was higher, 135 for males (based on 29 deaths) and over 200 for females (based on 9 deaths). Since the survival curves differed significantly by age (p=0.02), the difference in EDR by age may be regarded as also significant. I have not included the table in this underwriting note, because of the numerous assumptions involved, and the possibility that the reader might be misled into a false impression of accuracy of the many figures displayed.

It would be interesting to know how experienced medical directors will interpret these results from the standpoint of risk classification. Presented with an applicant who gives a history of spontaneous cardiac arrest, would you decline or consider at a very high rating? What selection criteria would you use? In my opinion, the excess mortality is an unacceptable risk when EDR exceeds 100 per 1000 per year. Clearly this would require declination of all such applicants within a year of the episode, and all applicants age 60 up after one year,

based on the limited follow-up data available. It is very questionable in my mind whether applicants under age 60 might be considered, with an EDR on the order of 80, implying the equivalent of a flat extra of $80 per $1,000, *not* on a temporary term of years. Most of these applicants would have associated heart disease, with a high prevalence of past myocardial infarction. How should the customary evidence of insurability be evaluated in the light of a history of cardiac arrest: history, blood pressure, pulse, electrocardiogram, chest X-ray, etc.? Should a portable monitoring electrocardiogram of ½ to 1 hour be required? If you have ideas on this as a problem of risk selection and would like to share them, how about a letter to the editor of *The Journal of Insurance Medicine?*

REFERENCES

1. M. S. Eisenberg, A. Hallstrom, L. Bergner, "Long-Term Survival After Out-of-Hospital Cardiac Arrest," *N. Engl. J. Med.*, 306 (1982): 1340-43.

2. G. Rockswold, B. Sharma, E. Rutz, et al., "Follow-up of 514 Consecutive Patients with Cardiopulmonary Arrest Outside the Hospital," *J. Am. Coll. Emerg. Phys.*, 8 (1979): 216-20.

3. R. R. Liberthson, E. L. Nagel, J. C. Hirschman, et al., "Prehospital Ventricular Fibrillation — Prognosis and Follow-up Course," *N. Engl. J. Med.*, 291 (1974): 317-21.

4. M. S. Eisenberg, L. Bergner, A. Hallstrom, "Paramedic Programs and Out-of-Hospital Cardiac Arrest: Factors Associated with Successful Resuscitation," *Am. J. Public Health,* 69 (1979): 30-38.

5. K. K. Kishpaugh, M. H. Ford, C. H. Castle, et al., "Myocardial Infarction: A Five-Year Follow-up of Patients," *West. J. Med.*, 134 (1981): 1-6.

6. R. B. Singer, "Mortality Follow-up Studies and Risk Selection: Retrospect and Prospect," *Trans. Assoc. Life Insur. Med. Dir. Amer.*, 62 (1978): 215-38.

TABLE 305K1-1

COMPARATIVE MORTALITY IN 3 SERIES OF CARDIAC ARREST CASES
AFTER SUCCESSFUL RESUSCITATION AND HOSPITAL DISCHARGE
(HOSPITAL DEATHS EXCLUDED)

Ref	FU Period	Average Age	No. of Entrants	Exposure Patient-yrs.	No. of Deaths Observed	No. of Deaths Expected	Mortality Ratio	Ave. Ann. Mort Rate Observed	Ave. Ann. Mort Rate Expected	Excess Death Rate
		$\bar{x}$	ℓ	E	d	d'	100(d/d')	$\bar{q}$	$\bar{q}'$	1000($\bar{q}-\bar{q}'$)
	EARLY EXPERIENCE, UP TO 1-2 YEARS									
1	0-1 Years	65	276	228.6	68	13.72	495%	0.297	0.060	237
2	Ave. 12.2 Months	63	47	47.7	12	2.62	460	0.255	0.055	200
3	Ave. 12.7 Months	63	42	44.6	20	2.45	815	0.448	0.055	393
	LATER EXPERIENCE, 1-4 YEARS									
1	1-4 Years	66	154	228.5	31	11.88	260%	0.136	0.052	84

1. 222 Males and 54 Females. q' first year estimated from survival curve, age/sex-matched U.S. population rates. q' for 1-4 years is a geometric mean from Figure 1.

2. Ambulatory discharge patients only (34 patients to chronic care facilities excluded), average age 63 years. Initial group 514 cardiac arrest cases, Hennepin County, Minnesota. $\bar{q}'$ adjusted approximation based on q' for Series 1, 1974-76 observations.

3. All patients discharged alive out of 301 cardiac arrest cases, Miami, 1970-73. Males 75% in 301 patients, mean age 63 years all patients. Cases other than ventricular fibrillation excluded. $\bar{q}'$ adjusted approximation based on $\bar{q}'$ for Series 1.

TABLE 305K1-2

FIRST-YEAR OBSERVED MORTALITY, KING COUNTY SERIES (1)

Interval Start-End	No. of Entrants	Withdrawn Alive	Interval No. Exposed to Risk	Deaths Observed	Interval Mortality Rate	Survival Rate		Exposure Pt.-yrs.
						Interval	Cumulative	
t to $t+\Delta t$	ℓ	w	$NER = \ell - w/2$	d	$q_i = d/NER$	$p_i = 1-q$	P	$E = NER \times \Delta t$
0-3 Months	276	(10)*	271	(43)*	0.159	0.841	0.841	67.8
3-12	223	44	201	25	0.124	0.876	0.737	150.8
0-12	276	54[†]	—	68[†]	—	—	0.737	228.6

* w approximated. d estimated from survival series in Figure 2.

[†] w and d from data on Figure 1.

TABLE 305K1-3

FOUR-YEAR OBSERVED MORTALITY, KING COUNTY SERIES (1)

Interval Start-End	No. of Entrants	Withdrawn Alive	Exposure Pt.-yrs.	Deaths Observed	Interval Mortality Rate	Survival Rate	
						Annual	Cumulative
t to $t+\Delta t$	ℓ*	w[†]	$E = \ell - w/2$	d*	$q = d/E$	$p = 1-q$	P
0-1 Years	276	54	228.6**	68	0.297	0.703	0.703
1-2	154	51	128.5	17	0.132	0.868	0.610
2-3	86	37	67.5	9	0.133	0.867	0.529
3-4	40	15	32.5	5	0.154	0.846	0.448
1-4	154	—	228.5	31	0.136	0.864	0.637

* ℓ and d from data on Figure 1.

[†] Calculated from data on Figure 1.

** Based on NER data 0-3 and 3-12 months.

MORTALITY ANALYZED BY MAXIMAL EXERCISE TEST (BRUCE PROTOCOL): SEATTLE HEART WATCH EXPERIENCE

Richard B. Singer, M.D. and Robert A. Bruce, M.D., F.A.C.C.

References:

1. R. A. Bruce, "Strategies for Risk Assessment of Ischemic Heart Disease and Total Mortality," *Trans. Assoc. Life Insur. Med. Dir. Amer.*, 73 (1989): 53-67.

2. R. A. Bruce, L. D. Fisher, "Strategies for Risk Evaluation of Sudden Cardiac Incapacitation in Men in Occupations Affecting Public Safety," *J. Occup. Med.*, 21 (1989): 124-33.

3. R. A. Bruce, Additional life table data in personal communication (1989).

Objective of Abstract: To present detailed tables of comparative mortality in men followed in the Seattle Heart Watch Registry, according to diagnosis, age and results of symptom-limited maximal exercise testing in community practice, with standard mortality derived from recent life insurance select tables.

Subjects Studied: Three diagnostic cohorts of men examined on a voluntary basis by dozens of physicians in the Seattle, Washington metropolitan area, 1971-81, with consent by physician and patient for follow-up in the Seattle Heart Watch Registry. In addition to a careful history, examination and other screening procedures, all of the men received a multistage treadmill test of maximal exercise according to the Bruce protocol, results of which were classified as low risk, moderate risk or high risk according to diagnostic group, selected risk factors and defined abnormal responses to exercise, either physical or in the exercise ECG. The first cohort consisted of 4,105 healthy men, mean age 44.6 years, with normal physical examination and resting ECG, not receiving any medical treatment. The second cohort consisted of 1,396 men, mean age 50.0 years, with a prior diagnosis of hypertension whether treated or not. The third cohort consisted of 2,371 men with chronic coronary heart disease, mean age 53.6 years. Patients with acute manifestations such as acute MI and unstable angina, and patients with overt congestive heart failure were excluded, but patients with a history of resuscitation from

cardiac arrest were included, together with the major categories of angina pectoris and history of acute MI. A fourth cohort of 537 men with atypical chest pain was excluded from this abstract because of the limited experience, with only 2 deaths. Results on 889 women similarly examined in the same time period have also been omitted because of the limited experience when classified into the diagnostic and risk groups. Results are therefore reported on a total of 7,872 men in the three diagnostic cohorts described above.

Follow-up: Continued until 1981, with a mean duration of 4.9 years and a maximum of 9.5 years. Questionnaires were mailed to each participant every 6 months for patients and every year for healthy persons to ascertain occurrence of cardiac events. Additional follow-up to next of kin, physician or hospital was carried out as necessary. Medical records, death certificates and narrative comments from next of kin, when obtained, were reviewed by a panel of cardiologists to classify cause of death (sudden, other cardiac or non-cardiac) and specified cardiac events. Follow-up was 94.5% complete.

Results: Expected deaths and mortality rates have been derived from the male 1975-80 Basic Select Tables, which represent the experience from the first to the 15th year after issue, for policyholders with standard insurance issued following the customary medical screening procedure. Actuarial methods were used to calculate exposure in person-years (converted from person-months), from which observed mean annual mortality rates have been derived and compared with the age-matched expected rates (q'). Age-matched expected deaths have also been derived as the product of q' and the appropriate exposure. All mean annual mortality rates, aggregate exposures, observed and expected deaths shown in the tables are for all durations combined.

The age distribution by diagnostic cohort and quinquennial age groups is given in Table 319K1-1, with mean ages for each age group as well as the total. A similar distribution is shown in Table 319K1-2 for the three risk groups in each of the diagnostic cohorts, all ages combined (detailed data by combination of diagnosis, risk group *and* age have been used in the derivation of

Source: R. B. Singer, R. A. Bruce, "Mortality Analyzed by Maximal Exercise Test (Bruce Protocol): Seattle Heart Watch Experience," *J. Ins. Med.*, 22 (1990): 212-16. Reproduced with permission of authors and publisher.

expected deaths and rates, but have been omitted to conserve space). The mean age of 44.6 years and the percentage of patients age 55 and up in the healthy men increase in the cohort with hypertension (mean age 50.0 years), and increase again in the cohort of men with coronary heart disease (CHD), the mean age becoming 53.6 years with about 47% of patients age 55 or older. The mean age in each quinquennial cell differs little from the central age, but the differences appear to reflect the shape of the distribution curve. In Table 319K1-2 it is apparent that the mean age increases as the risk classification increases from low to moderate to high, regardless of the diagnostic cohort. The patterns of mean age and age distribution are what the clinician would anticipate from the diagnostic groupings and the increase in complications associated with increasing severity of any chronic disease process. However, these cohorts are not, and were not intended to be, random samples of the respective populations of healthy men, hypertensive men and men with CHD. Men with older ages, especially over 65, are underrepresented in all cohorts.

The comparative mortality experience for healthy men (Table 319K1-3) shows overall mortality lower than expected with a mortality ratio of 83% when the risk factors are ignored. There were 4 risk factors not related to the exercise test: (1) family history of myocardial infarction (MI) or sudden cardiac death (SCD) in parents or siblings; (2) elevated cholesterol, 250 mg./dl. or higher; (3) blood pressure >140 mm. Hg. systolic; (4) history of smoking cigarettes. These are "minor" or possibly ratable impairments for insurance applicants. The abnormal exercise responses for healthy men were defined as chest pain or exercise duration <6 minutes (Bruce protocol), or maximal heart rate <90% of value predicted for age, ST segment depression of 1 mm. or more. Low-risk men were restricted to those who had none of the above risk factors, and their overall mortality ratio of 58% of standard reflects the absence of minor impairments and the selective effect of the normal exercise test, a test that is not part of the routine insurance screening, except for applications involving very large amounts. Less than half of the healthy men were in the low-risk category, but 55% were classified as moderate-risk because they had at least one risk factor with or without a single abnormal response in the exercise test. There was no excess mortality in any of the age groups, and the overall mortality ratio was only 91%. Just 44 of the 4,105 healthy men, about 1%, had a high degree of risk, as indicated by two or more abnormal responses to exercise with at least one additional risk factor. There were 5 observed versus only 0.91 expected deaths, giving a mortality ratio of 550% and an excess death rate of 22 per 1000 per year. The risk classification

has therefore selected out a very small group of ostensibly healthy mean who have a significantly increased mortality. (95% Confidence Limits for 5 observed deaths by the Poisson distribution lie in the range from 1.6 to 11.7 deaths; the lower Limit is in relative excess of the 0.91 expected deaths, hence $p<0.025$ for a single-tailed difference). The presence of two or more of the abnormal responses to maximal exercise represents a very sensitive risk factor for a high degree of excess mortality in ostensibly healthy men. The classification "healthy" included a resting ECG without major abnormalities, and this helps to explain why the mortality observed was lower than standard life insurance mortality in both the low-risk and the moderate-risk groups. No more than one abnormal response to exercise was permitted in the latter group, in which other "minor" risks probably predominated. The mortality experience was favorable in spite of the risk being classified as moderate, although it was significantly greater than in the low-risk group.

The risk classification employed also made a useful separation in men with hypertension: the overall mortality ratio was 156% in the low-risk group (36% of the total), 190% in the men with moderate risk, and 305% in the men with a high-risk classification. Again, low risk signifies absence of abnormal response to maximal exercise and absence of any other risk factor. Moderate risk signifies, for the hypertensive men, a non-exercise risk factor or factors, but *no* abnormal response in the exercise test, and high risk signifies presence of at least one abnormal response to exercise and one or more other risk factors.

In contrast to the healthy men, fully 37% of the hypertensive men were in the high-risk group. There was a consistent age pattern of increasing excess mortality (both mortality ratio and excess death rate) with advancing age in the younger men to age 50-59, but the excess mortality was invariably lower in the oldest group, age 60 and up. There were only 14 deaths in an exposure of 896 patient-years in the oldest age group, but the sharp drop from a mortality ratio of 275% in men age 50-59 to 127% in men age 60 and up is an interesting finding. These results are for men with all risk groups combined.

Men with chronic CHD made up 30% of the total. The exposure was sufficient, with the high mortality observed, to permit splitting of the under 50 age group into two, under 40 and age 40-49. There were 85 deaths in the men with low risk, 128 in those with moderate risk, and 195 in those with high risk. The CHD cohort was divided fairly evenly: 37% in the low-risk category, 36% in the moderate-risk, and 27% in the high-risk. Different criteria were used for classification of risk in the men with CHD. Low risk was defined by the absence of exertional myocardial ischemia and left ventricular dysfunction; moderate risk was defined by ST depression of 1 mm. or more, or occurrence of chest pain during the test, in the absence of all factors used to indicate the high-risk group. The patient was classified at high risk if there was cardiac enlargement at rest, or the duration of exercise was less than 3 minutes (less than stage II), or the peak exercise systolic pressure was less than 130 mm. Hg. The risk classification again provided a smoothly graded progression of excess mortality. The overall mortality ratio was 435% in the men with low risk, 595% in those with moderate risk, and 1,340% in those with high risk; the corresponding excess death rates were 18, 29 and 97 extra deaths per 1000 per year, respectively. Mortality ratios decreased with increasing age, but within a very high range, from 1,900% down to 255% in the low-risk group, 2,600% to 335% in the moderate-risk and 6,000% to 975% in the men classified as at high risk. This progression is due in large part to the increase in mean expected annual mortality, q', with increasing age. The excess death rate is relatively constant with age in the low-risk and moderate-risk groups; in the high-risk group the EDR increased from about 75 per 1000 under age 50, to 92 per 1000 in the 50-59 age group, to 112 per 1000 in the oldest age group. It is of interest that the increase in EDR with advancing age is of such magnitude in the high-risk group that it produces a similar pattern when all risk groups are combined (bottom part of Table 319K1-5), a pattern, incidentally, that is characteristic of the late mortality experience in most series of post-MI patients.

Comment: These results demonstrate the potential usefulness of a method of risk classification based primarily on a standardized maximal exercise test in the separation of three distinct diagnostic male cohorts into categories with widely differing comparative mortality over a follow-up in the range of 1 to 9 years. The risk prevalence data in each cohort should be studied with as much care as the mortality results. Only 1% of healthy men had a high-risk classification. Although excess mortality was very high, and the elevation was statistically significant, the overall mortality experience was still favorable with respect to male select mortality, even when the high-risk deaths (5 out of 58 deaths) were included. However, this prevalence increases with age, and the test may be very useful in the screening of older individuals, such as airline pilots, whose sudden incapacitation while on duty is a matter of public safety concern (see reference 2). Treadmill exercise tests with a protocol leading to maximal exercise are now widely used in medical underwriting, but this test is a costly underwriting requirement. The results in Table 319K1-3 will permit the medical director to reassess the cost-benefit analysis to see if his company's present amount limit for such a test as a routine requirement is too high, too low, or about right. The much larger prevalence of high-risk response in hypertensive men raises a question as to the desirability of using the maximal exercise test as an additional requirement in rated or even borderline hypertension, when the amount of the application would justify the cost. This question is also worthy of analysis by the medical director. Finally, the clearcut grading of excess mortality in men with chronic CHD, according to the results of a maximal exercise test, is another challenge to the medical director on his company's selection policy with regard to this common impairment. The post-MI mortality experience in the *1983 Medical Impairment Study* includes a large exposure, but only 330 deaths as compared with 411 in this Seattle Heart Watch cohort. The overall mortality ratio and EDR in the insurance experience are intermediate, between the corresponding levels seen in the low-risk and moderate-risk groups. However, it should be noted that most of these post-MI cases are being under-rated. It is likely that judicious use of a maximal exercise test might remove the high-risk applicants from the basic CHD rating schedule, to place them in a higher rated category or declined, if this seems indicated.

MAXIMAL EXERCISE TEST

TABLE 319K1-1

AGE DISTRIBUTION BY DIAGNOSIS — 7,872 MEN WITH MAXIMAL EXERCISE TEST

Age-Yrs.	Healthy Men			Hypertensive Men			Men with CHD		
	No.	% Distr.	Ave. Age	No.	% Distr.	Ave. Age	No.	% Distr.	Ave. Age
<35	501	13.2%	30.1	67	4.8%	30.0	40	1.7%	30.2
35-39	684	16.7	37.2	113	8.1	37.3	77	3.2	37.4
40-44	853	20.8	42.1	190	13.6	42.1	206	8.7	42.3
45-49	820	20.0	46.9	233	16.7	47.2	395	16.7	47.2
50-54	689	16.8	51.8	332	23.8	52.0	530	22.4	52.0
55-59	382	9.3	56.7	244	12.5	57.0	551	23.2	57.1
60-64	140	3.4	61.6	144	10.3	61.6	390	16.4	61.7
65 up	36	0.9	68.6	73	5.2	69.9	182	7.7	68.9
All	4,105	100.0	44.6	1,396	100.0	50.0	2,371	100.0	53.6

TABLE 319K1-2

DISTRIBUTION BY DIAGNOSIS AND RISK GROUP — 7,872 MEN WITH MAXIMAL EXERCISE TEST

Risk	Healthy Men			Hypertensive Men			Men with CHD		
	No.	% Distr.	Ave. Age	No.	% Distr.	Ave. Age	No.	% Distr.	Ave. Age
Low	1,792	43.6%	44.0	502	36.0%	51.1	880	37.1%	51.3
Moderate	2,269	55.3	45.0	379	27.1	48.0	863	36.4	53.7
High	44	1.1	53.1	515	36.9	50.3	628	26.5	56.6
All	4,105	100.0	44.6	1,396	100.0	50.0	2,371	100.0	53.6

TABLE 319K1-3

COMPARATIVE MORTALITY BY AGE AND RISK GROUP — 4,105 HEALTHY MEN
ALL DURATIONS COMBINED (RISK BASED IN PART ON MAXIMAL EXERCISE TEST)

Risk Group	Age Group	No. Alive at Start	Exposure Man-yrs.	No. of Deaths		Mortality Ratio	Ave. Ann. Mort. Rate per 1000		
				Observed	Expected*		Observed	Expected	Excess
		ℓ	E	d	d'	100(d/d')	q	q'	(q–q')
Low	<50	1,283	6,855	6	14.11	43%	0.9	2.1	−1.2
	50-59	335	2,308	8	11.41	70	3.5	4.9	−1.4
	60 up	74	328	3	3.66	82	9.1	11.2	−2.1
	All	1,792	9,491	17	29.18	58	1.8	3.1	−1.3
Moderate	<50	1,564	8,801	20	18.56	108	2.3	2.1	0.2
	50-59	612	3,387	12	16.72	72	3.5	5.1	−1.6
	60 up	93	408	4	4.38	91	9.8	10.7	−0.9
	All	2,264	12,596	36	39.66	91	2.8	3.1	−0.3
High	All	44	186	5	0.91	550	27	4.9	22
All	<40	1,185	6,189	6	7.43	81	1.0	1.2	−0.2
	40-49	1,673	9,527	20	25.14	80	2.1	2.6	−0.5
	50-59	1,071	5,800	24	28.67	84	4.1	4.9	−0.8
	60 up	176	756	8	8.30	96	10.6	11.0	−0.4
	All	4,105	22,272	58	69.76	83	2.5	3.1	−0.6

* Expected deaths calculated on 1975-80 Male Basic Select Tables.

TABLE 319K1-4

COMPARATIVE MORTALITY BY AGE AND RISK GROUP — 1,396 HYPERTENSIVE MEN
ALL DURATIONS COMBINED (RISK BASED IN PART ON MAXIMAL EXERCISE TEST)

Risk Group	Age Group	No. Alive at Start	Exposure Patient-yrs.	No. of Deaths Observed	No. of Deaths Expected*	Mortality Ratio	Ave. Ann. Mort. Rate per 1000 Observed	Ave. Ann. Mort. Rate per 1000 Expected	Ave. Ann. Mort. Rate per 1000 Excess
		ℓ	E	d	d′	100(d/d)′	q	q′	(q–q′)
Low	<50	210	1,063	3	2.50	120%	2.8	2.4	0.4
	50-59	195	965	11	5.06	215	11.4	5.2	6.2
	60 up	97	417	6	5.29	113	14.4	12.7	1.7
	All	502	2,445	20	12.85	156	8.2	5.3	2.9
Moderate	<50	188	1,278	4	2.93	137	3.1	2.3	0.8
	50-59	166	919	12	4.63	260	13.1	5.0	8.1
	60 up	25	164	2	1.86	108	12.2	11.3	0.9
	All	379	2,361	18	9.46	190	7.6	4.0	3.6
High	<50	205	744	5	1.59	315	6.7	2.1	4.6
	50-59	215	777	15	4.14	360	19.3	5.3	14.0
	60 up	95	315	6	3.85	141	19.0	13.5	5.5
	All	515	1,836	26	9.88	305	14.2	5.2	9.0
All	<40	180	897	1	1.11	91	1.1	1.2	–0.1
	40-49	423	2,188	11	5.96	185	5.0	2.7	2.3
	50-59	576	2,661	38	13.83	275	14.3	5.2	9.1
	60 up	217	896	14	11.00	127	15.6	12.3	3.3
	All	1,396	6,642	64	31.89	200	9.6	4.8	4.8

* Expected deaths calculated on 1975-80 Male Basic Select Tables.

TABLE 319K1-5

COMPARATIVE MORTALITY BY AGE AND RISK GROUP — 2,371 MEN WITH CHD
ALL DURATIONS COMBINED (RISK BASED IN PART ON MAXIMAL EXERCISE TEST)

Risk Group	Age Group	No. Alive at Start	Exposure Patient-yrs.	No. of Deaths Observed	No. of Deaths Expected*	Mortality Ratio	Ave. Ann. Mort. Rate per 1000 Observed	Ave. Ann. Mort. Rate per 1000 Expected	Ave. Ann. Mort. Rate per 1000 Excess
		ℓ	E	d	d′	100(d/d)′	q	q′	(q–q′)
Low	<40	61	256	6	0.315	1,900%	23	1.2	22
	40-49	287	1,329	27	3.69	730	20	2.8	17
	50-59	385	1,700	38	8.78	435	22	5.2	17
	60 up	147	600	17	6.66	255	28	11.1	17
	All	880	3,885	88	19.45	450	23	5.0	18
Moderate	<40	35	117	4	0.151	2,600	34	1.3	33
	40-49	204	833	28	2.38	1,180	34	2.9	31
	50-59	432	1,876	66	9.98	660	35	5.3	30
	60 up	192	823	30	8.93	335	36	10.9	25
	All	863	3,649	128	21.44	595	35	5.9	29
High	<40	21	53.6	14	0.066	6,000	75	1.2	74
	40-49	110	312	25	0.91	2,700	80	2.9	77
	50-59	264	773	76	4.36	1,740	98	5.6	92
	60 up	233	722	90	9.23	975	125	12.8	112
	All	628	1,861	195	14.57	1,340	105	7.8	97
All	<40	117	427	14	0.53	2,600	33	1.2	32
	40-49	601	2,474	80	6.98	1,150	32	2.8	29
	50-59	1,081	4,349	180	23.12	780	41	5.3	36
	60 up	512	2,145	137	24.82	550	64	11.6	52
	All	2,371	9,395	411	55.45	740	44	5.9	38

* Expected deaths calculated on 1975-80 Male Basic Select Tables.

SUMMARY DATA
(EXPOSURES, DEATHS, MORTALITY RATIOS AND EXCESS DEATH RATES)
FOR THE SEPARATE STANDARD AND SUBSTANDARD EXPERIENCE
OF THE 1979 BLOOD PRESSURE STUDY

Richard B. Singer, M.D.

The 1979 Blood Pressure Study presented mortality results for nearly 3.8 million standard polices and nearly 600,000 policies issued on a substandard basis because of elevated blood pressure without any other ratable impairment (Table 320K1-1, taken from the table on page 32 of the published Study). These numbers of policies in Table 320K1-1 include cases with and without minor impairments, regardless of treatment (specified in only a small fraction of policies), issued 1950 through 1971, and exposed from anniversaries in 1954 through 1972. The "S" Tables show mortality ratios for the combined standard and substandard experience, weighted in the ratio of 4 standard to 1 substandard, and the corresponding un-weighted numbers of deaths. The "D" tables give similarly weighted mortality ratios and unweighted observed deaths for the combined standard and substandard experience in more detailed age groups, and (unweighted) mortality ratios and observed deaths for the separate substandard experience. Expected deaths are not shown in the tables, but can easily be calculated from the observed deaths and the mortality ratios. However, no data are given in the published volume for exposures and excess death rates corresponding to the mortality ratios. Such data are included in three large volumes of computer printout made available to me through the Blood Pressure Study Committee, its Chairman, Ed Lew, and John Avery, Director of the Center of Medico-Actuarial Statistics of MIB, Inc. One printout contains data for the separate standard experience (nowhere given in the published volume), another contains data for the substandard experience, and the third contains data for the un-weighted combined experience.

After consultation with the Editor, it seemed worth-while to us to present to readers of the *Journal of Insurance Medicine* these unpublished results of the separate

Source: R. B. Singer, "Summary Data (Exposures, Deaths, Mortality Ratios and Excess Death Rates) for the Separate Standard and Substandard Experience of the 1979 Blood Pressure Study," *J. Ins. Med.,* 18, no. 3 (1986): 17-23. Reproduced with permission of author and publisher.

TABLE 320K1-1

1979 BLOOD PRESSURE STUDY
DISTRIBUTION OF REPORTED POLICIES
BY AGE, SEX AND ACTION

MALES

Age	Std Issue		SStd Issue*	
	Number	%	Number	%
15-19	67,771	2.0%	9,301	1.9%
20-29	722,080	21.9	86,333	17.4
30-39	1,221,620	37.0	141,683	28.6
40-49	927,392	28.1	165,342	33.3
50-59	320,404	9.7	79,990	16.1
60-69	43,919	1.3	13,463	2.7
Total	3,303,186	100.0	496,112	100.0

FEMALES

Age	Std Issue		SStd Issue*	
	Number	%	Number	%
15-19	18,764	4.0%	2,008	2.1%
20-29	77,791	16.4	7,850	8.3
30-39	102,977	21.6	11,879	12.5
40-49	177,193	37.2	36,277	38.2
50-59	84,691	17.8	29,361	31.0
60-69	14,434	3.0	7,494	7.9
Total	475,850	100.0	94,869	100.0

MALES & FEMALES COMBINED
NUMBER OF POLICIES

Age	Std	SStd*	Total	SStd Issue* % of Total
15-19	86,535	11,309	97,844	11.6%
20-29	799,871	94,183	894,054	10.5
30-39	1,324,597	153,562	1,478,159	10.4
40-49	1,104,585	201,619	1,306,204	15.4
50-59	405,095	109,351	514,446	21.3
60-69	58,353	20,957	79,310	26.4
Total	3,779,036	590,981	4,370,017	13.5

* Rated for elevated blood pressure alone.

standard experience, and the unpublished exposures and excess death rates for the substandard experience. Results have been condensed into three tables, two for men in blood pressure groups A-D, age 15-39 (Table 320K1-2), age 40-69 (Table 320K1-3), and substandard groups E-H, both age groups (Table 320K1-4). Each table contains the data for exposures, observed and expected deaths, mortality ratios and excess death rates, according to the eight lettered blood pressure groups as defined on page 8 of the *Blood Pressure Study 1979*, except that the standard experience for the hypertensive groups D-H has been combined because of the very small proportion of policies issued standard at these higher blood pressure levels. The experience has been given by the five duration intervals, 0-2, 2-5, 5-10, 10-15, and 15-22 years, as well as by all durations combined, because the duration trends are of interest. (Duration intervals are here defined by the times of the beginning and end of each interval, not by the number of each full year of follow-up, as used in the tables of the *Blood Pressure Study 1979*.)

Some preliminary explanation should be made of two potentially confusing features of the results published in the *Blood Pressure Study 1979*: (1) the weighting method used for the combined standard and substandard experience, constituting the bulk of the tables, and (2) the rationale in the progressively graded blood pressure groups lettered from A to H. On page 6 of the volume it is stated that the 4 to 1 weighting "was because in many companies it was common practice to prepare medico-actuarial records for only a sample of their standard issues, whereas virtually all companies prepared medico-actuarial records for their entire substandard issues. To reflect the actual proportions of standard and substandard business in the total issue it was, therefore, necessary to weight the standard and substandard issues appropriately." The logic of a weighting process is easy to understand, but the appropriateness of the constant 4 to 1 ratio is not, because the derivation of the ratio is never explained. It is clear that the sampling percentage of standard issues must have varied widely from one contributing company to another, from more than a 25% sample to considerably less than 25% (Table 1, page 5 of the volume). The ratio of substandard issues to the total issues actually submitted varies widely, of course, by age at issue, as shown in Table 320K1-1, and by blood pressure category, as shown in Tables 320K1-2 to 320K1-4. The potential bias and uncertainty introduced by a constant weighting ratio have always made me uneasy, because of the presumed variability of this ratio for different subsets of the total experience, according to blood pressure or other category. The proportion of substandard to total policies reported by the contributing companies does vary widely by age (Table 1, page 5, *Blood Pressure*

Study 1979), and by blood pressure (see exposure data, standard vs. substandard in Tables 320K1-2 and 320K1-3). This is acknowledged in section 5, page 59 of the *Blood Pressure Study 1979*: "The use of the 4 to 1 ratio in combining standard and substandard mortality data gives in some instances too great a weight to the standard experience; in such situations the mortality ratios may be slightly understated. This appears to have been the case in certain high blood pressure classifications." My personal preference has always been to present the standard and substandard mortality results separately, as in the 1951 and the 1983 Impairment Studies. It is for this reason I am glad that these additional data permit a close examination of the separate standard and substandard experience by all major blood pressure categories where the volume is large enough to permit a meaningful comparison. Incidentally, the numbers of observed deaths in the published tables are unweighted totals, so the Committee has been careful to avoid bias in the calculation of confidence limits for the mortality ratios from the numbers of deaths as shown in the tables.

Various of my medical director friends have expressed puzzlement over the Committee's choice of limits for the lettered blood pressure classes. Although this is not explained in the book and I was not involved in the decision process, I think the logic of the selection of these categories is made clear by an inspection of the systolic/diastolic pressure grid in Figure 320K1-1. Each cell of the grid contains the number of unweighted deaths, standard and substandard combined, except that each of the lettered categories (separately boxed) contains two or more of the basic cells of the grid. The eight special categories are identifiable by their letter, and weighted mortality ratios, men all ages combined, are entered above the numbers of deaths. Although less than half of the cells are utilized in the lettered categories, the latter include 78% of the observed deaths. In the grid, systolic pressures are 10 mm. apart and diastolic pressures only 5 mm. There is a very obvious progression of systolic/diastolic pressure combination from group A, the lowest normotensive group (under 128/83) to group F, the most severe hypertensive group (over 167/97). Approximate mean pressures for the intervening categories are 133/83 for group B, 143/88 for group C, 153/93 for group D, and 163/98 for group E. Group G comprises cases of predominantly systolic hypertension (maximum diastolic pressure 87 mm.), and group H, those with predominantly diastolic hypertension (maximum systolic pressure 147 mm.).

Even though at least two adjacent diastolic cells have been combined in each of the lettered categories it is obvious that there is no overlap of categories, and no blood pressure combination is counted more than once.

FIGURE 320K1-1

DISTRIBUTION OF DEATHS
MEN AGE 15-69 WITH AND WITHOUT MINOR IMPAIRMENTS
STANDARD AND SUBSTANDARD DEATHS COMBINED (UNWEIGHTED)

(diastolic)	(98)–108	108–118	118–128	128–138	138–148	148–158	158–168	168–178	178–(188)
68				558	110	25	15	0	3
73				3,111	481	73	14	15	3
78			A 84%	3,773	830	152	31	8	1
83			37,492	B	3,641	G	G	38	13
88	6	183	2,317	22,127 (B 111%)	C	154% 1,953		44	13
93	5	34	472	2,739	7,920 (C 140%)	D	548	111	34
98	1	1	15	H	H	176% 2,444	E	108	36
103	1	1	7	159% 1,475		524	226% 866	F	
108	0	0	0	10	47	114	116	269% (F)	
113	0	0	0	0	10	29	50	439	
	2	1	1	2	1	4	4		

Mortality ratios based on weighted totals, 4 standard to 1 substandard.

All other 20,486	112%	
Total deaths 95,202	100%	

Fringe BP Classes: < 98 systolic   80 deaths
(not shown)   >187 systolic   85 deaths
   All diastolic classes are shown

8 BP categories A-H, see Table S13, p. 96
Other BP cells, see Table S3, p. 75

When mortality results by the lettered categories are examined, this progression of increasing systolic/diastolic pressure for groups A through F should be kept in mind, as well as the systolic hypertension in group G and diastolic hypertension in group H. A basically simple classification, isn't it?

Results for the younger men, age 15-39, are given in Table 320K1-2, with the standard and substandard data side by side, groups A-C, and substandard group D aligned with standard groups D-H combined because of the small number of standard issues at these hypertensive blood pressure levels. In groups A and B the overwhelming predominance of the volume of standard experience is evident, as would be anticipated for these normotensive policyholders. Equally striking is the excess mortality in the much smaller but not insignificant substandard experience, with mortality ratios over 200%, all durations combined. Even though there were only 33 deaths in the substandard group A, the 95% confidence limits for the 202% mortality ratio are 137% to 285%, so the difference from the 87% mortality ratio in the standard group is highly significant. In the very large standard group A, with over 13,000 deaths, the confidence limits are narrow, only 84% to 88%, illustrating how much the confidence limits are affected by these extreme variations in the size of the groups under comparison. As would be expected, the size of the standard groups decreases with increasing blood pressure, while the size of the substandard groups increases to a maximum of 83,474 policy-years in group C, then diminishes in group D. The combined standard exposure in groups D-H gives only 92 deaths and less than 27,000 policy-years of exposure, about half that of substandard group D alone, and only one-eighth that of substandard groups D-H combined (see Table 320K1-4).

In standard group A, with blood pressure under 128/83, the mortality experience is highly favorable at all durations; almost two-thirds of the standard exposure was concentrated in this "low normotensive" blood pressure category. Mortality ratios in the standard groups, all durations combined, increased from 87% in group A to 116% in group B to 166% in group C, and then decreased to 163% in groups D-H. Since most of the policyholders in groups D-H had "high borderline" or "definite" hypertension by the customary American Heart Association definitions, these cases must have been carefully underwritten to achieve a mortality ratio slightly lower than in group C. In groups B and C there appears to be a definite trend for the mortality ratio and excess death rate to increase with duration, a trend that is more pronounced in the corresponding substandard groups. I am sure the mortality ratio of 166% in the standard group C is much higher than the minimal rating not imposed if the underwriting manual calls for at the borderline blood pressure level of 140/90, and the ratio of 224% is even higher than any minimal rating that was imposed in the substandard group C. However, those responsible for setting underwriting standards for blood pressure can console themselves that the standard class C exposure constituted less than 2% of the total exposure for all standard issues in the blood pressure study. It is less consoling to note that exposure in the two borderline hypertension groups C and D is about one-third of the exposure of all policies rated for blood pressure alone, and I am confident that the average rating imposed in these two groups is substantially less than the average mortality ratio of about 230%. For all durations combined there is a slight but consistent increase in the excess death rate from substandard group A through D, but the range of mortality ratio is only 202% and 244%.

In men age 40-69 results are generally similar in blood pressure groups A-D to results for the younger men, as is evident in Table 320K1-3. Exposure is smaller in the older men, especially in those issued standard insurance; however, in all categories numbers of deaths are larger, sometimes markedly so. For example, there were 2,027 deaths in substandard group D in men, as compared with only 191 in substandard group D in men age 15-39 (Table 320K1-2). In general, mortality ratios in the substandard groups A-D in Table 320K1-3 averaged about 50 percentage points less than the ratios in the corresponding groups in the younger men. Excess death rates were higher in men age 40-69 but they showed the same trend to increase with duration. As in the younger men, the standard group A experience for men age 40-69 was very favorable at all duration intervals, with a mortality ratio of 82% overall. The standard mortality ratio was 109% in the higher normotensive group B in Table 320K1-3, 134% in group C, and only 138% in groups D-H combined, based on 944 deaths in these policyholders issued standard insurance despite blood pressure at definite or borderline hypertensive levels. In standard groups B, C, and D-H the excess death rates tended to increase with duration as they did in Table 320K1-2.

The explanation for the blood pressure rating imposed in the currently normotensive groups A and B must be a history of past hypertension, with or without treatment. Such cases made up over 10% of the substandard exposure in Table 320K1-2, and over 6% in Table 320K1-3. Justification for imposing a rating is evident in the significant increase in mortality ratio in all of these normotensive groups. History of hypertension was apparently not reported with sufficient frequency to permit a separate analysis of the mortality. The mortality is very different in the standard and substandard normotensive groups A and B, and differences are also evident in groups C-H. To me, these differences are compelling reasons for separate presentation and analysis of the standard and substandard experience.

Substandard experience for men with definite hypertension, separate groups D through H, is given in Table 320K1-4. The highest mortality ratios were found in group F cases, those with blood pressures exceeding 167/97: 456% in men age 15-39 and 267% in men age 40-69. While mortality ratios were lower in all of these groups in the older men, excess death rates were approximately twice as high as in the men under age 40. Excess death rates increased with increasing duration in all blood pressure groups and rose to more than 40 per 1000 per year in both F groups at 15-22 years duration. In groups G and H, those with systolic and diastolic hypertension, respectively, mortality ratios were about the same as the overall ratios for the substandard experience: over 200% in men under 40, and under 200% in men age 40 and up. Systolic hypertension alone appeared to be more prevalent than isolated diastolic hypertension, but the increase in mortality was nearly the same in both groups. As judged from the difference in expected mortality rates at durations 0-2 years, the men age 40-69 with systolic hypertension (group G) had an older average age than the men with diastolic hypertension (group H).

Overall mortality has been given in the bottom of the table for the residual blood pressure cells not included in the lettered categories, and for the total substandard experience. The mortality ratio was close to 200% in the residual blood pressure cells, 228% for the total substandard issues reported for men age 15-39, and 192% for men age 40-69. In the standard experience (data not shown in Table 320K1-4) the mortality ratios were 111%

in the residual blood pressure cells and about 92% overall, regardless of age group.

Because of lack of time I have not prepared similar results for the much smaller mortality experience among women. The printouts also contain results by the detailed individual blood pressure cells, but not for decennial age groups. The results described above at least provide a summary of the mortality experience by separate standard and substandard categories.

REFERENCE

1. *Blood Pressure Study 1979* (Boston, Soc. Actuaries and Assoc. Life Ins. Med. Dir. Amer., 1980).

1979 BLOOD PRESSURE STUDY

TABLE 320K1-2

MORTALITY IN MEN AGE 15-39 BY DURATION AND BLOOD PRESSURE CLASS, SEPARATE STANDARD AND SUBSTANDARD.

Duration Years	STANDARD					SUBSTANDARD†				
	Exposure Policy-yrs.	No. of Deaths		Mortality Ratio	Excess Death Rate	Exposure Policy-yrs.	No. of Deaths		Mortality Ratio	Excess Death Rate
		Observed	Expected*				Observed	Expected*		
	E	d	d′	100(d/d′)	1000(d-d′)/E	E	d	d′	100(d/d′)	1000(d-d′)/E
A. NORMOTENSIVE (LOWER) SYSTOLIC <128, DIASTOLIC <83										
0-2	1,784,658	972	1,176	83%	−0.2	4,195	8	2.80	285%	1.3
2-5	2,211,561	2,252	2,406	94	−0.1	3,750	4	4.21	95	−0.1
5-10	2,602,415	3,631	4,122	88	−0.2	2,971	11	5.09	216	2.2
10-15	1,543,311	3,596	4,297	84	−0.5	928	8	2.73	293	6.2
15-22	778,136	3,303	3,766	88	−0.6	334	2	1.55	129	2.8
All	8,920,081	13,754	15,767	87	−0.2	12,178	33	16.35	202	1.4
B. NORMOTENSIVE (UPPER) SYSTOLIC 128-137, DIASTOLIC 78-87										
0-2	470,814	342	322	106%	0.0	9,397	9	6.47	139%	0.3
2-5	596,303	686	655	105	0.1	9,133	20	10.69	187	1.1
5-10	638,951	1,339	1,120	120	0.3	7,436	40	13.35	300	3.7
10-15	354,666	1,302	1,121	116	0.5	2,395	17	7.82	217	4.0
15-22	165,450	1,146	926	124	1.3	734	12	4.20	286	11.3
All	2,199,184	4,815	4,144	116	0.3	29,095	98	42.47	231	1.9
C. BORDERLINE (LOWER) SYSTOLIC 138-147, DIASTOLIC 83-92										
0-2	46,754	50	33.0	152%	0.4	25,702	26	18.12	143%	0.3
2-5	56,690	111	68.6	162	0.7	25,177	55	30.51	180	1.0
5-10	63,605	183	120.5	152	1.0	22,580	101	42.81	236	2.6
10-15	33,893	204	117.3	174	2.6	7,703	71	26.62	267	5.8
15-22	13,890	160	87.1	184	5.3	2,312	43	14.16	303	12.7
All	214,832	708	426.4	166	1.3	83,474	296	132.22	224	2.0
D-H. BORDERLINE OR HYPERTENSION**						**D. BORDERLINE (UPPER) SYSTOLIC 148-157, DIASTOLIC 88-97**				
0-2	4,799	9	3.36	268%	1.1	13,377	28	9.49	295%	1.4
2-5	6,318	10	7.56	132	0.4	13,258	45	16.17	278	2.2
5-10	8,046	32	14.96	214	2.1	12,480	55	23.80	231	2.5
10-15	4,891	24	16.36	147	1.6	5,289	49	18.37	267	5.9
15-22	2,395	17	14.23	119	1.2	1,671	14	10.51	133	2.4
All	26,449	92	56.47	163	1.3	46,075	191	78.23	244	2.5

* Basis of expected deaths: 1954-72 Standard Select and Ultimate Tables.

† Rated for elevated blood pressure only.

** Group E 158-167/93-102; Group F 168up/98up; Group G 148-167/78-87; Group H 128-147/93-102.

1979 BLOOD PRESSURE STUDY

TABLE 320K1-3

MORTALITY IN MEN AGE 40-69 BY DURATION AND BLOOD PRESSURE CLASS, SEPARATE STANDARD AND SUBSTANDARD

Duration Years	STANDARD					SUBSTANDARD[†]				
	Exposure Policy-yrs.	No. of Deaths		Mortality Ratio	Excess Death Rate	Exposure Policy-yrs.	No. of Deaths		Mortality Ratio	Excess Death Rate
		Observed	Expected*				Observed	Expected*		
	E	d	d′	100(d/d′)	1000(d-d′)/E	E	d	d′	100(d/d′)	1000(d-d′)/E
A. NORMOTENSIVE (LOWER) SYSTOLIC <128, DIASTOLIC <83										
0-2	911,625	1,671	1,994	84%	−0.4	4,251	24	10.96	219%	3.2
2-5	1,113,307	4,107	4,963	83	−0.8	3,756	32	19.04	168	3.6
5-10	1,210,283	7,328	8,915	82	−1.3	2,652	41	21.03	195	7.7
10-15	608,227	5,997	7,605	79	−2.6	659	12	8.46	142	6.1
15-22	251,596	4,490	5,397	83	−3.6	179	3	3.41	88	−0.4
All	4,095,038	23,593	28,874	82	−1.3	11,497	112	62.90	178	4.3
B. NORMOTENSIVE (UPPER) SYSTOLIC 128-137, DIASTOLIC 78-87										
0-2	465,177	1,130	1,149	98%	0.0	12,155	54	31.25	173%	1.9
2-5	563,662	3,107	2,855	109	0.4	11,504	116	59.01	197	5.0
5-10	595,082	5,414	4,966	109	0.8	8,383	122	68.01	179	6.5
10-15	278,818	4,421	3,908	113	1.8	1,911	47	25.34	185	11.6
15-22	106,899	2,789	2,531	110	2.4	445	14	9.92	141	10.3
All	2,009,638	16,861	15,409	109	0.7	34,398	353	193.58	182	4.6
C. BORDERLINE (LOWER) SYSTOLIC 138-147, DIASTOLIC 83-92										
0-2	105,635	391	310	126%	0.8	40,109	171	99.1	173%	1.8
2-5	130,260	997	794	126	1.6	41,226	360	207.2	174	3.7
5-10	137,905	1,845	1,387	133	3.3	35,078	519	284.8	182	6.7
10-15	61,969	1,464	1,035	141	6.9	9,700	235	128.6	183	11.0
15-22	21,005	821	580	142	11.5	2,660	113	59.6	190	20.0
All	456,504	5,518	4,106	134	3.1	128,773	1,398	779.4	179	4.8
D-H. BORDERLINE OR HYPERTENSION**					**D. BORDERLINE (UPPER) SYSTOLIC 148-157, DIASTOLIC 88-97**					
0-2	14,388	72	51.0	141%	1.5	41,526	226	125.0	181%	2.4
2-5	17,899	170	130.8	130	2.2	42,866	471	263.2	179	4.9
5-10	19,644	337	232.8	145	5.3	38,206	747	380.2	196	9.6
10-15	9,367	231	183.3	126	5.1	12,569	398	202.9	196	15.6
15-22	2,943	134	85.4	157	16.5	3,438	185	92.8	199	27.0
All	64,241	944	683.3	138	4.1	138,605	2,027	1,064.1	190	7.0

* Basis of expected deaths: 1954-72 Standard Select and Ultimate Tables.

[†] Rated for elevated blood pressure only.

** Group E 158-167/93-102; Group F 168up/98up; Group G 148-167/78-87; Group H 128-147/93-102.

1979 BLOOD PRESSURE STUDY

TABLE 320K1-4

MORTALITY IN MEN RATED FOR HYPERTENSION, BY AGE AND DURATION

Duration Years	AGE 15-39					AGE 40-69				
	Exposure Policy-yrs.	No. of Deaths		Mortality Ratio	Excess Death Rate	Exposure Policy-yrs.	No. of Deaths		Mortality Ratio	Excess Death Rate
		Observed	Expected*				Observed	Expected*		
	E	d	d′	100(d/d′)	1000(d-d′)/E	E	d	d′	100(d/d′)	1000(d-d′)/E

E. DEFINITE HYPERTENSION, SYSTOLIC 158-67, DIASTOLIC 93-102

Duration	E	d	d′	100(d/d′)	1000(d-d′)/E	E	d	d′	100(d/d′)	1000(d-d′)/E
0-2	3,281	3	2.35	128%	0.3	14,698	108	46.3	233%	4.2
2-5	3,154	15	3.91	384	3.7	14,242	232	93.0	250	9.8
5-10	2,959	19	5.76	330	4.6	11,797	284	125.8	226	13.5
10-15	1,172	14	4.10	341	8.9	3,497	127	61.6	206	18.8
15-22	423	7	2.71	258	11.3	831	39	22.7	172	20.0
All	10,989	58	18.81	308	3.6	45,065	790	349.4	226	9.8

F. DEFINITE HYPERTENSION, SYSTOLIC 168 up, DIASTOLIC 98 up

Duration	E	d	d′	100(d/d′)	1000(d-d′)/E	E	d	d′	100(d/d′)	1000(d-d′)/E
0-2	1,306	5	0.93	532	3.5	8,445	76	27.1	281	5.9
2-5	1,153	6	1.45	414	4.4	7,200	136	47.2	288	12.4
5-10	932	5	1.86	267	3.9	4,994	136	52.4	260	16.8
10-15	331	6	1.18	508	16.1	1,069	39	17.7	221	20.0
15-22	112	6	0.71	845	52	251	17	7.0	244	42.0
All	3,834	28	6.14	456	5.8	21,959	404	151.4	267	11.5

G. SYSTOLIC HYPERTENSION, SYSTOLIC 148-167, DIASTOLIC 78-87

Duration	E	d	d′	100(d/d′)	1000(d-d′)/E	E	d	d′	100(d/d′)	1000(d-d′)/E
0-2	12,878	11	8.50	129	0.2	26,513	164	92.2	178	2.7
2-5	13,008	30	14.34	209	1.2	28,338	383	203.8	188	6.3
5-10	12,393	50	20.64	242	2.4	26,236	560	305.6	183	9.7
10-15	5,083	32	15.24	210	3.4	8,492	272	161.0	169	13.1
15-22	1,537	15	8.25	182	4.7	2,104	131	67.4	194	30.0
All	44,899	138	66.9	206	1.6	91,683	1,510	830.0	182	7.4

H. DIASTOLIC HYPERTENSION, SYSTOLIC 128-147, DIASTOLIC 93-102

Duration	E	d	d′	100(d/d′)	1000(d-d′)/E	E	d	d′	100(d/d′)	1000(d-d′)/E
0-2	13,948	23	10.16	226	1.0	26,518	106	61.9	171	1.7
2-5	12,612	37	15.93	232	1.7	24,993	197	118.9	166	3.1
5-10	10,537	57	21.12	270	3.5	20,662	280	160.0	175	5.8
10-15	3,860	35	14.15	247	5.5	6,402	148	82.8	179	10.3
15-22	1,213	26	8.26	314	15.0	1,670	86	37.2	231	30.0
All	42,170	178	69.5	256	2.6	80,245	817	460.9	177	4.4

ALL BLOOD PRESSURE COMBINATIONS OUTSIDE GROUPS A-H

Duration	E	d	d′	100(d/d′)	1000(d-d′)/E	E	d	d′	100(d/d′)	1000(d-d′)/E
All	109,152	330	161.7	204	1.5	169,107	2,469	1,248.8	198	7.2

TOTAL EXPERIENCE, RATED FOR HYPERTENSION

Duration	E	d	d′	100(d/d′)	1000(d-d′)/E	E	d	d′	100(d/d′)	1000(d-d′)/E
All	381,866	1,350	592.1	228	2.0	721,332	9,880	5,140.3	192	6.6

*Basis of expected deaths: 1954-72 Standard Select and Ultimate Tables.

COMPARATIVE MORTALITY IN THE ASPIRIN COMPONENT OF THE PHYSICIANS' HEALTH STUDY

Richard B. Singer, M.D.

References:

1. Steering Committee of the Physicians' Health Study Research Group, "Final Report on the Aspirin Component of the Physicians' Health Study," *N. Engl. J. Med.*, 321 (1989): 129-35.
2. C. H. Hennekens, Personal communication of additional data (August, 1990).

Objective of the Study: "To determine whether low-dose aspirin (325 mg. every other day) decreases cardiovascular mortality and whether beta carotene reduces the incidence of cancer."[1]

Subjects Studied: A total of 22,071 U.S. male physicians age 40-84 years was accepted as volunteer participants in the study. Letters of invitation and other forms were mailed in 1982 to 261,248 physicians identified on a computer tape received from the American Medical Association. Of 112,538 replies received by December 31, 1983 there were 59,285 physicians willing to participate in the trial, as outlined below. Volunteers were excluded from the trial if they had a history of myocardial infarction (MI), stroke or transient ischemic attack, cancer (except nonmelanoma skin cancer), current liver or renal disease, peptic ulcer or gout; contraindications to aspirin consumption; current use of aspirin, other platelet-active drugs or nonsteroidal anti-inflammatory agents; or current use of a Vitamin A supplement. After the exclusion process 33,233 physicians were enrolled in a "run-in phase" and were given calendar packs containing aspirin and beta carotene placebo (taken on alternate days). After 18 weeks all preliminary participants were screened by questionnaire, and about one-third were excluded because they had changed their mind, demonstrated inadequate compliance (took less than 67% of their pills), or reported a reason for exclusion. Thus, the final accepted pool of 22,071 physicians was then randomized into four categories on a double-blind basis: aspirin and beta carotene, aspirin and beta carotene

placebo, aspirin placebo and beta carotene, and placebo for both agents. The number of physicians randomized to aspirin was 11,037, and the number to aspirin placebo, 11,034. This large sample resulted in virtually identical distributions of base-line characteristics in the two treatment groups reported here. Age distribution in terms of exposure is shown in Table 338K1-1 for quinquennial age groups,[2] in greater detail than in the published article.

Follow-up: In addition to their 12 calendar packs per year (aspirin or placebo on odd days and beta carotene or placebo on even days of the month) all participants were sent an annual questionnaire about their compliance with the treatment regimen and the development of an MI or other relevant conditions or symptoms. Reported diagnoses were confirmed in 95.6% of MIs, 95.2% of strokes, and 94.8% of all deaths, as a result of examination of medical records by an expert End Points Committee, after authorization was obtained and the records secured. The decision was made by the Data Monitoring Board in December, 1987 to terminate the Aspirin Component of the study, because of a highly significant ($p<0.00001$) reduction of risk of MI observed in the aspirin group, and for other cogent reasons, but the beta carotene Component continues as of the date of this abstract. The cutoff date for the Aspirin Component was January 25, 1988, at which time the mean follow-up was 60.2 months for all participants (range of 45.0 to 77.8 months). At this date 99.7% of surviving physicians were providing information in the completed questionnaires they returned, and the vital status of *all* of the 22,071 physician-entrants had been determined.

Expected Mortality: The volunteer response and the selection process resulted in a cardiovascular and a total mortality that was markedly below that of the age-matched U.S. male white population (1985 Abridged U.S. Life Tables). From these rates (right-hand column) and the exposures shown in Table 338K1-1 the 227 deaths in the placebo group were associated with a total of about 834 expected deaths, producing a mortality ratio of 27%. It was therefore considered appropriate to use select mortality rates instead of population rates from the total study group, which was clearly not a random sample of the population nor a random sample of physicians as

Source: R. B. Singer, "Comparative Mortality in the Aspirin Component of the Physicians' Health Study," *J. Ins. Med.*, 22 (1990): 279-83. Reproduced with permission of author and publisher.

an occupational group. The 1975-80 Intercompany Basic Select Tables are the latest available, but it was considered desirable to adjust these rates downward, because of the continuing secular trend for a decrease in both cardiovascular and total mortality. There was an 8-year interval between the mid-point of the Select experience and the mid-point of the Physicians' Health Study experience. The decrease was estimated by taking the ratio of the rate for each quinquennial age group, at duration 3 years, in the 1975-80 male table, to the corresponding rate in the 1965-70 table. This ratio, always a decimal less than 1, was a ratio for an interval 10 years between the mid-points of the observation periods for these two tables. The decrease from 1977-78 to 1985-86 has been estimated as this ratio raised to the power 0.8 (8 years/10 years). This is the factor f shown in Table 338K1-1, except that 0.66, age 55-59, has been substituted for an even lower factor at age 50-54, because this would have given an adjusted rate, q', that would have been lower than the 2.1 per 1000 for the preceding age group, 45-49. The highest age group in the Select Tables is 70 years and up; this has been assumed to be equivalent to age 70-74. Rates in the Ultimate Tables have been used for age groups 75-79 and 80-84, with the adjustment factor, f, derived as shown above. The select rate shown in Table 338K1-1 is therefore the third policy year rate in the 1975-80 Select Tables for males, adjusted for a downward secular change as described. These rates have been applied to the age-matched exposure data supplied by Dr. Hennekens to derive the quinquennial expected deaths for the aspirin and placebo groups. The data in Table 338K1-1 have been appropriately combined to give the results for the larger age groups shown in Table 338K1-2.

Results: Total deaths were almost equal, 217 in the aspirin group, and 227 in the placebo (Table 338K1-2). However, the 139 MIs in the aspirin group were very significantly lower than 239 total MIs in the placebo group ($p < 0.00001$). Some of the mortality and morbidity data have been developed in Tables 338K1-2 through 338K1-5, but for detailed results of the aspirin vs. the placebo group the reader is referred to the published report.[1]

Comparative mortality by age is shown for the aspirin and placebo groups separately in Table 338K1-2, all durations combined. Overall, the mortality experienced in both groups of these selected physicians was very close to the adjusted select mortality for the corresponding time period in the mid-1980s: the mortality, all ages combined, was 102% in the placebo group and 98% in the aspirin group. There was no consistent pattern of mortality variation with age. In most of the age groups the

differences in mortality ratio from the "expected" 100% were not statistically significant, some ratios being above and some below 100%. Excess death rates were sometimes positive, sometimes negative, and all differences below age 70-84 were very small, less than 1 per 1000 per year. In one age class, 60-69 years in the aspirin group, the 58 observed deaths had an upper 95% Confidence Limit of 75.0 deaths by the Poisson distribution. Both the select d' of 75.7 and the matching observed d of 76 deaths in the placebo group were just above this limit, and the reduced mortality is this age group is barely significant at the 95% level (p slightly <0.05). However, it would be imprudent to rely on the reduced mortality of this isolated age group, because of the scattering of the mortality differences in the other age groups. Furthermore, the authors of this elaborate clinical trial also made adjustments for differences in baseline characteristics and minor age differences, and the Poisson significance testing that I have used on the unadjusted data does not always correspond to the significance test results reported by the authors after such adjustment. Also, it is possible that the Poisson test is not the most appropriate for use in a clinical trial, in which the deaths observed in the placebo group may not correspond, in their random properties, to the expected deaths as derived from the exposure and age-matched rates from a large standard population.

In Table 338K1-3 deaths analyzed by cause in the aspirin group are compared directly with those in the placebo group. There were only two causes with notable differences. The 10 acute MI deaths in the aspirin group were significantly fewer than the 28 in the placebo group, both the Poisson test, and the test used in the report ($p=0.004$). The larger number of sudden deaths in the aspirin group, 22 vs. 12 in the placebo group, was a difference not statistically significant in Table 3 of the report ($p=0.09$), although the Poisson test gives a lower 95% Confidence Limit of 13.8, which does exceed the 12 deaths observed in the placebo group. Differences were minimal for all other causes, and for the total deaths, as already noted. Both fatal and nonfatal cases of MI and stroke have been similarly compared in Table 338K1-4. Because the exposure data by quinquennial age group were so closely matched in the aspirin and placebo groups (Table 338K1-1), I have assumed that any error in direct comparison of the observed events and rates is minimal. The important result of this clinical trial lies in the great reduction of nonfatal and total MIs, 139 total in the aspirin vs. 239 in the placebo group ($p<0.00001$). The incidence of fatal MI was also significantly reduced in the aspirin group, although the acute MI fatality rate was only about 10% overall. With regard to stroke, the incidence was higher in the aspirin than in the placebo group for all categories observed. The highest morbidity ratio, 192%, occurred in the relatively small category of hemorrhagic stroke, but the authors, after adjusting the rates, reported a *p* value of 0.06 for this difference, not significant at the 95% confidence level. Most of the strokes were classified as ischemic, differences were relatively small, and only 15 of 217 total strokes were fatal. Some severity categories reported in the article have not been included in Table 338K1-4. It should be noted that, with a common exposure value in a table of comparative mortality by cause, the excess death rates by cause are directly additive to the total. There is no similar direct relation for the mortality or morbidity ratio.

Incidence rates of total MI have been estimated in Table 338K1-5. Exposures are not exact, but have been approximated from the total exposures shown in Tables 338K1-5 and 338K1-2, and the age distribution in Table 338K1-2 relative to the total. The aspirin exposure data have been used for the placebo group, because the differences are very small. As expected, the incidence of MI increases significantly with advancing age, and the reduced incidence, aspirin vs. placebo, is seen in all age groups except the youngest. At ages 50 and up the reduction in MI incidence is highly significant, as it is for the total aspirin group.

Comment: The reader is referred to Table 5 of the article for details of side effects reported by the physicians while on the trial regimen. Gastrointestinal symptoms were common, and similar in frequency in both groups, although duodenal ulcer occurred in 46 cases in the aspirin group, as compared with 27 in the placebo (*p*=0.03). Bleeding problems, however, arose in 27.0% of the aspirin group, significantly more often (*p*<0.001) than the 20.4% cumulative incidence in the placebo group; easy bruising, melena and epistaxis were the most prominent manifestations. A single death due to gastrointestinal bleeding was confirmed in the aspirin group. Side effects of aspirin appear to be dose-related, and the authors note the relatively low incidence of serious side effects in this trial, with only 325 mg. taken on alternate days, as compared with higher doses used in previous trials. The beneficial effect of small doses of aspirin in reducing the incidence of MI is due to its effect on platelet enzymes that results in inhibition of platelet aggregation. This beneficial effect of aspirin found in previous trials on post-MI patients has thus been conclusively demonstrated in this large group of physicians with no history of overt coronary disease.

The remarkably low overall mortality in this large cohort of physicians doubtless is related to the selection process based on the factors of medical history, almost all of which involved an increased mortality risk thereby excluded. Self-selection may have been involved also, in the act of volunteering to participate in the study. Readers should understand that the cohort studied is by no means a representative sample of all physicians, or of the population at large. Age-specific incidence rates for MI in the placebo group (Table 338K1-5) are lower than corresponding rates for men in the Framingham Study (see the morbidity Abstract #345K1 in the *Journal of Insurance Medicine,* volume 20, no. 3, 1988). The Framingham experience was observed in a considerably earlier period, 1950 to 1970, but the Framingham cohort was not selected as rigorously as these physicians were. Mortality in the Framingham cohort was much closer to that of the matched U.S. white population than was the case in the Physicians' Health Study, with a mortality ratio of roughly 80% as compared with the 27% obtained by using the U.S. white male rates shown in Table 338K1-1. It is of interest to medical underwriting for life insurance that the selection process, equivalent to a partial nonmedical history form, has operated with such efficiency in the subjects age 50 and older. Of course these physicians had no motive to conceal adverse medical history, as applicants for insurance must always have.

ASPIRIN COMPONENT OF PHYSICIANS' HEALTH STUDY

TABLE 338K1-1

ADJUSTED BASIC SELECT MALE MORTALITY RATES PER 1000, EXPOSURES AND EXPECTED DEATHS, PLACEBO AND ASPIRIN GROUPS, BY QUINQUENNIAL AGES

Age	3rd Yr. Select Rate/1000*	Factor, Adj. 1978 to 1985[†]	Adj. Mean Rate/1000	Placebo		Aspirin		1985 US WM Rate per 1000
				Exposure Man-yrs.	Expected Deaths	Exposure Man-yrs.	Expected Deaths	
	q'	f	$(f)(q')$	E	d'	E	d'	q'**
40-44	1.86	0.80	1.5	12,084	18.1	12,113	18.2	3.6
45-49	2.77	0.76	2.1	10,526	22.1	10,511	22.1	5.8
50-54	3.35	(0.66)	2.2	10,034	22.1	9,961	21.9	9.6
55-59	5.24	0.66	3.5	8,605	30.1	8,664	30.3	15.6
60-64	8.24	0.70	5.8	6,202	36.0	6,259	36.3	24
65-69	13.04	0.77	10	3,955	39.6	3,939	39.4	37
70-74	17.27[††]	0.76	13	2,746	35.7	2,730	35.5	56
75-79	(27)[††]	(0.82)[††]	22	514	11.3	502	11.1	86
80-84	(44)[††]	(0.85)[††]	35	212	7.4	216	7.5	130

* 1975-80 3rd year Select Rate, Males (mean observation period, 60.2 months).

[†] Adjustment for secular decrease, 8 years (1977 to 1985 midpoints of observation periods), based on 92% of 10-year rates for male q', 1975-80/1965-70, except 0.66 used age 50-54 instead of anomalous smaller factor.

** Mean annual q' per 1000 from 1985 U.S. Abridged Life Tables, white male population, for comparison with select q'.

[††] Tabular rate 70 up assumed to be 70-74. Use factor 1.55 for 5-year increase in q' from age 70-74 to 75-79, and from age 75-79 to 80-84. For ages 75-79 and 80-84 use ratio of *ultimate* rate, 1975-80/1965-70, adjusted to 8 years.

TABLE 338K1-2

MORTALITY BY AGE, PLACEBO AND ASPIRIN GROUPS, ALL DURATIONS COMBINED, COMPARED WITH 1975-80 INSURANCE SELECT MALE RATES, ADJUSTED TO 1985 MIDPOINT OF OBSERVATION

Age	No. Alive at Start	Exposure Man-yrs.	No. of Deaths		Mortality Ratio	Mean Annual Mortality Rate per 1000		
			Observed	Expected*		Observed	Expected	Excess
	ℓ	E	d	d'	$100(d/d')$	$\bar{q}$	$\bar{q}'$	$(\bar{q}-\bar{q}')$
PHYSICIANS RANDOMIZED TO PLACEBO								
40-49	4,524	22,606	27	40.2	67%	1.2	1.8	−0.6
50-59	3,725	18,629	62	52.2	119	3.3	2.8	+0.5
60-69	2,045	10,157	76	75.6	101	7.5	7.4	+0.1
70-84	740	3,472	62	54.4	114	18	16	+2
All 40-84	11,034	54,864	227	222.4	102	4.1	4.0	+0.1
PHYSICIANS RANDOMIZED TO ASPIRIN								
40-49	4,527	22,624	28	40.3	70%	1.2	1.8	−0.6
50-59	3,725	18,625	64	52.2	123	3.4	2.8	+0.6
60-69	2,045	10,198	58	75.7	77	5.7	7.4	−1.7
70-84	740	3,468	67	54.1	124	19	16	+3
All 40-84	11,037	54,895	217	222.3	98	3.9	4.0	−0.1

* Basis of expected deaths: 3rd year Select Table male rates, adjusted (see Table 338K1-1).

ASPIRIN COMPONENT OF PHYSICIANS' HEALTH STUDY

TABLE 338K1-3

MORTALITY BY CAUSE, ASPIRIN VS. PLACEBO RATE, ALL DURATIONS COMBINED, WITH ASPIRIN EXPOSURE OF 54,895 PERSON-YEARS USED FOR BOTH GROUPS

| Cause of Death | No. of Deaths* | | Mortality Ratio | Mean Annual Mortality Rate per 1000 | | |
| | Aspirin | Placebo | | Aspirin | Placebo | Excess |
	d	d'	100(d/d')	$\bar{q}$	$\bar{q}'$	$(\bar{q}-\bar{q}')$
Confirmed CV	81	83	98%	1.48	1.51	−0.03
Acute MI	10	28	36	0.18	0.51	−0.33
Other Cor. HD	24	25	96	0.44	0.46	−0.02
Sudden Death	22	12	183	0.40	0.22	+0.18
Stroke	10	7	143	0.18	0.13	+0.05
Other CV	15	11	136	0.27	0.20	+0.07
Confirmed Non-CV	124	133	93	2.26	2.42	−0.16
Cause unconfirmed	12	11	109	0.22	0.20	+0.20
Total deaths	217	227	96	3.95	4.14	−0.19

* For statistical significance of differences, see text.

TABLE 338K1-4

CV INCIDENCE RATES, ASPIRIN VS. PLACEBO, ALL DURATIONS COMBINED, ASPIRIN GROUP EXPOSURE 54,560 EXPOSURE-YEARS FOR MI, 54,650 FOR STROKE (PLACEBO EXPOSURE MATCHED WITHIN 0.05%)

| Cardiovascular Morbid Event | No. of Events | | Morbidity Ratio | Mean Annual Event Rate per 1000 | | |
| | Aspirin | Placebo | | Aspirin | Placebo | Excess |
	n	n'	100(n/n')	$\bar{r}$	$\bar{r}'$	$(\bar{r}-\bar{r}')$
Fatal MI	10*	26	38%	0.18	0.48	−0.30
Nonfatal MI	129†	213	61	2.36	3.89	−1.53
Total MI	139†	239	58	2.54	4.37	−1.83
Fatal Stroke	9	6	150	0.16	0.11	+0.05
Nonfatal Stroke	110	92	120	2.01	1.68	+0.33
Total Stroke	119	98	121	2.17	1.79	+0.38
Ischemic Stroke	91	82	111	1.66	1.50	+0.16
Hemorrh. Stroke	23	12	192	0.42	0.22	+0.20
Type not known	5	4	125	0.09	0.07	+0.02

* Significantly fewer than 26 Placebo MIs, $p=0.007$.

† Significantly fewer than Placebo MIs, $p<0.00001$.

ASPIRIN COMPONENT OF PHYSICIANS' HEALTH STUDY

TABLE 338K1-5

TOTAL MI EVENT RATES BY AGE GROUP, ASPIRIN VS. PLACEBO, ALL DURATIONS COMBINED

Entry Age	No. Alive at Start	Exposure Estimated[†]	No. of MI Events*		Morbidity Ratio	Est. Mean Annual MI Rate per 1000		
			Aspirin	Placebo		Aspirin	Placebo	Excess
	ℓ	E	n	n′	100(n/n′)	r̄	r̄′	(r̄–r̄′)
40-49	4,527	22,475	27	24	112%	1.20	1.07	+0.13
50-59	3,725	18,510	51	87	59	2.76	4.70	−1.94
60-69	2,045	10,130	39	84	46	3.85	8.29	−4.44
70-84	740	3,445	22	44	50	6.38	12.77	−6.39
All 40-84	11,037	54,560	139	239	58	2.55	4.38	−1.83

* For statistical significance of differences, see text.

[†] Estimated from Aspirin MI and total death exposures, and proportionate death exposures by age. Placebo and Aspirin exposures approximately equal.

OUTCOME OF SUSPECTED ACUTE MI WITH HOSPITALIZATION, BUT MI NOT CONFIRMED BY SERUM ENZYMES OR Q WAVES IN THE ECG

Richard B. Singer, M.D.

A *prospective* study by Schroeder et al.[1] confirms previous reports, mostly retrospective in character,[2-5] that patients with acute MI strongly suspected on clinical grounds are at high risk for coronary death and subsequent MI, even though serial ECGs did *not* show abnormal Q waves and serum creatine phosphokinase (CPK) never became abnormal. A series of 189 patients admitted to the CCU of Stanford Medical Center was identified from consecutive acute chest pain cases under age 70 and resident within 10 miles of the center. Serial ECGs and CPK measurements were made at admission and 6, 12, 24, 48, and 72 hours later. The chest pain was diagnosed as noncardiac in 16 patients, none of whom died during a minimum follow-up of two years (average 27.8 months). Myocardial infarction (MI) was diagnosed on the basis of elevation of CPK to more than 200 IU with an elevated MB fraction that returned to normal within three days, associated with ST-T abnormalities in the ECG, or new Q waves over 0.04 seconds in width, or both. MI was thus diagnosed in 84 patients (22 subendocardial and 62 transmural), six of whom died in the hospital, but MI was "ruled out," in the terminology of the authors, in 89 patients, with only one hospital death. The latter were diagnosed as ischemic chest pain without MI; since the pain was prolonged these patients might also be designated as having acute coronary insufficiency (ACI), or unstable angina, or intermediate coronary syndrome, in whom evidence of MI failed to develop within 72 hours of admission to a CCU.

To compare experience following these two types of acute coronary events we will make use of first-year mortality rates. Since we are dealing with hospitalized patients, sudden deaths and also those occurring prior to being hospitalized are automatically excluded. These constitute a substantial fraction of the acute mortality observed in epidemiological studies of MI (Abstract #301 in *Medical Risks*). Because the mortality risk in MI is highest in the first 24 hours and decreases day by day, thereafter, another substantial fraction of the first year

mortality occurs during the period of hospitalization. This fraction of early mortality *has* been included in the demographic and mortality data shown in Table 340K1-1 for the first year after hospital admission, not only for the data of Schroeder et al., but for some other series considered to be comparable.

Although in-hospital mortality is lower in ACI than in Acute MI, there is little difference among the survivors who are discharged. In 4 of the 5 ACI series the range of first-year mortality, q, is 0.068 to 0.140. The report of Dussia et al. from Emory[3] provides a careful "taxonomic" classification of the acute chest pain admissions in the CCU, but there were 41 deaths within 48 hours out of 466 cases, and these were not assigned to the MI or ACI cases. I have made an arbitrary assignment of 11 cases to the ACI group and 30 to the MI cases with data as tabulated. If we postulate that all such early in-hospital deaths should be regarded as acute MI, the q would be $18/131=0.137$ for the ACI group, instead of 0.204 as shown in the table, while q for the patients with MI would be somewhat larger, 0.309 instead of 0.283. A q of 0.137 would be more in keeping with the average first-year mortality of 0.119 for the 648 patients with ACI but no MI in the upper part of the table.

After age 40 post-MI mortality increases with increasing age. Distribution of patients by age is not available for the individual studies shown in Table 340K1-1, except the 1974 retrospective analysis of Stanford CCU admissions with ACI.[2] No age or sex data are given for the Emory patients.[3] Presumably all ages and both sexes were included, whereas only patients under 70 were included in the prospective Stanford material.[1] Age differential may explain why the MI cases at Emory showed a first-year mortality rate about twice as high as the Stanford MI cases — 0.283 versus 0.143. The impact of age is seen in the four pooled groups of MI patients at the bottom of Table 340K1-1. First-year mortality is at least three times higher in patients age 65 and up than in patients under 65, for both males and females. There is little difference in q between males and females on either side of the dividing age, 65, although the *average* age is five years older for the females. First-year mortality is thus close to 50 per 100 for MI patients age 65 and up and 15 per 100 for those under age 65. The mortality in any series of patients

Source: R. B. Singer, "Outcome of Suspected Acute MI with Hospitalization, but MI Not Confirmed by Serum Enzymes or Q Waves in the ECG," *J. Ins. Med.*, 12, no. 1 (1981): 14-15. Reproduced with permission of author and publisher.

including all ages can be expected to increase with the proportion of older patients: with two-thirds under age 65 and one-third age 65 up, q would be approximately 26 per 100.

Because of the generally incomplete age data I have not attempted to compare mortality rates in the table with those in the U.S. population. However, expected rates for the four pooled series were, respectively, 0.013, 0.009, 0.084, and 0.069 in the order given at the bottom of the table. The corresponding excess death rates per 1000 were, in the same order, 143, 152, 387, and 482. If we assume a q' of 0.030 for the ACI total cases the EDR would come to approximately 90 per 1000, and the mortality ratio to 0.12/0.03, or about 400 percent.

From the underwriting standpoint it is clear that scant reassurance should be derived from a report of normal serum enzymes and absent Q waves in an applicant giving a history of hospital admission for acute coronary insufficiency or other severe chest pain episode strongly suspicious of ACI, less than a year prior to application. Excess mortality is very high and probably continues to be high after one year. Sudden death, death from MI and recurrent or initial MI can be anticipated in such patients,[1,2] and almost 40 percent of the VA series were found to have 3-vessel disease. It would be unwise, in my opinion, to reduce the waiting period or the rating schedule for "best" MI cases to any substantial degree for applicants with an ACI history but with MI "ruled out."

TABLE 340K1-1

FIRST-YEAR MORTALITY AFTER MI OR ACUTE CORONARY ATTACK WITHOUT MI

Ref.	Series	Sex	Age	No. of Cases	No. of 1st Year Deaths			Mort. Rate
					Hosp.	To 1 Yr.	0-1 Yr.	
				ℓ	d_H	d_1	d	$q=(d/\ell)$
ACUTE CORONARY ATTACK WITHOUT MI								
1	Stanford (1980)	M64, F24	<70 (57.3)	89	1	6	7	0.080
2	Stanford (1974)	M116, F54	29-88	170	1	16	17	0.100
3	Emory (1976)	No data	No data	142*	15*	14	29	0.204
4	VA (1978)	M121, F26	<70 (52.7)	147	4	6	10	0.068
5	Mass. Gen (1972)	M64, F36	39-87 (62)	100	1	13	14	0.140
	Total			648	22	55	77	0.119
ACUTE MI								
1	Stanford (1980)	M66, F12	<70 (56.3)	84	6	6	12	0.143
3	Emory (1976)	No data	No data	300*	50*	35	85	0.283
†	Pooled 4 series	Male	<65 (51.4)	2,100	—	—	313	0.156
†	Pooled 2 series	Female	<65 (56.5)	149	—	—	24	0.161
†	Pooled 4 series	Male	65 up (71.4)	293	—	—	138	0.471
†	Pooled 3 series	Female	65 up (76.4)	227	—	—	125	0.551

* Includes 41 deaths within 48 hours in CCU, arbitrarily allocated by RBS 30 to MI group and 11 to Acute Cororary Attack without MI.

† RBS compilation of 7 reports, experience 1950-72, abstracted in *Medical Risks* or *J. Ins. Med.*

REFERENCES

1. J. S. Schroeder, I. H. Lamb, M. Hu, "Do Patients in Whom Myocardial Infarction Has Been Ruled Out Have a Better Prognosis After Hospitalization Than Those Surviving Infarction?" *N. Engl. J. Med.*, 303 (1980): 1-5.

2. M. G. Lopes, A. P. Spivak, D. C. Harrison, J. S. Schroeder, "Prognosis in Coronary Care Unit Noninfarction Cases," *JAMA*, 228 (1974): 1558-62.

3. E. E. Dussia, D. Cromartie, J. McCraney, G. Mead, N. K. Wenger, "Myocardial Infarction With and Without Laboratory Documentation — One Year Prognosis," *Am. Heart J.*, 92 (1976): 148-51.

4. "Unstable Angina Pectoris: National Cooperative Study Group to Compare Surgical and Medical Therapy. II. In-Hospital Experience and Initial Follow-up Results in Patients with One, Two, and Three Vessel Disease," *Am. J. Cardiol.*, 42 (1978): 839-48.

5. K. R. Krauss, A. M. Hutter, Jr., R. W. DeSanctis, "Acute Coronary Insufficiency — Course and Follow-up," *Circulation*, 45, Supplement I (1972): pp. I-66 thru I-71.

RECURRENT MI IN POST-MI PATIENTS: THE FRAMINGHAM EXPERIENCE 1950-1970

Richard B. Singer, M.D.

References:

1. P. Sorlie, *Section 32. Cardiovascular Diseases and Death Following Myocardial Infarction and Angina Pectoris: Framingham Study, 20-Year Follow-up* (Bethesda, MD, National Institutes of Health, DHEW Publication No. [NIH] 77-1247 ,1977).

2. C. Gillespie, P. Sorlie, *The Framingham Study. Section 33. An Index to Previous Sections 1-32* (Bethesda, MD, National Heart, Lung and Blood Institute, NIH Publication No. 79-1671, 1978).

Object of Abstract: To present comparative morbidity data, in a prototype abstract, for recurrent myocardial infarction (MI) in post-MI patients, derived from the Framingham Study experience after 20 years of follow-up, 1950 to 1970. Mean annual incidence rates by age and sex have been calculated for the post-MI patients from Table II-10, and for the MI-free Framingham Study population from Table IV-7 in the *Section 32* report.[1] These morbid event results are presented in the usual life table format.

Subjects Studied: Residents of Framingham, Massachusetts, 2,336 men and 2,873 women, followed with biennial cardiovascular examinations from the central year of initiation of follow-up, 1950 (the earliest examinations were started in 1948, but a biennial schedule was kept according to each subject's date of initial examination). For details of the study design consult the appropriate references in *Section 33*.[2] The diagnosis of acute MI as a morbid event depended primarily on the characteristic serial electrocardiographic (ECG) changes, although a hospital report of prolonged ischemic chest pain with elevated serum enzyme levels was accepted after 1955.[1] MI is a type of acute morbid event that can usually be defined and dated with accuracy. A description of the tables and details of the definitions and methods are given in the text of *Section 32*.[1]

Follow-up: Biennial examinations were supplemented by additional information from hospital and physician records and from death certificates. Subjects who moved away from Framingham were regularly followed. It is stated that "loss to follow-up was extremely low with less than two percent completely unaccounted for."[1]

Results: First MI incidence rates, or morbid event rates, are summarized by mean attained age and sex for the MI-free Framingham Study population in Table 345K1-1. These provide "expected" MI event rates as number of MIs per 1000 person-years at risk. Subjects were withdrawn from risk because of initial MI or death from any cause. The symbol n, for number of morbid events, is substituted for deaths, d, in the conventional life table. Similarly, the event rate (incidence rate of MI), r, is substituted for the familiar symbol for mortality rate, q. Since Table 345K1-1 provides results for MI morbidity in the MI-free population it is an expected morbidity table; the symbols n' and r' have been used, as d' and q' are used for expected deaths and expected mortality rate. The annual life table data in Table IV-7 of *Section 32* have been combined to provide aggregate mean rates for durations 0-5, 5-10, 10-15 and 15-20 years of follow-up. The age groups are also quinquennial. The central age, duration 0-1, for the youngest group, age 30-34 years, is age 32. At duration 15-20 years a mean of 18 years must be added to get a mean attained age of 50 years. To these data can be added the data for the entry age/duration groups 35-39/10-15, 40-44/5-10, and 45-49/0-5, because all of these correspond to a mean attained age of 50 years. The results for age 35 and age 75 are based on only a single age/duration grouping, but the others contain pooled data from two, three or four groupings. It can be seen that during the 20 years of follow-up 262 first MIs occurred in the men and 93 in the women. Morbid event rates per 1000, r', increased with age and were much higher in men than in women of the same attained age. Table 345K1-1 also contains Poisson 95% confidence limits for r', based on n' and E, and graduated values of r', taken from a smooth curve drawn as an approximate best fit to the observed values of r'.

The 30-day mortality of acute MI is high, of course, and only the 30-day survivors are available for follow-up to determine the morbid event rate for a recurrent or second MI. The same principle of grouping results by quinquennial age at first MI and quinquennial duration

Source: R. B. Singer, "Recurrent MI in Post-MI Patients: The Framingham Experience 1950-1970," *J. Ins. Med.*, 20, no. 3 (1988): 51-53. Reproduced with permission of author and publisher.

periods has been followed for the post-MI patients as for the MI-free population. In Table II-10 there are annual data to 15 years for 10 age groups, since the age at which MI occurred represents an attained age up to as much as 20 years of follow-up added to the entry age. Only ℓ and n are given, but from these both w and E are readily calculated for single years of follow-up, and these data can be grouped into five years of follow-up, and these data can be grouped into five-year aggregates as was done in Table 345K1-1. From the ℓ values at 30 days, 5, 10 and 15 years it is also possible to calculate mean age. The numbers of acute MI survivors are small enough (162 men and 38 women) to result in very small numbers of n in the age groups shown in Table 345K1-2 or the duration groups in Table 345K1-3. If random variation is not the cause, the results appear to show an MI event rate for post-MI female patients of 63 excess MIs per 1000 per year, a rate about three times larger than the 20 per 1000 in male post-MI patients (Table 345K1-3). All of the 13 recurrent MIs in women occurred within five years of the first infarction. In the men the distribution was such that the excess MI rate per 1000 showed very little change with age (Table 345K1-2) or duration since first MI (Table 345K1-3). It is not possible to interpret any age or duration trend in the excess event rate (shall we abbreviate this as EER?) in women, as the total number of recurrent MIs was only 13.

Comment: Many questions require consideration and eventual answer before the application of comparative morbidity results of this sort can rest on a firm basis. These observations from the Framingham Study are more than 20 years old. Are they representative of current MI morbidity, not only in Massachusetts but in other states? Will it be practical to develop expected morbidity tables that depend on disease as well as age and sex? Intercompany health insurance studies of specific diseases in terms of specified morbid events could provide expected morbidity rates by age and sex on the most important problems in health insurance underwriting that involve special class action. However imperfect these MI results may be, at least they do provide actual data in life table format, data that can be studied, analyzed, and used experimentally for health insurance underwriting.

TABLE 345K1-1

FRAMINGHAM "EXPECTED" FIRST MI RATE BY ATTAINED AGE AND SEX

Attained Mean Age*	No. Alive at Start*	Exposure Person-yrs.	No. MI Events	MI Morbid Event Rate per 1000		
				Rate	95% C.L.[†]	Graduated**
$\bar{x}$	ℓ	E	n′			r′
FRAMINGHAM SERIES MEN						
35	384	1,904	3	(1.6)	—	1.3
40	819	4,073	7	1.7	0.7-3.5	1.9
45	1,225	6,057	20	3.3	2.0-5.1	3.3
50	1,549	7,479	37	4.9	3.5-6.8	4.9
55	1,498	7,096	54	7.6	5.7-9.4	6.7
60	1,273	5,985	59	9.9	7.5-12.7	9.0
65	818	3,754	40	10.7	7.6-14.5	11.5
70	455	2,062	29	14.1	9.4-20.2	14.5
75	167	706	13	18.4	9.8-31.4	18.0
FRAMINGHAM SERIES WOMEN						
35	443	2,209	0	(0)	—	—
40	1,025	5,103	1	(0.2)	—	(0.3)
45	1,526	7,600	3	(0.4)	—	(0.4)
50	1,962	9,598	10	1.0	0.5-1.9	0.7
55	1,922	9,319	7	0.8	0.3-1.5	1.1
60	1,699	8,230	17	2.1	1.2-3.3	2.1
65	1,172	5,270	28	5.3	3.5-7.7	3.9
70	699	3,261	21	6.4	4.0-9.8	5.7
75	299	1,322	6	4.5	1.7-9.9	7.5

* Central attained age for quinquennial entry age groups 30-34 through 55-59, and quinquennial duration periods, 0-5, 5-10, 10-15 and 15-20 years starting in 1950. Thus "age 50" includes entry age (duration) groups 30-34 (15-20), 35-39 (10-15), 40-44 (5-10), and 45-49 (0-5). Survivors in each of 6 entry age groups are therefore counted 4 times for "Number Alive at Start." Total exposure divided into 24 5-year periods by the indicated mean attained age.

[†] Poisson 95% Confidence limits for r′, based on MI events, n′, as counted.

** Graduated graphically from approximate best-fit smooth curve, r′ vs $\bar{x}$.

TABLE 345K1-2

COMPARATIVE MORBIDITY FOR SECOND MI IN POST-MI PATIENTS BY AGE AND SEX

Mean Age after MI	No. 30-Day Survival	Exposure Patient-yrs.	No. of 2nd MI Events		Morbidity Ratio	Mean Annual MI Rate per 1000		
			Observed	Expected		Observed	Expected*	Excess
$\bar{x}$	ℓ	E	n	n′	100(n/n′)	r	r′	(r–r′)
MALE MI 30-DAY SURVIVORS (DURATION TO 10 YEARS)								
50	75	318.5	8	1.59	505%	25	5	20
60	106	403.0	13	3.63	360	32	9	23
67	74	243.5	8	3.40	235	33	14	19
All Ages	(255)†	965.0	29	8.62	335	30	9	21
FEMALE MI 30-DAY SURVIVORS (DURATION TO 10 YEARS)								
53	8	26.5	3	0.024	(12,500%)	(113)	0.9	(112)
62	21	78.5	6	0.236	2,500	76	3.0	73
72	24	78.0	4	0.51	785	51	6.5	45
All Ages	(53)†	183.0	13	0.77	1,690	71	4.2	67

* Basis of expected MI rates: Framingham Series 1950-72 (See Table 345K1-1).

† Some patients counted more than once because of age/duration overlap.

TABLE 345K1-3

COMPARATIVE MORBIDITY FOR SECOND MI IN POST-MI PATIENTS BY DURATION AND SEX

Duration Start-End	No. Alive at Start	Exposure Patient-yrs.	No. of 2nd MI Events		Morbidity Ratio	Mean Annual MI Rate per 1000		
			Observed	Expected		Observed	Expected*	Excess
I to t+?	ℓ	E	n	n′	100(n/n′)	r	r′	(r–r′)
MALE MI 30-DAY SURVIVORS, ALL AGES COMBINED								
30d-5yrs.	162	660.5	19	5.94	320%	29	9	20
5-10	96	311.0	10	3.11	320	32	10	22
10-15	32	109.0	3	1.31	230	28	12	16
30d-15yrs.	162	1,080.5	32	10.35	310	30	9.6	20
FEMALE MI 30-DAY SURVIVORS, ALL AGES COMBINED								
30d-5yrs.	38	132.0	13	0.55	2,400%	98	4.2	94
5-15	15	60.5	0	0.34	0	0	5.6	–6
30d-15yrs.	38	192.5	13	0.89	1,460	68	4.6	63

* Basis of expected MI rates: Framingham Series 1950-72 (See Table 345K1-1)

MYOCARDIAL INFARCTION IN EUROPEAN INSUREDS

Manfred Fessel

References:

1. M. Fessel, "Comparison Between the Mortality Expected and that Actually Experienced by Life Insurance Companies, for Selected Impairments," *Annals of Life Insurance Medicine 9* (Proceedings of the 16th International Congress of Life Assurance Medicine, The Hague 1989), (1990): 39-45.

2. M. Fessel, Unpublished exposures and other data furnished (1990).

Subjects Studied: European male policyholders reassured and followed up at Swiss Reinsurance Company in Zurich, Switzerland. The experience is reported for cases with a history of myocardial infarction coded as their main impairment; the coexistence of hypertension, over or underweight or any other secondary impairments was not excluded. The policyholders observed have been insured in the years from 1956 through 1985 and traced to the end of 1985 or to prior termination.

Follow-up: Reinsurance policy records formed the basis of entry, of counting policies, exposure and death claims, and of follow-up information.

Results: Comparative experience is given in Tables 345K2-1 to 345K2-5, using a modification of Swiss Re's internal European mortality table SR 73/77 as basis of expected mortality. It is important to note that SR 73/77 is an aggregate, not a select mortality table, when comparing Swiss Re's results with American insurance experience.

There were overall 426 entrants into this study (more exactly: 426 policies issued on European males with a history of myocardial infarction, reassured with Swiss Re), showing a mortality ratio of 575% and an EDR of 29 per 1000. The average duration per policy observed was slightly more than five years.

As can be seen from Table 345K2-1 (experience by rating at policy issue), the actual mortality was significantly worse than expected, e.g. the mortality ratio of risks accepted with a rating of 200-250% was more than 200% higher (465%)! A very substantial extra mortality

of around 600% was also found for lives underwritten with a rating of 300% up and for "other" risks, the latter comprising applicants for which the extra mortality risk had been compensated by means of flat extra premiums or an artificial age increase, a method still used in the Netherlands.

The experience by age at policy issue, as shown in Table 345K2-2, is, for the two age groups 20-44 and 45-54, consistent with that known from other studies on insured lives with a history of myocardial infarction. By increasing ages at issue, the mortality ratios decrease (from 640 to 515%), whereas the EDRs increase (from 16 to 25 per 1000). The very unfavourable experience, however, for ages at entry 55 up (MR 635%, EDR 72 per 1000) was frightening and due to a number of bad risks inadequately underwritten by some ceding companies.

Table 345K2-3 gives the comparative experience by policy duration for all ages combined. The mortality ratios and EDRs gradually increase from 425 to 715% and from 15 to 44 per 1000, respectively, for durations 0-2 to 5-10 years. For policy durations of more than 10 years, the mortality ratio (550%) and the EDR (41 per 1000) are well in excess of those for durations 5 or less.

Table 345K2-4 shows Swiss Re's experience with insureds after myocardial infarction by duration since infarction at issue. The mortality ratios and EDRs seem to be quite independent from the number of years elapsed since infarction at entry. The traditional method of offsetting the increased risk due to infarction by means of a combination of percentage extra mortality and additional temporary extra premiums had been based on the results of clinical studies of infarction patients which showed significantly higher mortality ratios during the first years after infarction. However, life insurance companies require a recovery period after the infarction of several months, before insurance cover will be granted. The selection, which then takes place, eliminates those applicants who, on the basis of their clinical findings, have a particularly high risk of reinfarction or suffer fatal complications from the initial infarction. For those who are considered insurable, the mortality in the first years after infarction is hardly any worse than that of those where a long time elapsed between infarction and application. This reasoning has been confirmed by the results of our

Source: M. Fessel, "Myocardial Infarction in European Insureds," *J. Ins. Med.,* 22 (1990): 284-86. Reproduced with permission of author and publisher.

Table 345K2-3 and 345K2-4 and those of other studies of insured lives.

An unfavourable prognostic factor in applicants with a history of myocardial infarction is the coexistence of hypertension. As is shown in Table 345K2-5 the mortality ratio of insureds after infarction with normal blood pressure (systolic = ≤142 mm. Hg. and diastolic = ≤92 mm. Hg.) amounts to 525%, whereas the mortality ratio of those with both increased systolic as well as diastolic pressures was 350% higher (875%)! For applicants with either elevated systolic or diastolic pressures (but not both), the mortality ratio was in between (615%). We therefore conclude that the extra mortality for applicants presenting with a history of myocardial infarction and with hypertension exceeds by far the simple addition of the extra mortalities of the two individual impairments.

Comment: It is challenging to compare the results of this study with those of insureds after myocardial infarction covered by the *Medical Impairment Study 1983* (Volume I, p. 64-65, males — substandard lives). This comparison is particularly interesting in that both studies use a history of myocardial infarction (without further subdivision) as their selection criterion, and because the two periods of

observation are comparable. There are, however, some important differences between the two studies to be borne in mind:

- The exposure in the MIS for this impairment is more than five times that of Swiss Re's with a correspondingly higher significance of the resulting mortality ratios.
- The coexistence of other rateable impairments has been excluded from MIS but allowed in Swiss Re's study, leading to higher mortality rates in the latter.
- On the other hand, using an aggregate mortality table as comparative mortality, as done by Swiss Re, produces lower mortality ratios than the select rates applied in American studies, especially for higher ages at entry.

Taking all this into account, the two studies show quite similar mortality ratios for the total experience (MIS 505%, Swiss Re 575%) as well as by ages at issue, with the exception of Swiss Re's unfavourable experience for ages at issue 55 up, as commented above. In both studies there was no distinct pattern for the mortality ratios by policy duration, and in both studies these ratios were universally much higher than anticipated.

SWISS RE IMPAIRMENT STUDY 1989

TABLE 345K2-1

EUROPEAN MALE INSUREDS WITH A HISTORY OF MYOCARDIAL INFARCTION, 1956-85
COMPARATIVE EXPERIENCE BY RATING AT POLICY ISSUE

Rating	No. of Entrants	Exposure Policy-yrs.	Number of Claims		Mortality Ratio	Mean Ann. Mort. Rate per 1000		
			Observed	Expected*		Observed	Expected	Excess
	ℓ	E	d	d'	100(d/d')	$\bar{q}$	$\bar{q}'$	$(\bar{q}-\bar{q}')$
100-175%	32	183.5	5	1.81	275%	27	9.9	17
200-250	84	520.5	18	3.89	465	35	7.5	27
300 up	212	1,093.0	39	5.63	695	36	5.2	31
Other	98	453.0	16	2.26	710	35	5.0	30
Total	426	2,250.0	78	13.59	575	35	6.0	29

* Basis of expected claims: Swiss Re 1973-77 Aggregate Table, European Males, modified.

TABLE 345K2-2

EUROPEAN MALE INSUREDS WITH A HISTORY OF MYOCARDIAL INFARCTION, 1956-85
COMPARATIVE EXPERIENCE BY AGE AT POLICY ISSUE

Age at Issue	No. of Entrants	Exposure Policy-yrs.	Number of Claims		Mortality Ratio	Mean Ann. Mort. Rate per 1000		
			Observed	Expected*		Observed	Expected	Excess
	ℓ	E	d	d'	100(d/d')	$\bar{q}$	$\bar{q}'$	$(\bar{q}-\bar{q}')$
20-44	129	772.0	15	2.34	640%	19.4	3.0	16
45-54	216	1,174.5	37	7.15	515	32	6.1	25
55-84	81	303.5	26	4.11	635	86	13.5	72
Total	426	2,250.0	78	13.59	575	35	6.0	29

* Basis of expected claims: Swiss Re 1973-77 Aggregate Table, European Males, modified.

TABLE 345K2-3

EUROPEAN MALE INSUREDS WITH A HISTORY OF MYOCARDIAL INFARCTION, 1956-85
COMPARATIVE EXPERIENCE BY DURATION, ALL AGES COMBINED

Duration Start-End	Exposure Policy-yrs.	Number of Claims		Mortality Ratio	Mean Ann. Mort. Rate per 1000		
		Observed	Expected*		Observed	Expected	Excess
t to $t+\Delta t$	E	d	d'	$100(d/d')$	$\bar{q}$	$\bar{q}'$	$(\bar{q}-\bar{q}')$
0-2 yrs.	579.0	11	2.60	425%	19.0	4.5	15
2-5	809.0	23	4.33	530	28	5.4	23
5-10	621.0	32	4.48	715	52	7.2	44
10-30	241.0	12	2.18	550	50	9.0	41
Total	2,250.0	78	13.59	575	35	6.0	29

* Basis of expected claims: Swiss Re 1973-77 Aggregate Table, European Males, modified.

TABLE 345K2-4

EUROPEAN MALE INSUREDS WITH A HISTORY OF MYOCARDIAL INFARCTION, 1956-85
COMPARATIVE EXPERIENCE BY DURATION SINCE INFARCTION AT ISSUE

Duration since Infarction at Issue	No. of Entrants	Exposure Policy-yrs.	Number of Claims		Mortality Ratio	Mean Ann. Mort. Rate per 1000		
			Observed	Expected*		Observed	Expected	Excess
	ℓ	E	d	d'	$100(d/d')$	$\bar{q}$	$\bar{q}'$	$(\bar{q}-\bar{q}')$
0-5 yrs.	254	1,340.0	41	7.06	580%	31	5.3	26
5-10	103	514.0	21	3.98	530	41	7.7	33
10 up	38	214.0	7	1.42	495	33	6.6	26
Unknown	31	182.0	9	1.13	795	49	6.2	43
Total	426	2,250.0	78	13.59	575	35	6.0	29

* Basis of expected claims: Swiss Re 1973-77 Aggregate Table, European Males, modified.

TABLE 345K2-5

EUROPEAN MALE INSUREDS WITH A HISTORY OF MYOCARDIAL INFARCTION, 1956-85
COMPARATIVE EXPERIENCE BY BLOOD PRESSURE READINGS

Blood Pressure (mm. Hg.) Syst. Diast.	No. of Entrants	Exposure Policy-yrs.	Number of Claims		Mortality Ratio	Mean Ann. Mort. Rate per 1000		
			Observed	Expected*		Observed	Expected	Excess
	ℓ	E	d	d'	$100(d/d')$	$\bar{q}$	$\bar{q}'$	$(\bar{q}-\bar{q}')$
≤142 ≤92	284	1,564.5	45	8.57	525%	29	5.5	23
≥143 ≥93	37	163.5	7	0.80	875	43	4.9	38
Other	105	522.0	26	4.22	615	50	8.1	42
Total	426	2,250.0	78	13.59	575	35	6.0	29

* Basis of expected claims: Swiss Re 1973-77 Aggregate Table, European Males, modified.

FOLLOW-UP OF PATIENTS WITH CARDIAC CATHETERIZATION, HARTFORD HOSPITAL

Robert K. Palmer, M.D.

References:*

1. R. K. Palmer, "Hartford Hospital Cardiac Catheterization Mortality Study," CIGNA Report No. 33751 (no date).
2. R. K. Palmer, Personal communication to editors (1991).

Objective of Abstract: To present in standard abstract format the comparative mortality experience of patients undergoing cardiac catheterization at the Cardiac Laboratory of the Hartford Hospital, Hartford, 1971 through 1981.

Subjects Studied: This study was undertaken by the Medical Department of the CIGNA Insurance Company, Hartford, Connecticut. With the cooperation of the physicians and staff of the Cardiac Laboratory, Hartford Hospital, medical records were abstracted of all 5,306 patients who had a cardiac catheterization in the 11-year period from January 1, 1971 through December 31, 1981. The annual number of patients catheterized increased from 186 in 1971 to 739 in 1981. Male patients constituted 76.2% of the total, with a mean age of 56.4 years; female patients constituted 23.8%, with a mean age of 58.4 years. The age distribution by sex is shown in Table 354K1-1. A scoring system, 0-9, was used for severity of obstruction in the three main coronary arteries: one point each artery for 50-69% reduction in diameter, two points for 70-89% reduction, and three points for reduction of 90% or more. As shown in Table 354K1-2, obstruction was less severe in women than in men; 40.3% of the women had no significant obstruction (less than 50% reduction in diameter in all arteries, or 0 score), but only 13.5% of men were so classified. Impairment of left ventricular function was assessed by means of ejection fraction (EF) and left ventricular end-diastolic pressure (LVEDP). Other risk fac-

tors, such as history of smoking or history of MI, were also recorded; the distribution of these is given in Table 354K1-3.

Follow-up: This was carried out from entry to death of the patient, loss to FU, or end of FU in 81.3% of the total number catheterized. Most of this attrition was due to inability to trace a patient for any FU; a few patients were excluded because of incomplete ventriculography reports. The aggregate experience of the traced subjects consisted of 26,989 person-years. Subjects with a 0 point score (no significant coronary obstruction) accounted for nearly 20% of the exposure but only 5% of the 631 deaths.

Expected Mortality: In this abstract insurance select mortality has been chosen for the derivation of expected deaths: the 1978 CIGNA Best Estimate Select rates, matched by age, sex and duration to subjects observed in each group or subgroup. To allow for the downward trend in mortality, the 1978 rates have been decreased 2% for each successive calendar year of the period of exposure. Although all traced patients were included, it was observed in this as in previous studies of catheterized patients (see *1990 Medical Risks* monograph) that selection bias does occur prior to referral of patients for cardiac catheterization. It appears that physicians do not refer CHD patients with associated high-risk conditions such as advanced cancer. On the other hand, patients with hypertension, diabetes and similar risk factors are referred (Table 354K1-3). As a consequence, Group Life Insurance tables were used for expected deaths of catheterized patients in the tables of the *1990 Medical Risks* monograph, because these appeared to be better suited to the degree of selection manifest in such patient groups. The standard select rates for individual insurance utilized here provide even lower expected deaths, but are preferable to the high expected death values derived from population rates: the mortality ratio was 147% for patients with no coronary obstruction in Table 354K1-4, but only 55% with U.S. population rates (see tables in the original report, reference 1).

Results: Comparative mortality by severity of obstruction score is shown in Table 354K1-4, all ages, all durations, and male and female patients combined. Numbers of

---

* Editors' note: As part of a panel discussion of "Insurance Company Experience with Coronary Bypass Surgery," Dr. Palmer presented some of these results at the Annual Meeting of the Medical Section of the American Council of Life Insurance, June 18, 1986. No tables were published in the *Proceedings* of this Medical Section meeting, but copies of the report (ref. 1) were distributed.

patients followed have been estimated from the numbers catheterized as shown in Table 354K1-2 (numbers of patients untraced assumed to be proportionate to number followed). Subjects with 0 score or no significant coronary obstruction were predominantly female and younger than patients with significant obstruction. A modest degree of excess mortality was observed in the patients with 0 score: mortality ratio (MR) of 147% and excess death rate (EDR) of 2.4 per 1000 per year. The presence of this in spite of the elimination of subjects with less than 50% coronary obstruction is probably due to the presence of other risk factors such as high blood pressure, factors that are eliminated in the usual insurance selection process with a medical or paramedical examination. In mild coronary obstruction there was little change in excess mortality from score 1 to score 4, and the aggreagate EDR was 11.1 per 1000. Patients with a more severe obstruction score of 5-9, who outnumbered those with mild obstruction by about 2 to 1, had considerably higher excess mortality, with an overall MR of 525% and annual EDR of 28 per 1000.

As would be anticipated, the mortality experience for patients treated with coronary bypass surgery (CBPS) was different from the experience in the medically treated patients, and this difference is detailed in Table 354K1-5. Each treatment group has been divided into severity groups, with respective scores of 1-4 (less severe) and 5-9 (more severe), with comparative mortality also shown by duration. Deaths within 30 days after operation were excluded from the CBPS experience. Patients in both severity groups had a lower mortality if they were treated surgically rather than medically. This difference was greater in the patients with more severe obstruction. For all durations combined EDR in the group with less severe disease was 13 per 1000 when they were medically treated, and 6.5 per 1000 after CBPS; in the groups with more severe obstruction the EDR values were 50 and 14 per 1000, respectively. Corresponding differences were observed in the mortality ratios. Patterns by duration differed according to both severity and treatment. In the less severe medically treated patients EDR changed very little with duration in the duration intervals 0-1, 1-5, and 5 years up. In the more severe surgically treated patients EDR rose sharply from 9-10 per 1000 under 5 years to 28 per 1000 in the exposure 5 years or more in duration. In the other two groups the lowest EDR was found at durations 1-5 years, and the highest at durations 5 years or more. This pattern is the one usually found in both CBPS and medically treated post-MI patients in the numerous studies reported in the *1990 Medical Risks* monograph.

The mortality experience by age and by sex in Table 354K1-6 shows EDRs that increase with advancing age and MRs that decrease. Excess mortality in this and some

of the following tables has been somewhat diluted by inclusion of patients without significant obstruction. However, the overall magnitude of this dilution may be assessed by comparing the excess mortality for all patients combined with excess mortality of patients after excluding those with no significant obstruction. Results for these two groups are given in the two bottom lines of Table 354K1-6. All male patients had an annual EDR of 19 per 1000, while female patients had a lower EDR of 12 per 1000. The MR was almost as high in women as in men, because of the lower female expected mortality rate.

Comparative mortality results by EF are given in Table 354K1-7, and by LVEDP in Table 354K1-8, starting with normal levels, then in order of ascending degrees of abnormality for these indexes of left ventricular function. There are 8 classes of EF ranging from >57% to <23%, the most abnormal, and 7 classes of LVEDP, from <13 mm. of Hg. to 37 mm. and up. These have been grouped into 4 categories to which letter designations have been given, A for normal and D for the most abnormal. The effectiveness of EF and LVEDP in grading excess mortality is shown by the progressive increase in EDR and MR with increasing abnormality of the index used. About 63% of the catheterized patients had a completely normal EF, >52%, with a relatively small excess mortality, EDR being only 7.9 per 1000 per year and MR 240%. In the Group D cases, about 8% of the total, with EF <28%, the annual EDR was 109 per 1000 and the MR 1,800%. The group D cases with a high LVEDP >32 had an even greater excess mortality with EDR of 131 per 1000 and MR of 2,000%. These results reflect very high mortality, indeed, in the minority of patients with the most abnormal ventriculographic indexes. Intermediate levels of mortality were found at the intermediate levels of EF and LVEDP. As in Table 354K1-6 two contrasting totals are given at the bottom of these tables: one for all patients, and the other for all patients excluding those with no coronary obstruction (in excess of 50% reduction in diameter).

The comparative experience when various additional risk factors were present or not present is summariazed in Table 354K1-9. Again, this experience is for the total series. In the groups without the additional risk factor the range of excess mortality is rather narrow, with MRs from 285% to 355%, and EDRs 12 to 15 per 1000 per year. This range is considerably wider when the additional risk factor is present. Mortality ratios vary from 480% in patients with hypertension to 1,600% in a small group of patients with congestive heart failure; the corresponding EDR values were 22 and 107 per 1000 respectively. A history of smoking produced a slightly higher excess mortality as a risk factor than hypertension did.

The final step in summarizing the Hartford Cardiac Catheterization Study for this abstract is given in Table 354K1-10, which provides a cross-comparison of excess mortality: a ratio of mortality ratios and a difference between excess death rates. This is done first for the medically treated patients vs. those treated with bypass surgery, from the results in Table 354K1-5, and next for the patients with a risk factor vs. those without the factor, from the results in Table 354K1-9. The exposures shown are for the combined medically and surgically treated patients classified by severity score, but only for patients *with* a particular risk factor, when a risk factor is the basis for the comparison. The smallest difference in EDR was 3 per 1000, for medically vs. surgically treated patients with less severe obstruction (severity score 1-4), and the next smallest was 8 per 1000 patients with vs. those without hypertension. The corresponding ratios of MRs were 1.57 and 1.37, respectively. The advantage of CBPS over medical treatment was much greater in patients with more severe obstruction (score 5-9). The maximum difference in excess mortality was found in the comparison of patients with CHF as a risk factor: difference in EDRs of 152 per 1000, and ratio of MRs of 4.43. The importance of severely impaired left ventricular function is also reflected in the results for the Group D patients, EF and LVEDP, in Tables 354K1-7 and 354K1-8. To avoid propagation of errors in Table 354K1-10, all mortality ratios from the original report[1] and the ratios of MRs have not been rounded off as they have been in accordance with the usual rules for rounding off in the other Abstract tables.

Acknowledgment: I would like to thank Richard B. Singer, M.D. for his considerable efforts in finalizing this mortality abstract.

TABLE 354K1-1

DISTRIBUTION OF 5,306 CATHETERIZED PATIENTS BY AGE AND SEX

Age	Male	Female
<41 yrs.	6.8%	5.6%
41-50	23.6	19.0
51-55	20.8	21.3
56-60	20.5	19.7
<61	71.7	62.6
61-65	18.2	17.2
66-70	8.1	12.1
71-80	3.8	7.9
>80	0.2	0.2
All	100.0	100.0
Mean Age	56.4 yrs.	58.4 yrs.

TABLE 354K1-2

DISTRIBUTION OF 5,306 CATHETERIZED PATIENTS BY SEX AND SEVERITY SCORE OF CORONARY ARTERY OBSTRUCTION*

Severity Score	Males	Females
NO OBSTRUCTION		
0	13.5%	40.3%
MILD OBSTRUCTION		
1	2.4%	3.7%
2	3.6	5.3
3	14.4	10.7
MODERATE TO SEVERE OBSTRUCTION		
4	7.4%	6.6%
5	10.6	7.2
6	13.8	7.8
7	10.3	6.3
8	13.0	6.2
9	11.0	5.9

* 1 point for narrowing of major artery diameter by 50-69%, 2 points for narrowing by 70-89%, 3 points for narrowing by 90-100%. Points are added for the three major arteries.

DISTRIBUTION OF 5,306 CATHETERIZED PATIENTS BY SEX AND OTHER RISKS

Factor	Male	Female
Smoking—Yes	41.6%	34.5%
—No	50.6	53.8
—Uncertain	7.8	11.7
History of Prior MI	44.8	24.0
Family History, CHD	19.1	22.3
Major ECG Abnorm.	52.4	44.2
Cerebrovascular or Per. Art. Dis.	8.1	9.0
Hypertension	35.4	43.1
History of CHF*	14.7	16.5
Hyperlipidemia	5.3	5.3
Diabetes mell.	10.4	13.7

* Congestive Heart Failure

COMPARATIVE MORTALITY BY SEVERITY SCORE FOR CORONARY OBSTRUCTION, 4,633 ENTRANTS WITH AVERAGE FOLLOW-UP OF 5.8 YEARS

Severity Score[†]	Dist. of Patients	Exposure Patient-yrs.	Number of Deaths		Mortality Ratio	Mean Annual Mort. Rate per 1000		
			Observed	Expected*		Observed	Expected	Excess
	%	E	d	d′	100(d/d′)	$\bar{q}$	$\bar{q}'$	($\bar{q}$–$\bar{q}'$)
927 ENTRANTS WITH NO SIGNIFICANT CORONARY OBSTRUCTION (<50%)								
0	20.0%	5,770	34	23.1	147%	6.4	4.0	2.4
1,274 PATIENTS WITH MILD CORONARY OBSTRUCTION								
1	2.8%	706	9	3.9	230%	12.7	5.6	7.1
2	4.0	1,175	16	7.5	215	13.6	6.3	7.3
3	13.5	3,787	55	19.3	285	14.5	5.1	9.4
4	7.2	2,036	48	11.8	405	23	5.7	17
1-4	27.5	7,704	128	42.5	280	16.6	5.5	11.1
2,432 PATIENTS WITH MODERATE TO SEVERE CORONARY OBSTRUCTION								
5	9.8%	2,570	78	15.0	520%	30	5.8	24
6	12.3	3,207	101	19.8	510	31	6.2	25
7	9.3	2,396	80	16.7	480	33	7.0	26
8	11.4	2,893	100	20.1	500	35	7.0	28
9	9.7	2,449	110	17.9	615	45	7.3	38
5-9	52.5	13,215	469	89.5	525	35	6.8	28
3,706 PATIENTS WITH CORONARY OBSTRUCTION OF 50% OR MORE								
1-9	80.0%	21,219	597	132.0	450%	28	6.2	22
All 4,633 CATHETERIZED PATIENTS WHO WERE TRACED								
0-9	100.0%	26,989	631	155.2	405%	23	5.7	17

* Basis of expected deaths: 1978 CIGNA Best Estimate Select Table, adjusted for 2% secular reduction in mortality per calendar year.

[†] Severity score: see footnote for Table 354K1-2.

TABLE 354K1-5

COMPARATIVE MORTALITY, CHD PATIENTS AFTER CARDIAC CATHETERIZATION, BY SEVERITY OF OBSTRUCTION, DURATION AND MEDICAL OR SURGICAL TREATMENT

Severity Score[†]	Interval Start-End	Exposure Patient-yrs.	Number of Deaths		Mortality Ratio	Mean Annual Mort. Rate per 1000		
			Observed	Expected*		Observed	Expected	Excess
	Yrs.	E	d	d'	100(d/d')	q̄	q̄'	(q̄–q̄')
MEDICALLY TREATED PATIENTS								
1-4	0-1	959	16	2.5	650%	16.7	2.6	14
	1-5	2,985	55	14.9	370	18.4	5.0	13
	5 up	1,419	29	12.1	240	20	8.5	12
	All	5,363	100	29.5	340	18.6	5.5	13
5-9	0-1	988	70	3.1	2,200	74	3.3	71
	1-5	2,500	114	15.4	740	46	6.1	40
	5 up	989	67	9.6	700	68	9.7	58
	All	4,437	251	28.1	715	57	6.7	50
1-9	Total	9,800	351	57.6	615	36	5.9	30
SURGICALLY TREATED PATIENTS (START 1 MONTH AFTER CBPS)**								
1-4	1mo.-1yr.	360	5	1.0	500%	13.9	2.8	11
	1-5	1,304	9	6.7	135	6.9	5.1	1.8
	5 up	644	14	5.2	265	22	8.1	14
	All	2,308	28	12.9	215	12.1	5.6	6.5
5-9	1mo.-1yr.	1,462	20	5.0	400	14.0	3.4	11
	1-5	5,129	78	32.5	240	15.2	6.3	8.9
	5 up	2,320	87	23.3	375	38	10.0	28
	All	8,911	185	60.8	305	21	6.8	14
1-9	Total	11,219	213	73.9	290	19.0	6.5	13

* Basis of expected deaths: 1978 CIGNA Best Estimate Select Table, adjusted for 2% secular reduction in mortality per calendar year.
† Severity score: see footnote for Table 354K1-2.
** 33 of 58 first-year deaths occurred within 30 days, giving an overall acute mortality rate of about 33/2021, or 1.6%. For long-term FU all 33 early deaths have been allocated to the 5-9 severity group.

TABLE 354K1-6

COMPARATIVE MORTALITY BY AGE OR SEX, 4,633 CATHETERIZED PATIENTS WITH FU, INCLUDING 20% WITH NO SIGNIFICANT CORONARY OBSTRUCTION

Age/Sex	Dist. of Exposure	Exposure Patient-yrs.	Number of Deaths		Mortality Ratio	Mean Annual Mort. Rate per 1000		
			Observed	Expected*		Observed	Expected	Excess
	%	E	d	d'	100(d/d')	q̄	q̄'	(q̄–q̄')
<50 yrs.	28%	7,614	116	16.4	710%	15	2.2	13
50-54	21	5,569	90	20.9	430	16	3.7	12
55-59	20	5,549	116	28.9	400	21	5.2	16
60-64	17	4,577	142	36.4	390	31	8.0	23
65 up	14	3,690	167	52.5	320	45	14.3	31
Male	76	20,565	521	125.8	415	25	6.1	19
Female	24	6,424	110	29.4	375	17	4.6	12
Total	100	26,989	631	155.1	405	23	5.7	17
EXCLUDING 20% OF PATIENTS WITH NO SIGNIFICANT CORONARY OBSTRUCTION								
M&F	79%	21,219	597	132.0	450%	29	6.2	23

* Basis of expected deaths: 1978 CIGNA Best Estimate Select Table, adjusted for 2% secular reduction in mortality per calendar year.

COMPARATIVE MORTALITY BY EJECTION FRACTION,
4,633 PATIENTS WITH AVERAGE FOLLOW-UP OF 5.8 YEARS,
INCLUDING 20% WITH NO SIGNIFICANT CORONARY OBSTRUCTION

Ejection Fraction	Dist. of Cath. Pts.	Exposure Patient-yrs.	Number of Deaths		Mortality Ratio	Mean Annual Mort. Rate per 1000		
			Observed	Expected*		Observed	Expected	Excess
%	%	E	d	d'	100(d/d')	$\bar{q}$	$\bar{q}'$	$(\bar{q}-\bar{q}')$
>57%	55.6%	15,951	209	88.0	235%	13.1	5.5	7.6
53-57	7.1	1,730	28	9.7	285	16.2	5.6	11
A>52	62.7	17,681	237	97.7	240	13.4	5.5	7.9
48-52	7.6	1,861	48	12.3	390	26	6.6	19
43-47	6.5	1,756	45	10.6	425	26	6.0	20
38-42	8.2	2,326	73	13.9	525	31	6.0	25
B38-52	22.3	5,943	166	36.9	450	28	6.2	22
33-37	5.6	1,366	59	7.9	750	43	5.8	37
28-32	5.5	906	43	5.7	750	47	6.3	41
C28-37	11.1	2,272	102	13.6	750	45	6.0	39
23-27	5.0	620	49	4.0	1,230	79	6.4	73
<23	2.9	473	77	3.1	2,500	163	6.6	156
D<28	7.9	1,093	126	7.1	1,800	115	6.5	109
All Pts.	100.0	26,989	631	155.2	405	23	5.7	17
CHD Pts.	80.0	21,219	597	132.0	450	28	6.2	22

* Basis of expected deaths: 1978 CIGNA Best Estimate Select Table, adjusted for 2% secular reduction in mortality per calendar year.

COMPARATIVE MORTALITY BY LEFT VENTRICULAR END-DIASTOLIC PRESSURE (LVEDP),
4,633 PATIENTS INCLUDING 20% WITH NO SIGNIFICANT CORONARY OBSTRUCTION

LVEDP mm. Hg.	Dist. of Cath. Pts.	Exposure Patient-yrs.	Number of Deaths		Mortality Ratio	Mean Annual Mort. Rate per 1000		
			Observed	Expected*		Observed	Expected	Excess
	%	E	d	d'	100(d/d')	$\bar{q}$	$\bar{q}'$	$(\bar{q}-\bar{q}')$
A<13	58.1%	16,317	273	90.4	300%	16	5.5	11
13-17	22.1	6,214	138	37.1	370	22	6.0	16
18-22	10.5	2,687	85	16.4	520	31	6.1	25
B13-22	32.6	8,901	223	53.5	415	25	6.0	19
23-27	4.4	955	48	5.8	830	50	6.1	44
28-32	2.7	467	39	3.1	1,260	84	6.6	77
C23-32	7.1	1,422	87	8.9	980	61	6.3	55
33-37	1.2	209	23	1.65	1,390	110	7.2	103
>37	1.0	140	25	0.71	3,500	179	5.1	174
D>32	2.2	349	48	2.36	2,000	138	6.8	131
All Pts.	100.0	26,989	631	155.2	405	23	5.7	17
CHD Pts.	80.0	21,219	597	132.0	450	28	6.2	22

* Basis of expected deaths: 1978 CIGNA Best Estimate Select Table, adjusted for 2% secular reduction in mortality per calendar year.

**COMPARATIVE MORTALITY BY SMOKING HISTORY AND OTHER RISK FACTORS,
4,633 PATIENTS INCLUDING 20% WITH NO SIGNIFICANT CORONARY OBSTRUCTION**

Risk Factor	Exposure Patient-yrs.	Number of Deaths Observed	Expected*	Mortality Ratio	Mean Annual Mort. Rate per 1000 Observed	Expected	Excess
	E	d	d′	100(d/d′)	$\bar{q}$	$\bar{q}′$	$(\bar{q}-\bar{q}′)$
Smokers	10,527	284	47.4	600%	27	4.6	22
Non-smokers	14,520	272	94.6	285	18.7	6.5	12
Prior MI Hist.	10,302	339	59.5	570	33	5.8	27
No Prior MI	16,009	280	92.0	305	17.5	5.7	12
Other Art.Scl.	1,884	111	13.6	820	59	7.1	52
None Found	23,809	477	133.9	355	20	5.6	14
Cong.Hrt.Fail.	757	86	5.4	1,600	114	7.1	107
No CHF	26,167	541	149.3	355	21	5.7	15
Hypertension	9,037	252	52.3	480	28	5.8	22
Normal BP	17,213	347	98.2	355	20	5.7	14

* Basis of expected deaths: 1978 CIGNA Best Estimate Select Table, adjusted for 2% secular reduction in mortality per calendar year.

**CROSS-COMPARISON OF EXCESS MORTALITY, 4,633 PATIENTS WITH CARDIAC CATHETERIZATION:
MEDICAL TREATMENT (HIGH RISK) VS. SURGICAL TREATMENT (LOW RISK) BY SEVERITY SCORE;
PRESENCE OF OTHER MEDICAL RISK FACTOR (HIGH RISK) VS. ABSENCE (LOW RISK)***

Risk Factor*	Exposure† Patient-yrs.	Ratio of Mortality Ratios HiRisk MR	LowRisk MR	Ratio of MRs	Difference Excess Death Rates HiRisk EDR	LowRisk EDR	Diff. in EDRs
	E	%	%	decimal	All rates per 1000		
RESULTS BY TREATMENT — MEDICAL = HIGH RISK, SURGICAL = LOW RISK							
Score 1-4	7,671	340%	217%	1.57	14	11	3
Score 5-9	13,348	717	306	2.34	50	14	36
Score 1-9	21,019	617	290	2.13	30	12	18
RESULTS BY RISK FACTOR — PRESENT = HIGH RISK, ABSENT = LOW RISK							
Smoking Hist.	10,527	599%	287%	2.09	22	12	10
Prior MI	10,302	570	304	1.88	27	12	15
Other Art.Scl.	1,884	818	256	2.30	52	14	38
Cong.Hrt.Fail	757	1,600	362	4.43	167	15	152
Hypertension	9,037	482	353	1.37	22	14	8

* High risk groups: medically treated patients with severity scores 1-4 and 5-9; patients with severity score 0-9 and one of these risk factors, cigarette smoking, hypertension, cerebro-vascular or peripheral vascular disease ("other Art.Scl.") or history of prior MI or congestive heart failure. Low risk groups: surgically treated patients (bypass surgery) with severity scores of 1-4 or 5-9; patients with severity score 0-9 but without each of the previously listed risk factors, considered in turn. For data and other details, see Tables 354K1-5 and 354K1-9.

† Exposures classified by severity score are for *both* medically and surgically treated patients. Other exposures are *only* for the patients *with* the specified risk factor.

Note: Mortality ratios are those given in the tables of the report,[1] not rounded off, as in Abstract Tables 354K1-4-9. The ratio of MRs is given as a decimal, and it also is not rounded off.

CHRONIC CORONARY HEART DISEASE, WITH ANGIOGRAPHY AND MEDICAL TREATMENT

Richard B. Singer, M.D.

Reference:

K. Bachmann, W. Niederer, H. Fuchs, H. Holzberger, "Prognosis of Coronary Heart Disease Patients Evaluated by Data Obtained by Invasive and Noninvasive Methods," in International Symposium, Bad Kroningen, October 22-23, 1982, *Prognosis of Coronary Heart Disease. Progression of Coronary Atherosclerosis* (Berlin and Heidelberg, Springer-Verlag, 1983), pp. 24-35.

Subjects Studied: Out of 5,251 patients with actual or suspected coronary heart disease (CHD) studied by angiography and ventriculography at the Erlangen University Polyclinic 1969-76, there were 1,387 found to have grade III stenosis (75% or more obstruction of one of more of the major coronary arteries). After exclusion of 351 patients with bypass surgery and 52 patients not followed up, there were 984 patients treated medically during their follow-up, 912 men age 28-81 years (mean age 52.5 years), and 72 women age 31-76 years (mean age 52.3 years). Most of the patients were recommended for medical treatment of their CHD, but 135 of the group refused the bypass surgery that was recommended, and received medical treatment only. Coronary artery lesions were subdivided according to the 1975 AHA classification as classes I (score 1-20), II (score 21-40), and III (score over 40). Ventricular function was graded according to the ejection fraction (EF): grades I, normal (EF 60% or greater), II (EF 30%-59%), and III (EF <30%).

Follow-up: Only 22 patients had delayed bypass surgery and these were excluded along with 30 patients who were lost to follow-up. The mean follow-up for the 984 patients included in the series was 40.1 months, with a range of 12 to 108 months.

Results: Although numerous graphs present actuarial survival rates to 5 years in the published report, only the 5-year survival rates have been used to derive a geometric mean annual survival rate, and from the complement of this, a mean annual observed mortality rate in each patient category. The corresponding mean annual expected mortality rate (q') has been derived from an empirical curve relating mean age to mean q', established by an intensive analysis of 8 or more series of CHD patients with angiography in which the age/sex distribution was available (to be reported in Abstract #642 of *1990 Medical Risks* monograph). Because of the shape of the curve of mortality rate against age, a tabular q' taken with the mean age always underestimates the weighted mean q' derived from the age/sex distribution. This distribution about the mean was found to be quite uniform from one series to another, despite variation in the mean age. As a consequence, the empirical curve gives a more accurate estimate of mean q' than would be obtained by entering a life table with the mean attained age. The U.S. 1979-81 Life Table rates for white males and females have been used as a reasonable comparison standard for these patients in West Germany.

Overall results, all severity grades combined, are shown in Table 354K2-1. Mean annual observed and expected mortality rates were 73 and 11.2 per 1000, respectively, giving an excess death rate (EDR) of 65 per 1000 and a mortality ratio of 650%. Mortality was slightly lower in the minority of patients who refused to have the bypass surgery that was recommended. Observed and excess mortality rates were nearly the same in males and females, but the MR was much higher in females, 1,490%, because of the sex difference in q'. Among patients under age 45 observed, excess mortality rates were less than half the levels found in patients age 45-59, but again the mortality ratio was higher in the younger patients because of the small q'. The data reflect the general tendency for EDR to increase, and of the MR to decrease with advancing age in CHD patients.

Univariate analysis of patients by severity is shown in Table 354K2-2, with the three stenosis classes in the upper part of the Table, and the three classes of ejection fraction, as the index of left ventricular function, in the lower part. As would be anticipated, the lowest mortality was observed in both Group I classes, those with the least severe stenosis score or a normal EF of 60% or more, and the highest mortality in the Group III classes, the most severe cases. Mortality ratios were under 400% in the Group I classes and EDRs were 30 or fewer extra deaths

Source: R. B. Singer, "Chronic Coronary Heart Disease, with Angiography and Medical Treatment," *J. Ins. Med.*, 18, no. 4 (1986): 19-21. Reproduced with permission of author and publisher.

per 1000 per year. The group with normal EF was much larger than the group with a stenosis score of 20 or less. In the most severe Group III classes the EDR was very high, 133 extra deaths per 1000 per year in patients with a stenosis score exceeding 40, and 257 per 1000 in patients with an EF less than 30%, and the mortality ratios were correspondingly high.

The authors also analyzed their experience according to the 9 possible combinations of the severity classes for stenosis and ventricular function. The resulting "Prognosis Index" is shown and defined in Table 354K2-3, with the related mortality results. A remarkably smooth increase in mortality was observed as increasing severity was marked by the order of the Prognosis Index categories. Among 246 patients with the lowest stenosis score and the best EF (60% or more) the MR was less than 200% and the EDR only 11 per 1000 per year. The highest mortality was found in a small group of patients unfortunate to have both stenosis and functional Class III severity, or a Prognosis Index of 6, an EDR of 336 per 1000 per year, and a MR of 2,300%. The combination of both stenosis and functional severity classes therefore serves as a powerful predictor of mortality and survival in CHD patients treated medically. The 5-year survival rate in the group with the worst Progosis Index was only 11.4%. It is of interest that impairment of left ventricular function, as measured by the EF, is associated with a higher mortality than the impairment defined by the corresponding class of the coronary stenosis score, a finding noted in several other studies of similar design.

Comment: Caution should be exercised in attempting to translate these mortality ratios into an underwriting classification, for several reasons. The mortality ratio gives anomalous results in comparison with observed mortality rates and EDRs when age and sex are varied, as described above. U.S. population rates are not identical with those of West Germany, although differences in this series of CHD patients are probably not large. More important is the lower expected mortality if insurance tables are used.

With the 1975-79 Group Life Insurance Tables, the overall mortality ratio would have been 880% instead of the 650% shown in Table 354K2-1, based on recent U.S. population rates. On the other hand, the EDR would be little affected, increased only from 62, as shown in the Table, to 65 extra deaths per 1000 per year. This problem was considered in the Panel Discussion of the original *Medical Risks* volume at the 1976 ALIMDA meeting.

It seems to me the most important underwriting lesson to be learned from results of this sort is the adverse effect on mortality of both angiographic and ventriculographic severity factors in CHD patients who have not had the benefit of bypass surgery. In the *1976 Medical Risks* volume the excess mortality in CHD patients selected for insurance issue was much lower than in other series, when comparisons were made in terms of EDR rather than mortality ratio. The same difference has been found in the more recent and more extensive studies abstracted for the *1990 Medical Risks*. The customary selection standards used in underwriting exclude many of the high-risk CHD patients that are part of a series referred for angiographic study and found to have 70% or more narrowing in at least one major coronary artery. In the Cleveland Clinic series (Abstract #307 in the *1976 Medical Risks*) the EDR averaged over 5 years was 74 per 1000 per year, as compared with the 62 per 1000 in Table 354K2-1. EDR values were somewhat lower in four additional series of medically treated CHD patients with angiography to be reported in the *1990 Medical Risks*, but the overall mean EDR was again much higher than the 5-year EDR in the CHD experience of the *1983 Medical Impairment Study*. If test results of angiography and ventriculography are available in an insurance applicant who has not had bypass surgery, any impairment beyond the "best" severity categories implies, in my opinion, a mortality higher than the average for insured CHD patients, and the mortality becomes very high indeed with multi-vessel disease and abnormal left ventricular function. The prognosis is much better with single-vessel disease, with stenosis less than 70%, and with normal ventricular function.

TABLE 354K2-1

COMPARATIVE 5-YEAR MORTALITY, CHRONIC CHD PATIENTS WITH 75% OR MORE STENOSIS OF 1-3 MAJOR CORONARY ARTERIES, BY ENTRY CLASS, SEX AND AGE

Category	Mean Age	No. of Entrants	5-Year Surv. Rate	Mean Ann. Mort. Rate per 1000*			Mortality Ratio
				Observed	Expected	Excess	
	$\bar{x}$	ℓ	P_5	$\check{q}$	q'	$\check{q}-q'$	$100(\check{q}/q')$
All Patients	52.5	984	0.685	73	11.2	62	650%
Selected for Medical Rx	est. 52.5	849	0.679	75	11.2	64	670
Bypass Recom., Not Done	est. 52.5	135	0.729	61	11.2	50	545
All Males	52.5	912	0.684	73	11.9	61	615
All Females	52.3	72	0.690	72	5.0	67	1,440
Age 30-44	est. 39.8	157	0.853	31	2.4	29	1,290
Age 45-59[†]	est. 52.4	479	0.705	68	8.5	60	800

* Observed rate derived from geometric annual mean of 5-year survival rate. Expected rate derived from empirical relation, mean q'
 to mean age, several series of CHD patients having age/sex distribution, with use of U.S. 1979-81 Life Tables, white male and female.
[†] No separate data for 213 patients 60 up.

TABLE 354K2-2

COMPARATIVE 5-YEAR MORTALITY, CHRONIC CHD PATIENTS BY CLASSIFICATION OF CORONARY STENOSIS (75% OR MORE) OR VENTRICULOGRAPH (BY EJECTION FRACTION)

Category**	Estimated Mean Age[†]	Patients Entered No.	of Total	5-Year Surv. Rate	Mean Ann. Mort. Rate per 1000*			Mortality Ratio
					Observed	Expected	Excess	
	$\bar{x}$	ℓ	%	P_5	$\check{q}$	q'	$\check{q}-q'$	$100(\check{q}/q')$
SEVERITY OF CORONARY STENOSIS								
I AHA Score ≤20	51.5	282	33.2%	0.833	36	11.7	24	310%
II AHA Score 21-40	52.5	414	48.8	0.673	76	12.8	63	595
III AHA Score >40	54.5	153	18.0	0.446	149	15.5	133	960
LEFT VENTRICULAR FUNCTION BY EJECTION FRACTION (EF)								
I EF 60% or more	52.3	527	62.0%	0.801	43	12.6	30	340%
II EF 30-59%	52.2	256	30.2	0.546	14	12.5	102	910
III EF <30%	53.3	66	7.8	0.206	271	13.8	257	1,960

* Observed and expected rates derived as in Footnote, Table 354K2-1.
[†] Estimated from age/sex data other series coronary stenosis. Age in EF classes derived from cor. sten. classes.
** AHA score based on degree of stenosis in segments of all major coronary arteries. EF = ejection fraction.

COMPARATIVE 5-YEAR MORTALITY, CHRONIC CHD PATIENTS BY PROGNOSIS INDEX:
COMBINATION OR CORONARY STENOSIS AND EJECTION FRACTION CLASSES

Category			Estimated Mean Age†	Patients Entered		5-Year Surv. Rate	Mean Ann. Mort. Rate per 1000*			Mortality Ratio
				No.**	of Total		Observed	Expected	Excess	
P.I.	Cor.	EF	$\bar{x}$	ℓ	%	P_5	$\check{q}$	q'	$\check{q}-q'$	$100(\check{q}/q')$
2	CI	I	51.5	246	25.0%	0.892	23	11.7	11	197%
3a	CII	I	52.5	291	29.6	0.777	49	12.8	36	385
3b	CI	II	51.5	71	7.2	0.711	66	11.7	54	565
4a	CIII	I	54.5	74	7.5	0.631	88	15.5	72	570
4b	CII	II	52.5	150	15.3	0.573	105	12.8	92	820
4c	CI	III	51.5	10	1.0	0.485	135	11.7	123	1,150
5a	CIII	II	54.5	76	7.7	0.364	183	15.5	167	1,180
5b	CII	III	52.5	39	4.0	0.254	240	12.8	227	1,880
6	CIII	III	54.5	27	2.7	0.114	352	15.5	336	2,300

* See Footnote Table 354K2-2.
† See Footnote Table 354K2-2.
** Estimated for Total Series from distribution in 849 patients selected for medical treatment.

224

COMPARATIVE MORTALITY IN PATIENTS WITH ACTUAL OR SUSPECTED CORONARY HEART DISEASE AFTER ANGIOGRAPHY AND TREADMILL TEST

John H. Reardon, M.D.

Reference:

D. B. Mark, M. A. Hlatkly, F. E. Harrell, K. L. Lee, D. B. Pryor, "Exercise Treadmill Score for Predicting Prognosis in Coronary Artery Disease," *Ann. Int. Med.*, 106 (1987): 793-800.

Subjects Studied: This study group included 2,842 individuals, median age 49. Some 70% were males. 2/3 had stable angina, and 1/3 had progressive anginal symptoms. There was a history of MI in 29%, and 22% had pathologic Q waves. At catheterization 27% had 3-vessel disease or left main coronary artery disease, 18% had 2-vessel disease, and 16% had 1-vessel disease (75% or greater stenosis of a major coronary artery). Some 39% of the study group had no significant coronary artery disease.

All patients had catheterization and treadmill test at Duke University Medical Center between Nov. 1965 and Jan. 1981. Patients were excluded if there was significant valvular disease or congenital heart disease. Patients were also excluded if treadmill results were uninterpretable due to resting ST abnormality or exercise induced LBBB or technical problems or if there was ST elevation in leads showing pathologic Q waves.

Scoring was as follows: Score = Exercise time (minutes) – (5 x ST deviation in mm.) – (4 x angina index). Angina index was valued as 0 = no angina, 1 = angina during exercise, 2 = angina as the cause for stopping exercise. A score of –11 or lower = high risk, –10 to +4 = moderate risk, and +5 or greater = low risk.

Follow-up: This was accomplished by clinic visit, mailed questionaires or telephone at 6 months and one year after cardiac catheterization and at one year intervals thereafter. Overall follow-up was 98% at all intervals, median follow-up was 5 years and 10% were followed to 10 years.

Source: J. H. Reardon, "Comparative Mortality in Patients with Actual or Suspected Coronary Heart Disease after Angiography and Treadmill Test," *J. Ins. Med.*, 21 (1989): 270-71. Reproduced with permission of author and publisher.

Results: The cumulative survival graphs accompanying the study were used to develop mortality tables for all three categories of exercise treadmill score (low, moderate, high risk). Mortality data were calculated for intervals of zero to five years and five to nine years post testing. Expected mortality rates were taken from the 1975-79 Group Life Insurance experience for males, and it was assumed the average age of the study group increased by one year for each calendar year. Table 354K3-1 clearly shows that even for this mixed group of subjects (ranging from 39% free of coronary artery disease to those with 3-vessel disease of 75% obstruction or more) a negative treadmill test (score +5 or higher) is associated with 0 excess mortality or 100% mortality ratio at 0-5 years, and at 5-9 years the death rate is 6 per thousand less than expected and the mortality ratio is 39%. Groups with moderate and high risk classification show increasing excess death rate and mortality ratios, being highest at 0-5 years for the high risk group. Table 354K3-2 shows the 5-year experience for just those subjects with 3-vessel disease (and no left main disease). Those patients with a high risk score (–11 or lower) had a mortality ratio of 960%, those with a low risk score (+5 or greater) had a mortality ratio of 425% and those with a very low risk score (+7 or greater) had a mortality ratio of 175%. Prognostic stratification is also present by treadmill scoring in subjects with 2-vessel and 1-vessel disease, although less marked. Thus the low risk treadmill score is a favorable prognostic finding even in the presence of severe 3-vessel disease. For the medical examiner, these findings suggest the treadmill test, in addition to being an indicator of CHD, is also a reliable means of assessing physical fitness and survival rate even in the face of CHD.

Table 354K3-1 shows for the low risk group, an excess death rate of 0 (mortality ratio 100%) during the first five years post testing and during the five to nine year interval an excess death rate of –6 (mortality ratio 40%). Excess death rate and mortality ratio are correspondingly higher for moderate and high risk classification.

In summary, scoring for ST changes, duration of exercise and angina enables you to place a TRD result into one of three categories predicting a risk that is consistent with a mortality rate below, slightly above or markedly higher than that of the general population.

Acknowledgment: Dr. Richard B. Singer has very graciously offered many helpful suggestions for the preparation of this abstract. He has also provided the values for the geometric average expected mortality rates from a different sample of Duke University patients angiographically studied and medically treated. These values were used in the development of Table 354K3-1.

TABLE 354K3-1

COMPARATIVE EXPERIENCE CHD PATIENTS AT DUKE MEDICAL CENTER BY TREADMILL TEST RISK SCORE AND DURATION

Interval	Cumulative Survival Rate Observed	Cumulative Survival Rate Expected	Survival Ratio	Interval Survival Rate	Mean Ann. Mortality Rate Observed	Mean Ann. Mortality Rate Expected	Excess Death Rate	Mortalilty Ratio
	P	P'	$100(P/P')$	P_i	$\check{q}$	$\check{q}'$	$1000(\check{q}-\check{q}')$	$100(\check{q}/\check{q}')$
LOW RISK, 968 PATIENTS — TEST SCORE >+5								
0-5 yr.	0.97	0.965	100.5%	0.97	0.007	0.007	0	100%
5-9	0.955	0.927	103.0	0.985	0.004	0.010	−6	40
MODERATE RISK, 1,497 PATIENTS — TEST SCORE −10 TO +4								
0-5 yr.	0.91	0.965	94.3%	0.91	0.019	0.007	12	270%
5-9	0.853	0.927	92.0	0.937	0.016	0.010	6	160
HIGH RISK, 377 PATIENTS — TEST SCORE <−11								
0-5 yr.	0.72	0.965	74.6%	0.72	0.064	0.007	57	915%
5-9	0.565	0.927	60.9	0.785	0.059	0.010	49	590

TABLE 354K3-2

COMPARATIVE 5-YEAR EXPERIENCE 3-VESSEL CHD (EXCLUDING LEFT MAIN OBSTRUCTION) PATIENTS AT DUKE MEDICAL CENTER BY TREADMILL TEST RISK SCORE

Risk Group	No. Patients	5-Year Survival Observed	5-Year Survival Expected*	Ratio	Mean Ann. Mortality Rate Observed	Mean Ann. Mortality Rate Expected	Excess Death Rate	Mortality Ratio
	ℓ	P	P'	$100(P/P')$	$\check{q}$	$\check{q}'$	$1000(\check{q}-\check{q}')$	$100(\check{q}/\check{q}')$
Very Low Score >7	49	0.93	0.961	96.8%	0.014	0.008	6	175%
Low Risk Score >5	85	0.84	0.961	87.4	0.034	0.008	26	425
High Risk Score <−10	177	0.67	0.961	69.7	0.077	0.008	69	960

* Based on 1975-79 Group Life Tables matched by sex and 4 male are groups in another Duke patients angiography and treatment sample.

POSITIVE EXERCISE ECG AND NEGATIVE THALLIUM — A STANDARD RISK?

B. Ross Mackenzie, M.D., FRCP(C), FACC

Introduction

Coronary artery disease is the leading cause of morbidity and mortality facing the medical director. Clinical information and resting electrocardiograms are often insufficient for the detection of asymptomatic coronary artery disease and in predicting the risk of a cardiac event in applicants with known coronary artery disease.

Many sophisticated tests have thus been developed to allow an early and more accurate diagnosis of coronary artery disease or for use in predicting coronary artery disease prognosis. Unfortunately, few, if any, of these tests are perfect. Results can be negative in applicants with disease and positive in applicants without disease. Therefore, medical directors often cannot be sure that a test result indicates the true state of the applicant.

This article will address a common medical underwriting situation facing medical directors: the applicant with a positive exercise electrocardiogram and negative thallium stress test. Recent advances in the thallium scintigraphy will be briefly reviewed. This will be followed by a discussion of the principles and pitfalls of the application of Bayes' Theorem to sequential testing in the noninvasive diagnosis of coronary artery disease using the exercise electrocardiogram and the thallium stress test. Finally, a practical approach using this common underwriting situation will be given.

Thallium Stress Testing

Thallium is a potassium analog that is usually administered intravenously at peak exercise or during infusion of a coronary vasodilator such as dipyridamole or adenosine. It is efficiently extracted by viable myocardium in proportion to its regional blood flow; thus its initial distribution is related to myocardial perfusion and viability.

After the administration of thallium an initial series of images is acquired within 30 minutes and a second series several hours later. Homogeneous distribution of thallium on the initial series of images is considered normal, the presence of one or more defects in thallium distribution in the first set but not in the second set of images is considered to represent ischemia (the phenomenon of defect resolution is called redistribution) and the presence of one or more defects on both sets of images is considered to represent scarred or nonviable myocardium.

Recent studies[1] have shown that myocardial thallium defects that are nonreversible on 4-hour redistribution studies may be associated with improvement in the uptake after successful revascularization or with evidence of viable myocardium as analyzed by positron emission tomographic assessment of glucose metabolism/myocardial blood flow relations. A less well understood pattern of thallium "reverse distribution" or "apparent worsening" is seen commonly after successful thrombolytic therapy for evolving myocardial infarction or successful angioplasty. It is felt to represent non-transmural myocardial fibrosis, most commonly subendocardial infarction in the presence of a non-flow limiting stenosis.

Thallium imaging after intravenous infusion of the coronary vasodilator dipyridamole has been demonstrated[2] to detect coronary artery disease and is diagnostically equivalent to perfusion studies performed after maximal exercise. In contrast to exercise stress testing, dipyridamole thallium scintigraphy is not dependent on the level of exercise achieved, patient motivation or concurrent antianginal medications. The coronary dilating effect of dipyridamole results in a substantial increase in regional blood flow to areas perfused by normal coronary vessels, but abnormal flow reserve is observed in areas supplied by stenotic vessels. This inhomogeneity of flow is detected by abnormal thallium uptake when the radionuclide is injected during peak vasodilative effect of the drug. Redistribution occurs in areas of viable, but hypoperfused myocardial regions comparable to what is observed in exercise scintigraphy.

Initially planar imaging,[3] employing multiple discrete views, much like the anterior and lateral views of the chest X-ray, was used. The utility of planar thallium imaging was enhanced by the development of quantitative techniques for assessing the initial distribution and subsequent washout of thallium. Unfortunately, planar imaging is inherently suboptimal for assessing myocar-

Source: B. R. Mackenzie, "Positive Exercise ECG and Negative Thallium — A Standard Risk?" *J. Ins. Med.*, 22 (1990): 257-61. Reproduced with permission of author and publisher.

dial perfusion because frequent overlap of normally and abnormally perfused myocardial regions limits its ability to detect, localize and size myocardial perfusion defects. Because of these limitations most laboratories today use Single Photon Emission Computed Tomography (SPECT) imaging, in which multiple view images are acquired circumferentially and then reconstructed by computer to a single three-dimensional image, identical in principle to X-ray computed tomography.

Direct comparisons have demonstrated superiority of SPECT over planar thallium imaging including enhancement of overall detection of exercise induced ischemia especially in the circumflex artery distribution, better prediction of extent of disease and more accurate localization of stenosed branches of coronary vessels responsible for a given perfusion defect. An important advance in the clinical utility of SPECT thallium has been the recent development of quantitative analysis for image interpretation which significantly improves on visual analysis of the tomographic slices. Display of the SPECT data in the form of a polar map or "bulls-eye" plot simplifies the interpretation of tomographic slices.

Probability and Sequential Testing

In the past few years a rational approach to the interpretation of noninvasive tests for the diagnosis and prognosis of coronary artery disease, has been developed on the basis of simple concepts of clinical epidemiology and biostatistics.[4] Uncertainty may be quantified as the probability that the applicant has coronary artery disease.[5] As a language for expressing uncertainty, probability has the advantage that it is governed by fundamental rules of logic. The effect of new information on diagnostic uncertainty (i.e., the extent to which diagnostic test results alter the probability of disease) can therefore be determined precisely. Interpretation of test results depends in part on other known information about an applicant. A positive test result in an applicant who has a low pretest probability of disease (for example, an asymptomatic 30 year old female insurance applicant) is considerably more likely to be falsely indicative of disease than an identical result in an applicant with a high pretest probability (for example, an applicant with typical angina). Thus the medical director's expectation prior to looking at the test results is the starting point for using noninvasive tests in underwriting the risk of coronary artery disease.

On the basis of both theoretical considerations and clinical studies, it is now clear that diagnostic information derived from exercise electrocardiograms and thallium perfusion imaging of persons with a low pretest prob-

ability of coronary artery disease is limited.[6] However, by applying easily obtained clinical information, one can change pretest likelihood of coronary artery disease and thereby greatly improve diagnostic information derived from a normal or abnormal test result. Probability analysis can further enhance diagnostic accuracy if one applies the principle that when the results of two test procedures are reasonably independent of one another, the post test likelihood of disease derived from the first test can be used as the pretest likelihood of disease for the second.

An important issue for medical directors is what level of post-test probability is required to rule in or rule out coronary artery disease for an individual applicant. A frequently used clinical threshold is in the range of 5-10% (i.e., <10% probability rules out disease and >90% confirms disease is present), but this level could and should be varied to suit the clinical and business implications of the application.

To establish the initial pretest likelihood of coronary artery disease, most medical directors use a table similar to that illustrated in Table 355K1-1.[7] By assessing the patient's age, gender and specific characteristics of symptoms, it is possible to roughly estimate the probability of coronary artery disease. This estimate can be further refined if one additionally considers such risk factors as: serum lipid status, smoking status, presence or absence of hypertension, diabetes and obesity, as well as the resting electrocardiogram (normal or abnormal).

The effectiveness of noninvasive tests for coronary artery disease is related to test sensitivity, test specificity and the prevalence of coronary artery disease in the population being tested. If the prevalence of coronary artery disease in the population at hand is known, two other determinations can be made: the positive and negative predictive values of the test (post-test likelihood). It is these latter factors that are more directly relevant to the underwriting of coronary artery disease risk. Positive predictive value is defined as the probability than an applicant with a positive test actually has coronary artery disease. Negative predictive value is defined as the probability that an applicant with a negative test does not have coronary artery disease. The precise values for sensitivity and specificity for the exercise electrocardiogram and thallium stress tests vary from center to center and are still evolving with advances in technology. Despite this, an analysis of published data has allowed construction of probability curves relating pretest (prevalence) and posttest (predictive value) likelihood of coronary artery disease for the exercise electrocardiogram and exercise thallium tests (Figure 355K1-1) and (Figure 355K1-2).[6]

PRETEST LIKELIHOOD OF CORONARY ARTERY DISEASE

Age	Sex	No Known Chest Pain	Non-Anginal Chest Pain	Atypical Pain Probably Not Angina	Atypical Pain Probably Angina	Typical Anginal Pain
35	M	1.9%	5.2%	10.4%	55.0%	73.6%
	F	0.3	0.8	1.6	10.0	25.8
40	M	3.6	9.8	20.0	61.0	81.5
	F	0.5	1.7	3.5	29.0	39.8
45	M	♥5.5	14.1	28.2	65.5	87.3
	F	1.0	2.8	5.6	35.0	55.2
50	M	7.7	18.0	36.0	67.4	♦89.8
	F	1.8	4.8	9.6	41.4	69.0
55	M	9.7	21.5	43.0	69.0	92.0
	F	3.3	8.4	16.0	49.4	79.4
60	M	11.1	25.2	50.4	70.0	93.4
	F	5.2	12.8	25.6	53.2	85.8
65	M	12.3	28.1	56.0	71.0	94.3
	F	7.5	18.6	37.0	56.0	90.6

♥ refers to example #1
♦ refers to example #2
Modified from references (6) and (7)

FIGURE 355K1-1

EXERCISE ELECTROCARDIOGRAPHY
ST SEGMENT RESPONSE

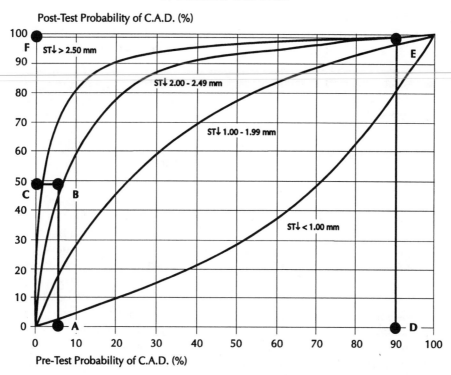

Family of ST depression curves and likelihood of Coronary Artery Disease. ST ↓ = S – T depression. A, B, and C refer to example #1 and D, E, and F refer to example #2. (Modified from references (6) and (7).)

THALLIUM PERFUSION SCAN
SENSITIVITY 85%, SPECIFICITY 90%

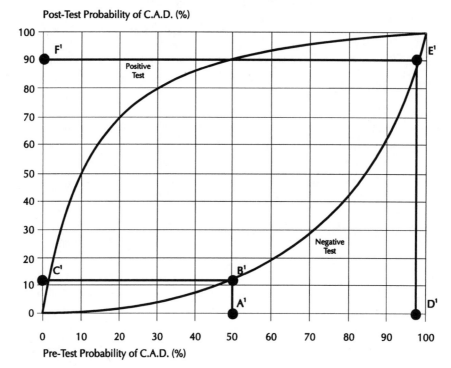

Thallium perfusion scanning and probability of Coronary Artery Disease.
A^1, B^1, and C^1 refer to example #1 and D^1, E^1, and F^1 refer to example #2. (Modified from reference (6).)

These likelihood curves are plotted with normal test results on the bottom and abnormal test results on the top. Their interpretation can be further refined by considering additional factors such as the severity of ST segment depression, the number of leads involved, duration of ST segment depression post exercise, peak workload, duration of exercise test, blood pressure response, arrhythmias and double product.

The reported sensitivity and specificity of exercise electrocardiograms are in the range of 60% to 85%[8] respectively. The high number of false positive responses observed in low prevalence population results from a wide variety of conditions that can affect the electrocardiogram. Some of these are technical: signal averaging of the ECG, inadequate skin preparation that results in noise or simply a wandering baseline. Patient related factors can be divided into those due to non-ischemic factors and those that are due to ischemia but a non-atheromatous process. Non-ischemic causes include: drugs, electrolyte abnormalities, hyperventilation, vasoregulatory asthenia, intraventricular conduction defects and WPW syndrome. Left ventricular hypertrophy or hypertension and mitral valve prolapse are common causes of false positive tests most likely on a ischemic basis. In addition there are less

common situations in which true ischemia might be present without atheromatous coronary artery disease, such as coronary spasm, left ventricular outflow tract obstruction, abnormal coronary vasodilator reserve and "syndrome X".

The sensitivity of thallium testing for coronary artery disease is in the range of 80-90% and the specificity has been traditionally high, at approximately 90%, although more recent reports[9] have indicated a slightly lower specificity perhaps due to post test referral bias in the population studied.

Some of the false positive thallium defects are most commonly artifactual due to shifting breast artifact, inaccurate patient positioning between stress and redistribution studies, diaphragmatic attenuation of the inferior wall and computer processing errors such as those resulting from over substraction of portions of the myocardium. Beyond these technical causes, false positive findings occur for similar nontechnical reasons as those for the exercise electrocardiogram. The causes of false positive thallium test, however, are not as numerous or frequent as for the exercise electrocardiogram.

During the last few decades a number of exercise ECG variables have been found to be useful prognostically including: depth of ST segment depression, slope of ST segment depression, duration of ST segment depression in recovery, time of onset of ST segment depression, exercise duration and exercise induced hypotension. Many investigators have found that an abnormal exercise ECG response in asymptomatic individuals is associated with roughly a fivefold increase in risk of cardiac events although the annual frequency in positive responders is relatively small. Thallium scintigraphy is a more expensive but also more powerful test of cardiac prognosis than is the exercise ECG because it is a more sensitive and specific marker of ischemia. Thallium scintigraphy gives results which reflect both the extent (proportion of myocardium at risk or number of diseased vessels) and severity (magnitude of ischemia within a given zone or severity of an individual stenosis) of coronary artery disease.[10] The number and location of perfusion abnormalities and presence of increased lung uptake represent important extent variables. Severe perfusion defects and slowly reversing defects represent important severity variables reflecting the presence of high grade (>90%) stenosis. Three variables have been found to provide independent prognostic information: 1) number of thallium defects, 2) magnitude of the initial reversible defect, and 3) thallium lung uptake.

Prognostic Implication of Negative Stress Thallium

Despite the recent advances in thallium scintigraphy, the method is not 100% sensitive and false negative results when compared with coronary angiography still occur. However, it is conceivable that the results of the thallium scintigraphy appropriately reflect the functional significance of disease. The medical director may then reasonably ask: is the technically correct negative thallium stress test able to predict a good prognosis? Some assurance may be gained from the studies looking at the prognostic significance of the negative thallium stress test in patients with chest pain. These studies[11] have consistently shown an excellent prognosis in this group of patients with yearly overall death rates of 0.2 to 0.5% and yearly myocardial infarction rates of 0.6 to 1.2%. This low cardiac event rate is comparable with that reported for patients with chest pain and angiographically normal coronaries. Further reassurance has been provided recently by the report of Fleg[12] et al. on silent ischemia detected by thallium scintigraphy and exercise ECG in asymptomatic low risk volunteers. A concordant positive exercise ECG and thallium stress test identified a small group of predominantly older subjects with a high risk for coronary events over the next 5 years. However, those with discordant results (positive exercise ECG and negative thallium) did not have an increased risk of cardiac events.

Practical Use of Probability Analysis

With the above background let us now approach the problem of the applicant with a positive exercise ECG and negative thallium stress test. The following example illustrates the concept. Suppose a 45 year old male who is asymptomatic presents with an exercise ECG associated with 2 mm. horizontal ST segment depression at peak exercise (9 minutes of standard Bruce protocol). A subsequent technically correct thallium stress test to a similar workload is negative.

The first step is to determine the pretest likelihood of coronary artery disease by using a table such as illustrated in Table 355K1-1. Using Table 355K1-1, we see the pretest likelihood of coronary artery disease in a 45 year old asymptomatic male would be approximately 5%. In practice, this figure might be adjusted slightly upward by the presence of other coronary risk factors.

The next step is to determine the post-test likelihood of coronary artery disease by using the exercise ECG results and applying them to the probability curves in Figure 355K1-1. This may be done by locating the pretest probability of coronary artery disease of 5% (point A) on the horizontal axis of Figure 355K1-1 and then locating the coinciding position on the –2.0 mm. ST segment depression curve (point B). The post-test probability of coronary artery disease may then be read off the vertical axis (point C) and in this example would be approximately 50%. A 50% likelihood of coronary artery disease falls in the intermediate probability range — not within the rule in or rule out thresholds of most medical directors as alluded to previously. At this point the medical director has several options given the 50% chance of coronary artery disease.

1. offer a rated policy based on your company's rating schedule.

2. postpone pending further evaluation by the attending physician.

3. ordering additional testing for cause — in this example an exercise thallium stress test.

Assuming that either of the latter 2 options is elected and the result is a negative thallium, the next step then will be to use this post-test probability of coronary artery disease as determined by the exercise ECG (50%) as the pretest likelihood for analyzing the thallium stress test result using the probability curves in Figure 355K1-2. Using the same procedure as with the exercise ECG, locate the 50% pretest probability of coronary artery disease on the horizontal axis (point A[1]) and then locate the coinciding position on the lower negative test curve (point B[1]). The post-test probability of coronary artery disease may then be read off the vertical axis (point C[1]) and is approximately 10%. This is within our threshold of confidence to exclude functionally significant coronary artery disease and we can with some confidence recommend a standard rating.

A further brief example is necessary to provide perspective and caution about using this approach. Suppose instead we are underwriting a 50 year old male with typical angina. Using Table 355K1-1, the pretest likelihood of coronary artery disease is approximately 90% (point D) and a subsequent positive exercise ECG with 2 mm. horizontal ST segment depression (point E) would increase the post-test probability of coronary artery disease (using Figure 355K1-1) to approximately 98% (point F). Although this is well within our threshold of diagnosing definite coronary artery disease, for purposes of illustration, let us suppose that the attending physician statement also includes a report of a negative thallium stress test. How does this affect our underwriting approach? Following the same principle utilized in the first example, we use the exercise ECG post-test probability of coronary artery disease (98%) (point D^1) as the pretest probability of coronary artery disease for the thallium stress test (Figure 355K1-2). We now see that a negative thallium (point E^1) only lowers the post-test probability of coronary artery disease to 90% (point F^1) which is still within our threshold of definite diagnosis of coronary artery disease. This applicant would then be rated according to your company rating schedule which has been developed to assign ratings for various levels of probability of coronary artery disease.

Conclusion

In this article I have attempted to review the recent advances in thallium stress testing and set forth the implications of probability analysis as applied to underwriting the insurance applicant with a positive electrocardiogram and negative stress thallium test. Several reservations[6] should be noted regarding the specifics of such analysis. The tables and figures are derived from data from an analysis of published reports. These data are often preliminary and incomplete and the results may vary from center to center. The resulting probability estimates are therefore only approximates. In addition many assumptions have been made in calculating the data. For example, the validity of using two tests in the same applicant to increase the reliability of the resulting diagnostic statements derives from the critical assumption that the tests are based on end points that are independent of one another. Although this assumption is probably not entirely valid, clinical experience utilizing the concept of sequential testing has confirmed its usefulness.

The noninvasive tests for coronary artery disease discussed above do not provide a yes or no statement regarding the presence of coronary artery disease. but rather offer a probability statement based on a continuum of risk. A working knowledge of probability analysis will make it easier for the medical director to decide about each applicant's future risk of coronary artery disease.

REFERENCES

1. E. H. Botvinick, "Late Reversibility: A Viability Issue," *J. Am. Coll. Cardiol.*, 15 (1990): 341-44.

2. G. A. Beller, "Dipyridamole Thallium-201 Scintigraphy: An Excellent Alternative to Exercise Scintigraphy," *J. Am. Coll. Cardiol.*, 14 (1989): 1642-44.

3. J. L. Ritche, M. D. Cerqueira, "Single Photon Computed Tomography (SPECT): 1989 and Beyond," *J. Am. Coll. Cardiol.*, 14 (1989): 1700-1.

4. R. E. Patterson, S. F. Horowitz, "Importance of Epidemiology and Biostatistics in Deciding Clinical Strategies for Using Diagnostic Tests: A Simplified Approach Using Examples from Coronary Artery Disease," *J. Am. Coll. Cardiol.*, 13 (1988): 1653-65.

5. H. C. Sox, Jr., "Noninvasive Testing in Coronary Artery Disease," *Postgrad. Med.*, 74 (1983): 319-36.

6. S. E. Epstein, "Implications of Probability Analysis on the Strategy Used for Noninvasive Detection of Coronary Artery Disease," *Am. J. Cardiol.*, 46 (1989): 491-98.

7. G. A. Diamond, J. S. Forrester, "Analysis of Probability as an Aid in the Clinical Diagnosis of Coronary Artery Disease," *N. Eng. J. Med.*, 300 (1979): 1350-58.

8. D. S. Berman, "The Detection of Silent Schemia: Cautions and Precautions," *Circulation*, 75 (1987): 101-5.

9. G. A. Diamond, "How Accurate is SPECT Thallium Scintigraphy?" *J. Am. Coll. Cardiol.*, 16 (1990): 1017-21.

10. A. Rozanski, D. S. Berman, "The Efficacy of Cardiovascular Nuclear Medicine Studies," *Semin. Nucl. Med.*, 17 (1987): 104-20.

11. F. J. T. Wackers, D. J. Russo, D. Russo, J. P. Clements, "Prognostic Significance of Normal Quantitative Planer Thallium-201 Stress Scintigraphy in Patients with Chest Pain," *J. Am. Coll. Cardiol.*, 6 (1985): 27-30.

12. J. L. Fleg, G. Gerstenblith, A. B. Zonderman, L. C. Becker, M. L. Weisfeldt, P. T. Costa, Jr., E. G. Lakatta, "Prevalence and Prognostic Significance of Exercise-Induced Silent Myocardial Ischemia Detection by Thallium Scintigraphy and Electrocardiography in Asymptomatic Volunteers," *Circulation*, 81 (1990): 428-36.

REOPERATION AFTER CORONARY BYPASS SURGERY (CBPS)

Richard B. Singer, M.D.

References:

1. F. D. Loop, D. M. Cosgrove, "Repeat Coronary Bypass Surgery: Selection of Cases, Surgical Risks, and Long-Term Outlook," *Mod. Concepts CV Dis.*, 55 (1986): 31-36.

2. W. C. Sheldon, F. D. Loop, "Coronary Artery Bypass Surgery: The Cleveland Clinic Experience, 1967-1982," *Postgrad. Med.*, 75 (1984): 108-21.

Subjects Studied: 1,500 consecutive patients with reoperation 1967-84 at the Cleveland Clinic, after initial coronary bypass surgery.[1] Patients have been divided into three time periods according to the year of reoperation. Mean age, sex, mean interval from initial operation to reoperation, and perioperative mortality are given in Table 358K1-1. Late mortality was observed in the first 1,000 of these 1,500 patients, with estimated mean age of 49.5 years at first CBPS and 55.1 years at reoperation, with 11.5% female patients, and estimated cutoff of entry at some time in 1982. Results after reoperation have been compared in this abstract with results for initial CBPS in 20,524 patients having first bypass with no associated cardiac surgery. This also is experience reported from the Cleveland Clinic, 1967-82.[2]

Follow-up: Was carried to 1984 for the first 1,000 reoperated patients, with a mean follow-up of 70.4 months, and survival rates were reported to 6 years in all patient categories shown. There were 23 patients lost to follow-up.

Results: For patients operated on in the 1970s the authors report a cumulative reoperation rate of 4% at 5 years and 14% at 10 years, with annual incidence rates at 5 and 10 years of 0.9% and 2.7%, respectively. Patients who eventually came to reoperation were younger than average for all patients at the time of their initial CBPS. Mean age at reoperation was 53.3 years during 1967-78, and this increased to 56.3 in the 1979-81 group, and to 58.0 in the 1982-84 group (Table 358K1-1); the interval between operations also increased from a mean of 4.1 to a mean of 7.0 years. The rise in mean age and proportion of females at reoperation parallels the rise observed at initial CBPS to 1982.[2] Perioperative mortality averaged 3.3% overall, somewhat higher than the 1.5% mortality rate observed in first CBPS operations at the Cleveland Clinic from 1967 through 1980. Not shown in the table is the increase in mortality with advancing age;[2] also, mortality is higher in females. During the period of observation from 1967 to 1984 graft closure, due to atherosclerosis, has tended to increase as the indication for reoperation while progressive sclerosis in the coronary arteries themselves has tended to decrease (Table 358K1-2). Blood use at reoperation and severe postoperative bleeding as a complication have decreased, with little change in the incidence of stroke as a complication. The incidence of perioperative myocardial infarction has decreased to 0.8% in initial operations, but has increased slightly to 8.0% in 1982-84 reoperations, thus widening the disparity between the initial operation and reoperation for this acute complication. The greater severity of impaired coronary circulation and higher mean age of the patients at reoperation during 1982-84 may account for this disparity.

Instead of U. S. population mortality rates, the 1975-79 Group Life Tables have been used as a more suitable standard for the estimate of comparative late mortality, as shown in Table 358K1-3. About half of the 966 survivors at hospital discharge had normal left ventricular function (LVF) on their preoperative ventriculogram, while the rest were classified into three different severity categories of abnormal function. The survival rate from hospital discharge to 6 years was obtained by dividing the overall 6-year survival (rates given at the end of the survival curve or in the text) by the perioperative survival rate (measured from the survival curve graphs). The geometric mean for this period of 5.95 years was used to derive a mean annual mortality rate for comparison with the rate expected from the 1975-79 Group Life Tables. Excess mortality over 6 years from reoperation in the total group was at a rather modest level: mortality ratio of 150% and excess death rate of 7 extra deaths per 1000 per year. When the patients were divided according to LVF those with normal function were found to have no excess mortality, while the excess death rate ranged from 9 extra deaths per 1000 per year in those with mild abnormality,

Source: R. B. Singer, "Reoperation after Coronary Bypass Surgery (CBPS)," *J. Ins. Med.*, 19, no. 1 (1987): 8-10. Reproduced with permission of author and publisher.

to 22 per 1000 in patients with moderate abnormality, to a high rate of 46 per 1000 in the small group with severe abnormality of LVF. Ventricular function was therefore a powerful severity discriminator for excess mortality after reoperation, as it is after initial CBPS. As compared with the overall reoperation rate, excess death rates were smaller for a 5-year period following initial CBPS: 5 per 1000 per year in the 1971-73 group, and only 2 per 1000 in the 1974-78 group.

Overall survival curves by number of vessels with 50% or greater narrowing showed 6-year rates of 93.4% for 1-vessel disease, and 89.8%, 82.1%, and 80.5% for 2-vessel, 3-vessel, and left main disease, respectively. Over 70% of patients were in New York Heart Association classes III or IV prior to reoperation, but improvement had occurred in most of these after reoperation, with only 13% still in classes III or IV, and 53% were angina-free (Class I). Graft patency, studied by angiography an average of 41 months after reoperation in 214 patients, was about 75% for saphenous vein grafts and 93% for internal mammary artery grafts.

From these results one may conclude that both perioperative mortality and late mortality to six years are higher for reoperation than for initial operation, but the differences are relatively small. Excess late mortality is confined to patients with abnormal LVF, and appears to be nil in those with normal function. Graft patency rates are similar to those observed after primary CBPS, and rates are considerably higher when the internal mammary artery is used. To quote the authors, "Angina relief is satisfactory after reoperation but is less than that achieved after the first operation, a finding attributed to diffuse coronary atherosclerosis and a higher prevalence of pre-reoperative left ventricular involvement." On the whole, results of reoperation are very nearly as good as those obtained with initial bypass surgery, when the operation is carried out with a high degree of technical proficiency. However, the reader should be cautioned that excess mortality tends to rise sharply with duration after 5 years in primary CBPS, as found in all studies with follow-up carried to 10 years or more, including the Cleveland Clinic experience.

REOPERATION AFTER CORONARY BYPASS SURGERY (CBPS) CLEVELAND CLINIC EXPERIENCE 1967-84

TABLE 358K1-1

CHARACTERISTICS AND PERIOPERATIVE MORTALITY OF REOPERATED CBPS PATIENTS

Operation Category	Time Period	Mean Age 1st Operation $\overline{x}_i$	Mean Interval $\overline{\Delta t}$(yrs.)	Mean Age Reoperation $\overline{x}_r$	Proportion Females %	No.Patients Operated ℓ_o	Perioperative Deaths d_o	Early Mortality Rate $q_o = 100(d_o/\ell_o)$
Reoperation	1967-78	49.1	4.1	53.3	8.7%	436	20	4.6%
Reoperation	1979-81	49.7	6.0	56.3	13.2	439	10	2.3
Reoperation	1982-84	52.2	7.0	58.0	14.7	625	20	3.2
Reoperation	1967-84	50.6	6.0	56.1	12.5	1,500	50	3.3
Reoperation (1st 1000 pts.)	1967-82	49.5	5.3	55.1	11.5	1,000	34	3.4
First CBPS	1967-80	54.3	—	—	11.9	20,524	313	1.5

INDICATIONS FOR AND COMPLICATIONS OF CBPS REOPERATIONS

Category	1967-68		1979-81		1982-84	
	No.	%	No.	%	No.	%
INDICATIONS						
Graft Closure	125	28.2%	157	35.8%	277%	44.3%
Cor. Art. Atherosclerosis	239	54.8	121	27.6	113	18.1
Combined Graft and Cor. Art.	74	17.0	161	36.7	235	37.6
COMPLICATIONS						
Bleeding Requiring Additional Operation	48	11.0%	28	6.4%	26	4.2%
Blood Usage (Mean No. Units)	8.0	—	2.5	—	2.0	—
Neurologic Deficit (Stroke)	8	1.8	8	1.8	16	2.6
Perioperative Infarction (MI)	29	6.7	28	6.4	50	8.0
Initial Operation — Perioperative MI	—	3.5	124	1.5	23(1982)	0.8

TABLE 358K1-3

COMPARATIVE LATE MORTALITY
SURVIVORS OF REOPERATION OR INITIAL OPERATION

Category	No. Surv. Hosp. Disch.	Cumulative Survival Rate			Mean Ann. Mort. Rate per 1000			Mortality Ratio
		Overall	to Hosp. Disch.	HD to t yrs.	Observed	Expected*	Excess	
	ℓ	P_t	p_o	$P=(P_t/p_o)$	q	q'	$q-q'$	$100(q/q')$
Reoperation 1967-82[†]								
Normal Left Ventr. Func.	476	0.888	0.968	0.917	14	14	0	100%
Mild Abn. LVF	263	0.859	0.985	0.872	23	14	9	164
Mod. Abn. LVF	179	0.755	0.948	0.804	38	(16)	22	240
Severe Abn. LVF	48	0.643	0.927	0.697	60	(14)	46	430
Total	966	0.85	0.966	0.880	21	14	7	150
Initial Oper.1971-73** 2979 HD to 5 yrs. d/E = 195/14089					14	9	5	156
1974-78** 4944 HD to 5 yrs. d/E = 308/22420					14	12	2	117

* Basis of expected mortality: 1975-79 Group Life rates adjusted to average age/sex/duration distribution
  for CBPS patients about the actual mean age.
[†] q derived from geometric mean annual survival rate to 6 years duration.
** q derived from observed late deaths and exposures to 5 years duration.

MORTALITY BY SEX AFTER CORONARY BYPASS SURGERY

Richard B. Singer, M.D.

References:

1. D. A. Killen, W. A. Reed, M. Arnold, et al., "Coronary Artery Bypass in Women: Long-Term Survival," *Ann. Thorac. Surg.*, 34 (1982): 559-63.

2. D. A. Killen, W. A. Reed, S. Wathanacharoen, et al., "Normal Survival Curve after Coronary Artery Bypass," *South. Med. J.*, 75 (1982): 906-12.

3. E. A. Lew, J. Gajewski, eds., *Medical Risks: Trends in Mortality by Age and Time Elapsed* (New York, Praeger, 1990). See Abstract #655.

Objectives of Abstract: To analyze the early and late mortality of a consecutive series of coronary bypass (CBPS) patients by sex and duration, all ages combined, and to supplement the experience reported in Abstract #655 (reference 3).

Subjects Studied: 2,628 patients with significant coronary artery obstruction and isolated CBPS performed between January 1971 and December 1976, at St. Luke's Hospital, Kansas City, Missouri. Significant obstruction was defined as 50% or more reduction of the internal diameter of a major coronary artery. Patients with cardiac surgery additional to coronary bypass and those with a history of prior bypass surgery were excluded; in other respects the series was consecutive. Of the total, 385 patients were women, and 2,243 were men. The range of age was 28 to 78 years for the series, and full age data for both sexes have been given only in reference 1, this article not being referred to in reference 2, published in the same year and used as the source for Abstract #655. Age distribution data for both sexes are shown in Table 358K2-1, estimated from measurement of the percentage distribution in the bar graphs of Figure 1, reference 1. Mean ages derived from these data are 53.9 years for the men and 57.8 years for the women. There was a tendency for men to have less 1-Vessel disease, only 16% as compared with 29% of the women. The corresponding prevalence of 3-Vessel disease was 52% in the male and 42% in the female patients.

Source: R. B. Singer, "Mortality by Sex after Coronary Bypass Surgery," *J. Ins. Med.*, 21 (1989): 267-69. Reproduced with permission of author and publisher.

Follow-up: Long-term mortality was based on life table data of 2,602 patients who survived 30 days after surgery, carried to December 1980, with only a single patient lost. Follow-up was complete on all patients to 3 years duration, the mean follow-up was 5.2 years and the maximum, 10 years. Because of withdrawals due to end of follow-up there were only 138 survivors at the end of 8 years; the results have therefore been restricted to those of the first 8 postoperative years.

Results: Expected deaths have been derived from the 1975-79 Group Life Tables, the standard chosen for all CBPS series in the new *Medical Risks* volume. The reason for using these instead of U.S. population tables is the evidence of bias in the referral of patients with coronary heart disease (CHD) to tertiary care medical centers for angiography as potential candidates for bypass surgery. The age/sex distribution shows fewer females and fewer patients over age 65 in the CBPS series than in series of patients with acute myocardial infarction or chronic CHD.

The probable reason is that patients with advanced cancer and other high-risk diseases are generally regarded by their physicians as unsuitable for referral for angiography. Some cardiothoracic surgeons affirm that they do not exclude any needful CHD patient from bypass because of age or associated medical condition, but their patients must come to them by referral. The lower group mortality has appeared to us to be a more appropriate standard than population tables. Derivation of the first-year mortality rates is shown in Table 358K2-1.

Perioperative mortality, within 30 days of operation, was extremely low in this series. The early mortality rate was only 0.9% in the men (21 deaths), and 1.3% in the women (5 deaths). These early deaths were excluded from the long-term mortality experience.

Comparative mortality by annual duration to 8 years is shown in Table 358K2-2 for male and female patients separately, with all ages and all degrees of CHD severity combined. The trend is for excess mortality to increase with duration. For individual years of duration sex differences in the observed mortality rates are not large and appear to be random (annual numbers of female deaths range from only 2 to 8). The expected mortality rates are smaller for the women than for the men, but the difference is less than might be anticipated because of the older ages in the female CBPS patients. Sex differences are more evident in Table 358K2-3, in which results are averaged over two periods, 1 month to 4 years, and 4 to 8 years. Both mortality ratio and EDR are distinctly higher in women than in men in the earlier period: ratios of 192% and 124% and EDRs of 10.2 and 2.8 per 1000, respectively. However, the sex differences in mortality ratio are minimal in the second period, and the higher EDR of 15 per 1000 is the same for both men and women. The values of mean annual q and q' in Table 358K2-3 should be examined with care to visualize the impact of both observed and expected rates on the magnitudes and changes in both MR and EDR.

Comment: Killen et al. used population mortality rates to compare survival curves, and emphasized "normal" survival for the men, survival for women about the same as for the men, but a higher expected survival curve for the women. In Table 358K2-3 it is evident that, with the lower expected mortality from the Group Life Tables,

there is slight excess mortality in the first 4 years in the men, but more in the women. Excess mortality is higher in both sexes at durations 4-8 years, a most important trend consistent with the many other CBPS abstracts in reference 3. The results presented here substitute an age/sex distribution for the age distribution that had to be assumed in Abstract #655, in which the life table data have been given for males and females combined, by duration in the lower half of Table 655B. This abstract should therefore be regarded as a supplement to Abstract #655. Neither in their reference 1 article nor in their correspondence with Dr. Gajewski about additional life table data did the authors mention the existence of the reference 2 article, which contained the overall age distribution for both sexes that we so badly needed. However, the assumed values of q' in Table 655B were within 10% of the accurately calculated values shown in the tables of this abstract. Readers of Table 655B, if they so desire, may adjust the EDR results to the accurate q' figures by subtracting 1 per 1000.

CORONARY BYPASS SURGERY MORTALITY EXPERIENCE
ST. LUKE'S HOSPITAL, KANSAS CITY, 1971-81

TABLE 358K2-1

APPROXIMATE AGE/SEX DISTRIBUTION* AND FIRST-YEAR EXPECTED DEATHS

Age Group	Males				Females			
	Approx.* No. Pts.	% Total Male	Expected Mort. Rate[†]	Expected Deaths	Approx.* No. Pts.	% Total Female	Expected Mort. Rate[†]	Expected Deaths
	ℓ_0	%	q'	d'	ℓ_0	%	q'	d'
28-29	7	0.3	0.0010	0.01	0	0.0	0.0005	0.00
30-39	88	3.9	0.0012	0.10	13	3.4	0.0007	0.01
40-49	553	24.7	0.0027	1.49	65	10.9	0.0013	0.08
50-59	948	43.2	0.0075	7.11	112	29.1	0.0032	0.36
60-69	580	25.9	0.0193	11.19	150	38.9	0.0081	1.22
70-78	67	3.0	0.0516	3.46	45	11.7	0.0240	1.08
All Ages	2,243	100.0	0.0104	23.36	385	100.0	0.0071	2.75

* Approximate distribution estimated from bar graphs, Figure 1, reference 1.
  Totals are exact reported data.
[†] Based on 1975-79 Group Life Tables.

TABLE 358K2-2

COMPARATIVE MORTALITY BY SEX AND DURATION, EARLY DEATHS EXCLUDED

Duration Start-End	No. Alive at Start	Exposure Patient-yrs.	Number of Deaths		Mortality Ratio	Mean Ann. Mort. Rate per 1000		
			Observed	Expected*		Observed	Expected	Excess
t to t+Δt	ℓ	E	d	d′	100(d/d′)	q	q′	(q–q′)
MALES								
1 mo.-1yr.	2,222	2,038	32	21.07	152%	15.8	10.4	5.4
1-2 yrs.	2,190	2,190	23	24.75	93	10.5	11.3	–0.8
2-3	2,167	2,167	39	26.87	145	18.0	12.4	5.6
3-4	2,128	1,960	29	26.47	110	14.8	13.5	1.3
4-5	1,764	1,480	37	21.76	170	25	14.7	10.3
5-6	1,163	944	30	15.11	199	32	16.0	16
6-7	676	532	19	9.31	205	36	17.5	18
7-8	349	238	12	4.56	265	57	19.1	38
FEMALES								
1 mo.-1yr.	380	347	6	2.46	245%	17.3	7.1	10.2
1-2 yrs.	374	374	7	2.88	245	18.7	7.7	11
2-3	367	367	5	3.08	162	13.6	8.4	5.2
3-4	362	332	8	3.05	260	24	9.2	15
4-5	294	250	5	2.50	200	20	10.0	10
5-6	201	165.5	4	1.80	220	24	10.9	13
6-7	126	93.0	3	1.11	270	32	11.9	20
7-8	57	40.5	2	0.53	375	49	13.0	36

* Based on 1975-79 Group Life Tables.

TABLE 358K2-3

COMPARATIVE MORTALITY BY SEX, AVERAGED OVER SUCCESSIVE 4-YEAR PERIODS

Sex	No. Alive at Start	Exposure Patient-yrs.	Number of Deaths		Mortality Ratio	Mean Ann. Mort. Rate per 1000		
			Observed	Expected*		Observed	Expected	Excess
	ℓ	E	d	d′	100(d/d′)	q	q′	(q–q′)
DURATION 1 MONTH TO 4 YEARS								
Male	2,222	8,345	123	99.2	124%	14.7	11.9	2.8
Female	380	1,420	26	11.5	225	18.3	8.1	10.2
DURATION 4-8 YEARS								
Male	1,764	3,195	98	50.7	193%	31	15.9	15
Female	294	549	14	5.9	235	26	10.8	15

* Based on 1975-79 Group Life Tables.

VALVE REPAIR FOR MITRAL INSUFFICIENCY WITHOUT STENOSIS

Richard B. Singer, M. D.

References:

1. W. Kirklin, "Mitral Valve Repair for Mitral Incompetence," *Mod. Concepts of CV Dis.*, 56 (Feb. 1987): 7-11.

2. E. A. Lew, J. Gajewski, eds., *Medical Risks: Trends in Mortality by Age and Time Elapsed* (New York, Praeger, 1990).

Subjects Studied: A series of 210 patients diagnosed at the Medical Center of the University of Alabama at Birmingham, 1967-85 as having mitral insufficiency without stenosis, and treated by surgical repair of the mitral valve (MVR) instead of mitral valve replacement. The largest group in the series consisted of 86 patients with isolated MVR, although a few of these also had tricuspid valve annuloplasty. The remaining patients had associated cardiac surgery: 63 patients with coronary bypass (CBPS); 31 patients with aortic valve replacement (AVR); 27 patients with repair of a congenital cardiac defect; two patients with pericardiectomy and one with removal of a myxoma. A long list of causes of the mitral insufficiency is given in reference 1. The insufficiency was considered as rheumatic in origin in only 26 patients; prolapse ascribed to myxomatous degeneration was found in 27 patients and isolated rupture of chordae in 39; "important" coronary artery disease was found in 39 patients, and insufficiency was ascribed to ischemic disease in 25 additional ones. Functionally, however, all patients were demonstrated to have mitral insufficiency without stenosis. Two additional series were reported for the period 1975-83: 101 patients with MVR, and 389 with mitral valve replacement (survival curves in Figure 3 of the article).

Limitations of Study: No data for age and sex distribution were given for the total series or any of the subgroups. The usual socioeconomic and geographical limitations that pertain to patients referred to a tertiary care medical center.

Follow-up: The survival curve for the total series was carried to a maximum of 13 years (17 survivors at that duration), with no mention of methods used or cases lost to follow-up. Maximum follow-up of 5 or 8 years was reported for the two series started in 1975.

Results: Early mortality was defined as deaths prior to hospital discharge (HD). The average duration of hospitalization was not given, but has been assumed to be 3 weeks or 0.06 year. Overall perioperative mortality prior to HD was 6.7%, and appears from the survival curves to have been considerably lower than the early mortality in the patients subjected to mitral valve replacement (no tabular data given). As shown in Table 369K1-1, the group of MVR patients with the lowest mortality rate of 3.7% consisted of those with isolated MVR, with or without tricuspid annuloplasty. The highest perioperative rate of 11.1% was experienced in the group with associated CBPS, and the rate was nearly as high when the associated surgery was aortic valve replacement.

Despite the complete lack of age/sex information, the author has provided an expected survival curve based on "an age-sex-race-matched general population," but the source tables are not cited. From this curve it has been possible to derive and graduate expected annual rates, q' or q̄', as shown in Table 369K1-2. Although the derivation is reasonably accurate for the first year, the reader should be cautioned that the annual increase of about 8% per year in q' may be much too high as compared with an increase of about 1% per year found for q', all ages combined, from data by age group and sex for a series of patients with mitral valve replacement in one of the abstracts in reference 2. The matching appears to have been done only for the entry-year distribution of patients by age, sex and race, not for the distribution of survivors at each year of follow-up. Although each survivor does have an advance of one full year in attained age with each year of elapsed duration, this is not true of the mean age, because mortality rates are consistently much higher at the older ages, with resultant flattening of the mean age and the mean q' duration curves. Values of q' as derived from the survival curve have been used in the table, but q' would be smaller at durations beyond the first year or two, and both Mortality Ratio and EDR would be proportionately larger than the results in the table.

Another methodological feature of Table 369K1-2 is reconstruction of annual life table data to 10 years from biennial data on the survival graph (Figure 1 of the article)

Source: R. B. Singer, "Valve Repair for Mitral Insufficiency Without Stenosis," *J. Ins. Med.*, 20, no. 1 (1988): 21-23. Reproduced with permission of author and publisher.

for distribution of the 52 late deaths, and the number of patients entering each biennium alive. This reconstruction, despite some random error, provides more detailed and more accurate results than it is possible to derive from geometric mean rates by estimate of the survival rate, P, at various durations on the observed survival curve. Tabular values of E, d, and d' may therefore be regarded as close approximations to the actual observed and calculated values. Comparative experience as given in the table indicates highest excess mortality in the first year after discharge from the hospital, with an EDR of 72 extra deaths per 1000 per year, and a Mortality Ratio of 760%. EDR reached a minimum of 17 per 1000 per year at duration 3-5 years, but rose to 27 per 1000 as mean annual rate over the last 5 years shown in the table. The Mortality Ratio of 255% at durations 5-10 years would be about 360% if the annual q' had increased only to 12 per 1000, as I have reason to believe (see above).

From Figure 2 of the article I have thought it wiser to fall back on the 5-year survival rates (most are given in the text), to obtain the interval survival rate from HD to 5 years by dividing P by the discharge survival rate, P_o (Table 369K1-1), and then to derive the geometric mean annual q̌'. This is a straightforward and reasonably accurate derivation. However, it would, on the basis of data in valve replacement series described in reference 2, be inaccurate to assume the same q̌' for each group, as previously derived for the total series. The latter q̌' has therefore been adjusted for an assumed age difference compatible with the age difference found in other series of patients with prosthetic replacement of a diseased mitral valve. Such crude approximations of 5-year late mortality by associated surgery group indicate the most favorable mortality in the isolated EDR group, with an EDR of 14 per 1000 per year; the highest EDR, 82 per 1000 per year, was found in the patient group in which aortic valve replacement was carried out in addition to MVR. However crude the actual Mortality Ratio and EDR results may be, it seems likely that the relative order for the groups is the actual one in each index of excess mortality. In contrast to these results for the various groups, the data for all MVR patients, on the bottom line, are much more accurate and do serve as a reliable basis for comparison.

Comment: In comparison with mitral valve replacement, repair of the mitral valve, where surgically feasible, offers a comparatively low perioperative and late mortality, a lower incidence of reoperation, and good functional results (74 of 111 survivors at end of follow-up were in NYHA Class I, 29 in Class II, and only 8 in Class III or IV). Another important advantage of valve repair is that there is no need for anticoagulation, which is needed for most types of prosthetic valve. Despite all of the changes in valve type and design, complication rates remain fairly high following valve replacement for severe hemorrhage, stroke and endocarditis (reference 2). Many of these complications are fatal, contributing to the high late mortality; even a nonfatal stroke may be severely disabling to the patient. For the minority of patients with mitral insufficiency but no stenosis, repair of the valve appears to offer many advantages over valve replacement, as emphasized by Kirklin, although repair is seldom used by most cardiac surgeons (reference 1).

From the underwriting standpoint it is my judgment that the better applicants with a history of valve replacement would be acceptable only at the highest rating levels, if acceptable at all. It appears reasonable to consider high but not the highest ratings for applicants with a history of isolated mitral valve repair who are doing well and free of complications. I use the term "high" rather than "moderate" because the expected mortality rates used here are based on population, not select insurance, tables. A method of translating mortality ratios from those based on population mortality to the familiar ones based on select insurance tables may be found in the panel discussion on the first volume of *Medical Risks* in the *1976 ALIMDA Proceedings,* or Methodology Article 003K1 in Chapter 3 of this volume.

VALVE REPAIR FOR MITRAL INSUFFICIENCY WITHOUT STENOSIS
EXPERIENCE OF UNIVERSITY OF ALABAMA AT BIRMINGHAM, 1967-85

TABLE 369K1-1

EARLY (IN-HOSPITAL) AND LATE DEATHS BY ASSOCIATED CARDIAC PROCEDURE

Type of Cardiac Surgery	No. Pts. Operated	No. Early Deaths	In-Hospital Mort. Rate	Hospital Surv. Rate	Pts. Discharged Alive	No. Late Deaths
	ℓ_o	d_o	$q_o=d_o/\ell_o(\%)$	$P_o=1-q_o$	$\ell=\ell_o-d_o$	d
Mitral Valve Repair (MVR) Isolated*	86	3	3.5%	0.965	83	22
MVR + Coronary Bypass	63	7	11.1	0.889	56	13
MVR + Aortic Valve Replacement	31	3	9.7	0.903	28	13
MVR + Repair, Cong. Heart Defect	27	1	3.7	0.963	26	4
MVR + Miscellaneous[†]	3	0	0.0	1.000	3	0
All Mitral Valve Repair	210	14	6.7	0.933	196	52

* Includes some cases with tricuspid valve annuloplasty.
[†] 1 case, removal of myxoma, 2 cases of pericardiectomy.

TABLE 369K1-2

MORTALITY BY DURATION (HOSPITAL DISCHARGE TO 10 YEARS) IN ALL PATIENTS WITH MITRAL VALVE REPAIR
(RECONSTRUCTED LIFE TABLE DATA FROM SURVIVAL GRAPHS AND OTHER RESULTS)

Interval Start	No. Alive at Start	Exposure Patient-yrs.	Number of Deaths		Mortalilty Ratio	Mean Annual Mortality Rate per 1000		
			Observed	Expected		Observed	Expected*	Excess
t to t+Δt	ℓ	E	d	$d'=(\bar{q}')(E)$	$100(d/d')$	$\bar{q}$	$\bar{q}'$	$\bar{q}-\bar{q}'$
HD-1 yr.	196	180	15	1.98	760%	83	11	72
1-3 yrs.	171	314	11	3.77	290	35	12	23
3-5	131	225	7	3.15	220	31	14	17
5-10	93	297	13	5.05	255	44	17	27

* Derived and graduated from cumulative survival curve of an "age-sex-race-matched general population" (Figure 1 in reference 1). Matching apparently done only for patients at entry, not for survivors at each duration, because progression of q' much higher by duration than in a mitral valve replacement series (2), with life table data by age group, sex and duration. The q' values derived for the table correspond closely to annual q' values in the 1979-81 U.S. Life Tables for the total population, starting at tabular age 57.

TABLE 369K1-3

MORTALITY IN PATIENTS WITH MITRAL VALVE REPAIR (HOSPITAL DEATHS EXCLUDED),
APPROXIMATE ESTIMATES BY ASSOCIATED CARDIAC SURGERY

Associated Cardiac Surgery* MVR=Mitral Valve Repair	Hosp. Dis. to Durt.	Age Diff.[†]	No. Alive at Start	Survival Rates		Mean Ann. Mort. Rate per 1000			Mortality Ratio
				From OP	From Hosp. Dis.	Observed**	Est. Exp.[††]	Excess	
	Yrs.	ΔX	ℓ	P	$Pi=P/p_o$	$\check{q}$	$\check{q}'$	$\check{q}-\check{q}'$	$100(\check{q}/\check{q}')$
Isolated MVR±TVA	5	−1	83	0.84	0.870	28	12	14	235%
MVR+CBPS	5	+4	56	0.66	0.742	59	17	42	350
MVR+AV Repl.	5	+1	28	0.55	0.609	96	14	82	685
MVR+Cong. Defect	3	−7	26	0.81	0.841	57	6	51	950
MVR+Miscell.	5	0	3	1.00	1.000	(0)	13	(−13)	(0)
All MVR Patients	5	0	196	0.738	0.791	46	13	33	355

* See categories in Table 369K1-1.
[†] Difference assumed on basis of other series (2). See text.
** Derived from geometric mean of interval survival rate, P.
[††] Adjusted from $\check{q}'$ for total series according to assumed age difference.

MORTALITY ASSOCIATED WITH
CHRONIC OBSTRUCTIVE PULMONARY DISEASE

Roger H. Butz, M.D.

References:

1. B. Burrows, et al., "The Course and Prognosis of Different Forms of Chronic Airways Obstruction in a Sample from the General Population," *N. Engl. J. Med.*, 317 (1987): 1309-14.

2. B. Burrows, Personal letter (1988).

Subjects Studied: Randomly selected households from 1970 census data in Tucson, Arizona were invited to participate in a "health study." Participants were limited to white, non-Mexican households. Some 3,500 subjects were enrolled while 18% refused. Among the subjects tested 207 persons showed a forced expiratory volume during the first second of less than 65% of predicted value on spirometric test (a rate of 5.9%). Because the study was to determine the results of obstructive airways disease, 12 were excluded because they had a history of prior lung resection or thoracoplasty, and 9 subjects because they were considered to have a restrictive rather than obstructive ventilatory impairment. An additional 17 subjects were excluded when their first follow-up spirometry showed an FEV (1.0) of more than 70% of the predicted volume. Another 49 subjects were under 40 years of age or over 74 years, and these were excluded.

The remaining 120 subjects, age 40-74, were divided into three groups, Group I being the 27 subjects considered to have features most characteristic of "chronic asthmatic bronchitis." They all reported a diagnosis of asthma, and all of them had either never smoked cigarettes *or* had clear evidence of atopy by positive allergy skin test. Group III consisted of the 45 subjects who reported never having had asthma *and* who had smoking histories *and* had negative allergy skin tests. Of those remaining, 45 were assigned to Group II which consisted of individuals not clearly matching either Group I or Group III. Three subjects could not be classified and were then excluded from the study. Characteristics of the groups upon enrollment were as shown in Table 466K1-1.

Source: R. H. Butz, "Mortality Associated with Chronic Obstructive Pulmonary Disease," *J. Ins. Med.*, 20, no. 4 (1988): 46-47. Reproduced with permission of author and publisher.

Follow-up: Observation was continued for a 10-year period to determine rate of progression of obstruction to airways and associated mortality. Some 49 deaths occurred during the 10 years (including one in the three unclassified subjects), and 8 subjects were lost to follow-up

Results: Comparative mortality was derived using 1975-79 Group Life Tables to determine age and sex-specific expected mortality rates using age and sex data by group, which were obtained from the author. It is assumed that the subjects agreeing to participate in the health study would have self-selected against that portion of the population already seriously ill or debilitated, thus having more similarity to a mortality expectation showing the "healthy worker" effect, i.e. group life tables rather than population based tables.

Calculation of the years of exposure involved the assumption that losses due to death and loss to follow-up were evenly distributed over the 10-year period. That assumption is borne out in general terms by the data in Table 466K1-2, although losses are not group-specific.

The findings (Table 466K1-3) demonstrate favorable overall mortality in Group I. Though similar in age and severity at enrollment, the other two groups show significant extra mortality. Both Group II and III are over half male while Group I is over 2/3 female. In addition to the differences in rates of atopic skin reactions, Groups II and III both had about half current smokers. Any association between the deaths and current smoking status is not stated. It is clear that the mortality rates in Groups II and III exceed the mortality expected among a group containing about 50% smokers.

The authors were able to obtain death certificates for 23 of the 24 who died from Group III. In 12 (52%) the primary cause of death listed was a respiratory disease. In another 6 (26%) airways obstruction was listed on the death certificate as a contributing cause. Among the 5 whose death certificates omitted any reference to respiratory disease, 2 were attributed to cerebrovascular accidents and 1 each to arteriosclerotic heart disease, carcinoma of the lung and carcinoma of the colon. In contrast, the 4 deaths in Group I were ascribed to myocardial infarction (2 cases), cerebrovascular accident and carcinoma of the lung.

Comment: It may be concluded that the presence of abnormal airways function due to an allergic state and in the absence of a smoking history was nearly insignificant as a cause of mortality in this group of subjects. Future mortality studies of insured lives should stratify by smoking history among those with evidence of obstructive airways disease.

TABLE 466K1-1

ENROLLMENT CHARACTERISTICS

	Group I	Group II	Group III
Number of Subjects	27	45	45
Mean Age	62±9	63±8	65±7
Males	8	26	29
Mean FEV (1.0)	51%	47%	47%
Allergy by Skin Test	68%	38%	0
Never Smoked	56%	13%	0
Current Smokers	7%	49%	51%
Serum IgE 100 I.U. +	36%	22%	5%
Eosinophile Ct. 5% +	26%	7%	3%

TABLE 466K1-2

COMPARATIVE MORTALITY BY DURATION, ALL SUBJECTS COMBINED (INCLUDING THE THREE UNCLASSIFIED)

Interval	No. Alive at Start	Withdrawn or lost	Exposure Person-yrs.	Number of Deaths Observed	Number of Deaths Expected*	Mortality Ratio	Mean Annual Mort. Rate Observed	Mean Annual Mort. Rate Expected	Mean Annual Mort. Rate Excess
	ℓ	w	E	d	d'	100(d/d')	$\bar{q}$	$\bar{q}'$	1000($\bar{q}-\bar{q}'$)
0-1 yr.	120	0	120.0	3	2.16	139%	0.0250	0.0180	7
1-2	117	0	117.0	5	2.21	225	0.0427	0.0189	24
2-3	112	2	111.0	2	2.31	87	0.0180	0.0198	–2
3-4	108	3	106.5	5	2.22	225	0.0469	0.0208	26
4-5	100	0	100.0	4	2.19	183	0.0400	0.0219	18
5-6	96	2	95.0	8	2.18	365	0.0842	0.0230	61
6-7	86	1	85.5	5	2.06	245	0.0585	0.0241	34
7-8	80	0	80.0	6	2.03	295	0.0750	0.0253	50
8-9	74	0	74.0	4	1.97	205	0.0541	0.0266	27
9-10	70	0	70.0	7	1.95	360	0.1000	0.0279	72
0-10 yrs.	120	8	959.0	49	21.28	230	0.0511	0.0219	29

* Expected deaths based on 1975-79 Group Life Table Experience.

TABLE 466K1-3

COMPARATIVE MORTALITY BY GROUP AND DURATION

Group	Interval	No. Alive at start	Exposure Person-yrs.	Number of Deaths		Mortality Ratio	Mean Annual Mort. Rate		
				Observed	Expected*		Observed	Expected	Excess
		ℓ	E	d	d′	100(d/d′)	$\bar{q}$	$\bar{q}'$	1000($\bar{q}$–$\bar{q}'$)
I	0-5 yrs.	27	129.5	2	1.94	103%	0.0154	0.0150	0
	5-10	24	117.0	2	2.25	89	0.0171	0.0192	−2
	0-10	27	246.5	4	4.19	96	0.0162	0.0177	−1
II	0-5 yrs.	45	209.0	6	4.08	147	0.0287	0.0195	9
	5-10	37	147.0	14	3.68	380	0.0952	0.0250	70
	0-10	45	356.0	20	7.76	260	0.0562	0.0229	33
III	0-5 yrs.	45	204.0	10	4.69	215	0.0490	0.0230	26
	5-10	33	130.5	14	3.85	365	0.1073	0.0295	67
	0-10	45	334.5	24	8.54	280	0.0718	0.0255	46

* Expected deaths based on 1975-99 Group Life Table Experience.

244

CYSTIC FIBROSIS MORTALITY

Roger H. Butz, M.D.

Cystic Fibrosis (CF) is an autosomal recessive genetic defect. The defect is carried by one in every twenty persons and the chances are one in four that a child of two persons who are carriers will have CF. The general location of the CF gene has been located and research continues to determine the exact location and nature of the problem. CF is the number one genetic disease causing disability and death in America, so the research effort is significant.

Cystic Fibrosis causes mucous glands to produce a thick, sticky mucus which clogs airways and pancreatic ducts. Digestive problems include a neonatal intestinal obstruction, meconium ileus, seen in 10% of all CF babies. Malabsorption and malnutrition from inadequate digestion of fats and proteins are also very common. The most serious problem is the recurrence of bronchial infections. Serious infections, often with Pseudomonas, can lead to death or to cumulative pulmonary damage and eventual respiratory failure.

Signs of CF are quite typical, but a definitive sweat test showing four of five times the normal salt content establishes the diagnosis. The link between the thick mucus and the defective transport of salt appears to be in the control of the viscosity of mucus by the swelling of the polymer gel network depending upon the salinity of the water in the airways.

During the past two decades the life expectancy of CF patients has nearly doubled. Now, more than half of patients will reach 25 years of age, an improvement of over five years in average survival during the past 10 years. Mortality is highest among females, and Table 563K1-1 details the results of a 10-year follow-up from about 14,000 patients followed at the 120 affiliated CF centers around the United States. This information is collected by the Cystic Fibrosis Foundation which maintains current year follow-up data for the preceding decade. Table 563K1-2 shows the outlook for males, which is somewhat better at every age. Obviously, mortality far exceeds insurable levels and tends to increase with advancing years, evidencing the cumulative damage occurring with the repeated respiratory infections and other complications.

The male/female difference in cumulative survival is depicted in Figure 563K1-1. Differences in excess death rates appear in Figure 563K1-2. These figures also graphically display the age-related growing rate of excess deaths for CF patients. In Figure 563K1-3, the annual mortality rate is plotted against age and demonstrates a nearly linear relationship. The graph simply shows an averaging of the quartile mortality rates, but actual calculation of a correlation coefficient demonstrates an r value of 0.876, a very linear relationship. The slope of the line relates to

Source: R. H. Butz, "Cystic Fibrosis Mortality," *J. Ins. Med.*, 20, no. 1 (1988): 14-15. Reproduced with permission of author and publisher.

TABLE 563K1-1

CYSTIC FIBROSIS IN FEMALES, 10-YEAR FOLLOW-UP 1976-85

Ages	E	d	d'	Mortality Ratio	Avg. Ann. Mortality Rate	Est. 10 Yr. Surv. Rate	EDR
1-4	1,145.5	10	0.55	1,800%	0.0087	0.916	8.3
5-9	1,355.8	23	0.32	7,200	0.0170	0.842	16.7
10-14	1,039.8	31	0.24	12,900	0.0298	0.739	29.6
15-19	828.1	40	0.38	10,500	0.0483	0.610	47.9
20-24	582.1	26	0.32	8,100	0.0447	0.633	44.1
25-29	304.0	22	0.18	12,200	0.0724	0.472	71.8
30+	233.9	14	—	—	—	—	—

E = Exposure in person-years
d = Actual deaths
d' = Expected deaths estimated from U.S. population mortality rates.
EDR = Excess death rate per 1000 per year.

an approximate annual *increase* in mortality rate of 0.2%, or a 2% increase in *annual* mortality rate each passing decade.

Temporal improvement in overall mortality is apparent on Figure 563K1-4. This compares cumulative survival for 1985 with the combined experience of the preceding decade.

The proportionate improvement is rather dramatic but still represents only the modest results of more effective antibiosis, pulmonary toilet, and nutrition, and does not represent a major breakthrough in the care of CF patients. This distressing problem awaits a major advance before individual, voluntary insurance can reasonably be underwritten for CF patients.

TABLE 563K1-2

CYSTIC FIBROSIS IN MALES, 10-YEAR FOLLOW-UP 1976-85

Ages	E	d	d'	Mortality Ratio	Avg. Ann. Mortality Rate	Est. 10 Yr. Surv. Rate	EDR
1-4	1,186.2	7	0.73	950%	0.0059	0.943	5.3
5-9	1,452.6	15	0.46	3,250	0.0103	0.902	10.0
10-14	1,194.4	23	0.42	5,500	0.0193	0.823	18.9
15-19	1,017.1	32	1.26	2,550	0.0315	0.726	30.2
20-24	703.5	32	1.22	2,600	0.0445	0.628	37.3
25-29	446.1	27	0.76	3,550	0.0605	0.536	58.8
30+	372.7	25	—	—	—	—	—

See footnotes to Table 563K1-1.

FIGURE 563K1-1

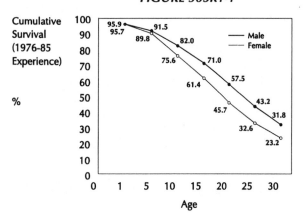

FIGURE 563K1-3

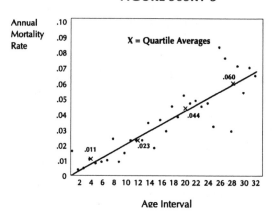

FIGURE 563K1-2

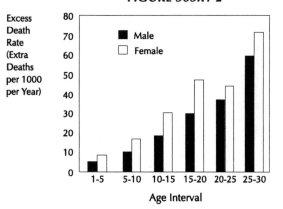

FIGURE 563K1-4

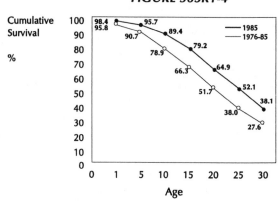

Morbidity Article 609K1

UPDATE — URINE HIV STATISTICS

Robert L. Stout, Ph.D.

Abstract

The introduction of any new test is followed by a period of assessment to determine if the method meets its initial claims. The claims about a new test normally related both to scientific validity, i.e., specificity, sensitivity, and to marketing — does the test provide a solution for a perceived problem? Urine-HIV testing was formally introduced with testing for Security Life of Denver in June 1989. Since that time, over 150,000 urine-HIV specimens have been tested at CRL. The prevalence of HIV positives in urine specimens is 60% higher than in serum (urine 0.1367% vs. serum 0.085%) for the insurance buying population. All urine positive applicants are requested to provide sera for confirmation testing. Ninety-seven (97%) percent of sera specimens submitted are positive by the standard double ELISA-Western Blot criteria.

Sensitivity of InsurScreen™

The sensitivity of the assay has been improved since its initial introduction. The sensitivity reported in the September, 1989 issue of this journal was 98.6%; currently it is 99.1%. During the last two years when an applicant was determined to be serum positive, the companion urine was tested for the presence of anti-HIV antibodies. A total of three hundred twenty-four samples have been tested with three hundred twenty-one found positive with urine (321/324=99.1%).

Specificity of InsurScreen™

The specificity of an assay is determined by the assay's ability to correctly identify negative specimens. In a population of 103,000 urine-HIV assays performed from January - August 1990, 102,860 were negative. Of the 140 initially reactive urine specimens, two (2) sera on subsequent testing were not positive; one (1) indeterminate, one negative. Therefore, the specificity of the assay is

$$\frac{103,000 - 140 = 102,860}{\text{negative urines}} \qquad \frac{102,860}{102,860 + 2} = 99.998\%$$

Source: R. L. Stout, "Update — Urine HIV Statistics," *J. Ins. Med.*, 22 (1990): 302-3. Reproduced with permission of author and publisher.

InsurScreen™

The following is a summary of urine and serum results on specimens tested for the insurance industry. This data show a 60% increase in urine reactive samples compared to sera. The data presented were acquired from January - August, 1990

Serum vs. Urine HIV

Population Statistics for HIV Infection in the Insurance Applicant Population for Serum and Urine Testing

	Number Tested	Positive	% Reactive
Serum	179,901	153	0.085
Urine	103,000	140	0.136

Nationwide the ratio of urine reactives to serum reactives is 160%. This represents the excess anti-selective pressure that is being applied against insurance companies. Recall that urine-HIV testing is done mainly in lower dollar policy applications. Serum results are mainly for application policy amounts in excess of $200,000.

Confirmation

Confirmation of InsurScreen™ Reactive Specimens by Serum Retest

	Number Tested	Positive	Indeterminate	Negative
Serum	68	66	1	1

InsurScreen™ is a screening assay to determine if follow-up testing is necessary. Thus, a serum sample is requested on all repeatedly reactive InsurScreen™ specimens. A total of 140 urines were reported as reactive to insurance companies' Medical Directors. Of the 140 reactive applicants, 68 (48.6%) have complied with the request to submit a blood sample for testing. Of the 68 sera retested, 66 (97%) were positive; 1 (1.5%) was indeterminate; and 1 (1.5%) was negative. There is frequently a long delay between the request for a serum sample and the time when the applicant consents to the request. The longest to date is 120 days. It was pointed out to me by Curtis Lashley, M.D., Jefferson Pilot, that agents may in many of these cases simply submit an application to another insurance company and hope for underwriting review before the initial MIB Code is reported on the first urine. This may create an additional anti-selective pressure on companies not testing in these lower policy amounts.

During the ongoing analysis of data comparing urine and serum reactive samples, it was noted that there was a disproportionate number of positive urines compared to sera. This may suggest anti-selective pressure being applied in the policy dollar amounts. The following data are an example of these findings.

High Risk States

InsurScreen™ Results by State for New York & California Applicants

	#Performed	Insurscreen Positive	Companion Serum Recorded	Companion Serum HIV Positive
CA	19,700	36 (0.183%)	16	15 (93.8%)
NY	5,133	16 (0.313%)	5	5 (100%)

The percent positive serum HIV found in California and New York are 0.111% and 0.126%, respectively. A serum is considered HIV positive only when it has passed through the HIV Testing Algorithm with a positive Western Blot. The higher incidence of positives found in urine vs. serum suggests anti-selection — applicants requesting lower dollar amount policies to bypass serum HIV testing. The following table indicates the degree of anti-selection taking place.

Anti-Selection

	State of CA	State of NY
Serum % Positive	0.111	0.126
Urine % Positive	0.183	0.312
Urine/Serum	0.183/0.111=165%	0.312/0.126=248%

The data summarized above provide the scientific verification for sensitivity (99.1%) and specificity (99.998%). While these criteria are important in the determination of reliability of an assay, they convey no information about acceptance in the market. The assay was originally conceived to simplify the testing of insurance applicants. It has proved to be a very favorable option with the broker and agent. The favorable response by the field force was described by Paula Romano, Director of Underwriting of The Prudential during her presentation at the IHOU Annual Meeting in Washington, DC in October 1990.

The Future

The testing of alternate samples, both urine and saliva, for the presence of antibodies to HIV will increasingly become the preferred assay for insurance risk assessment. It will allow insurance companies to test applicants at lower policy amounts providing greater protection to the insurer and its policy holders.

REFERENCES

1. D. M. Archibald, L. Zon, J. E. Groopman, M. F. McLane, M. Essex, "Antibodies to Human T-Lymphotrophic Virus Type III (HTLV-III) in Saliva of Acquired Immune Deficiency Syndrome (AIDS) Patients and in Persons at Risk for AIDS," *Blood,* 67 (1986): 831-34.

2. Y. Z. Cao, A. E. Friedman-Kien, J. Chuba, M. Mirabile, B. Hosein, "IgG Antibodies to Human Immunodeficiency Virus Type 1 (HIV-1) in the Urine of HIV-1 Seropositive Individuals (letter)," *Lancet,* 2 (1988): 869-70.

3. Y. Z. Cao, B. Hosein, W. Borkowsky, M. Mirabile, L. Baker, D. Baldwin, B. Poiesz, A. E. Friedman-Kien, "Antibodies to Human Immunodeficiency Virus Type 1 in the Urine Specimens of HIV-1 Seropositive Individuals," *AIDS Res. Hum. Retroviruses,* 5 (1989): 311-19.

4. L. Posnick, "HIV Urine Testing Eyed," *CCN,* 16 (1990): 1-6.

5. P. Skolnik, B. Kosloff, L. Bechtel, K. Huskins, T. Flynn, N. Karthas, K. McIntosh, M. Hirsch, "Absence of Infectious HIV-1 in the Urine of Seropositive Viremic Subjects," *J. Infect. Dis.,* 160 (1989): 1056-60.

CHILDREN WITH EXSTROPHY OF THE BLADDER

Richard B. Singer, M.D.

Reference:

M. T. Macfarlane, J. K. Lattimer, T. W. Hensle, "Improved Life Expectancy for Children with Exstrophy of the Bladder," *JAMA*, 242 (1979): 442-44.

Subjects Studied: The series consists of 163 patients with classical exstrophy of the bladder treated on the Pediatric Urological Service of the Babies Hospital, Columbia-Presbyterian Medical Center, New York. Infants with bladder exstrophy complicated by multiple serious congenital defects were excluded; death in such cases ordinarily occurred early in life. More cases were referred than diagnosed initially at Babies Hospital, and some had been treated medically for a period of months or years prior to referral. No age or sex distribution is given. No calendar period of operation is given. Earlier operations were uterosigmoidostomy, but for the past 20 years primary closure was the major type of surgery, with only 12 patients treated by primary conduit diversion.

Follow-up: Methods used are not given. Survival was calculated from birth "regardless of the age at which the patient entered into follow-up study at our institution." Out of 150 patients born at least 10 years prior to the end of follow-up 73% were traced; 63% of 88 patients with 20 or more years of potential follow-up were traced, and 53% of 32 patients with 30 years or more.

Results: In the derivation of expected survival and mortality for this abstract it has been assumed that follow-up begins at age 4 weeks instead of birth. This does not eliminate all retrospective "exposure," which should be eliminated completely because of the bias introduced by its use. However, it does eliminate that part of the first year of life which contributes most heavily to expected mortality. Observed data and derivation of expected deaths are shown in Table 611K1-1, and comparative mortality and survival in Table 611K1-2. Over half of the total exposure and three of six observed deaths were concentrated within the first ten years of life. The mortality ratio was only 146% because of the high expected mortality in the first year, even with the first four weeks excluded (compare q' values for the different attained age intervals). The mortality ratio was 410% in the second decade and 235% thereafter. The highest EDR was only 2.0 per 1000 per year in the second decade. With only 6 total deaths the overall excess mortality above the 2.98 expected deaths was significant at the 91% level but not the 95% level (single-tailed test *p*=0.09 by the Poisson distribution).

Comment: The authors cite two early reports from the Mayo Clinic on survival in patients with operation for bladder exstrophy and comment: "In 1925 the majority died. In 1978 practically all lived." These references and the quoted 20-year survival rates are shown in Table 611K1-3, together with the 20-year survival rate from Table 611K1-2. In an effort to provide comparative mortality data over a wide range of time, about 1910 to 1978, I have used two sets of U.S. Life Tables for each of the Mayo Clinic reports and calculated geometric mean annual survival rates and q̆ and q̆'. As above, deaths in the first 4 weeks of life have been excluded and equal numbers of male and female patients have been assumed. Because of the marked decrease in q̆' from the 1909-11 tables to the 1959-61, mortality ratios have not been calculated. The low survival rate in the earliest (1926) report is associated with an EDR of 42-43 per 1000 per year, and the somewhat better survival in the 1951 report with an EDR of 27-30 per 1000. On this geometric mean method the corresponding EDR of the Columbia-Presbyterian series is only 1.0 per 1000 per year. Although bladder exstrophy is very rarely encountered in underwriting I felt this limited experience was worth abstracting, because it contradicts the opinion I held until recently that mortality was still high enough to make declination necessary in all such applicants. On the basis of this 1979 report properly treated and managed cases of bladder exstrophy certainly appear to be acceptable on a rated basis.

Source: R. B. Singer, "Children with Exstrophy of the Bladder," *J. Ins. Med.*, 11, no. 1 (1980): 1-2. Reproduced with permission of author and publisher.

TABLE 611K1-1

OBSERVED DATA AND EXPECTED DEATHS IN CHILDREN WITH EXSTROPHY OF THE BLADDER

Attained Age Interval	No. Alive at Start	No. During Interval		No. Exposed to Risk		Expected Deaths	
		Last Seen Alive	Deaths	Start of Int.	Pt.-yrs.	Ave. Ann. Rate	No.
x to x+Δx	ℓ_x	w	d	E*=ℓ-w/ℓ	E[†]	q'**	d'=(E)(q')
1 mo.-5 yrs.*	163	25	3	150.5	733	0.00234	1.72
5-10 yrs.	135	27	0	121.5	608	0.00056	0.34
1 mo.-10 yrs.	163	52	3	—	1,341		2.06
10-15 yrs.	108	25	2	95.5	472	0.00044	0.21
15-20	81	38	0	62.0	310	0.00091	0.28
10-20	108	63	2	—	782		0.49
20-25 yrs.	43	18	0	34.0	170	0.00125	0.21
25-30	25	9	1	20.5	98	0.00129	0.13
30-35	15	8	0	11.0	55	0.00162	0.09
20-35	43	35	1	—	323		0.43

* Arbitrary assumption of age 4 weeks at start of "observation" instead of birth because many cases were first seen after age 2, involving retrospective "exposure," and cases with severe multiple congenital anomalies were excluded.

† Exposure, E, in patient-years estimated as [ℓ–(w+d)/2][Δt]. Distribution of deaths and withdrawals from observation within 5-year interval not given.

** Basis of expected mortality: U.S. Life Tables 1959-61 (total population).

TABLE 611K1-2

COMPARATIVE MORTALITY AND SURVIVAL EXPERIENCE

Attained Age Interval	Exposure Pt.-years	No. of Deaths	Ave. Ann. Mort. Rate		Mortality Ratio	Excess Death Rate	Cumulative Survival Rate		
			Observed	Expected*			Observed	Expected	Relative
x to x+Δx	E	d	$\bar{q}$	$\bar{q}'$	100(d/d')	1000($\bar{q}$–$\bar{q}'$)	P	P'	100(P/P')
1 mo.-10 yrs.	1,341	3	0.0022	0.0015	146%	0.7	0.9801	0.9862	99.4%
10-20 yrs.	782	2	0.0026	0.0006	410	2.0	0.9596	0.9795	98.0
20-35	323	1	0.0031	0.0013	235	1.8	0.9128	0.9594	95.1
All	2,446	6	0.0025	0.0012	200	1.3	0.9128	0.9594	95.1

* Basis of expected mortality: U.S. Life Tables 1959-61 (total population).

TABLE 611K1-3

TREND IN 20-YEAR SURVIVAL, CHILDREN WITH EXSTROPHY OF THE BLADDER, MAYO CLINIC COMPARATIVE MORTALITY VS. COLUMBIA-PRESBYTERIAN HOSPITAL (ABOVE)

Report (Date)	20-Year Survival*	Geom. Mean Ann. Rate		U.S. Life Tables[†]	Survival*	Geom. Mean Ann. Rate		Excess Death Rate
		Survival	Mortality			Survival	Mortality	
	P	$\check{p}$=$^{\Delta t}\sqrt{P}$	$\check{q}$=1–$\check{p}$		P'	$\check{p}'$=$^{\Delta t}\sqrt{P'}$	$\check{q}'$=1–$\check{p}'$	1000($\check{q}$–$\check{q}'$)
1. Mayo Clinic (1926)	0.33	0.950	0.050	White 1909-11	0.8453	0.9916	0.0084	42
				White 1919-21	0.8712	0.9931	0.0069	43
2. Mayo Clinic (1951)	0.52	0.968	0.032	White 1929-31	0.9122	0.9954	0.0046	27
				White 1939-41	0.9609	0.9980	0.0020	30
3. Columbia-Presb. (1979)	0.960	0.998	0.002	Total 1959-61	0.9795	0.9990	0.0010	1.0

* Excluding first month of life.

† 50% Male and 50% Female, White rates for Mayo, total population for Columbia-Presbyterian.

1. C. H. Mayo, W. A. Hendricks, *Surg. Gynecol. Obstet.*, 93 (1926): 129-33.

2. B. M. Harvard, G. J. Thompson, *J. Urol.*, 65 (1951): 223-34.

MORTALITY ASSOCIATED WITH POLYCYSTIC KIDNEY DISEASE

Ole Zeuthen Dalgaard, M.D.

Introduction

Autosomal dominant polycystic kidney disease (ADPKD, McKusick's catalog number 17390, 1986[1]) is one of the commonest monogenetic disorders, with an estimated frequency of about 1 in 1,000, essentially complete penetrance, but variable clinical presentation with onset at an average age of about 40 years.[2,3]

Source: O. Z. Dalgaard, "Mortality Associated with Polycystic Kidney Disease," *J. Ins. Med.*, 21 (1989): 263-66. Reproduced with permission of author and publisher.

The pathogenetic processes involved in the progressive development of renal cysts, leading to terminal uremia, are still unknown.

As for the general symptomatology, progressive clinical development, and age of diagnosis they have not changed significantly during the last 30 years (Tables 621K1-1 and 621K1-2).

In 60% of Dalgaard's 350 cases (1957) the clinical diagnosis had still not been made at the age of 45 years.[2] Bear et al. (1984) report similarly.[4]

TABLE 621K1-1

NUMBER OF INDIVIDUALS WITH POLCYSTIC KIDNEYS IN DIFFERENT AGE GROUPS, WHEN WARNING WAS GIVEN OF THE MALFORMATIONS FOR THE FIRST TIME BY ONE OR MORE OF THE VARIOUS SYMPTOMS (FROM DALGAARD 1957[2]).

Age	Pain and abdominal symptoms	Kidney Colic passage of calculi	Protein-uria	Hema-turia	Pyuria and bacteriuria	Kidney-tumour	Cardio-vascular symptoms hypertension	Uremia symptoms	Renal insuffi-ciency
5-9	1	—	—	—	—	—	—	—	—
10-14	—	—	2	1	—	—	—	—	—
15-19	6	2	3	—	4	1	—	—	—
20-24	9	6	4	5	4	2	1	—	—
25-29	13	6	10	6	10	3	2	—	—
30-34	15	10	10	15	7	5	3	—	—
35-39	18	8	6	11	10	7	5	2	—
40-44	23	4	7	13	5	6	8	2	—
45-49	16	3	5	10	5	3	4	6	1
50-54	18	5	5	12	3	5	9	2	—
55-59	6	1	4	3	1	1	8	5	2
60-64	3	—	1	3	1	1	5	1	—
65-69	1	—	1	—	—	—	3	1	—
70-74	2	—	1	1	—	—	5	1	1
75-79	1	—	—	—	—	—	1	1	—
Women	88	21	34	33	44	25	26	13	1
Men	44	24	25	47	6	9	28	8	3
Totals	132	45	59	80	50	34	54	21	4

PROBABILITY OF CLINICAL DIAGNOSIS OF ADULT POLYCYSTIC KIDNEY DISEASE

Age	Dalgaard 1957[2] %	Bear et al. 1984[4] %
25	5	3.8
35	17	16.4
45	40	41.0
55	70	69.4

However, the prognosis and life expectancy of affected individuals have improved due to the progress in the treatment of complications such as urinary tract infections and calculi, hypertension and cardiac insufficiency, let alone the development of hemodialysis and kidney transplantation. ADPKD currently accounts for 10% of kidney transplantations in Denmark. Furthermore, the development of ultrasonography has made early presymptomatic diagnosis possible, and recent advances in molecular biology now allow a still earlier evaluation of carrier status by DNA analysis. For embryos with ADPKD-gene prenatal diagnosis of ADPKD can be made in 95% of the cases.[5]

Gene Localization

The gene for ADPKD (locus-symbol PKD1) has recently been assigned to the short arm of chromosome 16, by demonstration of linkage to the TK-globin gene cluster, in a genetic distance of about 5 centimorgan.[6,7] This was accomplished by use of the highly polymorphic DNA marker 3' HVR.[8,9]

Subjects Studied

Some 242 adults with bilateral polycystic disease of the kidneys were ascertained from the hospitals of Greater Copenhagen during the period 1920-53.

For the deceased the death certificates and possible hospital records were traced.

The author examined the living and all their closer living family members in Denmark including clinical history, physical examination, blood pressure, urine examination, kidney function test and intravenous urography.

The total material comprises a clinical analysis of the course of the disease in 350 certain cases of ADPKD, 157 men and 193 women.

Table 621K1-1 shows the ages at which ADPKD was first manifest by one or more of the various symptoms, which seldom appear during the first two decades.

The mean age at onset of the disease established by one or more symptoms was 40.7 years, 41.6 years for males, 39.9 years for females, and varying from 8 to 77 years.

The mean age of the time of diagnosis was 47.2 years, one year earlier for the females than for the males and varying from 16 to 85 years.

In Bear et al. (1984)[4] the probability that cases with ADPKD has been diagnosed by the ages 25, 35, 45 and 55 years are nearly identical to my calculations of 1954 — 30 years earlier (Table 621K1-2).

Follow-up

At the time of follow-up 254 patients were deceased, the average age of death was 51.5 years, identical for males and females, in contrast to 71 years among the general Danish Population.

Some 59% died from uremia, 13% from cerebral hemorrhage, 6% from heart disease and 22% from other causes (Table 621K1-3).

In the case of the 96 living patients, 43 males and 53 females, the average age was 45.7 years and thus less than in the case of the deceased, due to the fact that almost a third were diagnosed by the author himself when they were at a young age, with limited exposure for risk of death up to 1953, the end of follow-up.

Results

At the suggestion of Richard B. Singer, M.D., all the 350 patients were considered as a cohort with mortality and survival by annual periods of attained age. With the retrospective exposure (Table 621K1-4) all the patients were age 20 at the time of entry into the life table as there were no deaths observed under that age.

The patients were separated into male and female cohorts.

Exposure was calculated in person-years from entry at age 20 until age of death for the 254 fatal cases or the age of follow-up for the 96 survivors.

Comparative mortality was derived from 1951-55 Mortality Table for the Danish Population, with calculation of d' as the product of E and age/sex-specific values of q'.

Mortality experience is extremely high, mortality ratios averaging 600% in that of the Danish Population for ages 30-39 years rising to more than 900% for ages 40-59 years, but diminishing to 350% for ages over 60 years. The higher mortality ratios in females are attributable to lower q' rates rather than higher observed q values.

A mortality ratio (MR) of 350% at ages 60 up is extremely high in terms of excess death rate (EDR).

Excess deaths per 1000 (EDR) for males are quite low under age 35, however increase from 16 for ages 35-39 to about 60 at ages 50 up.

TABLE 621K1-3

CAUSES OF DEATH IN RELATION TO AGE AT DEATH FOR 173 PATIENTS WITH POLYCYSTIC KIDNEYS (ONLY AUTOPSIES), DIVIDED INTO 10-YEAR GROUPS

Cause of Death	20-29	30-39	40-49	50-59	60-69	70-79	80-	in all	in all %
Uremia	1	10	33	37	18	4	1	104	60
Cerebral Hemorrhage	2	2	10	6	3	1		24	14
Heart death	0	1	1	4	1	2		9	5
Other causes	1	1	7	16	7	3	1	36	21
Totals	4	14	51	63	29	10	2	173	100

TABLE 621K1- 4

COMPARATIVE MORTALITY IN POLYCYSTIC KIDNEY DISEASE BY ATTAINED AGE 20 AND UP*

Attained Age	No. Alive at Age x[†]	Withdrawn Alive	Exposure Patient-yrs.	Number of Deaths		Mortality Ratio	Mean Ann. Mort. Rate per 1000		
				Observed	Expected*		Observed	Expected	Excess
x to x+Δx	ℓ	w	E	d	d'	100(d/d')	q=d/E	q'	(q–q')
				MALE PATIENTS					
20-29	156	4	1,537.0	3	2.00	150%	2.0	1.3	0.7
30-39	149	12	1,408.0	13	2.37	550	9.2	1.7	7.5
40-49	124	14	1,009.0	36	3.73	965	36	3.7	32
50-59	74	6	519.0	39	5.09	765	75	9.8	65
60-69	29	6	183.0	15	4.43	340	82	24	58
70-83	8	1	55.5	7	3.61	194	126	65	61
20-83	156	43	4,711.5	113	21.23	530	24	4.5	20
				FEMALE PATIENTS					
20-29	193	2	1,920.0	3	1.35	220%	1.6	0.7	0.9
30-39	188	17	1,742.5	15	2.44	615	8.6	1.4	7.2
40-49	156	10	1,318.0	45	4.09	1,100	34	3.1	31
50-59	101	16	725.0	45	5.22	860	62	7.2	55
60-69	40	5	248.5	24	4.55	530	97	18	79
70-79	11	3	50.5	8	2.39	335	158	47	111
20-79	193	53	6,004.5	140	20.04	700	23	3.3	20

* Basis of expected deaths: 1951-55 Danish Life Tables.
[†] Retrospective exposure to age 20 assumed valid: excess mortality very small < age 35.

For females the excess deaths per 1000 continue to increase at ages 50 up, exceeding 100 in the oldest age group.

Comments

The use of retrospective exposure prior to diagnosis can be justified in an inherited disease that is progressive in severity (homochronous). The method has been used in some types of congenital heart disease (see Abstract #332 in *Medical Risks 1976*).

The combination of a rather late development of incapacitating clinical manifestations, and a dominant mode of inheritance, explains the frequent propagation of the disease for many generations of affected families. When, furthermore, the incidence of ADPKD is as high as about 1 in 1,000, there is a sizeable need for preventive measures, if possible, for those families who desire to have only unaffected children.

Early detection of asymptomatic carriers became possible with the development of urography, and especially ultrasonography which is a harmless, non-invasive and fast procedure with a high degree of sensitivity. By this analysis polycystic kidneys, and liver, can be visualized 10-15 years before the onset of clinical symptoms, ie., the diagnosis can be established in about 85% of the actual carriers at the age of 25 years.[4]

DNA markers analysis has greatly improved the early delineation of carriers and non-carriers among at-risk individuals, including the early fetus, and has thus become a valuable tool for the prevention of propagating ADPKD in affected families.[10,11]

The high mortality rate of ADPKD patients is reflected in the policies recommended for Life Insurance Companies (Brackenridge 1985[12]). Applicants with known polycystic kidney disease must be declined. For applicants with a family history of ADPKD it is suggested that the insurance company should as a rule only consider individuals who have reached the age of thirty or more. Applicants with a recent normal ultrasonography can be considered for life insurance at the age of 25 years, with a temporary extra premium ceasing at the age of 35. If reliable ultrasound scanning is normal at or above age 35 years, the individual can be insured at standard premium rates.

One has to realize that the recent development in predictive DNA analysis for ADPKD, and other genetic diseases manifesting in adulthood, is bound to have an impact on insurance strategies.[13]

Acknowledgment: Thanks to Richard B. Singer, M.D. for invaluable help and guidance.

REFERENCES

1. V. A. McKusick, *Mendelian Inheritance in Man: Catalogs of Autosomal Dominant, Autosomal Recessive, and X-Linked Phenotypes.* 7th Edit. (Baltimore, The Johns Hopkins University Press, 1986).

2. O. Z. Dalgaard, "Bilateral Polycystic Disease of the Kidneys: A Follow-up of Two Hundred and Eighty-Four Patients and their Families," *Acta Med. Scand.,* 158 suppl. 328 (1957): 1-255.

3. O. Z. Dalgaard, *Polycystic Disease of the Kidneys: In Disease of the Kidneys,* M. B. Strauss, L. G. West, eds. (Boston, Little, Brown & Co., 1963), pp. 1223-58.

4. J. C. Bear, et al., "Age at Clinical Onset and at Ultrasonographic Detection of Adult Polycystic Kidney Disease: Data for Genetic Counseling," *Am. J. Med. Genet.,* 18 (1984): 45-53.

5. M. H. Breuning, et al., "Improved Early Diagnosis of Adult Polycystic Kidney Disease With Flanking DNA Markers," *Lancet,* ii (1987): 1359-61.

6. S. T. Reeders, et al., "A Highly Polymorphic DNA Marker Linked to Adult Polycystic Kidney Disease on Chromosome 16," *Nature,* 317 (1985): 542-44.

7. S. T. Reeders, et al., "Two Genetic Markers Closely Linked to Adult Polycystic Kidney Disease on Chromosome 16," *Brit. Med. J.,* 292 (1986): 851-53.

8. D. R. Higgs, et al., "Analysis of the Human TK-Globin Gene Cluster Reveals a Highly Informative Genetic Locus," (1986).

9. A. P. Jarman, et al., "Molecular Characterization of a Hypervariable Region Downstream of the Human α-Globin Gene Cluster," *EMBO J.,* 5 (1986): 1857-63.

10. S. T. Reeders, et al., "Prenatal Diagnosis of Autosomal Dormant Polycystic Kidney Disease with a DNA Probe," *Lancet,* ii (1986): 6-8.

11. O. Z. Dalgaard, S. Norby, "Autosomal Dominant Polycystic Kidney Disease in the 1980's," Symposium 28-29 October 1988 on the occasion of the 50 years anniversary of the University Institute of Medical Genetics, Copenhagen. To be printed in the Symposium Proceedings *Clinical Genetics* (1989).

12. R. D. C. Brackenridge, *Medical Selection of Life Risks: A Comprehensive Guide to Life Expectancy for Underwriters & Clinicians,* 2nd Edit. (Bath, Macmillan Publishers Ltd., 1985).

13. W. H. Alexander, "Insurance and Genetics," *J. Ins. Med.,* 20 (1988): 35-41.

DIABETES MELLITUS IN EUROPEAN INSUREDS

Manfred Fessel

References:

1. M. Fessel, "Comparison Between the Mortality Expected and that Actually Experienced by Life Insurance Companies, for Selected Impairments," *Annals of Life Insurance Medicine 9* (Proceedings of the 16th International Congress of Life Assurance Medicine, The Hague 1989), (1990): 39-45.

2. M. Fessel, Unpublished exposures and other data furnished (1990).

Subjects Studied: European male policyholders reassured and followed up at Swiss Reinsurance Company in Zurich, Switzerland. The experience is reported for cases with diabetes mellitus coded as their main impairment; the coexistence of hypertension, over or underweight or any other secondary impairments was not excluded. The policyholders observed have been insured in the years from 1956 through 1985 and prior to the end of 1985 or to prior termination.

Follow-up: Reinsurance policy records formed the basis of entry, of counting policies, exposure and death claims, and of follow-up information.

Results: Comparative experience is given in Tables 701K1-1 to 701K1-5, using a modification of Swiss Re's internal European mortality table SR 73/77 as basis of expected mortality. It is important to note that SR 73/77 is an aggregate, not a select mortality table, when comparing Swiss Re's results with American insurance experience.

There were overall 1,290 entrants into this study (more exactly, policies issued on European male diabetics reassured with Swiss Re), showing a mortality ratio of 250% and an EDR of 7.4 per 1000. The average duration per policy observed was slightly more than seven years.

As can be seen from Table 701K1-1 (experience by rating at policy issue), the actual mortality corresponded well with that assessed for insureds rated 200% up, but was somewhat higher than expected for those underwritten at standard rates or with an extra mortality of up to 75%.

The experience by age at policy issue shows the same picture as known from other studies on insured diabetics, i.e. decreasing mortality ratios with increasing age (Table 701K1-2). The main reason for this finding is the higher percentage of type I diabetes with its more unfavourable prognosis in the younger age groups. It is nevertheless interesting to note that the absolute extra mortality, expressed by the EDRs, is increasing with higher ages at issue.

Table 701K1-3 gives the comparative experience by policy duration for all ages combined. The mortality ratios observed do not fluctuate much by duration and show a decreasing tendency for higher durations, going down from 290% to 215%, whereas the EDRs again increase (from 5.9 to 8.6 per 1000). Looking through a number of other studies on insured diabetics gives the impression that no clear tendency for the course of mortality ratios by duration is ascertained (see also Comment).

Also not in line with clinical thinking is Swiss Re's experience by duration of diabetes at issue, as shown in Table 701K1-4. The mortality ratios seem to be quite independent of the number of years the diabetes had been diagnosed before application. There is no doubt that the probability of life-reducing complications of diabetes is greater the longer the duration of the disease. But on the other hand, the worse risks are already eliminated by the insurability criteria in the selection of diabetics with a long history of illness; those remaining do not necessarily have a less favourable prognosis than the group of applicants with recently diagnosed diabetes. Again, these considerations have been confirmed by other studies on insured diabetics.

A very unfavourable prognostic factor in the event of diabetes is the coexistence of hypertension. As is shown in Table 701K1-5, the mortality ratio for diabetics with normal blood pressure (systolic = 142 mm. Hg. and diastolic = 92 mm. Hg.) was only 181% (with an EDR of 3.7 per 1000), whereas the mortality ratio of those with an increased systolic and diastolic pressure rose to 505% (EDR 24 per 1000). For diabetics with elevated systolic or diastolic pressures (but not both) the mortality ratio was 310% and the EDR 11 per 1000. We therefore note that the extra mortality for applicants presenting with diabetes

Source: M. Fessel, "Diabetes Mellitus in European Insureds," *J. Ins. Med.*, 22 (1990): 217-19. Reproduced with permission of author and publisher.

and hypertension exceeds by far the simple addition of the extra mortality of the two individual impairments.

Comment: It is tempting to compare the results of this study with those of the diabetic lives covered by the *Medical Impairment Study 1983* (MIS) (Volume I, p. 96-97, males — substandard lives). This comparison is particularly interesting in that both studies use diabetes mellitus (without further subdivision according to type) as their selection criterion, and because the two periods of observation are comparable. There are, however, some important differences between the two studies to be borne in mind:

• The exposure in the MIS for diabetics is more then ten times that of Swiss Re's with a correspondingly higher significance of the resulting mortality ratios.

• The coexistence of other rateable impairments has been excluded from MIS but allowed in Swiss Re's study, leading to higher mortality rates in the latter.

• On the other hand, using an aggregate mortality table as comparative mortality, as done by Swiss Re, produces lower mortality ratios than the select rates applied in American studies, especially for higher ages at entry.

Taking all this into account, the two studies show quite similar mortality ratios for the total experience (MIS 220%, Swiss Re 250%) as well as by ages at issue. The actual mortality in both studies corresponded well with that expected by the underwriters. There was, however, a striking difference between the two studies in their experience by policy duration: Whereas the European diabetics showed a tendency of decreasing mortality ratios by duration (see above), the ratios in the MIS increased sharply from 125% for policy years 1-2, up to nearly 300% for policy years 11 or more.

SWISS RE IMPAIRMENT STUDY 1989

TABLE 701K1-1

EUROPEAN MALE INSUREDS WITH DIABETES MELLITUS, 1956-85
COMPARATIVE EXPERIENCE BY RATING AT POLICY ISSUE

Rating	No. of Entrants	Exposure Policy-yrs.	Number of Claims		Mortality Ratio	Mean Ann. Mort. Rate per 1000		
			Observed	Expected*		Observed	Expected	Excess
	ℓ	E	d	d'	100(d/d')	$\bar{q}$	$\bar{q}'$	$(\bar{q}-\bar{q}')$
100-175%	348	2,605.0	32	17.71	181%	12.3	6.8	5.5
200-250	479	3,833.5	47	19.04	245	12.3	5.0	7.3
300 up	392	2,532.0	32	7.89	400	12.6	3.2	9.4
Other	71	276.0	3	0.86	350	10.9	3.1	7.8
Total	1,290	9,246.5	114	45.59	250	12.3	4.9	7.4

* Basis of expected claims: Swiss Re 1973-77 Aggregate Table, European Males, modified.

TABLE 701K1-2

EUROPEAN MALE INSUREDS WITH DIABETES MELLITUS, 1956-85
COMPARATIVE EXPERIENCE BY AGE AT POLICY ISSUE

Age at Issue	No. of Entrants	Exposure Policy-yrs.	Number of Claims		Mortality Ratio	Mean Ann. Mort. Rate per 1000		
			Observed	Expected*		Observed	Expected	Excess
	ℓ	E	d	d'	100(d/d')	$\bar{q}$	$\bar{q}'$	$(\bar{q}-\bar{q}')$
20-44	747	5,495.5	48	13.34	360%	8.7	2.4	6.3
45-54	395	2,826.5	43	18.99	225	15.2	6.7	8.5
55-84	148	924.5	23	13.25	174	25	14.3	11
Total	1,290	9,246.5	114	45.59	250	12.3	4.9	7.4

* Basis of expected claims: Swiss Re 1973-77 Aggregate Table, European Males, modified.

TABLE 701K1-3

EUROPEAN MALE INSUREDS WITH DIABETES MELLITUS, 1956-85
COMPARATIVE EXPERIENCE BY DURATION, ALL AGES COMBINED

| Duration Start-End | Exposure Policy-yrs. | Number of Claims | | Mortality Ratio | Mean Ann. Mort. Rate per 1000 | | |
| | | Observed | Expected* | | Observed | Expected | Excess |
t to t+Δt	E	d	d'	100(d/d')	$\bar{q}$	$\bar{q}'$	$(\bar{q}-\bar{q}')$
0-2 yrs.	1,782.5	16	5.55	290%	9.0	3.1	5.9
2-5	2,733.5	30	10.49	285	11.0	3.8	7.2
5-10	2,743.0	36	14.58	245	13.1	5.3	7.8
10-30	1,987.5	32	14.97	215	16.1	7.5	8.6
Total	9,246.5	114	45.59	250	12.3	4.9	7.4

* Basis of expected claims: Swiss Re 1973-77 Aggregate Table, European Males, modified.

TABLE 701K1-4

EUROPEAN MALE INSUREDS WITH DIABETES MELLITUS, 1956-85
COMPARATIVE EXPERIENCE BY DURATION OF DIABETES AT ISSUE

| Duration of Diabetes at Issue | No. of Entrants | Exposure Policy-yrs. | Number of Claims | | Mortality Ratio | Mean Ann. Mort. Rate per 1000 | | |
| | | | Observed | Expected* | | Observed | Expected | Excess |
	ℓ	E	d	d'	100(d/d')	$\bar{q}$	$\bar{q}'$	$(\bar{q}-\bar{q}')$
0-5 yrs.	836	6,167.5	77	32.14	240%	12.5	5.2	7.3
5-10	170	1,249.5	15	6.38	235	12.0	5.1	6.9
10 up	217	1,394.5	14	5.19	270	10.0	3.7	6.3
Unknown	67	435.0	8	1.88	425	18.4	4.3	14
Total	1,290	9,246.5	114	45.59	250	12.3	4.9	7.4

* Basis of expected claims: Swiss Re 1973-77 Aggregate Table, European Males, modified.

TABLE 701K1-5

EUROPEAN MALE INSUREDS WITH DIABETES MELLITUS, 1956-85
COMPARATIVE EXPERIENCE BY BLOOD PRESSURE READINGS

| Blood Pressure (mm. Hg.) Syst. Diast. | No. of Entrants | Exposure Policy-yrs. | Number of Claims | | Mortality Ratio | Mean Ann. Mort. Rate per 1000 | | |
| | | | Observed | Expected* | | Observed | Expected | Excess |
	ℓ	E	d	d'	100(d/d')	$\bar{q}$	$\bar{q}'$	$(\bar{q}-\bar{q}')$
≤142 ≤92	804	5,748.5	47	25.99	181%	8.2	4.5	3.7
≥143 ≥93	97	561.0	17	3.36	505	30	6.0	24
Other	389	2,937.0	50	16.24	310	17.0	5.5	11
Total	1,290	9,246.5	114	45.59	250	12.3	4.9	7.4

* Basis of expected claims: Swiss Re 1973-77 Aggregate Table, European Males, modified.

IDIOPATHIC HEMOCHROMATOSIS: AN ASSESSMENT OF MORTALITY

John R. Iacovino, M.D.

The purpose of this paper is to assist the medical director and underwriter in the mortality assessment of Idiopathic Hemochromatosis (IH). Although a relatively rare disorder with a frequency of 1:10,000 in the United States, we will undoubtedly be requested to underwrite more cases with the advent of multiphasic screening. We must be knowledgeable in underwriting both those with established disease as well as those diagnosed on screening in an asymptomatic state. Finally, those applicants with a family history may have to be considered for insurability.

Hereditary transmission of IH is by an autosomal recessive gene.[1] Partial biochemical expression has been noted in heterozygotes whose gene frequency is 1:50 in the United States.[1] Fifty percent of siblings of a source case can have hypersideremia and thus are at risk for development of IH.[1] Disease susceptibility is linked to the major histocompatibility complex HLA (A3, B14) on the sixth chromosome; however, cases of an absent or variable HLA linkage have been described.[1] Alcohol can affect development and progression by both accelerating iron absorption from the gastrointestinal tract and a synergistic fibrogenic effect with iron.[1,2]

Laboratory diagnosis of IH can be difficult. Serum iron levels with a sensitivity of 68 percent and a positive predictive value of 61 percent are unreliable for screening probands as well as the detection of early stages of the disease. The serum ferritin and transferrin saturation have higher degrees of predictability, with the sensitivity and specificity being 85%-95% and 82%-88% respectively. The combination of ferritin and transferrin saturation is recommended for screening with a positive predictive value of 94%.[3] Conclusive diagnosis can only be established by a liver biopsy.

Serum iron is usually greater than 200 mcg./dL. in affected individuals. Total iron binding capacity is characteristically reduced and fully saturated. Plasma transferrin is greater than eight percent saturated. Serum ferritin is usually elevated above 200 mg./dL.; a level beyond 700 mg./dL. is essentially diagnostic of patients with superimposed cirrhosis.[3]

Source: J. R. Iacovino, "Idiopathic Hemochromatosis: An Assessment of Mortality," *J. Ins. Med.*, 17, no. 2 (1986): 9-11. Reproduced with permission of author and publisher.

Using liver function tests to screen for hepatic involvement in IH can be misleading, as up to two-thirds of cases, at presentation with an abnormal liver histology, can be normal.[4] Conversely, those without cirrhosis can have laboratory evidence of liver dysfunction.

The preponderance of current mortality from IH is related to the fibrogenic affect of iron deposition in the liver. In the past, 30 percent of the deaths were cardiac, usually cardiomyopathies with congestive heart failure at a young age; with treatment this complication has been reduced to 9 percent. At present, the leading cause of death in treated patients is the late development of hepatocellular carcinoma.[4]

The key to the mortality of IH is the presence of cirrhosis at biopsy. Cirrhosis is present in 40 to 80 percent of liver biopsies on initial evaluation in symptomatic patients[5] as well as in a number of those without symptoms. There is controversy in the literature concerning the reversibility of cirrhosis and its progenitor, fibrosis.[1,4,6,7] Clearly the latter, if mild and without nodular regeneration, can resolve in most cases with phlebotomy. However, often the histologic presentations of fibrosis and cirrhosis merge; thus one must not underwrite with the assumption of resolution. Moreover fibrosis can progress to cirrhosis during the phlebotomy period which can take from 6 months to 2 years (mean 18 months). Deironing cannot reduce the degree of cirrhosis once it is present but it can significantly improve mortality.[5] To prevent the development of cirrhosis, phlebotomy must continue for the lifetime of the patient; otherwise the iron will reaccumulate.

Hepatocellular carcinoma is currently the leading cause of death in IH comprising nearly 30 percent of the mortality in treated patients whereas in untreated patients the major cause of death is hepatic failure.[4] Hepatomas occur in about 30 percent of patients who have cirrhosis at presentation despite a adequate iron removal.[7] At an age greater than sixty five, 50 percent will die from hepatoma if cirrhosis was present on the initial biopsy.[1] Whether there is an increased incidence of extrahepatic malignancies is controversial.[4,8]

Complete deironing in the precirrhotic state is essential to remove the risk of hepatocellular carcinoma. Hepatomas do not appear to have an increased incidence when fibrosis and cirrhosis are absent on the biopsy;[2,9]

conversely all patients who did develop hepatomas had cirrhosis on their initial liver biopsy.[4] Total deironing of cirrhotic livers does not remove the risk of malignancy.[5,8] Hepatomas have developed up to 18 years after maintenance phlebotomy.[4] The mean interval from the completion of deironing to the development of hepatomas is 9 years with a range of 3 to 19 years.[9]

Mortality of IH can be reduced by phlebotomy. Sherlock noted a mean survival time with phlebotomy of 8.2 years, without treatment 4.9 years.[8] McLaren's group noted similar results with survival from the onset of symptoms of 7 years, treated and 4.4 years, untreated.[1]

A life table analysis by Bomford showed the 5- and 10-year survival after diagnosis at onset of symptoms to be 66 and 32 percent respectively in treated patients. This corresponds to a mean survival time for those treated of about 6 years, those untreated about 2 years.[4]

In each of the preceding, the mean age at which the patients became symptomatic and were initially diagnosed as having IH was about 55 years. All three study groups included subjects who had advanced disease on presentation.

Niederau[9] recently published the most comprehensive mortality study of IH. The mean age of his study group was 46 and mean follow-up was 10.5±5.6 years. Compared to previous studies the 10-year lower mean age was attributed to the inclusion of asymptomatic individuals as well as those identified by family screening; thus the group was similar to our applicant pool. Unfortunately, the population used for comparison was not totally applicable to an insurable group, it being similar to the United States general population.

Multiple group survival comparisons are available. The mortality rate of the IH patients, at each 5-year interval, was approximately twice that of the normal population. Those without cirrhosis were showed to have a standard mortality. The cirrhotic group was then compared to the noncirrhotic. The mortality ratios at 5, 10 and 15 years, were 400, 180 and 180 percent for those with cirrhosis. If we exclude, as an insurable risk, those diagnosed in the first 5 years then mortality is approximately 200% at 10 and 15 years after initial diagnosis. The group that could not be completely deironed in the first 18 months had the highest mortality at each interval.

Discussion

Idiopathic Hemochromatosis produces a reduction in survival, despite treatment, after onset of the histological demonstration of cirrhosis. As noted previously, liver function tests are unreliable in screening for the existence of liver disease. Total removal of iron from the involved liver will neither produce a reversal in the cirrhosis with its attendant mortality nor decrease the high risk of hepatocellular carcinoma in later years. Newer therapies such as the chelating agent desferrioxamine are not likely to be any more effective than phlebotomy.[1,7]

Underwriting of established IH requires an initial liver biopsy even in asymptomatic individuals with normal liver function tests. Since cirrhosis can develop during the acute phlebotomy period (up to two years) a repeat liver biopsy is highly advisable, in fact probably necessary at the completion of therapy. The follow-up biopsy is also required to document total iron removal. If the liver histology is normal then, provided maintenance phlebotomy is continued, this group appears to be a standard risk.[9] An exception to the follow-up biopsy might be the individual who has mild iron loading, has no fibrosis on the initial biopsy and whose deironing phlebotomy time is short as documented by laboratory studies.

For those applicants, who on screening have blood studies indicative of IH, a liver biopsy is also required to rule out asymptomatic hepatic involvement. A negative biopsy will place them in a standard mortality group, provided phlebotomy is initiated and maintained to prevent iron-induced cirrhosis.

The judgement of the medical director is tested in those cases where cirrhosis is present on the biopsy. Those who are overtly symptomatic with signs of cardiac or hepatic decompensation are obviously not insurable. Also those who cannot be deironed within one and one-half years have an unacceptable mortality.

It appears prudent to postpone any applicant with IH and cirrhosis for the first 5 years unless very mild disease is present. Somewhere between the fifth and tenth years those with asymptomatic, histologic cirrhosis become insurable at 200%. This rating assumes maintenance phlebotomies and is feasible due to the age of this group at diagnosis, about 55 years, and the long tail, about 10 years, until the potential development of hepatocellular carcinoma.

Cardiac abnormalities and Diabetes Mellitus contribute to the mortality of IH. However, both of these are almost invariably associated with large iron overloads and associated cirrhosis. By eliminating those with advanced hepatic disease their contribution to mortality should be minimal. Where diabetes is present, and unimproved by phlebotomy, an additional rating may be appropriate. One may also want to rate for associated electrocardiographic abnormalities. However, since further iron overload is prevented by continued phlebotomy neither problem is likely to progress in severity.

Acknowledgments

I wish to express my gratitude to John G. Hellstrom, M.D. whose criticism and suggestions were appreciated and to Carolyn Swanson and her word processor, without whose assistance this paper could not have been completed by the given deadline.

REFERENCES

1. G. D. McLaren, W. A. Muir, R. W. Kellermeyer, "Iron Overload Disorders: Natural History, Pathogenesis, Diagnosis and Therapy," *CRC Crit. Rev. Clin. Lab. Sci.,* 19, no. 3 (1984): 205-66.

2. J. W. Rowe, J. R. Wards, "Familial Hemochromatosis: Characteristics of the Precirrhotic Stage in a Large Kindred," *Medicine,* 56, no. 3 (1977): 197-211.

3. M. L. Bassett, J. W. Halliday, R. A. Ferris, L. W. Powell, "Diagnosis of Hemochromatosis in Young Subjects: Predictive Accuracy of Biochemical Screening Tests," *Gastroenterology,* 87 (1984): 628-33.

4. A. Bomford, R. Williams, "Long Term Results of Venesection Therapy in Idiopathic Hemochromatosis," *Q. J. Med.,* 180 (October 1976, New Series XLV): 611-23.

5. A. Cohen, C. Witzleben, E. Schwartz, "Treatment of Iron Overload," *Semin. Liver Dis.,* 4, no. 3 (1984): 228-38.

6. L. R. Weintraub, M. E. Conrad, W. H. Crosby, "The Treatment of Hematochromatosis by Phlebotomy," *Med. Clin. North Am.,* 50 (1966): 1579-90.

7. J. W. Halliday, M. L. Bassett, "Treatment of Iron Storage Disorder," *Drugs,* 215 (1980): 207-15.

8. S. Sherlock, "Hemochromatosis: Course and Treatment," *Annu. Rev. Med.,* 27 (1976): 143-49.

9. C. Niederau, R. Fischer, et al., "Survival and Causes of Death in Cirrhotic and Noncirrhotic Patients with Primary Hemochromatosis," *N. Engl. J. Med.,* 313 (1985): 1256-62.

A CARDIOVASCULAR SURVEY OF THE CHEST X-RAY IN NEARLY 5,000 LIFE INSURANCE APPLICANTS: NORMAL STANDARDS AND DISTRIBUTION CURVES FOR RELATIVE HEART DIAMETER

Ferris J. Siber, M.D., Arthur E. Brown, M.D., Richard B. Singer, M.D., and Frank I. Pitkin, M.D.

Introduction

Prior to 1960 one of us (AEB) undertook to preserve all chest X-rays on life insurance applicants for the purpose of subsequent review, with particular reference to the measurements of the heart and the thoracic aorta and other potential abnormalities of the chest film, as a special mortality study. Such a review was initiated in November, 1976, and the findings are presented in this report. An additional purpose of our study has been to make a careful analysis of the distribution of the observed transverse diameter of the cardiac silhouette in relation to that predicted from the Clark-Ungerleider table.[1,2] Percentage ratios, observed to predicted heart diameter, have been plotted and analyzed as distribution curves in standard and rated cases. In this way we can compare our curves with the original 1938 distribution curve obtained at the Equitable Diagnostic Laboratory by examination of a large group undifferentiated by selection criteria. All of the cases in our series also had the benefit of review of an electrocardiogram (ECG) so that standard insurance issue implies a satisfactory X-ray and ECG, as well as the usual selection criteria. Comparative mortality is being assessed with respect to insurance action and various combinations of X-ray and associated medical findings.

Radiography has long been the most widely used method for determining the size and configuration of the heart and great vessels. Quantitative measurements of the heart and aorta in the chest X-ray are supplemented by routine evaluation of the lung parenchyma as well as the bony structures, pleurae, diaphragm, the mediastinum and other tissues. The conventional chest X-ray is a P-A view taken with subject erect and in moderate inspiration, although a lateral view is highly desirable as a routine supplement to the P-A film. With a target-to-film distance of six feet and the sternum of the subject as close to the film as possible, magnification of the image over the true configuration is reduced to about 5±1%. The tables for measurements of the heart and aorta have been established with this technique, also employed for the X-rays reviewed in this series.

Cardiac enlargement on conventional radiography may reflect hypertrophy or dilation of the heart, usually of the left ventricle. Either of these is indicative of a significant abnormality. However, since heart size obviously depends on body size as well as the presence or absence of disease, some index dependent on body size is needed for comparison with the observed measurement. In 1919 Danzer proposed the cardio-thoracic ratio as an index of enlargement.[3] The transverse heart diameter as the standard measurement for the evaluation of cardiac enlargement was firmly established by the results of Hodges and Eyster in 1926.[4] The work of Ungerleider and Clark in 1938[1,2] established that the transverse diameter of the heart in a series of 1,460 subjects with chest X-rays taken at the clinic of the Equitable Life Assurance Society was correlated with height and weight, but not the age of the subject. The Clark-Ungerleider table was developed to give an average predicted value of the transverse cardiac diameter according to height and weight. This table has been in use for 40 years, especially in insurance medicine, to provide a predicted value with which the observed transverse cardiac diameter may be compared and thus a percentage ratio that is more reliable than the cardio-thoracic ratio. An upper normal limit of 50% has long been accepted for the latter. Ungerleider and Clark proposed 110% as an upper limit of normal for the use of their table. However, more liberal limits have been used in the medical departments of many insurance companies: these have generally been in the range of 112% to 118%. Wittenborg and Sossman concluded that an increase in heart size of 11% or more was "probably abnormal" and an increase of 15% or more was "definitely abnormal" in 97% of cases.[5] With ventriculography available as an adjunct of coronary arteriography we are

Source: F. J. Siber, A. E. Brown, R. B. Singer, F. I. Pitkin, "A Cardiovascular Survey of the Chest X-ray in Nearly 5,000 Life Insurance Applicants: Normal Standards and Distribution Curves for Relative Heart Diameter," *Trans. Assoc. Life Insur. Med. Dir. Amer.*, 63 (1979): 159-74. Reproduced with permission of authors and publisher.

now able to assess more accurately left ventricular volume and mass,[6] but volume can also be estimated from the regular chest film alone.[7,8] Upper limits of normal for heart volume have been estimated at 500-540 ml. per M^2 of body surface area in males, and 450-490 ml. per M^2 in females.[9]

Sheridan has validated a method for the quantitative assessment of the overall horizontal width of the thoracic aortic silhouette in the P-A chest film.[10] Sheridan noted that the transverse dimension of the aorta averages about 46% of the transverse cardiac diameter for a subject of given build and age, the latter having been found to be a significant factor, as average aortic width increases 1 mm. for every three years increase in age, in the range of 20-65 years. Comparison of the observed aortic width with that predicted from the Sheridan table, based on height, weight and age, gives the Sheridan Index, which is used in the same way as the percentage of observed to predicted heart diameter. Rodstein and Wolloch evaluated limits of normal for the Sheridan Index and reported that only 5% to 8% of otherwise normal subjects had a Sheridan Index exceeding 115%.[11] They concluded that measurement of the aortic width in conjunction with the Sheridan Index is a valuable indicator of abnormal tortuousity of the aorta and can be used in older subjects as well as those under age 65.

Material and Methods

Subjects studied were policyholders of the New England Mutual Life Insurance Company with an electrocardiogram (ECG) and chest X-ray interpreted in the period January 1, 1954 through December 31, 1966. During this period all files on applicants with an ECG were coded not only for ECG findings but also for insurance data, history and medical information including basic X-ray findings, when an X-ray was also interpreted.[12] The computerized ECG file was searched to produce a list of more than 8,000 names of applicants with an X-ray as well as an ECG. Applicants or policyholders with an X-ray but no ECG were not included in the ECG master file, and any extract from such a file probably underestimates the true prevalence of abnormal X-rays in an insured or applicant population. Because of potential difficulties in processing and matching we did not attempt to search the actuarial file of policyholders for X-ray cases without ECG, as the latter file is a numerical policy record without name identification. Many cases from the original list had to be excluded because the X-ray was a borrowed one, or was missing, or the folder could not be located. We were able to assemble 4,962 cases on applicants with both X-ray and ECG, a minimum of one year of follow-up exposure, and a prescribed set of coded information. The policy record used for follow-up was the policy with most recent available information, regardless of date of issue with respect to the application on which the X-ray was interpreted. In this way information was accumulated on some cases with declined, incomplete or cancelled applications, provided at least one year of policy follow-up information was available.

A distinct coding system was set up for this study, with the following fields of coded data entered on coding sheets for keypunching of 80-column IBM cards, which were, in turn, used as input for further data processing:

1. Date of Birth
2. Name
3. Number of policy applied for
4. Codes for application year, sex, age, amount and rating
5. Follow-up information
6. Blood pressure, medical findings and reasons for rating, including ECG
7. X-ray findings, including % observed to predicted heart diameter and width of aorta, and other features.

The X-ray interpretations were made by a single observer, a board-certified radiologist (FJS), thus eliminating inter-observer variation except for a small percentage of cases in which the X-ray was unavailable, but the interpretations sheet in the folder had been completed by a medical department staff member whose measurements and interpretation were found by comparison of other cases to correspond well with those of the radiologist. All X-ray coding was done by the radiologist, on the basis of personal review of the film, or use of an acceptable interpretation sheet containing complete measurements of heart, aorta, C/T ratio and other parts of the interpretation, in a selected minority of cases when the film could not be located or had been a loan. Other parts of the coding, follow-up and verification were carried out by staff members of the Medical Research Department.

Data on the coding sheets were keypunched and verified on 80 column IBM cards which were used as input for preparation of the tape used in the data processing, which was carried out by Theodore Yonge, of the Medical Research Department. Programs were developed to provide tabular output for a statistical analysis of the material, distribution of cases by age, sex, insurance action and measurements of heart and aorta, as a percentage of observed to predicted width. The Clark-Ungerleider table was used for predicted transverse diameter of the cardiac silhouette and the Sheridan table for predicted width of the aortic silhouette. A special program made available by the Research Department was used to develop data for normal distribution curves from the actual distribution curves for relative width of heart and aorta.

Mortality data processing is being carried out to produce number of cases, exposure, average rating (standard =1.00), observed and expected deaths, mortality ratio, and average annual rates, observed and expected, and the excess mortality rate, EDR. The 1965-70 intercompany standard ordinary tables, select and ultimate, were employed in the calculation of expected deaths, using rates specific for sex, quinquennial entry age, and individual years of policy duration. Detailed mortality calculations are still being carried out and, therefore, are not being reported at this time.

Results

Out of a total of 4,984 coded cases we excluded 11 outside the age limits of 20 to 74 years, 11 with incomplete coding, leaving 4,962 cases, for which the distribution is shown in Table 903K1-1 for age, sex and insurance action. Only 249 cases, 5.1% of the total, were females, who had a higher average age than the males, with 54% age 50-74, in contrast to only 36% age 50-74 in the men. The principal age break-down used in later figures and tables consists of a younger group, age 20-49, and an older group, age 50-74. Insurance issues to those age 20-49 were on a standard basis on 70.9%, with 19.1% rated for cardiovascular reasons (CV-rated) and 10.0% for reasons other than cardiovascular (other rated). This division of reason for rating has been followed in most of the data presented because the cases rated for X-ray or chest abnormalities other than cardiovascular were so few in number. It should be emphasized that CV-rated cases also included only a small number rated for in-

creased heart diameter or other CV findings in the X-ray. However, the pattern of mortality ratio in relation to heart diameter is quite different in the CV-rated cases from the patterns seen in the standard and other rated cases. The distribution of cases by insurance action in the subjects age 50-74 shows a much higher proportion of CV-rated cases, 31.9% instead of 19.1% in the younger applicants, and a smaller proportion of standard issues, 56.8% instead of 70.9%. This is consistent with the general trend for proportion of ratings to increase with age in all insurance applicants.

Distribution of relative heart diameters (HD) is shown in Figures 903K1-1 to 903K1-6. The HD is given as a percentage of observed diameter to that predicted in the Clark-Ungerleider table on the horizontal scale in all of these figures. The distribution is shown on the vertical scale as the percentage of total number for single values of HD, generally in the range of 70% to 118%. Relative frequency as a percent of total is more useful than the count of cases in comparing distribution curves, because the ordinates tend to be similar, which would not be true if the actual number of cases were used, as the totals vary widely from one age/rating group to another (Table 903K1-1). Observed points are connected by straight lines, and the actual distribution thus plotted can be compared with the computer-derived normal distribution curve, which is superimposed.

Despite their irregularity, the actual distribution curves conform closely to the shape of normal, "bell-shaped" curves. Coefficients of skewness (asymmetry about the mean) and kurtosis (flattening of the peak of the

TABLE 903K1-1

DISTRIBUTION OF CASES BY AGE, SEX AND INSURANCE ACTION

Age	Standard	CV-Rated	Other Rated	Total	Total Male	Total Female
20-24	30	12	5	47	42	5
25-29	79	36	12	127	122	5
30-34	254	64	32	350	341	9
35-39	431	104	62	597	577	20
40-44	814	170	97	1,081	1,051	30
45-49	610	211	105	926	880	46
20-49	2,218	597	313	3,128	3,013	115
%	70.9	19.1	10.0	100.0	96.3	3.7
50-54	386	198	76	660	627	33
55-59	397	202	70	669	622	47
60-64	180	122	43	345	315	30
65-69	71	46	15	132	114	18
70-74	8	16	4	28	22	6
50-74	1,042	584	208	1,834	1,700	134
%	56.8	31.9	11.3	100.0	92.7	7.3
20-74	3,260	1,181	521	4,962	4,713	249
%	65.7	23.8	10.5	100.0	94.9	5.1

curve) were calculated and generally found to be small in magnitude, indicating that the normal distribution curve makes a good fit with the observed data. This can be confirmed by visual inspection. The appearances of the curves and their normal distribution are similar to the features of the distribution of the single curve obtained by Ungerleider and Clark in their 1,460 cases.[1,2] However, there are small but statistically significant differences in the mean HD by age and by CV rating in our series of 4,962 X-rays, and also significant differences between our standard mean HDs and the 100% standard developed by Clark and Ungerleider.

The distribution of HD for 2,137 men age 20-49 in Figure 903K1-1 gives a mean of 96.5%, and for 959 men age 50-74 in Figure 903K1-2 the mean is 98.8%. The standard deviations (SD) of the two distributions in the men issued standard insurance are almost identical ±7.1% and ±6.9%. The standard error of the mean HD is obtained by dividing the SD by $\sqrt{n}$, where n is the total number of cases. Since these numbers are so large, the standard errors of the mean are correspondingly small, ±0.15% for the younger men and ±0.22% for the older men. Although the mean HD is only 2.3% higher for those age 50 up than it is for men under age 50, this difference is highly significant. A consistently higher HD was noted in the older men in both rated groups also. We can therefore conclude that heart diameters as measured by current radiological technique in applicants issued standard insurance (satisfactory ECG and other requirements as well as chest X-ray) are on the average 2.3% lower in men age 20-49 than in men age 50-74 with similar body build. Figures 903K1-3 and 903K1-4 provide the opportunity to compare HD in men and women issued standard insurance. The mean and SD are 97.2 ±7.1% for men (3,096 cases) and 97.0 ±7.7% for women (164 cases). This difference is not statistically significant, and we therefore confirm that no separate standards of normal are needed by sex.

The distribution curve for 1,121 men rated for CV reasons and shown in Figure 903K1-5 gives results for HD of 99.3±8.0%, the mean being 2.1% higher than the standard mean, again a difference that is statistically highly significant. A careful inspection of the curve will confirm that there is a scattering of cases with HD 117% or higher, whereas only two cases with such high HDs are found in the much larger number of standard cases in Figure 903K1-3. The mean HD for men issued standard insurance 97.2%, is also shown in Figure 903K1-5 as an additional dotted vertical line. The higher mean HD in the CV-rated cases signifies that heart diameters throughout the distribution curve tend to be 2.1% higher than they are in the curve for men issued standard insurance. The longer upper tail of the curve is to be expected, since the CV ratings for some of these men included debits for increased HD. What is somewhat surprising is the relatively small number of cases with diameters exceeding 115%, the upper 95% confidence limit with a mean of 99.3 and SD of ±8. There were only 16 such cases,

FIGURE 903K1-1

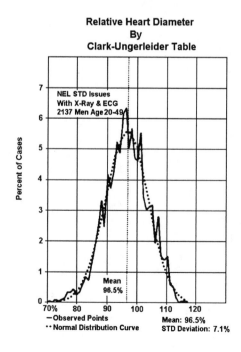

**Relative Heart Diameter
By
Clark-Ungerleider Table**

FIGURE 903K1-2

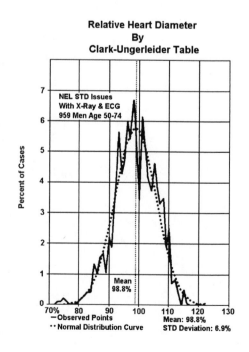

**Relative Heart Diameter
By
Clark-Ungerleider Table**

FIGURE 903K1-3

FIGURE 903K1-4

Relative Heart Diameter
By
Clark-Ungerleider Table

NEL STD Issues
With X-Ray & ECG
3096 Men Age 20-74

Mean
97.2%

— Observed Points
•• Normal Distribution Curve

Mean: 97.2%
STD Deviation: 7.1%

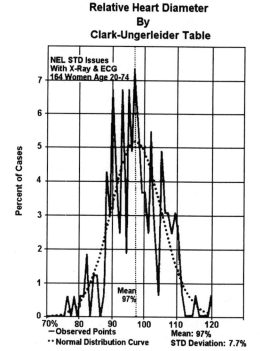

Relative Heart Diameter
By
Clark-Ungerleider Table

NEL STD Issues
With X-Ray & ECG
164 Women Age 20-74

Mean
97%

— Observed Points
•• Normal Distribution Curve

Mean: 97%
STD Deviation: 7.7%

FIGURE 903K1-5

Relative Heart Diameter
By
Clark-Ungerleider Table

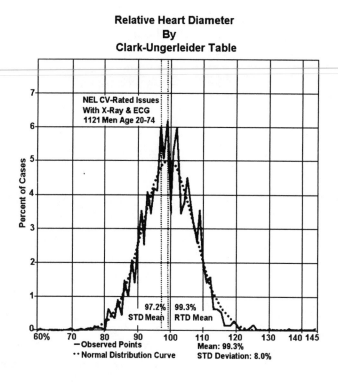

NEL CV-Rated Issues
With X-Ray & ECG
1121 Men Age 20-74

97.2%
STD Mean

99.3%
RTD Mean

— Observed Points
•• Normal Distribution Curve

Mean: 99.3%
STD Deviation: 8.0%

265

although 2.5% (half of the 5% outside the confidence limits) of 1,121 would predict 27 such cases. However, it makes better sense to use confidence limits derived from the standard cases, and 53 or 5.0% of the rated cases had an HD exceeding the upper standard limit (110.4% for men age 20-49 and 112.3% for men age 50-74). As will be seen later, borderline increase in heart diameter should be underwritten more conservatively when a ratable CV impairment is present.

The distribution of HD in cases rated for reasons that are noncardiovascular is shown in Figure 903K1-6. It does not differ from the standard distribution in Figure 903K1-3, the mean being 97.2±7.3%. Distributions in the rated cases therefore differ significantly, depending on whether the cause for the rating is cardiovascular or not. The other rated cases could be combined with the standard cases as far as the heart diameter distribution is concerned, but the curve for the CV-rated cases is distinctly and significantly shifted to the right, giving a higher mean and slightly wider confidence limits.

We have made an analysis of the distribution of aortic width measurements, expressed as the Sheridan Index. The mean for men issued standard insurance was 94.3± 8.6%. There was no significant difference in the mean with respect to age or rating for reasons other than

cardiovascular. However, the mean Index of 95.8±9.8% for the CV-rated cases was significantly different, even though the difference of 1.5% was smaller than the corresponding difference in heart diameter, (2.1%). All distribution patterns corresponded closely with the shape of the normal bell-shaped curve.

Computer processing of the mortality data is, unfortunately, far from completed at the time of final preparation of this manuscript. No tabular data can be presented on comparative mortality in the standard, CV-rated, and other rated groups, correlated with heart diameter, aortic width or specific CV reasons for rating. However, we do have preliminary mortality ratios by heart diameter for the standard issues, which we believe will be close enough to the final results to warrant quoting at this point in the text.

Our approach in evaluating the experience by relative heart diameter was to divide the group material into four parts, approximately the lowest sixth, a lower one-third below the mean, an upper one-third and the highest sixth above the mean. For heart diameter these four sub-groups, in order of ascending heart diameter, were those with an HD under 90%, next those with an HD 90-96% inclusive, then 97-104% inclusive, and finally 105% HD and up. The two larger sub-groups correspond approximately to cases falling within the limits of +1 SD and –1 SD on either side of the mean in the normal distribution curve. The smaller sub-groups were cases falling outside these limits of ±1 SD from the mean. This division was used in preference to division into quantities of equal size, or into a larger number of sub-groups of smaller size.

The mortality ratio in the total standard issues prior to subsequent checking procedures was 70% relative to the Intercompany 1965-70 Tables, Select and Ultimate, with separate male and female rates. By heart diameter the standard mortality ratios were 78% and 80% for the sub-groups below the mean HD, and 66% for the sub-group with HD from 97-104%, and finally, 61% for the sub-group with the highest relative heart diameters 105% and up. It should be emphasized that these are preliminary mortality ratios, obtained without benefit of all case validation procedures now in use. Somewhat different ratios may emerge from the final processing, but it is our current opinion that any differences will prove to be small in magnitude. Subject to this uncertainty it can be seen that there is *no* trend for the mortality ratio to increase with increasing relative heart diameter in the standard issues.

A similar set of preliminary mortality ratios was obtained on the rated issues, in relation to heart diameter. The average mortality ratio was about twice that observed among the standard issues, and here there was a definite

FIGURE 903K1-6

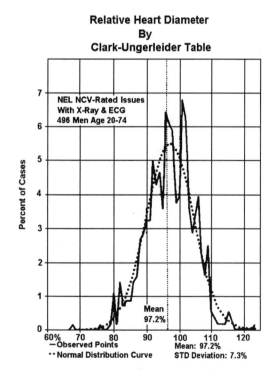

**Relative Heart Diameter
By
Clark-Ungerleider Table**

NEL NCV-Rated Issues
With X-Ray & ECG
496 Men Age 20-74

Percent of Cases

Mean
97.2%

60% 70   80   90   100 110   120
— Observed Points   Mean: 97.2%
•• Normal Distribution Curve   STD Deviation: 7.3%

upward trend in the provisional mortality ratio with increasing heart diameter. No ratios will be quoted on these results, which were obtained on all rated cases combined, about two-thirds CV-rated and one-third rated for other reasons (Table 903K1-1). The two rated groups are being analyzed separately in the tabulations now being processed. This distinctive pattern if confirmed for the CV-rated cases, will have an important bearing on the limit of heart diameter beyond which debits are justified when there is some other ratable CV impairment present.

Discussion

All medical directors are aware of the importance attached to relative heart diameter from the chest X-ray and Clark-Ungerleider table, especially if the observed diameter is more than 10% above the predicted, and if there is a ratable CV impairment present. In discussing this underwriting significance, Kiessling and Oliver[13] stressed the special problems encountered in insurance as opposed to clinical medicine: serial studies usually are not available; it is impractical to make additional studies; the clinical data are often incomplete, yet an underwriting decision cannot be postponed. It is, therefore, reassuring to confirm the normal distribution curve of relative heart diameter in a large population of insurance applicants who satisfied the orthodox requirements for standard issue, including review of a satisfactory ECG. Our series of 3,260 standard issue cases was more than twice as large as the series 1,460 home office examinees reported by Ungerleider and Clark who were life insurance applicants with blood pressure 110-145 mm. systolic and 60-100 mm. diastolic, after exclusion of 732 cases with blood pressure outside these limits, mostly applicants with hypertension. Ungerleider and Clark give no information on insurability of the 1,460 selected subjects, although they do state that applicants in the large group of 2,192 cases were "not necessarily accepted as insurance risks" (527 of these had a systolic pressure of 150 mm. or higher). In any mortality study it is of obvious importance to correlate the experience with insurance action and reasons for any rating imposed, a correlation that is being made in our series.

Although our distribution curve for standard issues resembles very closely the conformation of the curve in the Ungerleider and Clark Table, our mean heart diameter for a given build is 2.8% or 3.7 mm. below the corresponding average found by them and used in construction of their table of predicted values. There are two obvious factors among many possible ones that might account for the lower mean HD obtained very recently as compared with the mean obtained over forty years ago, a difference that is statistically of high significance. The first is technological and the second depends on selection of the group. There have been many changes in X-ray equipment and X-ray films in the past forty years, and it would scarcely be surprising if the apex of the heart can now be located somewhat more accurately in those situations where it tended to be obscured by a fat pad and that this point is inside the locus previously used in such cases. Our normal series differed from that of Ungerleider and Clark in that all were issued standard insurance, and all had a satisfactory ECG as part of the screening process, in addition to the X-ray itself; our series probably contained a smaller proportion of borderline blood pressure elevations. Standard radiological interpretation technique was employed in both series and interobserver variability was reduced to a minimum within our series. Since there is no way to compensate for possible interobserver differences in measurement technique between different series, perhaps the ideal solution for each company medical department would be to develop a similar distribution curve for heart diameter in standard issues in order to determine how much the normal mean differs from the mean tabular value as 100.0%.

What advice do we have for those who may wish to utilize the results presented here as more representative of current measurement standards than the Clark-Ungerleider table without going through all the work of developing a separate distribution curve and percentage mean value? We do not think it is necessary to construct a completely new table with different predicted diameters, each 2.8% lower than the present value, for any given combination of height and weight. Instead, the percentage of observed to predicted heart diameter can be obtained in the usual way and then 3% added to adjust for smaller mean predicted HD (2.8% below the tabulated value). If the effect of age is also to be included, this can be done quite simply by using an adjustment of +4% for applicants under age 45, +3% for those age 45-54, and +2% for those age 55 up. Such an approximation should be sufficiently close, and some medical directors may feel that the corrections are small enough to be ignored. It is of interest that Ungerleider and Clark did note a slight increase in heart diameter with age, but felt that no adjustment was needed under age 50, and they chose to ignore about 1% increase for older subjects, thus recommending use of their table for all ages. We believe the age difference is a little greater in magnitude than their estimate, and an adjustment taking account of the small age variation is simple to make.

The next question, one of great importance in underwriting, is what value to select as an upper limit of "normal." A value too high will result in standard insurance for some cases with significant hypertrophy and increased mortality risk even in the absence of some other known CV risk factor; that is, it will result in underwriting that it too liberal. An upper limit of normal that is too low will result in very conservative underwriting and will exclude too many cases that properly justify standard issue.

Ungerleider and Clark failed to give a standard deviation for their normal distribution curve. However, the ordinate of the normal curve at ±1 SD is very close to 0.6 of the maximum calculated value, which is 0.6 of 75, or 45 cases, in their figure. The SD corresponding to this ordinate is ±7.5%, very close to the SD of ±7.1% we obtained for our standard male cases, all ages combined. If we set 95% confidence limits to define the upper limit, 97.2+(1.96)(7.1) = 97.2+13.9 = 111% using the Clark-Ungerleider table unadjusted, or 114% using the average adjustment of +3% for ages 45-54. This is a purely statistical convention that excludes the highest 2.5% of a presumably normal population. When we examine the actual distribution of our cases in the "upper tail" of standard issues for men, we find only 40 cases with an HD over 111%, instead of the predicted 77. If we extend the upper limit to 15% above the mean, slightly more than +2 SD, there are only 21 cases excluded. The two highest values of relative HD are one at 117% and one at 122%. These are unadjusted values derived from the original predicted table; with the +3% adjustment recommended from our data, the possible upper limits against a true mean of 100% would be 114% for +2 SD, 115% for a percentage point above this, and 120% for a very liberal limit that would exclude only 2 cases in more than 3,000 men in the normal series. It is our opinion that the original limit suggested by Ungerleider and Clark, 111% or above (114% or above adjusted to our mean) is reasonably conservative, and it should be possible to go a little beyond this relative HD, in view of the favorable preliminary mortality ratio found in the upper sixth of our standard issue cases.

We further believe that limits based on the *standard* experience should be applied to the CV-rated cases. If we use the upper limit for HD of 111% unadjusted or 114% adjusted, we will exclude 53 cases, or the top 5.0% of CV-rated cases, twice the number predicted on the basis of the *normal* case distribution. As we have already indicated, the mean HD in the CV-rated cases is significantly elevated, 2.1% above the mean for the standard cases, and the two distributions are distinctly different. It would be improper to attempt to utilize an upper confidence limit for the CV-rated cases based on the group mean and SD of 99.3±8.0%. This would give an upper limit of 115% unadjusted, much too high, when the object of the limit is to distinguish as many "abnormally high" heart diameters as possible, in comparison with the *standard* distribution. The positive trend of mortality ratio to increase with relative HD found in our preliminary tabulation of all rated cases implies a need to be more conservative about the possible use of debits for only borderline increase HD. For example, a relative HD of 107% unadjusted or 110% adjusted we would regard as clearly within standard limits in a case with no ratable CV impairment. However, if such a case were ratable for blood pressure elevation, or a heart murmur or a history of old MI with good recovery, then serious consideration should be given to applying some debits for excess mortality that very likely will be demonstrated when our mortality processing is completed. If minimal debits are applied in a borderline range for CV-rated cases, for example from 105 to 111% unadjusted or 108 to 114% adjusted, it is only fair to add proportionately higher debits for those cases with definitely ratable heart diameters.

To sum up, our re-examination of the distribution of relative heart diameters in the cardiac silhouette of the chest X-ray confirms the essential validity of the Clark-Ungerleider table, if relatively minor adjustments are made for a lower mean diameter as a normal average, and a slight additional adjustment for age. No further correction is needed when the table is used for females. We have suggested upper limits of "normal" (satisfactory) heart diameter, and we believe that mortality results now being obtained will indicate the desirability of different limits and different schedules of debits, depending on the presence or absence of an associated ratable CV impairment.

Acknowledgments

We gratefully acknowledge assistance to this project provided in a variety of ways by the following individuals: Martha Langlois, Harris Lee, Hazel Martin, Helen Moynihan, Charles N. Walker, F.S.A., Theodore Yonge, and members of the Medical Department over the years.

REFERENCES

1. H. E. Ungerleider, C. P. Clark, "A Study of the Transverse Diameter of the Heart Silhouette with Prediction Table Based on the Teleoroentgenogram," *Trans. Assoc. Life Insur. Med. Dir. Amer.*, 25 (1938): 84-103.

2. H. E. Ungerleider, C. P. Clark, "A Study of the Transverse Diameter of the Heart Silhouette with Prediction Table Based on the Teleoroentgenogram," *Am. Heart J.*, 17 (1939): 92-102.

3. C. S. Danzer, "The Cardiothoracic Ratio: An Index of Cardiac Enlargement," *Am. J. Med. Sci.*, 157 (1919): 513.

4. F. J. Hodges, J. A. E. Eyster, "Estimation of Transverse Cardiac Diameter in Man," *Arch. Intern. Med.*, 37 (1926): 707-14.

5. M. D. Wittenborg, M. C. Sossman, "Heart Measurements by X-Ray," *Mod. Concepts Cardiovasc. Dis.*, 16 (1947).

6. H. T. Dodge, "Determination of Left Ventricular Volume and Mass," *Radiol. Clin. North Am.*, 9 (1971): 459-67.

7. M. H. Schreiber, "The Volume of the Heart — A Roentgenographic Determination," *Ariz. Med.*, 21 (1964): 551.

8. P. M. Chikos, M. M. Figley, L. Fisher, "Correlation Between Chest Film and Angiographic Assessment of Left Ventricular Size," *Am. J. Roentgenol.*, 128 (1977): 367-73.

9. P. Amundsen, "The Diagnostic Value of Conventional Radiological Examination of the Heart in Adults," *Acta Radiol. Suppl.*, 181 (1959).

10. J. T. Sheridan, "The Transverse Diameter of the Cardiac Silhouette," *Trans. Assoc. Life Insur. Med. Dir. Amer.*, 28 (1941): 49-73.

11. M. Rodstein, L. Wolloch, "The Determination of Aortic Size by Use of the Sheridan Index in the Elderly — A Study of 300 Individuals 65 years of Age and Older," *Trans. Assoc. Life Insur. Med. Dir. Amer.*, 51 (1967): 341-49.

12. R. B. Singer, "An Analysis of Electrocardiographic Abnormalities in Insurance Applicants: Bundle Branch Block and Related Defects," *Proc. Medical Section. Am. Life Convention*, 50th Annual Meeting, (1962), pp. 114-44.

13. C. E. Kiessling, L. W. Oliver, Jr., "Enlarged Hearts in Normal Individuals," *Trans. Assoc. Life Insur. Med. Dir. Amer.*, 53 (1969): 306-11.

MORTALITY IN 4,100 INSURANCE APPLICANTS WITH ECG AND CHEST X-RAY: RELATION TO CARDIOVASCULAR AND OTHER RISK FACTORS, INCLUDING RELATIVE HEART DIAMETER

Richard B. Singer, M.D., Ferris J. Siber, M.D.,
Arthur E. Brown, M.D., and Frank I. Pitkin, M.D.

Introduction

In 1979 we reported an analysis of the measurements of relative heart diameter and aortic width in 4,984 chest X-rays made on life insurance applicants 1954 through 1966.[1] All available chest X-rays on cases having both ECG and X-ray were re-interpreted by one of us (FJS), with coding of insurance data, measurements and other X-ray data, and associated medical data. We found normal, bell-shaped distribution curves for both heart diameter and aortic width in all groups studied. The mean heart diameter in men issued standard insurance was 96.5% in those age 20-49, with a standard error of ±0.15%, and 98.8% in those age 50-74, with a standard error of ±0.21%, with use of the Clark-Ungerleider table for diameter expected from height and weight.[2] Observed heart diameters were significantly different by age and significantly lower than the 100.0% based on the table values. There was no sex difference, but in men rated for cardiovascular reasons the mean diameter of 99.2% was significantly higher than the 97.2%, all ages combined, in standard cases. A mean aortic width of 94.3% of the value predicted in the Sheridan table[3] was found in men issued standard insurance. For further discussion of the findings the reader is referred to the full report.

Of the cases originally coded we found 4,143 with a minimum follow-up of one year and no essential codes missing, and these constituted the data base for the mortality study to be described. Because our ECG file was used as the source for a list of cases with both chest X-ray and ECG, we found a disappointingly low prevalence of 0.8% for cases rated because of a cardiovascular or other abnormality in the chest X-ray: 18 for aortic width or calcification, 8 for heart enlargement, and 6 for other findings. Accordingly this mortality study is focussed on the associated cardiovascular findings in both the stand-ard and rated cases, with special attention to the correlated measurements of heart diameter and aortic width.

Material and Methods

The 841 cases excluded from the original group of 4,984 were mainly for lack of any follow-up data, with much smaller numbers because of incomplete coding or age outside the limits set. We thus had 4,143 applicants age 20 through 74 years, almost all of whom had life insurance issued by the New England Mutual Life Insurance Company from 1954 through 1966. Follow-up for exposure and death information was carried out through policy records to July 1, 1978; in a small number of cases where the policy was not issued or not taken the record of another policy was used. Reasons for rating, medical findings, and X-ray findings were coded in addition to the usual personal and follow-up information and rating, if any. Relative measurements of heart diameter and aortic width were remade by a single observer, a board-certified radiologist (FJS), and were coded as a percentage of the predicted values from the Clark-Ungerleider and Sheridan tables, respectively. The input was prepared in the form of 80-column IBM punched cards and transferred to magnetic tape. Programs for sorting, counting and life table calculations were prepared by Theodore Yonge. The 1965-70 Select and Ultimate Intercompany tables were employed in the program for the calculation of expected deaths; separate male and female rates were used. The tabular data presented are for all durations combined. Follow-up ranged from 1 to 24 years, with an average of about 12 years.

Results

In Figure 903K2-1 we give the age distribution of all cases in the bar graphs and of the females separately in the linear graph, and in Table 903K2-1 we give the distribution by insurance action, the average age and proportion of females in each group, standard or rated. Since only 5.0% of the applicants were female, the percentage age distribution for both sexes combined is virtually the same as that for men alone. Rated cases

Source: R. B. Singer, F. J. Siber, A. E. Brown, F. I. Pitkin, "Mortality in 4,100 Insurance Applicants with ECG and Chest X-ray: Relation to Cardiovascular and Other Risk Factors, Including Relative Heart Diameter," *Trans. Assoc. Life Insur. Med. Dir. Amer.*, 65 (1981): 180-93. Reproduced with permission of authors and publisher.

tended to be older than those issued standard insurance, and females tended to be older than males. More detailed tabular data by age, sex and insurance action are given in the previous report[1] for the somewhat larger series from which these 4,143 cases were drawn.

Mortality data are presented in Table 903K2-2 for the 3,054 standard issues, classified first by age, then by sex. Mortality ratios for New England Life standard experience, medical and nonmedical combined, cluster in the range of 80-85% of concurrent intercompany standard mortality from 1954 to 1978, with random fluctuations for individual years and age groups with smaller numbers of deaths. The addition of a satisfactory ECG and chest X-ray to the usual medical requirements for standard issue would be expected to produce an even lower mortality than standard. Such a result is found in Table 903K2-2 at ages 40 up, with mortality ratios between 74% and 69% for the three age groups and for the men, all ages combined. However, the mortality ratio for the standard females was 109%, and for all cases age 20-39, 94%. There were 17 deaths in females and 25 in entrants under age 40, so these differences from 85% of the expected numbers of deaths are not significant at the 95% confidence level. On the other hand, the observed deaths for ages 40-74 combined are significantly lower than 85% of the combined expected deaths. This standard experience on 3,054 cases produced 38,921 exposure-years, with an average follow-up of 12.7 years, and 256 observed deaths.

Results are given in Table 903K2-3 for comparative mortality by presence or absence of minor impairments in the standard cases, and for single or multiple reasons for rating in cases rated for noncardiovascular (NCV) reasons only. Standard cases with no minor impairment codes, all ages and both sexes combined, had the lowest mortality ratios, 70% and 69%. Those with a single cardiovascular code had an "average" New England Life standard mortality ratio of 85%, but those with a NCV code still showed a low ratio of 81%. About 5% of the standard cases had more than one minor CV or minor NCV code; mortality ratios were 99% and 143%, respectively, although the numbers of deaths were small. The overall mortality ratio of 99% for the 269 cases with major (rated) NCV impairments shows no excess mortality in the presence of satisfactory ECG and X-ray (there were six cases rated for chest X-ray other than heart and aorta, with no deaths). Again, results were quite different depending on whether single or multiple reasons for rating were present: with only one rated NCV code the mortality ratio was only 79%; with more than one the ratio was 209%.

To assess the results by relative heart diameter we have divided the material in each group into four divi-

sions: two below the average of 97% for all ages with standard issue and two at 97% or above. The divisions are under 90% (about one-sixth of the total of standard cases), 90-96% (one-third), 97-104% (also one-third), and the final sixth at 105% and up. This division based on the heart diameter distribution in standard cases is also used in the rated cases. There is no upward trend in mortality ratio whatsoever, with increasing heart diameter in the standard cases or the cases rated for NCV reasons (Table 903K2-4). The ratios are actually higher for the groups with relative heart diameter below the mean.

Table 903K2-5 presents a different picture for the 820 cases rated for CV reasons. Excess mortality does show an upward trend with increasing heart diameter, whether measured by mortality ratio or the extra deaths per 1000 years of exposure, EDR. The 820 cases rated for CV reasons have been broken down into two age groups, under 50 and 50-74; the upward trend is evident in both the younger and older applicants. Relatively minor degrees of increased heart diameter by the Clark-Ungerleider table appear to contribute substantially to excess mortality of CV-rated cases, just as heart diameters well below the average appear to have a favorable effect on mortality.

When the Sheridan Index of aortic width is used to subdivide the material into four groups of a size similar to the heart diameter groups, there is no evidence of a trend for excess mortality to increase with increasing width of the aorta in CV-rated cases (lower half of Table 903K2-6). However, the 18 cases rated for abnormal aorta did show a mortality ratio of 374%, based on 7 deaths; some of these were rated not for increased width, but for calcification or a combination of these. The absence of any trend in the standard cases (upper part of Table 903K2-6) is similar to what was observed with heart diameter (Table 903K2-4).

Comparative mortality in the CV-rated cases has been further analyzed by reason for rating, with results shown in Table 903K2-7. Again a difference is observed depending on whether single or multiple reasons for rating are involved. There were 636 cases rated for CV reasons without any NCV rating; excess mortality was relatively low, with an EDR of 4.3 per 1000 and mortality ratio of 143%. Among the 184 cases rated for NCV as well as CV reasons the mortality ratio of 228% and EDR of 12 per 1000 were substantially higher. These CV-rated cases have been subdivided into four major categories of CV reason for rating, with hypertension showing a ratio of 118% and valvular and coronary heart disease as single impairments combined only 119%. A small number of cases with stroke or arterial disease alone produced a higher excess mortality, with ratio of 203% and EDR of

18 per 1000. Cases with abnormal ECG, or arrhythmia or other rated CV impairment had a mortality ratio of 130%. Collectively the 576 cases of single CV reason for rating were found to have a mortality ratio of 130%, much lower than the ratio of 245% in 254 cases rated for multiple CV reasons; the EDRs were 3.0 and 14 per 1000 respectively. Thus multiple reasons for rating, either CV or a combination of CV and NCV, resulted in a substantial increase in excess mortality.

Table 903K2-8 shows excess mortality in the CV-rated cases analyzed by ECG pattern code. These codes were assigned in a priority order, so that no separate code was used for any combination of patterns. Minor T wave abnormalities (low amplitude) and disturbances of rhythm and conduction showed the lowest excess mortality, with major (inverted) T waves, ST deviations, and Q wave and other QRS abnormalities giving much higher mortality ratios, from 225% to 307%, and corresponding EDRs in the range of 12 to 21 per 1000. The 546 cases bearing an ECG abnormal pattern code showed a mortality ratio of 192%, in sharp contrast to absence of excess mortality (ratio 101% in 272 cases with no pattern code. It is clear that a normal or virtually normal ECG (minor changes in the ECG were not assigned a pattern code) has a favorable impact on the long-term mortality of CV-rated cases.

Discussion

We were unable to find any published clinical reports of mortality in relation to CV abnormalities of the chest X-ray and associated conditions. However, we are aware of three published studies of life insurance company experience dealing with heart enlargement in the chest X-ray. Bolt and Bell reported little or no extra mortality in 70 otherwise normal applicants to the New York Life Insurance Company whose chest X-ray showed a relative heart diameter exceeding 112% by the Clark-Ungerleider table.[4] Kiessling and Oliver, at the 1969 ALIMDA meeting, presented data on 55 male employees of the Prudential Home Office, whose chest X-rays taken initially from 1933 through 1964 showed a relative heart diameter of 113% or more despite a normal ECG and normal clinical status otherwise.[5] With an average follow-up of 19.8 years 16 deaths were observed, giving a mortality ratio of 122% versus 13 expected deaths calculated from the 1955-60 Basic Intercompany Table for males. The 1955-60 Basic Table gives mortality rates undoubtedly too low for the selected experience prior to 1950; if a larger figure for expected deaths were used, the mortality ratio might well be 100% or less. There is no evidence of significant excess mortality in this small series, and the results are therefore consistent with our findings of a favorable mortality ratio of 68% in 525

standard cases with heart diameter of 105% and up (48 observed deaths, Table 903K2-4). At a cutoff of 113% we would have had a very much smaller number of standard cases to include, as shown in our previous report.[1] Further evidence of the benign character of heart diameters of 111% or more in an otherwise satisfactory application is provided by unpublished New England Life experience.[6] With 761 standard policies so coded 1958-74 the mortality ratio was only 58%, based on 17 observed death claims and expected claims calculated from the 1965-70 Basic Select Tables.

Two insurance studies also provide evidence on the degree of excess mortality in rated issue cases with the chest X-ray showing increased heart diameter, 111% or more. The 1972 New York Life study used as a source of data in *Medical Risks: Patterns of Mortality and Survival*[7] showed a mortality ratio of 230% in an exposure of 744 policy years, cases rated for this degree of heart enlargement as the single major impairment (11 death claims). A higher mortality ratio of 309% was observed in rated issues of the 1958-74 New England Life experience.[6] This was based on a smaller number, 479 policies with heart diameter 111% or more, but with a considerably longer duration and 46 death claims. Unlike the New York Life study, rated issues in the New England Life experience represent an undifferentiated total, regardless of the reason for rating or number of reasons. This ratio of 309% with relative heart diameter of 111% or more is substantially greater than the ratio of 169% for the CV-rated cases reported in Table 903K2-5, with relative heart diameter of 105% and up (all ages combined, total 43 deaths). The two series are so different in methodology that a disparity of this magnitude is not unexpected. It does suggest the need for caution in rating cases with other CV reasons and heart enlargement in the chest X-ray, even when the Clark-Ungerleider relative diameter is only 111%. These cases with the increased heart diameter code in our 1958-74 rated experience constituted one of the few groups in which the mortality ratio exceeded the average table rating percentage. The mortality ratio tended to decrease with increasing age or duration.

Our results for mortality in relation to heart diameter (Tables 903K2-4 and 903K2-5) do provide some useful underwriting information, despite the absence of significant data at diameters of 111% or more. In cases not rated for any CV reason there was only random variation of mortality ratio with heart diameter; this was true within the entire range of heart diameters for both standard issues and for cases rated for NCV reasons (Table 903K2-4). The second feature of potential importance is the apparent trend for excess mortality to increase as relative heart diameter increases (Table 903K2-5). The absence of significant excess mortality in CV-rated cases with small heart diameter (under 90%) suggests the feasibility of giving credits against the rating in such cases, especially if the rating is for a single impairment only. The reason for this qualification is the much more favorable mortality ratio of 130% for single CV impairment cases seen in Table 903K2-7, as compared with ratios over 200% for both CV and NCV second impairments. This seems to be true for coronary disease, hypertension, abnormal ECGs collectively, and other CV impairments except for the small group of cases of stroke and other arterial disease combined. It should be emphasized that cases of coronary disease as a single impairment did not have an abnormal ECG, so it is *not* suggested that credits be given for a relative heart diameter in coronary disease, hypertension or other CV impairments unless the underwriter also has the reassurance of a satisfactory current ECG. The results in Table 903K2-8 indicate that low T waves were associated with the most favorable mortality of all the ECG pattern codes. Not all of the 546 CV-rated cases with ECG pattern codes were rated for the ECG, which was a minor impairment in about one-quarter of them. More of the ECG-rated cases fell in the 254 multiple than in the 211 single-reason for rating codes, the proportion being about 80% of the total in each code. There were more cases rated for coronary disease and abnormal ECG than for coronary disease alone, but unfortunately we could not separate this or any other combination of cases with multiple CV-reasons for rating as a separate category for comparative mortality.

In our previous report on the distribution pattern of relative heart diameter in these carefully evaluated chest X-rays we emphasized the small but significant shift of the curve for CV-rated cases to the right (large diameters) of the curve for standard issues. The mean diameter for the standard cases was 97.2% and for the CV-rated, 99.3%. Furthermore, only 2.1% of standard cases had a relative heart diameter exceeding 110%, about the number expected by adding twice the standard deviation of +7.1% to get an upper "normal" limit of 111%. In contrast, 5.6% of the CV-rated cases had a relative heart diameter exceeding 110% by the Clark-Ungerleider table. Cases with CV disease, especially heart disease, develop moderate to marked heart enlargement in a minority of cases. It is reasonable to infer from analysis of the distribution of heart diameters and of the mortality results presented here that slight degrees of heart "enlargement," within heart diameter limits that are normal for standard cases, may have prognostic importance for cases with a ratable CV impairment. The limit of 105% we selected as the starting point for the group with largest heart diameters is 1 standard deviation above the mean for the standard issue and NCV-rated cases. This may be too low to consider as a dividing line for extra debits to

be added because of heart diameter to CV-rated cases, especially if there is only a single CV impairment and the ECG is satisfactory. On the other hand, 110% by the Clark-Ungerleider table may be too high a dividing line, especially when one considers that this corresponds to a diameter of 113% of the mean, by our estimate of the mean, which may represent the type of measurement that is generally being made of the cardiac silhouette with better X-ray techniques that are now available as compared to more than 40 years ago. In our opinion the most important finding in this study is the potentially adverse underwriting significance of heart diameters in this borderline zone between the "true mean" for cases without known CV disease (97% of the Clark-Ungerleider predicted mean) and a limit for "definite" enlargement, such as any diameter over 110%.

Turning now to the handful of cases coded as being rated for abnormality of heart or aorta in the chest X-ray we can mention again that only 8 cases were rated for heart enlargement. The deaths in the cases rated for CV abnormality of the X-ray were restricted to the 18 with abnormal aorta. In only three cases rated for aortic calcification with no widening of the aorta there were two deaths and a mortality ratio over 700%. The 15 cases with widened or tortuous aorta also showed excess mortality, with a ratio of 311%, based on 5 deaths. Random variation because of small numbers may contribute to this apparently unfavorable experience, because the degree of the excess mortality is not confirmed in the individual mortality studies by policy previously referred to,[6,7] and in a report presented at the 1963 ALIMDA meeting.[8] In the New York Life Single Impairment study policies coded for tortuous aorta were found to have a mortality ratio of 123% (5 death claims), and those coded for aortic calcification, a ratio of 265% (15 death claims). Some standard issues were included in the tortuous aorta cases, but not in those with aortic calcification. In the New England Life experience with coded policies we found many more cases of widened aorta (over 110% by the Sheridan table) than we did of aortic calcification. The mortality ratio for the aortic calcification code was 79% in the standard cases (20 death claims), and only 183% in all rated cases, regardless of reason (16 death claims). For the widened aorta code we had a standard mortality ratio of 78% (37 death claims), and a ratio on all rated cases of 222% (69 death claims). In both codes the mortality ratio for rated cases was less than the average initial table rating imposed. This experience with 1958-74 policies is consistent with the results of Table 903K2-6, which show a below-average mortality for all aortic width categories in the standard cases, and no mortality trend in the CV-rated cases. Bell et al. combined New York Life insurance experience with data from the Prudential

Home Office employee file to give a series of 153 cases in which the mortality ratio was 112%, based on 23 deaths. Other known CV disease was excluded.[8] The authors noted several papers in the literature which suggest an anatomic factor — the area of attachment of the ligamentum arterio sum — as a frequent benign cause of calcification of the thoracic aorta, not indicative of widespread arteriosclerosis. In view of all of this evidence we feel that the apparently high excess mortality in the 18 cases rated for widened or calcified aorta is of very doubtful significance. It seems to us much more likely that aortic tortuosity and calcification are less adverse as abnormal findings in the chest X-ray than is heart enlargement in CV-rated cases.

Acknowledgments

We gratefully acknowledge assistance to this project provided in a variety of ways by our medical colleagues and the following individuals: Martha Langlois, Harris Lee, Hazel Martin, Helen Moynihan, Charles N. Walker, F.S.A. and Theodore Yonge.

REFERENCES

1. F. J. Siber, A. E. Brown, R. B. Singer, F. I. Pitkin, "A Cardiovascular Survey of the Chest X-ray in Nearly 5,000 Life Insurance Applicants: Normal Standards and Distribution Curves for Relative Heart Diameter," *Trans. Assoc. Life Insur. Med. Dir. Amer.*, 63 (1979): 159-74.

2. H. E. Ungerleider, C. P. Clark, "A Study of the Transverse Diameter of the Heart Silhouette with Prediction Table Based on the Teleoroentgenogram," *Trans. Assoc. Life Insur. Med. Dir. Amer.*, 25 (1938): 84-103.

3. J. T. Sheridan, "The Transverse Diameter of the Frontal Aortic Silhouette," *Trans. Assoc. Life Insur. Med. Dir. Amer.*, 28 (1941): 49-73.

4. W. Bolt, M. F. Bell, "Cardiac Enlargement of Undetermined Cause in Asymptomatic Adults," *Am. Heart J.,* 50 (1955): 331-36.

5. C. E. Kiessling, L. W. Oliver, Jr, "Enlarged Hearts in Normal Individuals," *Trans. Assoc. Life Insur. Med. Dir. Amer.*, 53 (1969): 306-11.

6. R. B. Singer, Unpublished Study of New England Life Mortality Experience, 1958-74 Standard and Rated Policy Issues with Impairment Code, Followed to 1975 Policy Anniversary (various reports 1978).

7. Data from "New York Life Single Impairment Study — 1972" in Mortality Abstract 399, in *Medical Risks: Patterns of Mortality and Survival*, R. B. Singer, L. Levinson, eds. (Lexington, MA, Lexington Books, 1976).

8. M. F. Bell, R. S. Schaaf, T. P. Jernigan, "The Prognostic Import of Calcification of the Aortic Knob," *Trans. Assoc. Life Insur. Med. Dir. Amer.*, 58 (1963): 33-41.

FIGURE 903K2-1

AGE DISTRIBUTION 4,143 CASES FOLLOWED UP

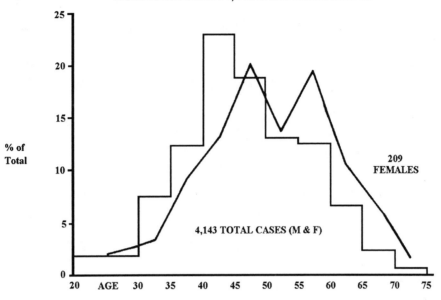

TABLE 903K2-1

DISTRIBUTION OF CASES BY RISK CLASS,
WITH AVERAGE AGE AND PROPORTION OF FEMALES

Risk Class	Distribution		Average Age	Proportion of Females
	Number	Proportion		
	ℓ	%	x	%
Standard	3,054	73.7	45.6	5.0
Rated Cardiovascular				
CV Alone	636	15.4	48.1	5.5
CV and Non CV	184	4.4	49.4	3.8
Total CV	820	19.8	48.4	5.1
Rated Non CV Alone	269	6.5	47.1	4.9
Total with Follow-up	4,143	100.0	46.2	5.0

TABLE 903K2-2

COMPARATIVE MORTALITY BY AGE AND SEX
CASES NOT RATED FOR CARDIOVASCULAR (CV) DISEASES

Age/Sex		No. of Cases	Exposure Person-yrs.	Number of Deaths		Mortality Ratio
				Observed	Expected*	
		ℓ	E	d	d'	100(d/d')
Age	20-39	743	9,695	25	26.5	94%
	40-49	1,342	17,842	83	117.3	71
	50-59	728	9,029	98	133.1	74
	60-74	241	2,715	50	72.6	69
Males		2,900	36,916	239	333.9	72
Females		154	2,005	17	15.6	109
Male and Female All Ages		3,054	38,921	256	349.5	73

* Basis of expected deaths: 1965-70 Select and Ultimate Tables, separate male and female rates.

275

TABLE 903K2-3

COMPARATIVE MORTALITY BY ASSOCIATED IMPAIRMENT CODE
CASES NOT RATED FOR CV DISEASE

Associated Code	No. of Cases	Exposure Person-yrs.	Number of Deaths		Mortality Ratio
			Observed	Expected*	
	ℓ	E	d	d′	100(d/d′)
3,054 STANDARD ISSUE CASES					
Minor CV—None	2,467	31,609	200	285.4	70%
Single	514	6,422	47	55.6	85
Multiple	73	890	9	9.10	99
Minor NCV—None	2,439	30,899	188	271.6	69
Single	554	7,240	58	71.5	81
Multiple	61	782	10	7.00	143
269 CASES RATED FOR NCV REASONS ONLY					
Major NCV—Single	233	2,731	20	25.40	79%
Multiple	36	407	9	4.31	209
All Cases	269	3,138	29	29.71	98

* Basis of expected deaths: 1965-70 Select and Ultimate Tables, separate male and female rates.

TABLE 903K2-4

COMPARATIVE MORTALITY BY RELATIVE HEART DIAMETER
CASES NOT RATED FOR CARDIOVASCULAR DISEASE

Relative Heart Diameter	No. of Cases	Exposure Person-yrs.	Number of Deaths		Mortality Ratio
			Observed	Expected*	
	ℓ	E	d	d′	100(d/d′)
3,054 STANDARD ISSUE CASES					
Under 90%[†]	414	5,292	32	39.0	82%
90-96%	1,012	12,674	89	104.2	85
97-104%	1,113	14,283	91	135.7	67
105% and up	525	6,817	48	72.6	68
269 CASES RATED FOR NCV REASONS ONLY					
Under 90%[†]	39	467	4	4.46	90%
90-96%	73	861	5	6.89	73
97-104%	115	1,333	15	12.80	117
105% and up	35	365	4	4.29	93

* Basis of expected deaths: 1965-70 Select and Ultimate Tables, separate male and female rates.

[†] Ratio (%) of observed diameter to diameter predicted from Clark-Ungerleider table.

TABLE 903K2-5

COMPARATIVE MORTALITY BY AGE AND RELATIVE HEART DIAMETER
ALL CASES RATED FOR CARDIOVASCULAR DISEASE

Relative Heart Diameter	Exposure Person-yrs.	Number of Deaths		Mortality Ratio	EDR
		Observed	Expected*		
	E	d	d′	100(d/d′)	1000(d–d′)/E
440 CASES AGE 20-49, MALE AND FEMALE COMBINED					
Under 90%†	709	4	3.80	105%	0.3
90-96%	1,342	12	6.97	172	3.7
97-104%	1,976	13	8.96	145	2.0
105% and up	1,164	11	5.54	199	4.7
380 CASES AGE 50-74, MALE AND FEMALE COMBINED					
Under 90%†	280	6	4.82	124%	4.2
90-96%	871	19	13.18	144	6.7
97-104%	1,631	46	28.20	163	11
105% and up	1,163	32	19.85	161	10

* Basis of expected deaths: 1965-70 Select and Ultimate Tables, separate male and female rates.

† Ratio (%) of observed diameter to diameter predicted from Clark-Ungerleider table.

TABLE 903K2-6

COMPARATIVE MORTALITY BY RELATIVE AORTIC WIDTH
AND CARDIOVASCULAR RATING, ALL AGES COMBINED

Aortic Width (Sheridan Index)	Exposure Person-yrs.	Number of Deaths		Mortality Ratio	EDR
		Observed	Expected*		
	E	d	d′	100(d/d′)	1000(d–d′)/E
3,054 STANDARD CASES (NO CV OR OTHER RATING)					
Under 87%†	7,143	59	71.6	82%	−1.8
87-94%	12,608	83	106.0	78	−1.8
95-102%	11,360	66	100.6	66	−3.0
103% and up	7,838	52	73.1	71	−2.7
820 CASES RATED FOR CV REASONS					
Under 87%†	1,377	30	13.9	216%	12
87-94%	2,665	34	23.8	143	3.8
95-102%	2,794	36	25.4	142	3.8
103% and up	2,300	43	26.3	164	7.3

* Basis of expected deaths: 1965-70 Select and Ultimate Tables, separate male and female rates.

† Ratio (%) of observed aortic width to predicted width in Sheridan Table, adjusted for difference from age 43.

TABLE 903K2-7

COMPARATIVE MORTALITY BY REASONS OF RATING
ALL CV-RATED CASES

Reason for Rating	No. of Cases	Exposure Person-yrs.	Number of Deaths		Mortality Ratio	EDR
			Observed	Expected*		
	ℓ	E	d	d′	100(d/d′)	1000(d–d′)/E
Valv. Cor. Ht. Dis.	83	1,042	10	9.09	110%	0.9
Hypertension	241	2,603	31	26.19	118	1.8
Stroke or Art. Dis.	27	308	11	5.41	203	18
ECG, Arrhythmia, etc.	211	2,551	33	25.34	130	3.0
All Single CV	566	6,542	86	66.37	130	3.0
Multiple CV	254	2,540	60	24.45	245	14
All CV without NCV	636	7,064	102	71.5	143	4.3
Both CV and NCV	184	2,018	44	19.3	228	12.2
Total CV-Rated	820	9,082	146	90.8	161	6.1

* Basis of expected deaths: 1965-70 Select and Ultimate Tables, separate male and female rates.

TABLE 903K2-8

COMPARATIVE MORTALITY BY ECG PATTERNS
ALL CASES RATED FOR CARDIOVASCULAR DISEASES

ECG Pattern	No. of Cases	Exposure Person-yrs.	Number of Deaths		Mortality Ratio	EDR
			Observed	Expected*		
	ℓ	E	d	d′	100(d/d′)	1000(d–d′)/E
No pattern code	272	3,191	31	30.7	101%	0.1
Total pattern codes	546	5,867	115	59.8	192	9.4
Q and QS Wave(s)	72	728	23	8.02	287	21
QRS Axis & Other†	61	582	17	5.89	289	19
ST Segment	53	504	12	3.91	307	16
Low T Waves (Minor)	171	1,879	27	19.86	136	3.8
Inverted T Waves (Major)	93	992	22	9.78	225	12
3 Rhythm & Cond. Codes**	92	1,135	13	11.53	113	1.3

* Basis of expected deaths: 1965-70 Select and Ultimate Tables, separate male and female rates.

† Excluding BBB and wide QRS patterns.

** BBB and wide QRS patterns, arrhythmias and abnormal AV conduction.

A STUDY OF 6,000 CHEST X-RAYS OBTAINED
FOR INSURANCE PURPOSES

M. Iréne Ferrer, M.D.

Investigation into the usefulness of chest X-rays obtained on insurance applicants is important, especially with regard to cost effectiveness. The present study was undertaken to obtain clinical information on a large, relatively healthy group of insurance applicants and, where possible, insurance data. All chest films were read by the author at the Equitable Life Assurance Society of America. The findings were divided into pulmonary and cardiovascular abnormalities. A previous survey of 4,962 chest X-rays was done but only heart diameter was evaluated.[1]

Results

6,000 chest X-rays were obtained on 6,000 applicants during the years 1975 and 1976. There was a large predominance of males — 88% of the applicants, a 7:1 ratio of males to females. An 11% incidence of abnormal X-rays was noted (660 of 6,000 X-rays).

Of the original 6,000 cases with chest X-rays, 4,209 (70%) were available for detailed study. Of the original 660 abnormal cases, 463 (70%) were also available and these form the data base of the abnormalities. There were 470 abnormalities found in 463 abnormal films as seven films had two abnormalities. Table 904K1-1 presents the pulmonary and cardiac diagnoses of the abnormalities. There were 312 cases, or 67% with pulmonary findings and 158 cases, or 33%, with cardiovascular abnormalities.

Pulmonary Diseases

The most common pulmonary abnormality — noted in 36.7% of the abnormal films — was bilateral enlargement of the hilar nodes (Table 904K1-1). Of the 170 cases with this finding, 141 (83%) had calcification in the nodes. This latter finding, or course, strongly suggests that the etiology of the calcified nodes was tuberculosis. Second in frequency in the pulmonary abnormalities was previous parenchymal pulmonary tuberculosis which was found in 55 cases, or 11.8%. If one adds these two groups together as tuberculosis, it is an impressive figure,

— 225 cases or 49% of the 463 abnormal X-rays and 72% of all the pulmonary abnormalities. Thus, in a set of 4,209 applicants with chest films, 225 cases (5.3%) had findings consistent with previous tuberculosis.

Diffuse pulmonary fibrosis was not rare — 39 cases, or 8.4%, were seen in the 463 abnormal chest films. Pulmonary fibrosis and emphysema, emphysema alone and chronic obstructive pulmonary disease (COPD) grouped together, occurred in 17 films (3.7% of the total 463) and kyphoscoliosis seen in 13 (2.8%). As shown in Table 904K1-1, smaller groups of abnormalities included nodular fibrotic disease, cancer of the lung, histoplasmosis, pleural effusion, thoracoplasty, diaphragmatic hernia, and bronchiectasis.

Cardiovascular Abnormalities

In 158 cases with cardiovascular abnormalities (Table 904K1-1) the most common was an enlarged heart which was noted in 78 cases (16.8% of 463 abnormal films). Cardiac enlargement was diagnosed when the heart's transverse diameter was 50% or more than the chest transverse diameter, — a figure recently reconfirmed as valid.[1] Almost as common — occurring in 14.0% of the abnormal films, were the 65 cases of calcification of the aortic knob. Surgical wires in the chest area from prior cardiac surgery, and dilated aorta were next, 8 and 6 cases respectively. There was one X-ray typical of congenital heart disease (interatrial septal defect with large pulmonary flow).

Thus in a group of 4,209 applicants with chest films available, cardiac enlargement was seen in 1.9% and calcified aortic knob in 1.5%.

Electrocardiographic Findings

In the 463 cases with abnormal chest X-rays, 262 also had an electrocardiogram taken and 73 of these ECGs were abnormal. The same male predominance, as seen in the overall study, prevailed as there were 70 men and 3 women with abnormal tracings. The 73 abnormal tracings, comprising 28% of 262 ECGs taken, were analyzed and tabulated (Table 904K1-2). In the 73 abnormal tracings, 81 abnormalities were seen as two deviations occasionally occurred in one ECG. The types of electrocardiographic abnormalities are listed in Table 904K1-2.

Source: M. I. Ferrer, "A Study of 6,000 Chest X-rays Obtained for Insurance Purposes," *J. Ins. Med.*, 14, no. 2 (1983): 12-14. Reproduced with permission of author and publisher.

The two most common ones were diffusely low T waves, occurring in 27 instances (37%), and combined ST-T abnormalities which were seen 11 times (15%). Complete right bundle branch block in 9 cases (12%), left ventricular hypertrophy with strain in 6 (8%), 5 cases of inferior myocardial infarction, 4 with incomplete right bundle branch block, 3 with anteroseptal myocardial infarction, 3 with ST depressions were also noted. One or two cases with premature beats of atrial, junctional or ventricular origin, two with prolonged PR, and one case each of complete heart block, intra-atrial block (wide P), pre-excitation of WPW type, left anterior fascicular block, complete the list.

Thus in 41 instances, or 56% of the abnormal ECGs, ST-T abnormalities were seen. Excluding the three children in the group of 262 applicants with electrocardiograms (ages 8, 10 and 10 years), the age range of the 259 adults was 23 to 75 years. The individuals age ranges seen with each abnormality are listed in Table 904K1-2.

Insurance Aspects

A study was made of 206 cases out of the total 463 with abnormal chest X-rays in whom detailed insurance information was obtainable. Of these 206, 86 (41.7%) had chest films taken because of age and amount requirements, and 120 (58.3%) had films taken because they were medically indicated from information on the applications.

Of 206 cases with abnormal films 150 (73%) had pulmonary findings — 77 of these had enlarged hilar nodes (a relatively unimportant finding as far as a rating is concerned), and 73 had other more important pulmonary findings. There also were 56 cases of cardiovascular abnormalities (27%).

Of 86 applicants (out of the 206 reviewed for insurance data) that had films because of age and amount requirements, 8, or 9.3%, were rated or declined because of X-ray findings alone. Of the 120 who had chest films taken because they were medically indicated, 23 (or 19.2%) were rated or declined because of X-ray findings alone. Of the total 206 abnormal cases, 31 applicants, or 15%, received insurance ratings or were declined based solely on the abnormal chest X-rays. The 206 abnormal cases were culled from a total of 2,527 cases who had films taken. It is evident therefore that there were 31 out of 2,527 X-rays taken, an incidence of 1.2% of all the X-rays taken, that proved to be important to insurance evaluation.

TABLE 904K1-1

DIAGNOSES IN 463 ABNORMAL CHEST X-RAYS

Diagnosis	Number (%)
PULMONARY (312 CASES)	
Bilateral enlarged hilar nodes	170 (36.7)
with calcification	141
without calcification	29
Pulmonary Tbc	55 (11.8)
Pulmonary Fibrosis	39 (8.4)
Pulmonary Fibrosis and Emphysema including COPD	17 (3.7)
Kyphoscoliosis	13 (2.8)
Nodular fibrotic disease	6 (1.3)
Cancer of lung	4 (0.86)
Histoplasmosis	2 (0.43)
Pleural effusion	2 (0.43)
Thoracoplasty	2 (0.43)
Diaphragmatic hernia	1 (0.22)
Bronchiectasis	1 (0.22)
CARDIAC (158 CASES)	
Enlarged Heart	78 (16.8)
Calcified Aortic Knob	65 (14.0)
Congenital Heart Disease	1 (0.22)
Dilated Aorta	6 (1.3)
Surgical wires in chest from cardiac surgery	8 (1.72)

TABLE 904K1-2

FINDINGS IN 73 ABNORMAL ELECTROCARDIOGRAMS

ECG Diagnosis	Number	Age Range (Years)
Diffuse T wave abnormality	27	31-74
ST-T abnormality	11	38-75
RBBB	9	10-62
LVH with strain	6	28-64
Inferior myoc. infarct.	5	50-57
Incomplete RBBB	4	49-57
Anteroseptal myoc. infarct.	3	50-55
ST depressions	3	33-58
Prolonged PR interval	2	30, 64
JPCs	2	53, 57
VPCs	2	47, 68
RBBB and LAFB (MLAD)	2	23, 32
APCs	1	59
Complete heart block	1	37
Intra-atrial block	1	54
WPW	1	41
LAFB (MLAD)	1	66

Abbreviations:
  RBBB = Right Bundle Branch Block
  JPCs = Junctional Premature Contractions
  LAFB (MLAD) = Left Anterior Fascicular Block (Marked Left Axis Deviation)
  VPCs = Ventricular Premature Contractions
  APCs = Atrial Premature Contractions
  LVH = Left Ventricular Hypertrophy

Discussion

This study provides some interesting clinical information on insurance applicants who had chest X-rays taken. Eleven percent of the films were abnormal, with pulmonary diseases twice as common (67% of the abnormal films) as the cardiovascular abnormalities (33%). Evidence of prior pulmonary tuberculosis was found to be frequent and occurred in 49% of the abnormal chest films and in 5.3% of all the chest X-rays (i.e. including normals) reviewed.

In almost 17% of the abnormal chest X-rays, cardiomegaly was noted and this represented about 2% of all the applicants who had films. Calcified aortic knobs were not uncommon in this group — a finding actuaries might review.

In reviewing electrocardiographic findings, 28% of the tracings were abnormal — a figure to be stressed in evaluating these applicants. The non-specific ECG abnormalities of ST and T waves accounted for 52% of the deviations, while the more serious ECG defects (complete right bundle branch block, left ventricular hypertrophy, myocardial infarction — 23 of 73) made up 32% of the total deviations from normal.

The study of insurance ratings and their origins indicated that ratings and declines are much more common (19.2% versus 9.3%) in the group where the X-rays were medically indicated as contrasted to those taken for age and amount — a difference to be expected. However, only 15% of the abnormal chest films produced negative insurance results, i.e. a rating or decline. Furthermore it was shown that only 1.2% of all the chest X-rays taken proved to be important in affecting an insurance decision. This suggests that chest X-rays may not be very cost effective.

Conclusions

1. A survey of 6,000 chest X-rays obtained for insurance purposes, revealed an 11% incidence of abnormal films.

2. Pulmonary findings were twice as frequent as cardiovascular findings, with evidence of previous tuberculosis being seen quite often.

3. Two percent of these applicants had enlarged hearts.

4. Of the abnormalities found on electrocardiograms, 32% were of a serious nature.

5. Only 15% of the abnormal chest films affected ratings or declines and only 1.2% of the entire group of chest X-rays reviewed for insurance data had any value in insurance evaluations — a point to be made when considering cost effectiveness.

Acknowledgments

The author wishes to thank William A. Canfield, Vice President, Underwriting; Wilson M. Lee, Manager, Research Section; Maribelle L. Denegall, Research Assistant, of the Equitable Life Assurance Society of America for their help in analyzing the insurance data.

REFERENCES

1. F. J. Siber, A. E. Brown, R. B. Singer, F. I. Pitkin, "A Cardiovascular Survey of the Chest X-ray in Nearly 5,000 Life Insurance Applicants: Normal Standards and Distribution Curves for Relative Heart Diameter," *Trans. Assoc. Life Insur. Med. Dir. Amer.*, 63 (1979): 159-74.

ASYMPTOMATIC HYPERCALCEMIA: RATABLE HYPERPARATHYROIDISM OR BENIGN ANOMALY OF SERUM CHEMISTRY?

Richard B. Singer, M.D.

Limits of normal values for common constituents of blood or plasma have always intrigued my interest since the years long ago when I taught biochemistry to medical students. It is an oversimplification to determine the mean ±2 standard deviations from a series of values on supposedly normal subjects without critical evaluation of the subjects as to their physiological status and absence of occult disease that might affect the variable under study. Yet this is the way many normal limits are determined, and normal ranges are apt to be carried over from one text or reference book to another without critical examination of the source, conditions and reliability of the data. All physicians know that a blood glucose level cannot be interpreted without knowledge of the time relation of the blood sample to the last meal (or test dose of glucose). But do all physicians remember that most glucose determinations these days are carried out with an automated machine such as the Autoanalyzer, and that serum used in these machines gives results about 15 per cent higher than in whole blood? Solutes such as glucose and urea are distributed between serum (or plasma) and red cells in accordance with the water content, which is considerably higher in serum (93 per cent) than in the red cells (about 72 per cent). To test you, the reader, a little further, are you aware that blood volume is 10 per cent or more higher when a subject is recumbent for at least one-half hour than when up and about? Normal limits for constituents to which the capillary wall is impermeable (red cells, plasma proteins) should therefore be at least 10 per cent lower for bed patients than for office patients under customary procedures for blood sampling.

These reflections were brought to mind when I read an interesting epidemiological report, "Primary Hyperparathyroidism" in the January 24, 1980 number of the *New England Journal of Medicine*.[1] The authors used records of residents of Rochester, Minnesota from the Rochester-Olmsted Epidemiology Project (for details see the article) to obtain the annual incidence of primary hyperparathyroidism in the period 1/1/65 to 12/31/76. The average population at risk was 50,000. Through June 1974 serum calcium was available only on specific physician request, and 39 cases were confirmed, with an average annual incidence rate of 7.8 per 100,000 unadjusted, or 8.8 adjusted to the age distribution of the U.S. population. However, serum calcium became available on July 1, 1974 as part of a 12-channel serum chemistry panel carried out on most hospitalized and clinic patients. From that date until the end of 1976, a much shorter period, 51 cases were documented, with an annual incidence of 37.1 per 100,000 (42.1 age-adjusted as before). Incidence rates increased with age, and were higher in females than in males, as shown in the table below. For older patients, age 60 up, the annual incidence since July 1974 was estimated to be 92 per 100,000 in men and more than twice this rate, 188 per 100,000 in women. Criteria used for diagnosis were one or more of: histological evidence in parathyroid tissue (adenoma or hyperplasia); serum calcium over 10.1 mg. per deciliter (dl.) and pathognomonic X-ray signs, and/or elevated serum immuno-reactive parathyroid hormone (iPTH); hypercalcemia for more than one year without another cause despite careful evaluation.

Annual Incidence Rates for Primary Hyperparathyroidism

Age/Sex	No. of Cases	Rate per 100,000
1/1/65 to 6/30/74		
Under 40	7	2.0
40-59	15	16.5
60 up	17	25.6
All male	13	5.7
All female	26	9.5
Total	39	7.8
7/1/74 to 12/31/76		
Under 40	6	6.4
40-59	17	68
60 up	28	154
All male	11	92
All female	40	188
Total	51	37.1

Source: R. B. Singer, "Asymptomatic Hypercalcemia: Ratable Hyperparathyroidism or Benign Anomaly of Serum Chemistry?" *J. Ins. Med.*, 11, no. 2 (1980): 4-6. Reproduced with permission of author and publisher.

The distribution of serum calcium values was not affected after the start of routine calcium measurements. The normal range was 8.9 to 10.1 mg./dl. Of the 84 cases with calcium values recorded (the other six cases were diagnosed at autopsy) 48 percent did not exceed 10.5 mg./dl., 31 percent were in the range 10.6-11.0, 12 percent 11.1-11.5, and only 9 percent from 11.6-13.0. Of the 39 cases diagnosed prior to July, 1974, 32 had one or more complications or concomitants of primary hyperparathyroidism, whereas this was true in fewer than one half (25 of 51 cases) of those diagnosed more recently, when routine serum calcium measurements were available. This difference was statistically significant ($p<0.005$). The percentage of cases with hypercalcemia, above 10.1, as the principal diagnostic determinant, either confirmed over a year or with elevated immuno-reactive hormone, but without clinical manifestations, therefore, rose from 18 to 51 percent after the start of routine serum calcium determination. The most frequent clinical finding was urinary tract stone, found in 51 percent of cases before July, 1974, but in only 4 percent of subsequent cases. The percentage differences were much smaller and not statistically significant for other less frequent findings such as hypercalciuria, osteoporosis, or parathyroid bone disease, and complications such as history of psychiatric disorder, peptic ulcer, or pancreatitis. The relative risk of definite hypertension was found to be 1.98 in primary hyperparathyroidism versus its prevalence in 450 matched case controls. The difference was statistically significant for definite hypertension, but not for definite and borderline hypertension combined.

How should one handle the underwriting of an insurance applicant with a medical report giving an abnormally elevated serum calcium of 11.0 mg./dl., for example? Should this be handled as a case of primary hyperparathyroidism, thus excluding the possibility of standard issue? Assuming the absence of a definite diagnosis of primary hyperparathyroidism supported by other definite clinical confirmation, what can the medical underwriter do to come to a reasonable classification? I doubt if skeletal X-rays or metabolic studies such as urinary calcium output per day could be requested and paid for as part of an underwriting work-up, even for a very large amount application. However, other useful things could be required by the underwriter. A current serum calcium could be obtained, and perhaps an assay of iPTH as well, if justified by the amount of insurance. The medical history should be carefully rechecked for depression, psychosis, severe neurosis, peptic ulcer, pancreatitis, and especially renal stone. Any of these conditions would greatly increase the probability that the high serum calcium does represent primary hyperparathyroidism and should be rated accordingly. Further, urine speci-

mens should be carefully re-examined, and renal function assessed, if possible, with renal function tests (unfortunately this is rarely done on insurance applicants), or blood urea nitrogen or serum creatinine. What if the recheck serum calcium is still elevated, say 10.5 to 11.0 mg./dl., but all other findings are negative? Should we rate for the high serum calcium as an isolated abnormality of serum chemistry? My own inclination would be to regard this as a relatively minor risk factor and consider the applicant as borderline standard if there are no other major risk factors present and not more than one or two minor ones.

This liberal attitude is based partly on the knowledge that unexplained deviations from "normal" standards in apparently healthy persons are much more common than we suppose. For example, biochemical profiles on 1,000 periodic health examinations at the Metropolitan were analyzed and reported in the *Statistical Bulletin*.[2] Out of the 1,000 Technicon Autoanalyzer reports 748 were negative (within normal limits). Of the 252 positive or abnormal profiles there were 24 leading to a new confirmed diagnosis (11 cases of disease and 13 of a pathophysiological biochemical syndrome such as hypercholesterolemia), 38 confirmatory of a pre-existing disease, but 190 "unclassified, without any clear-cut diagnostic significance." Two of the 24 new positives were diagnosed as hyperparathyroidism, so many other serum constituents in addition to calcium were involved. To quote the report: "Most of the findings in the unclassified positive cases were slightly outside the normal limits as defined by previous studies. No clinical evidence of disease was found nor had disease developed in the course of the two ensuing years. *Most of the unclassified positive findings appear to be the result of the statistical criteria chosen to define the 'normal' range.*" The medical director and senior underwriter of any company that uses a biochemical profile as a routine supplement to their paramedical examination should realize they may anticipate about 20 percent "unclassified positive" results, which outnumber confirmed positives at least four to one. This may lead to delay and expense in trying to distinguish true from (probably) false "positives," or to carelessness in the handling of significant abnormalities. To me, these are both undesirable consequences of using the biochemical profile as a screening substitute for a full physician's examination. Perhaps others disagree, and readers of the *Journal of Insurance Medicine* might like to hear more about actual underwriting experience with paramedical examinations supplemented by a biochemical profile.

One other encouragement to adopt a liberal attitude on isolated hypercalcemia may be found in an earlier report from the Mayo Clinic, entitled "Treatment of Primary Hyperparathyroidism."[3] The authors, Purnell et al., recommended four treatment categories based on more than 500 patients managed at the Mayo Clinic. There were 475 patients surgically treated for primary hyperparathyroidism (abnormal parathyroid found in 90 percent, none found in 10 percent), 14 patients were re-explored because of unsuccessful initial operation and 22 patients had to be treated medically. However, the remaining group of 147 patients consisted of asymptomatic and uncomplicated hyperparathyroidism, on whom follow-up was initiated by Dr. Keating in 1968. These patients had a serum calcium under 11.0 mg./dl., but an abnormal iPTH initially, without any of the other diagnostic criteria for hyperparathyroidism. After five years of intensive follow-up 29 patients had been surgically explored with successful resection of parathyroid lesions in all but two, 27 had dropped out of regular re-examination, 6 had died of causes "not directly attributable" to hyperparathyroidism, and 85 were in apparently good health. No patient developed a hypercalcemic crisis. This can be regarded,

I think, as a generally favorable experience in an exposure of roughly 685 patient-years with only 6 apparently unrelated deaths in an older age group (see preceding table), and no deaths in the 29 patients who did come to parathyroid surgical exploration.

The Mayo Clinic reports therefore provide encouragement to adopt a liberal underwriting attitude towards asymptomatic insurance applicants with elevated serum calcium 10.2-11.0 mg./dl. if they have none of the other findings that corroborate a diagnosis of primary hyperparathyroidism. A persistently elevated serum calcium above 11.0 perhaps should be treated with more caution. Serum calcium is only one of the constituents in the biochemical profiles so frequently done these days. Collectively, "positive" results of one or more constituents on routine screening may occur in 25 percent of active, working individuals, and most, but not all, of these are probably without clinical or underwriting significance.

REFERENCES

1. H. Heath, III, S. F. Hodgdson, M. A. Kennedy, "Primary Hyperparathyroidism-Incidence, Morbidity and Potential Economic Impact in a Community," *N. Engl. J. Med.*, 302 (January 24, 1980): 189-93.

2. Anon., "Detecting Diseases by Biochemistry of Blood," *Stat. Bull.*, 52 (Sept. 1971): 5-7.

3. D. C. Purnell, D. A. Scholz, L. H. Smith, et al., "Treatment of Primary Hyperparathyroidism," *Am. J. Med.*, 56 (1974): 800-9.

MORTALITY ASSOCIATED WITH SERUM ALBUMIN LEVEL

Richard B. Singer, M.D.

Reference:

A. Phillips, A. G. Shaper, P. H. Whincup, "Association Between Serum Albumin and Mortality from Cardiovascular Disease, Cancer and Other Causes," *Lancet* II (Dec. 16, 1989): 1434-36.

Object of the Study: To identify possible mortality association with any serum biochemical factors measured by the Technicon SMA 12/60 Autoanalyzer in a prospective study of British men age 40-59 years.

Subjects Studied: In the British Regional Heart Study 7,735 men age 40-59 were drawn at random from the age/sex registers of a single general practice in each of 24 towns in England, Scotland and Wales, in 1978-80. Data collected included completion of a health and lifestyle questionnaire by a research nurse, blood pressure, forced expiratory volume at 1 second (FEV1), and a blood sample for analysis of serum total cholesterol and about 20 hematological and biochemical factors. All blood samples were sent to the Wolfson Research Laboratories, Birmingham, and were analyzed within 12-36 hours of venipuncture, with use of the Technicon SMA 12/60 Autoanalyzer for determination of the biochemical factors, including serum albumin. In addition to age, serum albumin, serum total cholesterol, blood pressure, smoking history, and FEV1, men were classified into one of the Register General's six social classes, and by the presence or absence of "pre-existing disease." The latter was considered present if the subject reported prior diagnosis by a doctor of any of the following: angina, heart attack, coronary thrombosis, myocardial infarction, "other heart trouble," high blood pressure, stroke, diabetes, peptic ulcer, gout, gall bladder disease, thyroid disease, arthritis, bronchitis, asthma, or other condition requiring surgery; pre-existing disease was also considered present if the subject reported current regular treatment by a physician for any condition. Mean age and age distribution data are not given in the article, but age was one of the factors used for the statistical adjustment of the crude mortality rates derived from the follow-up observations.

Follow-up: Subjects were followed up to 1988 for mortality through each general practice and through death certificates obtained from the National Health Services Central Registry. Serum albumin data were missing in 45 subjects, so the total group was reduced to 7,690 men. Follow-up was 99% complete. Average follow-up was 9.2 years (range 8.2-10.2 years).

Statistical Methods: Mortality results are presented in the form of mean annual mortality rates per 1000 per year, both tabular and graphical, for three cause of death categories (CV, cancer, all other) and total deaths, for six subgroups of serum albumin concentration, for the total group and for subdivisions by a combination of other factors and serum albumin. Mortality rates are given as crude rates (presumably d/E for each cell, all durations combined, although neither details nor data are given), and rates adjusted for mortality effects of variations in age, social class, town of residence, cigarette smoking habit, systolic blood pressure, serum total cholesterol, and FEV1. Mortality rate adjustments were made by use of a multiple logistic regression model. A measure called the "standardized relative odds," associated with a standard deviation, is presented for serum albumin, a decimal less than one, since the association of mortality rate with albumin concentration is an inverse one. Statistical significance of this odds ratio and correlation coefficients is given in the form of conventional p values. Numbers of entrants are given for the serum albumin subgroups. Numbers of deaths and entrants are given for some other risks factor divisions and for the total group, permitting approximation of a few crude mortality rates not specified in the article. In the absence of age data, the "expected" mortality rate for use in the abstract table on mortality rate associated with serum albumin has been derived from ℓ, d, and mean follow-up (FU) of 9.2 years for the total group, the derived E value being adjusted for 99% FU.

Results: There were significant cross-correlations observed between serum albumin concentration and other mortality risk factors. Table 983K1-1 shows correlation coefficients and whether the association is direct or inverse for the measures of age, serum total cholesterol, systolic blood pressure and FEV1. All of the correlation coefficients are highly significant ($p<0.0001$). Serum albumin decreases with increasing age (inverse association), but increases with the numerical units for the other

Source: R. B. Singer, "Mortality Associated with Serum Albumin Level," *J. Ins. Med.*, 22 (1990): 57-59. Reproduced with permission of author and publisher.

three variables. However, the mortality association is more complex, because mortality increases with age, blood pressure and cholesterol, but increases as FEV1 *decreases*. The need for adjustment of the crude mortality rate in each albumin subgroup is obvious. The mean serum albumin concentration also changed significantly with social class number and from town to town.

The range of serum albumin concentration was 30 to 57 grams per Liter, with a mean of 44.6 and an SD of ±2.55 g./L. Table 983K1-2 shows the distribution of serum albumin concentration in the 7,690 men, with adjusted mean annual mortality rate per 1000 ($\bar{q}$), and comparative mortality derived from the total group mortality, $\bar{q}=\bar{q}'=d/E$. The value for d is given as 643 deaths in one of the tables, and includes 323 CV, 224 cancer, and 96 other deaths. The value for E is a close estimate, derived as the product of a mean duration of 9.2 years and 99% of the total ℓ of 7,690 (because FU was reported to be only 99% complete). The E values for the individual subgroups of albumin concentration are rough approximations, enclosed in parentheses, because the mean FU duration in each subgroup without doubt varied somewhat about the mean duration of 9.2 years for the total. It is also possible to estimate d as $E/\bar{q}$, but these are also rough approximations, not comparable to the exact total of 643 deaths for the entire series. It is evident that adjusted mortality decreased with increasing albumin concentration, from 20.3 deaths per 1000 per year for the 2.4% of men with serum albumin under 40 g./L., down to an annual minimum of 5.0 per 1000. The range of unadjusted (crude) mean annual mortality rate was even greater, from 26.2 to 4.4 per 1000. Because of the age and other adjustments the value of the crude mean annual $\bar{q}$ of 9.2 per 1000 per year found for the total group is equal precisely to the constant value of adjusted $\bar{q}'$, 9.2 per 1000, in each of the albumin subgroups. Since this use of an aggregate $\bar{q}'$ results in some subgroups with excess mortality and some with mortality below the aggregate mean, the range of mortality ratio was from 220% to 54%, and the range of EDR (excess death rate) from +11.1 to a minimum of −4.2 per 1000 per year, indeed a wide range of mortality rate. The standardized odds ratio was reported as 0.66, with a highly significant *p* value <0.0001. Adjusted rates for deaths in each of the cause categories were also reported, and showed a similar inverse association with albumin concentration; the respective *p* values were <0.0001 or 0.0001. Tables similar to Table 983K1-2 have not been constructed for these cause of death results. The authors excluded the experience of the first 5 years, and on the experience from 5 to 10.2 years they found a *p* value still >0.0001 for the 369 total deaths remaining, 0.003 for the 158 CV deaths,

0.0002 for the 143 cancer deaths, but only 0.13 for the 48 other deaths. The highly significant association therefore persisted after 5 years duration for the CV, cancer and total adjusted mortality rates, but not for all other causes of death.

It was also possible to derive crude mortality rates for two other risk factors: smoking and pre-existing disease. These are compared with crude mortality rates in three categories of serum albumin concentration in Table 983K1-3. For "expected" mortality the lowest rate has been used for each risk factor, about 4.4 per 1000 per year in all of them. Mortality ratios on this basis were 305% for 2,556 men with serum albumin <44 g./L. versus men with the highest serum albumin, 280% for 3,161 current smokers versus men who never smoked, and 260% for men with pre-existing disease versus those without this factor. Only 33% of the men did not have evidence of pre-existing disease as defined in this study. With this division of serum albumin concentration the maximum excess mortality, both MR and EDR, is greater for the serum albumin than for it is for current smokers, a point stressed by the authors.

Comment: I am grateful to Ed Lew for ferreting out this interesting recent article and sending me a photocopy. Such a strong inverse association between serum albumin and mortality was an unexpected finding, for which no plausible hypothesis was offered. Serum albumin is synthesized in the liver; low levels may be found in a long list of conditions involving nutritional problems and debilitating diseases. As the authors point out, a low serum albumin is usually noted by a physician as an incidental finding adding little or nothing to the differential diagnosis of a patient, because of its nonspecific character. The authors also stress that this unexpected finding must be treated with caution because no confirmation is yet available, no causal hypothesis has been proven or even suggested, and a coincidental association has not been ruled out. Also, there is no evidence as to whether a similar association is found in women. In spite of these reservations the findings reported here raise intriguing questions for life insurance medicine, because results of an SMA biochemical profile, including the serum albumin, are frequently available to the underwriter, who, through the results of this abstract, now possesses knowledge that relative mortality is higher when serum albumin is low but within a range previously regarded as normal. There is an urgent need for confirmation and further study. Let us hope that Mr. Woodman's committee developing plans for an intercompany study of test results on life insurance policyholders will include serum albumin as one of the biochemical factors to be investigated.

TABLE 983K1-1

SERUM ALBUMIN ASSOCIATION WITH OTHER RISK FACTORS IN BRITISH REGIONAL HEART STUDY, SAMPLE OF MEN AGE 40-59

Risk Factor or Category	Serum Alb. Change with Risk Factor	Correl. Coeffic.	Statist. Signif.
	Increase	(r)	(p)
Age (40 to 59)	Decrease	−0.22	<0.0001
Serum total Chol.	Increase	+0.22	<0.0001
Systolic BP	Increase	+0.09	<0.0001
FEV1 (Forced Exp. (Vol. at 1 Sec.)	Increase	+0.20	<0.0001

TABLE 983K1-2

MEAN ANNUAL MORTALITY RATE IN BRITISH REGIONAL HEART STUDY, SAMPLE OF MEN AGE 40-59, BY SERUM ALBUMIN. RATE ADJUSTED FOR AGE AND OTHER RISK FACTORS*

Serum Albumin	No. of Men	Distribution	Exposure (Estimated)	No. of Deaths	Mean Adj. Ann. Mort. Rate per 1000			Mort. Ratio
					Observed	Total	Excess	
g/L	ℓ	%	E	d	$\bar{q}$	$\bar{q}'$	$(\bar{q}-\bar{q}')$	$100(\bar{q}-\bar{q}')$
30-39.9	187	2.4	(1,700)**	No data	20.3	9.2	11.1	220%
40-41.9	654	8.5	(5,950)**	"	11.6	9.2	2.4	126
42-43.9	1,715	22.3	(15,610)**	"	11.4	9.2	2.2	124
44-45.9	2,416	31.4	(21,980)**	"	8.7	9.2	−0.5	95
46-47.9	1,854	24.1	(16,940)**	"	7.8	9.2	−1.4	85
48-57	864	11.3	(7,860)**	"	5.0	9.2	−4.2	54
Total	7,960	100.0	70,040††	643	9.2†	9.2†	(0)	(100)

* Adjusted for differences from distributions in the total group with respect to age, social class, town of residence, smoking habits, systolic blood pressure, serum total cholesterol, and FEV1.

† Basis of expected mortality: $\bar{q}'=\bar{q}=d/E$.

** Approximate estimate (E)=(0.99ℓ)(9.2). Average duration is an approximation of the 9.2 years for the total group. Follow-up 99% complete.

†† E estimated as (9.2)(0.99ℓ), rounded off. Average duration is 9.2 years.

TABLE 983K1-3

CRUDE MORTALITY RATES ASSOCIATED WITH SERUM ALBUMIN, SMOKING HISTORY, AND PRE-EXISTING DISEASE. LOWEST MORTALITY CLASS USED AS STANDARD

Category	No. of Men	Estimated Exposure*	Estimated No. Dths.†	Mean Ann. Mort. Rate per 1000			Mort. Ratio
				Observed	Lowest	Excess	
	ℓ	E	d	$\bar{q}$	$\bar{q}'$	$(\bar{q}-\bar{q}')$	$100(\bar{q}-\bar{q}')$
Serum Alb.							
<44g/L	2,556	23,260	312	13.4	4.4	9.0	305%
44-47.9	4,270	38,920	297	7.6	4.4	3.2	173
48-57.9	864	7,860	34	4.4	4.4	(0)	(100)
Smoking Hist.							
Current	3,161	28,790	361	12.5	4.5	8.0	280
Ex-smoker	2,701	24,600	208	8.5	4.5	4.0	189
Never48-57	1,812	16,500	74	4.5	4.5	(0)	(100)
Pre-existing Disease							
Yes	5,095	46,410	528	11.4	4.4	7.0	260
No	2,595	23,610	115	4.4	4.4	(0)	(100)

* Approximate estimate, E=(9.2)(0.99ℓ)

† d = reported data for smoking history and pre-existing disease. For serum albumin subgroups, approximate d estimated as 1000E/$\bar{q}$.

THE PROTECTIVE VALUE OF PROSTATE SPECIFIC ANTIGEN (PSA) TESTING

Richard L. Bergstrom, F.S.A.

Introduction

The purpose of this paper is to estimate the protective value of Prostate Specific Antigen (PSA) testing in the underwriting process for individual life insurance.

Selected life insurance pricing assumptions and data published in other external resources are used to measure the estimated present value (over a ten-year period) of excess prostate cancer mortality in male age groups 50-59 and 60-69. Assumed incidence rates of applicants testing positive for PSA values greater than 20 ng./ml. (based on actual test data from Home Office Reference Laboratory) are then used to calculate a return on investment (ROI), which is the discount rate which equates the cost of testing to the expected savings in mortality realized from the testing results. The approach for this study parallels that used in a research paper submitted to HORL in 1989 entitled "A Report on The Protective Value of Laboratory Testing."[1]

Assumptions

Mortality

One of the most important assumptions in this study is the mortality associated with prostate cancer. Survival rates from the National Cancer Institute's Surveillance, Epidemiology, and End Results (SEER) program, were used in developing an appropriate mortality table. The SEER program is population based and has maintained a substantial number of clinical patients with 10 years of follow-up medical surveillance. These results were published in the *CA-A Cancer Journal for Clinicians*, January/February 1989.[2]

Table 984K1-1 shows the SEER Survival Rates for prostate cancer.

TABLE 984K1-1

SEER SURVIVAL RATES FOR PROSTATE CANCER

Age Group	5-Year Rates Observed	Relative	10-Year Rates Observed	Relative
55-59	65.2%	71.6%	43.6%	55.1%
60-64	64.2	73.8	38.9	54.8
65-69	59.0	72.3	33.3	55.0

Source: R. L. Bergstrom, "The Protective Value of Prostate Specific Antigen (PSA) Testing," *J. Ins. Med.*, 22 (1990): 300-1. Reproduced with permission of author and publisher.

The observed survival rate (at five or 10 years) provides an estimate of the proportion of the original group of patients who survived the selected length of time. The observed rate does not account for survival "free-of-disease," but only for survival overall. The relative survival rate is an estimate of the chance of escaping death due to cancer (for five or 10 years). The relative rate, the ratio of the observed survival rate to a general-population survival rate, is an indirect adjustment for deaths due to causes other than cancer.

The mortality associated with the above SEER Survival Rates can be closely approximated by using U.S. population mortality plus 55 extra deaths per 1000. Table 984K1-2 shows survival rates under this assumption:

TABLE 984K1-2

1980 U. S. POPULATION MORTALITY PLUS 55 DEATHS PER 1000 PER YEAR

Age	5-Year Rates Projected	Relative	10-Year Rates Projected	Relative
55	69.7%	75.0%	46.5%	56.2%
65	62.9	74.6	36.1	55.4

For our analysis, standard insured mortality is assumed to be 95% of the 1975-80 Select and Ultimate Table, Male, age last birthday. Standard insured mortality plus 55 extra deaths per 1000 per year is assumed for applicants who would otherwise be standard, but have PSA values above 20 ng./ml.

Incidence Rates

As the PSA test is relatively new to life insurance company underwriting practices, a large base of tested data regarding incidence rates for PSA values in excess of 20 ng./ml. currently does not exist. However, using what data is available from HORL's historical database, initial test results of PSA values provide a starting point for calculating preliminary protective values. Thus the HORL data indicate that about 0.3% of 50-59 year-old males and about 0.7% of 60-69 year-old males are reasonable initial assumptions.

Persistency

The following lapse rates were used in projecting death claims:

TABLE 984K1-3

Duration	Lapse Rate
1	25%
2	15
3	12
4	10
5 & over	8

Present Value of Mortality Differences

Using the above assumptions, we developed the present values of death benefits for both standard insureds and for insureds with prostate cancer. Table 984K1-4 shows present values of death benefits for males ages 50-59 and 60-69 over a 10-year period:

TABLE 984K1-4

PRESENT VALUE AT 8% OF DEATH BENEFITS PER $1,000 APPLIED FOR

	Male Ages 50-59	Male Ages 60-69
Prostate Cancer Mortality	$206.85	$225.78
Less: Standard Mortality	21.65	49.40
Excess mortality cost of Prostate Cancer	$185.20	$176.38

Certain literature indicates that males over age 50 with a PSA value ≥10 ng./ml. are at high risk of having or developing prostate cancer. However, in order to present a conservative estimate of the cost benefit associated with testing all males over age 50 for PSA, we assumed that applicants with PSA values below 20 ng./ml. will exhibit standard insured mortality and that applicants with PSA values above 20 ng./ml. will exhibit prostate cancer mortality.

According to a paper entitled "PSA as a Marker for Prostatic Cancer" by Daniel W. Chan, Ph.D (Associate professor of laboratory medicine at Johns Hopkins), published in *Laboratory Management*, the specificity of PSA values greater than 20 ng./ml. in detecting prostate cancer was 100%.[3] Thus, no false positives have been assumed in this study. Note that the sensitivity for PSA values greater than 20 ng./ml. is 21% in Chan's paper. This means that among 100 people having the disease, only 21 test positive at a level greater than 20 ng./ml. Because the sensitivity increases as the PSA test cutoff level is reduced, additional protective value (not assumed in this study) could be achieved by obtaining additional underwriting information (medical exams, APS, etc.) for applicants with PSA values from 10-20 ng./ml. or even lower.

Using the excess mortality cost of prostate cancer from Table 984K1-4, it is possible to develop the present value of mortality savings from PSA screening for several amounts of insurance for age groups 50-59 and 60-69. These values are derived by multiplying Table 984K1-4 values by the assumed incidence rate and by the face amounts applied for.

TABLE 984K1-5

PRESENT VALUE AT 8% OF MORTALITY SAVINGS FROM PSA SCREENING

Amount of Insurance	Ages 50-59	Ages 60-69
$ 25,000	$13.89	$30.87
50,000	27.78	61.73
100,000	55.56	123.47
150,000	83.34	185.20

The values derived above are directly dependent on the assumed incidence rates of applicants testing positive for PSA values in excess of 20 ng./ml. As incidence data provided by HORL were based (necessarily) on a limited number of test results, actual results achieved by a life insurance company may vary from those illustrated in this paper.

Return on Investment

In the previous section, values shown were in terms of the present value of mortality savings for various amounts of insurance applied for. This section describes what that means in terms of return on the investment to an insurance company per dollar of cost.

If one views the cost of testing as an investment, with future returns on the investment equal to potential mortality savings over a period of time, it is possible to determine an interest rate (i.e., an ROI) which equates both sides of the equation.

Table 984K1-6 illustrates the return on investment (ROI) over 10 policy years from PSA testing at various policy sizes for age groups 50-59 and 60-69, assuming a marginal PSA testing cost of $10 per applicant and a $0 collection cost, since presumably PSA testing will be performed in addition to a routine blood chemistry profile.

TABLE 984K1-6

RETURN ON INVESTMENT FROM PSA SCREENING

Male Age Group	Policy Size			
	$25,000	$50,000	$100,000	$150,000
50-59	18%	60%	157%	276%
60-69	74	193	531	1,026

As the reader can see from Table 984K1-6, a company utilizing PSA testing on applications as low as $25,000 is still receiving an ROI of 18% at age group 50-59. The ROI increases substantially at older ages and for larger policy sizes, since the value of the test increases substantially whereas the cost remains the same. The reader should be aware that the above values assume that the prostate condition could not be uncovered by a company's standard underwriting procedures. This is obviously not true in 100% of the cases. However, even if the identification of a prostate condition is found solely by utilizing the PSA test in only 50% of all applicants, the ROI values are still quite substantial. For example, if the savings attributable to the test is only 50%, the values shown above for a policy size of $50,000 would then correspond to a policy size of $100,000. Similarly, values shown for a policy size of $25,000, would then be appropriate for a policy size of $50,000. Further, such values would increase if the duration of study were extended beyond 10 years.

Summary

The protective value an insurer will actually receive will be dependent on its own underwriting practices, products, markets, etc. However, this study illustrates that a substantial return on investment might be obtained when all males applicants over the age of 50 are tested for PSA values.

REFERENCES

1. R. L. Bergstrom, *A Report on the Protective Value of Laboratory Testing*, August 1989.

2. M. H. Myers, L. A. G. Ries, "Cancer Patient Survival Rates: SEER Program Results for 10 Years of Follow-up," *CA-A Cancer Journal for Clinicians* (Jan./Feb. 1989): 21-32.

3. D. W. Chan, "PSA as a Marker for Prostatic Cancer," *Laboratory Management*, 26, no. 1 (Jan., 1988): 35-39.

IS PSA GOOD FOR INSURANCE?

William H. Alexander, M.D.

Dear Editor:

In my opinion, some life insurance and reinsurance companies appear to be moving towards acceptance of and even promotion of Prostate Specific Antigen (PSA) testing on a routine basis for older age male applicants. This is unfortunate, since it will propel others, even if they disagree about the use of such tests, to follow their lead or risk adverse selection. We are told that PSA is what the top-notch urologists recommend and that PSA has proven itself cost-effective for insurance purposes, that it is a test well worth performing. Why am I unconvinced? Why are my "senses" assaulted by the marketing of this test to the life insurance industry?

First of all, my *business* sense tells me not to remove these and other oft-screened individuals from the standard pool. *Medical* sense tells me *not* to perform a tumor marker screen on this asymptomatic population — it is inappropriate and the workup done on the false positives is potentially harmful. An *ethical* sense tells me not to simply dismiss abnormal values *once* found, even if under the magical 10ng.% level — this will be dangerous

for some too. Finally, *common* sense demands that issues such as consent and counseling, industry public image, and equity for the insurance buying applicant should *not* be made subordinate to the quest for "cost effectiveness."

Why does the pressure to do apolipoprotein and fructosamine levels, urine amphetamine and adulterant screens, and now PSA determinations make me feel like we are riding successive waves of some laboratory marketing typhoon and that the next wave or the one after that will crash us all down upon the public shoals and regulatory shores?

The public talks of "discrimination;" we in the industry prefer the term "equitable risk selection." Equity can not mean profitability, solely; common sense can not lose out to dollars and cents, always; and corporate Medical Directors must retain some medical sense too, including a "sense" of advocacy for the person behind the application.

Very truly yours,

William H. Alexander, M.D.
Stamford, CT

Source: W. H. Alexander, "Is PSA Good for Insurance?" *J. Ins. Med.*, 22 (1990): 310. Reproduced with permission of author and publisher.

CONTRIBUTOR INDEX

SUBJECT INDEX

REFERENCE LIST

CONTRIBUTOR INDEX

SUBJECT INDEX

Note: Three numerical entries are used in this index. A **number** without any accompanying letters (e.g., 111) gives the **page** number on which the subject entry may be found. A **number preceded by the acronym "cd"** gives the classification **code** or range of codes for the subject entry (e.g., Accidental death, cd050-059). Many of these codes in the alphabetical Subject Index are not given in the numerical list on pages 104-107, the Appendix of Chapter 5. The final locator is the **abstract or article number**, which always has a 3-digit number followed by a capital letter and a single digit as described in Chapter 5 (e.g., 086K1 for the mortality abstract on AIDS). Most abstract/article codes are followed by the page number in parentheses, to facilitate location of the entry. All abstract/article codes in Part II are also given in the Table of Contents, arranged in numerical order. Coded articles or abstracts in Part I, the Chapter text, also have the code given in the Table of Contents, but the arrangement is not always in numerical order. Each main subject entry is in boldface type. Subheadings are given in normal type. Some entries contain a cross-reference instruction: "See," or "See also." Subheadings are used for more detailed indexing of each abstract or article, under a paraphrase of the title as the main heading.

REFERENCE LIST

References as cited by contributor, Alphabetical by First Author
Page number location in brackets.

A

H. O. Adami, B. Malker, L. Holmberg, I. Persson, B. Stone, "The Relation Between Survival and Age at Diagnosis in Breast Cancer," *N. Engl. J. Med.,* 315 (1986): 559-63.
[174]

J. S. Aikins, J. C. Kunz, E. H. Shortliffe, R. J. Fallat, "PUFF, An Expert System for Interpretation of Pulmonary Function Data," *Comput. Biomed. Res.,* 16 (1983): 199-208.
[44]

D. Albanes, D. Y. Jones, A. Schatzkin, et al., "Adult Stature and Risk of Cancer," *Cancer Res.,* 48 (1988): 1658-62.
[88]

W. H. Alexander, "Insurance and Genetics," *J. Ins. Med.,* 20 (1988): 35-41.
[254]

Professional Liability in the '80s: Report I, (AMA Special Task Force on Professional Liability and Insurance, 1984).
[144]

P. Amundsen, "The Diagnostic Value of Conventional Radiological Examination of the Heart in Adults," *Acta Radiol. Suppl.,* 181 (1959).
[269]

R. P. Anderson, L. I. Bonchek, G. L. Grunkemeier, et al., "The Analysis and Presentation of Surgical Results by Actuarial Methods," *J. Surg. Res.,* 16 (1974): 224-30.
[88]

Annegers, et al., "The Incidence, Causes and Secular Trends of Head Trauma in Olmsted County, Minnesota, 1935-74," *Neurology,* 30 (1980): 912-19.
[144]

Anon., "Detecting Diseases by Biochemistry of Blood," *Stat. Bull.,* 52 (Sept. 1971): 5-7.
[284]

D. M. Archibald, L. Zon, J. E. Groopman, M. F. McLane, M. Essex, "Antibodies to Human T-Lymphotrophic Virus Type III (HTLV-III) in Saliva of Acquired Immune Deficiency Syndrome (AIDS) Patients and in Persons at Risk for AIDS," *Blood,* 67 (1986): 831-34.
[248]

M. G. Arrigoni, L. B. Wollner, P. E. Bernatz, "Atypical Carcinoid Tumors of the Lung," *J. Thorac. Cardiovasc. Surg.,* 64 (1972): 413-21.
[163]

J. R. Avery, "Center for Medico-Actuarial Statistics of MIB, Inc.," *J. Ins. Med.,* 24 (1992): 117-25.
[3]

B

J. W. Bachman, G. S. McDonald, P. C. O'Brien, "A Study of Out-of-Hospital Cardiac Arrests in Northeastern Minnesota," *JAMA,* 266 (1986): 477-83.
[121]

K. Bachmann, W. Niederer, H. Fuchs, H. Holzberger, "Prognosis of Coronary Heart Disease Patients Evaluated by Data Obtained by Invasive and Noninvasive Methods," in International Symposium, Bad Kroningen, October 22-23, 1982, *Prognosis of Coronary Heart Disease. Progression of Coronary Atherosclerosis* (Berlin and Heidelberg, Springer-Verlag, 1983), pp. 24-35.
[221]

A. K. Bahn, *Basic Medical Statistics* (New York, Grume and Stratton, 1972).
[64]

M. A. Baker, "Determining Prognosis for Cancer Patients," *Trans. Assoc. Life Insur. Med. Dir. Amer.,* 70 (1986): 19-26.
[157]

J. N. Baldwin, O. F. Grimes, "Bronchial Adenomas," *Surg. Gynecol. Obstet.,* 124 (1967): 813-18.
[163]

D. S. Bana, A. Leviton, W. V. Slack, D. E. Geer, J. R. Graham, "Use of a Computerized Data Base in a Headache Clinic," *Headache,* 21 (1981): 72-74.
[43]

G. O. Barnett, "The Application of Computer-Based Medical-Record Systems in Ambulatory Practice," *N. Engl. J. Med.,* 310 (1984): 1643-50.
[44]

REFERENCE LIST (continued)

M. L. Bassett, J. W. Halliday, R. A. Ferris, L. W. Powell, "Diagnosis of Hemochromatosis in Young Subjects: Predictive Accuracy of Biochemical Screening Tests," *Gastroenterology*, 87 (1984): 628-33.
[260]

T. Bayes, "An Essay Toward Solving a Problem in the Doctrine of Chances," *Philos. Trans. R. Soc. Lond.*, 53 (1763): 370-75.
[49]

J. C. Bear, et al., "Age at Clinical Onset and at Ultrasonographic Detection of Adult Polycystic Kidney Disease: Data for Genetic Counseling," *Am. J. Med. Genet.*, 18 (1984): 45-53.
[254]

J. R. Beck, "Who Takes Lead in Promoting Medical Informatics," *Comp. News Physic.*, (July 1986): C-10.
[43]

J. B. Beckwith, N. F. Palmer, "Histopathology and Prognosis of Wilms' Tumor," *Cancer*, 41 (1978): 1937-48.
[173]

M. F. Bell, R. S. Schaaf, T. P. Jernigan, "The Prognostic Import of Calcification of the Aortic Knob," *Trans. Assoc. Life Insur. Med. Dir. Amer.*, 58 (1963): 33-41.
[274]

G. A. Beller, "Dipyridamole Thallium-201 Scintigraphy: An Excellent Alternative to Exercise Scintigraphy," *J. Am. Coll. Cardiol.*, 14 (1989): 1642-44.
[232]

B. T. Benham, "The Promise of Technology," *Best's Rev.*, 88 (1987): 40-46.
[43]

R. L. Bergstrom, *A Report on the Protective Value of Laboratory Testing*, August 1989.
[290]

D. S. Berman, "The Detection of Silent Schemia: Cautions and Precautions," *Circulation*, 75 (1987): 101-5.
[232]

H. L. Bleich, R. F. Beckley, G. L. Horowitz, et al., "Clinical Computing in a Teaching Hospital," *N. Engl. J. Med.*, 312 (1985): 756-64.
[44]

Blood Pressure Study 1979 (Boston, Soc. Actuaries and Assoc. Life Ins. Med. Dir. Amer., 1980).
[3, 103, 121, 196]

W. Bolt, M. F. Bell, "Cardiac Enlargement of Undetermined Cause in Asymptomatic Adults," *Am. Heart J.*, 50 (1955): 331-36.
[274]

A. Bomford, R. Williams, "Long Term Results of Venesection Therapy in Idiopathic Hemochromatosis," *Q. J. Med.*, 180 (October 1976, New Series XLV): 611-23.
[260]

E. H. Botvinick, "Late Reversibility: A Viability Issue," *J. Am. Coll. Cardiol.*, 15 (1990): 341-44.
[232]

C. A. Boyle, et al., "Postservice Mortality Among Vietnam Veterans," U.S.P.H.S. Centers for Disease Control, Atlanta, GA 30337 (1987).
[125]

M. B. Bracken, et al., "Incidence of Acute Traumatic Hospitalized Spinal Cord Injury in the United States, 1970-77," *Am. J. Epidemiol.*, 113 (1981): 615-22.
[144]

R. D. C. Brackenridge, W. J. Elder, eds., *Medical Selection of Life Risks*, 3rd Edit. (New York, Stockton Press, 1992).
[121]

R. D. C. Brackenridge, *Medical Selection of Life Risks: A Comprehensive Guide to Life Expectancy for Underwriters & Clinicians*, 2nd Edit. (Bath, Macmillan Publishers Ltd., 1985).
[254]

T. Bray, et al., "Cost of Orthopedic Injuries Sustained in Motorcycle Accidents," *JAMA*, 254 (1985): 2452-53.
[144]

N. E. Breslow, J. B. Beckwith, "Epidemiological Features of Wilms' Tumor: Results of the National Wilms' Tumor Study," *J. Natl. Cancer Inst.*, 68 (1982): 429.
[173]

N. E. Breslow, P. A. Norkool, A. Olshan, A. Evans, G. J. D'Angio, "Second Malignant Neoplasms in Survivors of Wilms' Tumor: A Report From the National Wilms' Tumor Study," *J. Natl. Cancer Inst.*, 80 (1988): 1326-31.
[173]

M. H. Breuning, et al., "Improved Early Diagnosis of Adult Polycystic Kidney Disease With Flanking DNA Markers," *Lancet*, ii (1987): 1359-61.
[254]

R. A. Bruce, "Strategies for Risk Assessment of Ischemic Heart Disease and Total Mortality," *Trans. Assoc. Life Insur. Med. Dir. Amer.*, 73 (1989): 53-67.
[187]

R. A. Bruce, L. D. Fisher, "Strategies for Risk Evaluation of Sudden Cardiac Incapacitation in Men in Occupations Affecting Public Safety," *J. Occup. Med.*, 21 (1989): 124-33.
[187]

L. D. Budnick, B. P. Chaiken, "The Probability of Dying of Injuries by the Year 2000," *JAMA*, 254 (1985): 3350-52.
[144]

1959 Build and Blood Pressure Study, Vol. 1 (Compiled and published by the Society of Actuaries, 1959).
[103]

1959 Build and Blood Pressure Study, Vol. 2 (Compiled and published by the Society of Actuaries, 1960).
[103]

Build Study 1979 (Boston, Soc. Actuaries and Assoc. Life Ins. Med. Dir. Amer., 1980).
[3, 103]

D. Burger, C. G. Moorman-Voestermans, H. Mildenberger, J. Lemerle, P. A. Voute, M. F. Tournade, C. Rodary, J. F. Delemarre, B. Sandstedt, D. Sarrazin, J. M. V. Burgers, P. Bey, M. Carli, J. deKraker, "The Advantages of Preoperative Therapy in Wilms' Tumor: A Summarized Report on Clinical Trials Conducted by the International Society of Pediatric Oncology (SIOP)," *Z. Kinderchir*, 40 (1985): 170-75.
[173]

J. M. V. Burgers, M. F. Tournade, P. Bey, D. Burger, M. Carli, J. F. M. Delemarre, D. Harms, B. Jereb, J. deKraker, J. Lemerle, C.G.M. Moorman-Voestermans, H. Perry, A. Rey, B. Sandstedt, D. Sarrazin, P. A. Voute, J. M. Zucker, "Abdominal Recurrences in Wilms' Tumors: A Report from the SIOP Wilms' Tumor Trials and Studies," *Radiotherapy Oncology*, 5 (1986): 175-82.
[173]

G. N. Burrow, "Book Reviews," *N. Engl. J. Med.*, 317 (1987): 987-88.
[43]

B. Burrows, et al., "The Course and Prognosis of Different Forms of Chronic Airways Obstruction in a Sample from the General Population," *N. Engl. J. Med.*, 317 (1987): 1309-14.
[242]

C

N. Callaghan, A. Garrett, T. Goggin, "Withdrawal of Anticonvulsant Drugs in Patients Free of Seizures for Two Years," *N. Engl. J. Med.*, 318 (1988): 942-46.
[88]

Y. Z. Cao, A. E. Friedman-Kien, J. Chuba, M. Mirabile, B. Hosein, "IgG Antibodies to Human Immunodeficiency Virus Type 1 (HIV-1) in the Urine of HIV-1 Seropositive Individuals (letter)," *Lancet,* 2 (1988): 869-70.
[248]

Y. Z. Cao, B. Hosein, W. Borkowsky, M. Mirabile, L. Baker, D. Baldwin, B. Poiesz, A. E. Friedman-Kien, "Antibodies to Human Immunodeficiency Virus Type 1 in the Urine Specimens of HIV-1 Seropositive Individuals," *AIDS Res. Hum. Retroviruses,* 5 (1989): 311-19.
[248]

W. P. Castelli, R. J. Garrison, P. W. F. Wilson, R. D. Abbott, S. Kalousdian, W. B. Kannel, "Incidence of Coronary Heart Disease and Lipoprotein Cholesterol Levels — The Framingham Study," *JAMA*, 256 (1986): 2835-39.
[54]

R. D. Cebul, J. R. Beck, "Applications in Ambulatory Screening and Preadmission Testing of Adults," *Biochem. Profiles,* 106 (1987): 403-13.
[49]

The Centers for Disease Control Vietnam Experience Study, "Postservice Mortality Among Vietnam Veterans," *JAMA,* 257 (1987): 790-95.
[125]

D. W. Chan, "PSA as a Marker for Prostatic Cancer," *Laboratory Management,* 26, no. 1 (Jan., 1988): 35-39.
[290]

M. E. Charlson, A. R. Feinstein, "A New Clinical Index of Growth Rate in the Staging of Breast Cancer," *Am. J. Med.*, 69 (1980): 527-36.
[75]

P. M. Chikos, M. M. Figley, L. Fisher, "Correlation Between Chest Film and Angiographic Assessment of Left Ventricular Size," *Am. J. Roentgenol.*, 128 (1977): 367-73.
[269]

C. H. Cissley, *Systems and Data Processing in Insurance Companies,* Revised Edition (Atlanta, GA, FLMI Insurance Education Program, Life Management Institute, LOMA 1, 1982).
[43]

W. B. Clark, L. Midanik, "Alcohol Use and Alcohol Problems Among U.S. Adults: Results of the 1979 National Survey, in Alcohol Consumption and Related Problems," *Alcohol and Health Monograph 1* (Rockville, MD, National Institute on Alcohol Abuse and Alcoholism, 1982).
[50]

G. L. Clifton, "Spinal Cord Injury in the Houston-Galveston Area," *Tex. Med.*, 79 (1983) 55-57.
[144]

J. W. Clouse, P. R. M. Thomas, R. C. Griffith, C. A. Perez, T. J. Vietti, B. Fineberg, "The Changing Management of Wilms' Tumor Over a 30-Year Period (1949-78)," *Cancer*, 56 (1985): 1484-89.
[173]

A. Cohen, C. Witzleben, E. Schwartz, "Treatment of Iron Overload," *Semin. Liver Dis.*, 4, no. 3 (1984): 228-38.
[260]

M. F. Collen, C. D. Flagle, "Full-Text Medical Literature Retrieval by Computer," *JAMA*, 254 (1985): 2768-74.
[44]

S. M. Collins, D. J. Skorton, "Computers in Cardiac Imaging," *J. Am. Coll. Cardiol.*, 9 (1987): 669-77.
[44]

T. Colton, *Statistics in Medicine* (Boston, Little Brown, 1974).
[64]

T. Colton, "Critical Reading of the Medical Literature," *Statistics in Medicine* (Boston, Little Brown, 1974), pp. 315-22.
[81]

D. G. Covell, G. C. Uman , P. R. Manning, "Information Needs in Office Practice: Are They Being Met?" *Ann. Intern. Med.*, 103 (1985): 596-99.
[43]

M. W. Cowell, W. H. Hoskins, *AIDS, HIV Mortality and Life Insurance, a Joint Special Report of the Society of Actuaries* (Itasca, IL, Soc. Actuaries, 1987).
[121]

J. R. Cox, Jr., C. Zeelenberg, "Computer Technology: State of the Art and Future Trends," *J. Am. Coll. Cardiol.*, 9 (1987): 204-14.
[43]

J. D. Curb, N. O. Borhani, T. P. Blaszkowski, et al., "Long-term Surveillance for Adverse Effects of Antihypertensive Drugs," *JAMA*, 253 (1985): 3263-68.
[88]

D

G. J. D'Angio, N. Breslow, B. Beckwith, A. Evans, E. Baum, A. deLorimier, D. Fernbach, E. Hrabovsky, B. Jones, P. Kelalis, H. B. Othersen, M. Tefft, P. R. M. Thomas, "The Treatment of Wilms' Tumor: Results of the National Wilms' Tumor Study," *Cancer*, 38 (1976): 633-46.
[173]

O. Z. Dalgaard, "Bilateral Polycystic Disease of the Kidneys: A Follow-up of Two Hundred and Eighty-Four Patients and their Families," *Acta Med. Scand.*, 158 suppl. 328 (1957): 1-255.
[254]

O. Z. Dalgaard, *Polycystic Disease of the Kidneys: In Disease of the Kidneys*, M. B. Strauss, L. G. West, eds. (Boston, Little, Brown & Co., 1963), pp. 1223-58.
[254]

O. Z. Dalgaard, S. Norby, "Autosomal Dominant Polycystic Kidney Disease in the 1980's," Symposium 28-29 October 1988 on the occasion of the 50 years anniversary of the University Institute of Medical Genetics, Copenhagen. To be printed in the Symposium Proceedings *Clinical Genetics* (1989).
[254]

A. L. Dannenberg, W. B. Kannel, "Remission of Hypertension — The 'Natural History' of Blood Pressure Treatment in the Framingham Study," *JAMA*, 257 (1987): 1477-83.
[88]

C. S. Danzer, "The Cardiothoracic Ratio: An Index of Cardiac Enlargement," *Am. J. Med. Sci.*, 157 (1919): 513.
[269]

W. S. Davis, *Computers and Business Information Processing* (Reading, MA, Addison-Wesley Publishing Company, 1981).
[43]

B. de Camargo, M. L. de Andrea, E. L. F. Franco, "Catching up with History: Treatment of Wilms' Tumor in a Developing Country," *Med. Pediatr. Oncol.*, 15 (1987): 270-76.
[173]

L. F. DeCaro, R. Paladugu, J. R. Benfield, L. Lovisatti, H. Pak, R. L. Teplitz, "Typical and Atypical Carcinoids Within the Pulmonary APUD Tumor Spectrum," *J. Thorac. Cardiovasc. Surg.*, 86 (1983): 528-36.
[163]

Statistical Abstract of the United States (Washington, D.C., U.S. Department of Commerce, 1986).
[144]

A. W. DeTore, "Medical Informatics in Insurance Medicine: An Introduction to Computers for Insurance Medical Directors," *J. Ins. Med.*, 20, no. 1 (1988): 3-9.
[50]

A. W. DeTore, "The Evaluation of Abnormal Laboratory Results," *J. Ins. Med.*, 20, no. 2 (1988): 5-9.
[64]

M. J. DeVivo, et al., "The Prevalence of S.C.I.: A Re-estimation Based on Life Tables," *S.C.I.: Digest*, 1 (1980): 3-11.
[144]

M. J. DeVivo, P. L. Kartus, S. L. Stover, R. D. Rutt, P. R. Fine, "Seven-Year Survival Following Spinal Cord Injury," *Arch. Neurol.*, 44 (1987): 872-75.
[180]

G. A. Diamond, J. S. Forrester, "Analysis of Probability as an Aid in the Clinical Diagnosis of Coronary Artery Disease," *N. Engl. J. Med.*, 300 (1979): 1350-58.
[49, 64, 232]

G. A. Diamond, "How Accurate is SPECT Thallium Scintigraphy?" *J. Am. Coll. Cardiol.*, 16 (1990): 1017-21.
[232]

H. T. Dodge, "Determination of Left Ventricular Volume and Mass," *Radiol. Clin. North Am.*, 9 (1971): 459-67.
[269]

A. C. Doyle, "The Copper Beeches," *The Adventures of Sherlock Holmes* (New York, Harper & Brothers, 1892).
[43]

A. C. Doyle, *The Sign of Four* (London, Ward Lock, 1890).
[49]

E. E. Dussia, D. Cromartie, J. McCraney, G. Mead, N. K. Wenger, "Myocardial Infarction With and Without Laboratory Documentation — One Year Prognosis," *Am. Heart J.*, 92 (1976): 148-51.
[207]

E

M. S. Eisenberg, A. Hallstrom, L. Bergner, "Long-Term Survival After Out-of-Hospital Cardiac Arrest," *N. Engl. J. Med.*, 306 (1982): 1340-43.
[185]

M. S. Eisenberg, L. Bergner, A. Hallstrom, "Paramedic Programs and Out-of-Hospital Cardiac Arrest: Factors Associated with Successful Resuscitation," *Am. J. Public Health*, 69 (1979): 30-38.
[185]

R. C. Elser, "Apolipoproteins, Lipoproteins and Coronary Heart Disease," *Roche Labtrends*, 2 (1988): 1-8.
[54]

P. S. Entmacher, "Medical Information Bureau," *JAMA*, 233 (1975). 1370-72.
[3]

S. E. Epstein, "Implications of Probability Analysis on the Strategy Used for Noninvasive Detection of Coronary Artery Disease," *Am. J. Cardiol.*, 46 (1989): 491-98.
[232]

J. Erickson, P. Staun Olsen, A. C. Thomsen, "Gamma-Glutamyltranspeptidase, Aspartate Aminotransferase, and Erythrocyte Mean Corpustular Volume as Indicators of Alcohol Consumption in Liver Disease," *Scand. J. Gast.*, 19 (1984): 813-19.
[50]

A. E. Evans, N. Breslow, P. Norkool, G. J. D'Angio, "Complications in Long-Term Survivors of Wilms' Tumor," *Proceedings of AACR*, 27 (1986): 204 Abstract #808.
[173]

F

A. R. Feinstein, *Clinical Biostatistics* (St. Louis, Mosby, 1977).
[64]

A. R. Feinstein, D. M. Sosin, C. K. Wells, "The Will Rogers Phenomenon — Stage Migration and New Diagnostic Techniques as a Source of Misleading Statistics for Survival in Cancer," *N. Engl. J. Med.*, 312 (1985): 1604-8.
[75]

A. R. Feinstein, "An Additional Basic Science for Clinical Medicine: IV. The Development of Clinimetrics," *Ann. Int. Med.*, 99 (1983): 843-48.
[75]

A. R. Feinstein, J. A. Pritchett, C. R. Schimpff, "The Epidemiology of Cancer Therapy. IV. The Extraction of Data from Clinical Records," *Arch. Int. Med.*, 123 (1969): 571-90.
[75]

A. R. Feinstein, R. I. Horwitz, "Double Standards, Scientific Methods, and Epidemiologic Research," *N. Engl. J. Med.*, 307 (1982): 1611-17.
[99]

M. Fessel, "Comparison Between the Mortality Expected and that Actually Experienced by Life Insurance Companies, for Selected Impairments," *Annals of Life Insurance Medicine 9* (Proceedings of the 16th International Congress of Life Assurance Medicine, The Hague 1989), (1990): 39-45.
[211, 255]

R. A. Figlin, S. Piantadosi, R. Field, Lung Cancer Study Group, "Intracranial Recurrence of Carcinoma after Complete Surgical Resection of Stage I, II, and III Non-Small-Cell Lung Cancer," *N. Engl. J. Med.*, 318 (1988): 1300-5.
[88]

P. R. Fine, et al., "Spinal Cord Injuries: An Epidemiologic Perspective," *Paraplegia,* 17 (1980): 237-50.
[144]

J. L. Fleg, G. Gerstenblith, A. B. Zonderman, L. C. Becker, M. L. Weisfeldt, P. T. Costa, Jr., E. G. Lakatta, "Prevalence and Prognostic Significance of Exercise-Induced Silent Myocardial Ischemia Detection by Thallium Scintigraphy and Electrocardiography in Asymptomatic Volunteers," *Circulation,* 81 (1990): 428-36.
[232]

R. J. Flemma, D. C. Mullen, M. L. Kleinman, et al., "Survival and 'Event-Free' Analysis of 785 Bjork-Shiley Spherical Disc Valves at 10-16 Years," *Ann. Thor. Surg.,* 45 (1988): 258-72.
[88]

R. H. Fletcher, S. W. Fletcher, E. H. Wagner, *Clinical Epidemiology: The Essentials* (Baltimore, MD, Williams and Wilkins, 1982).
[49]

R. G. Fraser, J. A. P. Pare, *Diagnosis of Diseases of the Chest*, 1st ed. (Philadelphia, W. B. Saunders Company, 1970), pp. 724-30.
[163]

B. A. Friedman, J. B. Martin, "Hospital Information Systems: The Physician's Role," *JAMA*, 257 (1987): 1792.
[44]

Y. F. Friedman, C. Franklin, S. Freels, et al., "Long-term Survival of Patients with AIDS, Pneumocystis Carinii Pneumonia, and Respiratory Failure," *JAMA*, 266 (1991): 89-92.
[145]

G

J. Gajewski, R. B. Singer, "A Mortality Study of Atrial Fibrillation in an Insured Population," *JAMA*, 245 (1981): 1540-44.
[3]

R. S. Galen, S. R. Gambino, *Beyond Normality* (New York, Wiley, 1975).
[64]

R. M. Gardner, B. J. West, T. A. Pryor, K. G. Larson, H. R. Warner, T. P. Clemmer, J. F. Orme, Jr., "Computer-Based ICU Data Acquistion as an Aid to Clinical Decision-Making," *Crit. Care Med.*, 10 (1982): 823-30.
[44]

E. A. Geiser, D. J. Skorton, eds., "Seminar on Computer Applications for the Cardiologist, Introduction," *J. Am. Coll. Cardiol.*, 8 (1986): 930-32.
[43]

W. O. Geisler, et al., "Survival After Traumatic Transverse Myelitis," *Paraplegia,* 14 (1977): 262-75.
[144]

H. George, "Analyzing and Underwriting The Blood Chemistry Profile," *Lincoln National Management Services.*
[64]

C. Gillespie, P. Sorlie, *The Framingham Study. Section 33. An Index to Previous Sections 1-32* (Bethesda, MD, National Heart, Lung and Blood Institute, NIH Publication No. 79-1671, 1978).
[208]

J. N. Gitlin, "Teleradiology," *Radiol. Clin. North Am.*, 24 (1986): 55-68.
[44]

D. M. Goldberg, "Structural, Functional, and Clinical Aspects of Gamma-Glutamyltransferase. CRC Critical Reviews," *Clin. Lab. Sci.*, 12 (1980): 1-58.
[50]

D. J. Gordon, J. L. Probstfield, R. J. Garrison, J. D. Neaton, W. P. Castelli, J. D. Knoke, D. R. Jacobs, S. Bangdiwala, H. A. Tyroler, "High-Density Lipoprotein Cholesterol and Cardiovascular Disease — Four Prospective American Studies," *Circulation,* 79 (1989): 8-15.
[54]

H. M. Greenberg, E. M. Dwyer, Jr., eds., *Sudden Cardiac Death* (New York, vol. 382 of Ann. N.Y. Acad. Sci., 1982).

M. R. Griffin, et al., "Traumatic Spinal Cord Injury in Olmsted County, Minnesota, 1935-81," *Am. J. Epidemiol.,* 121 (1985): 884-95.
[144]

P. F. Griner, et al., "Selection and Interpretation of Diagnostic Tests and Procedures," *Ann. Intern. Med.,* 94 (1981) (4, Part 2): 453-600.
[64]

G. L. Grunkemeier, D. R. Thomas, A. Starr, "Statistical Considerations in the Analysis and Reporting of Time-Related Events," *Am. J. Cardiol,* 39 (1977): 257-58.
[88]

H

S. I. Hajdu, S. J. Winawer, W. P. Myers, "Carcinoid Tumors," *Am. J. Clin. Pathol.,* 61 (1974): 521-28.
[163]

J. W. Halliday, M. L. Bassett, "Treatment of Iron Storage Disorder," *Drugs,* 215 (1980): 207-15.
[260]

R. B. Haynes, K. A. McKibbon, D. Fitzgerald, G. H. Guyatt, C. J. Walker, D. L. Sackett, "How to Keep Up With the Medical Literature: V. Access by Personal Computer to the Medical Literature," *Ann. Intern. Med.,* 105 (1986): 810-24.
[44]

R. B. Haynes, C. J. Walker, "Computer-Aided Quality Assurance," *Arch. Intern. Med.,* 147 (1987): 1297-1301.
[44]

"Mistakes Doctors Make," *HEF News,* Health Education Foundation, Vol. 7, No. 4, Winter 1984.
[144]

H. Heath, III, S. F. Hodgdson, M. A. Kennedy, "Primary Hyperparathyroidism-Incidence, Morbidity and Potential Economic Impact in a Community," *N. Engl. J. Med.,* 302 (January 24, 1980): 189-93.
[284]

J. Herlitz, A. Halmarson, B. W. Karlson, et al., "Long-Term Morbidity in Patients Where the Initial Suspicion of Myocardial Infarction Was Not Confirmed," *Clin. Cardiol.,* 11 (1988): 209-14.
[88]

D. H. Hickman, E. H. Shortliffe, M. S. Bischoff, A. C. Scott, C. D. Jacobs, "The Treatment Advice of a Cancer Chemotherapy Protocol Advisor," *Ann. Intern. Med.,* 103 (1985): 928-36.
[44]

D. R. Higgs, et al., "Analysis of the Human TK-Globin Gene Cluster Reveals a Highly Informative Genetic Locus," (1986).
[254]

D. H. Hindert, et al., *Structured Settlements and Periodic Payment Judgments* (New York, Law Journal Seminars Press, 1984).
[144]

C. A. Hinz, "Computer Tests Track Decisions in Making," *Am. Med. News,* 6 (March): 1.
[44]

F. J. Hodges, J. A. E. Eyster, "Estimation of Transverse Cardiac Diameter in Man," *Arch. Intern. Med.,* 37 (1926): 707-14.
[269]

C. Hogstedt, L. Aringer, A. Gustavsson, "Epidemiologic Support for Ethylene Oxide as a Cancer-Causing Agent," *JAMA,* 255 (1986): 1575-78.
[88]

Home Office Reference Laboratory, *Laboratory Bulletin,* 88-06.
[54]

A. F. Hoskin, et al., *Accident Facts, 1985 Edition* (Chicago, National Safety Council, 1985).
[144]

K. W. Hunter, Jr., "Technological Advances in Bedside Monitoring: Biosensors," *Arch. Pathol. Lab. Med.,* 111 (1987): 633-36.
[44]

I

1951 Impairment Study (Compiled and published by the Society of Actuaries, 1954).
[3, 103]

Medical Impairment Study Committee, "1983 Medical Impairment Study: Provisional Results," *J. Ins. Med.,* 14 (1983): 8-23.
[50]

Medical Impairment Study 1983, Volume I (Boston, Soc. Actuaries and Assoc. Life Ins. Med. Dir. Amer., 1986).
[3, 103, 121]

J. A. Ingelfinger, et al., *Biostatistics in Clinical Medicine* (New York, Macmillan, 1987).
[64]

Insurance Facts, *1985-86 Property/Casualty Fact Book* (New York, Insurance Information Institute, 1985).
[144]

J

J. Jagger, et al., "Epidemiologic Features of Head Injury in a Predominantly Rural Population," *J. of Trauma,* 24 (1984): 40-44.
[144]

A. P. Jarman, et al., "Molecular Characterization of a Hypervariable Region Downstream of the Human α-Globin Gene Cluster," *EMBO J.,* 5 (1986): 1857-63.
[254]

M. L. Johnson, "Record Linkage," *Arch. Dermatol.,* 122 (1986): 1383-84.
[44]

K

W. D. Kalsbeek, et al., "The National Head and Spinal Injury Survey: Major Findings," *J. of Neurosurg.,* 53 (1980): S19-S31.
[144]

A. Kay, "Computer Software," *Sci. Am.,* 251 (1984): 53.
[43]

K. A. Kealey, ed., *Survival Rates for U.S. Comprehensive Cancer Center Patients, Admissions 1977-82* (Seattle, Centralized Cancer System Statistical Analysis and Quality Control Center, 1985).
[121, 157]

D. P. Kiel, D. T. Felson, J. J. Anderson, et al., "Hip Fracture and the Use of Estrogens in Postmenopausal Women — The Framingham Study," *N. Engl. J. Med.,* 317 (1987): 1169-74.
[88]

C. E. Kiessling, L. W. Oliver, Jr., "Enlarged Hearts in Normal Individuals," *Trans. Assoc. Life Insur. Med. Dir. Amer.,* 53 (1969): 306-11.
[269, 274]

D. A. Killen, W. A. Reed, M. Arnold, et al., "Coronary Artery Bypass in Women: Long-Term Survival," *Ann. Thorac. Surg.,* 34 (1982): 559-63.
[236]

D. A. Killen, W. A. Reed, S. Wathanacharoen, et al., "Normal Survival Curve after Coronary Artery Bypass," *South. Med. J.,* 75 (1982): 906-12.
[236]

T. H. Kim, G. S. Zaatari, E. S. Baum, N. Jaffe, B. Cushing, R. L. Chard, Jr., G. T. Zwiren, J. B. Beckwith, "Recurrence of Wilms' Tumor After Apparent Cure," *J. Pediatr.,* 107 (1985): 44-49.
[173]

L. C. Kingsland, III, D. A. B. Lindberg, G. C. Sharp, "Anatomy of a Knowledge-Based Consultant System: AI/RHEUM.," *MD Comp.,* 3 (1986): 18-26.
[44]

W. Kirklin, "Mitral Valve Repair for Mitral Incompetence," *Mod. Concepts of CV Dis.,* 56 (Feb. 1987): 7-11.
[239]

K. K. Kishpaugh, M. H. Ford, C. H. Castle, et al., "Myocardial Infarction: A Five-Year Follow-up of Patients," *West. J. Med.,* 134 (1981): 1-6.
[185]

M. W. Kita, "Morbidity and Mortality Abstraction — Finding Suitable Articles," *J. Ins. Med.,* 22 (1990): 287-88.
[99]

M. R. Klauber, et al., "The Epidemiology of Head Injury," *Am. J. Epidemiol.,* 113 (1981): 500-9.
[144]

W. L. Kleinsasser, "Insurance Medicine — The Future," *J. Ins. Med.,* 17 (1986): 8-10.
[44]

R. A. Korpman, "Using the Computer to Optimize Human Performance in Health Care Delivery," *Arch. Pathol. Lab. Med.,* 111 (1987): 637-45.
[43]

R. Kramer, "Adenoma of Bronchus," *Ann. Otol. Rhinol. Laryngol.,* 39 (1930): 689-92.
[163]

K. R. Krauss, A. M. Hutter, Jr., R. W. DeSanctis, "Acute Coronary Insufficiency — Course and Follow-up," *Circulation,* 45, Supplement I (1972): pp. I-66 thru I-71.
[207]

L

R. T. H. Laennec, *Traité de l'auscultation médiate et des maladies des poumons et du coeur*, Third Edition, Vol. 1: 250 (Paris, Chaude, 1831).
[163]

R. M. Lawson, L. Ramanathan, G. Hurley, K. W. Hinson, S. C. Lennox, "Bronchial Adenoma: Review of an 18 Year Experience at the Brompton Hospital," *Thorax,* 31(1976): 245-53.
[163]

W. K. Lelbach, "Leberschaden bei Chronischem Alcoholismus," *Acta. Hepatosplenol.,* 14 (1967): 9-39.
[50]

J. Lemerle, P. A. Voute, M. R. Tournade, et al., "Preoperative Versus Postoperative Radiotherapy, Single Versus Multiple Courses of Actinomycin-D, in the Treatment of Wilms' Tumor," *Cancer,* 38 (1976): 647-54.
[173]

J. Lemerle, P. A. Voute, M. F. Tournade, "Effectiveness of Preoperative Chemotherapy in Wilms' Tumor: Results of an International Society of Pediatric Oncology (SIOP) Clinical Trial," *J. Clin Oncol.,* 1 (1983): 604-9.
[173]

G. F. Lemp, S. F. Payne, D. Neal, et al., "Survival Trends for Patients with AIDS," *JAMA,* 263 (1990): 402-6.
[145]

M. Lenauer, B. Posner, R. K. Stone, J. Hughes, R. B. Halpern, J. O'Brien, "Effects of the Pediatric Protocol System on Ambulatory Care in New York City Municipal Hospitals (Abstract)," *Med. Decis. Making,* 6 (1986): 267.
[44]

A. J. Levi, D. M. Chalmers, "Recognition of Alcoholic Liver Disease in a District General Hospital," *Gut,* 19 (1978): 521-25.
[50]

E. A. Lew, J. Gajewski, eds., *Medical Risks: Trends in Mortality by Age and Time Elapsed* (New York, Praeger, 1990).
[3, 69, 88, 99, 103, 121, 236, 239]

F. P. Li, W. R. Williams, K. Gimibrere, F. Flamant, D. M. Green, A. T. Meadows, "Heritable Fraction of Unilatral Wilms' Tumor," *Pediatrics,* 81 (1988): 147-49.
[173]

R. R. Liberthson, E. L. Nagel, J. C. Hirschman, et al., "Prehospital Ventricular Fibrillation — Prognosis and Follow-up Course," *N. Engl. J. Med.,* 291 (1974): 317-21.
[185]

D. A. B. Lindberg, "Medical Informatics and Computers In Medicine," *JAMA,* 256 (1986): 2120-22.
[43]

F. D. Loop, D. M. Cosgrove, "Repeat Coronary Bypass Surgery: Selection of Cases, Surgical Risks, and Long-Term Outlook," *Mod. Concepts CV Dis.,* 55 (1986): 31-36.
[233]

M. G. Lopes, A. P. Spivak, D. C. Harrison, J. S. Schroeder, "Prognosis in Coronary Care Unit Noninfarction Cases," *JAMA,* 228 (1974): 1558-62.
[207]

M

M. T. Macfarlane, J. K. Lattimer, T. W. Hensle, "Improved Life Expectancy for Children with Exstrophy of the Bladder," *JAMA,* 242 (1979): 442-44.
[249]

P. R. Manning, D. W. Petit, "The Past, Present, and Future of Continuing Medical Education," *JAMA,* 258 (1987): 3542-46.
[44]

D. B. Mark, M. A. Hlatkly, F. E. Harrell, K. L. Lee, D. B. Pryor, "Exercise Treadmill Score for Predicting Prognosis in Coronary Artery Disease," *Ann. Int. Med.,* 106 (1987): 793-800.
[225]

E. Matsunaga, "Genetics of Wilms' Tumor," *Hum. Genet.,* 57 (1981): 231.
[173]

J. B. McCabe, "Decision Making in Laboratory Test Studies," *Emerg. Med. Clin. North Am.,* 4 (1986): 1-14.
[49]

B. C. McCaughan, N. Martini, M. S. Bains, "Bronchial Carcinoids," *J. Thorac. Cardiovasc. Surg.,* 89 (1985): 8-17.
[163]

F. W. McFarlan, J. L. McKenney, *Corporate Information Systems Management: The Issues Facing Senior Executives* (Homewood, IL, R. D. Irwin, 1983).
[43]

V. A. McKusick, *Mendelian Inheritance in Man: Catalogs of Autosomal Dominant, Autosomal Recessive, and X-Linked Phenotypes.* 7th Edit. (Baltimore, The Johns Hopkins University Press, 1986).
[254]

G. D. McLaren, W. A. Muir, R. W. Kellermeyer, "Iron Overload Disorders: Natural History, Pathogenesis, Diagnosis and Therapy," *CRC Crit. Rev. Clin. Lab. Sci.,* 19, no. 3 (1984): 205-66.
[260]

W. W. McLendon, "Technological Revolutions in Modern Pathology and Laboratory Medicine," *Arch. Pathol. Lab. Med.,* 111 (1987): 581-83.
[44]

B. J. McNeil, H. Sherman, "Primer on Certain Elements of Medical Decision Making," *N. Engl. J. Med.,* 293 (1975): 211-15.
[64]

M. A. Merrilees, P. J. Scott, R. M. Norris, "Prognosis After Myocardial Infarction: Results of 15 Year Follow-up," *Brit. Med. J.,* 288 (1984): 356-59.
[69]

L. Mesard, "Survival after Spinal Cord Trauma: A Life Table Analysis," *Arch. Neurol.,* 35 (1978): 78-83.
[144]

H. Meyer, "Electronic Processing: New System Speeds Up Bill Collections," *Am. Med. News,* 6 (March 1987): 10.
[44]

V. Mike, A. T. Meadows, G. J. D'Angio, "Incidence of Second Malignant Neoplasms in Children: Results of an International Study," *Lancet,* 2 (1982): 1326-31.
[173]

R. A. Miller, H. E. Pople, Jr., J. D. Myers, "INTERNIST-I, An Experimental Computer-Based Diagnostic Consultant for General Internal Medicine," *N. Engl. J. Med.,* 307 (1982): 468-76.
[44]

F. M. Mims, III, ed., *Consumers Guide: Easy to Understand Guide to Home Computers* (USA Publications International, 1982).
[43]

Report of the Secretary's Task Force on Black and Minority Health, *Morbidity and Mortality Weekly Report,* 35 (1986): 109-12.
[144]

Leads from the MMWR, "Deaths Associated with Fires, Burns, and Explosions, New Mexico, 1978-83," *JAMA,* 254 (1985): 2538-41.
[144]

C. G. Moertel, T. R. Fleming, E. T. Creagan et al., "High-Dose Vitamin C versus Placebo in the Treatment of Patients with Advanced Cancer Who Have Had No Prior Chemotherapy," *New Engl. J. Med.,* 312 (1985): 137-41.
[164]

R. D. Moore, J. Hidalgo, B. W. Sugland, et al., "Zidovudine and the Natural History of the Acquired Immunodeficiency Syndrome," *N. Engl. J. Med.,* 324 (1991): 1412-16.
[145]

H. J. Morowitz, "Past, Present, Future," *Hosp. Prac.,* 22 (1987): 209-13.
[44]

Specialized Mortality Investigation (Compiled and published by the Actuarial Society of America, predecessor of the Society of Actuaries, 1903).
[3]

H. Müller, *Zur entstehungsgeschichte der bronchial-erweiterrungen,* (E. Germany, Ermsleben Halle, 1982).
[163]

E. Munoz, "Economic Costs of Trauma, United States, 1982," *J. of Trauma,* 24 (1984): 237-44.
[144]

E. A. Murphy, *The Logic of Medicine* (Baltimore, Johns Hopkins Press, 1976).
[64]

M. H. Myers, L. A. G. Ries, "Cancer Patient Survival Rates: SEER Program Results for 10 Years of Follow-up," *CA-A Cancer Journal for Clinicians,* 39 (1989): 21-32.
[121, 290]

N

A. M. Nahum, J. Melvin, eds., *The Biomechanics of Trauma* (Norwalk, Appleton Century Crofts, 1985).
[144]

J. Naisbitt, *Megatrends: Ten New Directions Transforming Our Lives* (New York, Warner Books, 1984).
[43]

H. K. Naito, "The Clinical Significance of Apolipoprotein Measurements," *J. Clin. Immunoassay,* 9 (1986): 11-20.
[54]

"Unstable Angina Pectoris: National Cooperative Study Group to Compare Surgical and Medical Therapy. II. In-Hospital Experience and Initial Follow-up Results in Patients with One, Two, and Three Vessel Disease," *Am. J. Cardiol.,* 42 (1978): 839-48.
[207]

C. Niederau, R. Fischer, et al., "Survival and Causes of Death in Cirrhotic and Noncirrhotic Patients with Primary Hemochromatosis," *N. Engl. J. Med.,* 313 (1985): 1256-62.
[260]

R. M. Norris, P. W. T. Brandt, D. E. Caughey, et al., "A New Coronary Prognostic Index," *Lancet,* 1 (1969): 174-78.
[69]

R. M. Norris, D. E. Caughey, C. J. Mercer, et al., "Coronary Prognostic Index for Predicting Survival After Recovery from Acute Myocardial Infarction," *Lancet,* 2 (1970): 485-88.
[69]

R. M. Norris, D. E. Caughey, C. J. Mercer, et al., "Prognosis After Myocardial Infarction. Six-year Follow-up," *Brit. Heart J.,* 36 (1974): 786-90.
[69]

O

1967 Occupation Study (Compiled and published by the Society of Actuaries, 1967).
[103, 121]

R. H. Ochs, G. G. Pietra, "Neoplasms of the Lung Other Than Bronchogenic Carcinoma," A. P. Fishman, *Pulmonary Diseases and Disorders* (New York, McGraw-Hill, 1980), pp. 1439-41.
[163]

N. Okike, P. E. Bernatz, L. B. Woolner, "Carcinoid Tumors of the Lung," *Ann. Thorac. Surg.,* 22, no. 3 (1976): 270-77.
[163]

M. R. Oreskovich, et al., "Geriatric Trauma: Injury Patterns and Outcome," *J. of Trauma,* 24 (1984): 565-69.
[144]

P

R. S. Paffenbarger, Jr., R. T. Hyde, A. L. Wing, C. H. Hsieh, "Physical Activity, All-Cause Mortality, and Longevity of College Alumni," *N. Engl. J. Med.,* 314 (1986): 605-13.
[128]

R. K. Palmer, "Hartford Hospital Cardiac Catheterization Mortality Study," CIGNA Report No. 33751 (no date).
[214]

R. E. Patterson, S. F. Horowitz, "Importance of Epidemiology and Biostatistics in Deciding Clinical Strategies for Using Diagnostic Tests: A Simplified Approach Using Examples from Coronary Artery *Disease*," *J. Am. Coll. Cardiol.,* 13 (1988): 1653-65.
[232]

T. W. Pendergrass, "Congenital Anomalies in Children with Wilms' Tumor: A New Survey," *Cancer,* 37 (1976): 403.
[173]

B. S. Peters, E. S. Beck, D. G. Coleman, et al., "Changing Disease Pattern in Patients with AIDS in a Referral Centre in the United Kingdom: the Changing Face of AIDS," *Brit. Med., J.,* 302 (1991): 203-207.
[145]

A. Phillips, A. G. Shaper, P. H. Whincup, "Association Between Serum Albumin and Mortality from Cardiovascular Disease, Cancer and Other Causes," *Lancet* II (Dec. 16, 1989): 1434-36.
[285]

Steering Committee of the Physicians' Health Study Research Group, "Final Report on the Aspirin Component of the Physicians' Health Study," *N. Engl. J. Med.,* 321 (1989): 129-35.
[200]

R. J. Pokorski, "Overview of Test Theory," BIM Triennial Course, The Wigwam, Litchfield Park, Arizona, 1988.
[64]

R. J. Pokorski, "Mortality Methodology and Analysis Seminar," *J. Ins. Med.,* 20, no. 4 (1988): 20-45.
[99]

R. A. Polacsek, "The Fourth Annual Medical Software Buyer's Guide," *MD Comp.,* 4 (1987): 23-135.
[43]

L. Posnick, "HIV Urine Testing Eyed," *CCN,* 16 (1990): 1-6.
[248]

D. C. Purnell, D. A. Scholz, L. H. Smith, et al., "Treatment of Primary Hyperparathyroidism," *Am. J. Med.,* 56 (1974): 800-9.
[284]

R

D. F. Ransohoff, A. R. Feinstein, "Problems of Spectrum and Bias in Evaluating the Efficacy of Diagnostic Tests," *N. Engl. J. Med.,* 299 (1978): 926-30.
[49]

P. Rausmussen, "Use of the Laboratory in Patient Management," *Am. Fam. Prac.,* 35 (1987): 214-23.
[49]

S. T. Reeders, et al., "A Highly Polymorphic DNA Marker Linked to Adult Polycystic Kidney Disease on Chromosome 16," *Nature,* 317 (1985): 542-44.
[254]

S. T. Reeders, et al., "Two Genetic Markers Closely Linked to Adult Polycystic Kidney Disease on Chromosome 16," *Brit. Med. J.,* 292 (1986): 851-53.
[254]

S. T. Reeders, et al., "Prenatal Diagnosis of Autosomal Dormant Polycystic Kidney Disease with a DNA Probe," *Lancet,* ii (1986): 6-8.
[254]

J. A. Reggia, D. R. Tabb, T. R. Price, M. Banko, R. Hebel, "Computer-Aided Assessment of Transient Ischemic Attacks," *Arch. Neurol.,* 41 (1984): 1248-54.
[44]

S. Ridgway, "Computers Leap Beyond Billing to Patient Care," *Med. World News,* 22 (1987): 30-40.
[44]

R. K. Riegelman, "Diagnostic Discrimination of Test," *Studying a Study and Testing a Test — How to Read the Medical Literature* (Boston, Little Brown and Company, 1981).
[54]

R. K. Riegelman, *Studying a Study and Testing a Test* (Boston, Little Brown, 1981).
[64]

R. K. Riegelman, R. P. Hirsch, "Questions to Ask in Studying a Study," *Studying a Study and Testing a Test: How to Read the Medical Literature,* 2nd ed., (Boston, Little Brown, 1989), pp. 75-77.
[81]

J. L. Ritche, M. D. Cerqueira, "Single Photon Computed Tomography (SPECT): 1989 and Beyond," *J. Am. Coll. Cardiol.,* 14 (1989): 1700-1.
[232]

A. H. Roberts, "Chapter 12. Life Expectancy and Causes of Death." In *Severe Accidental Head Injury* (London, Macmillan Press, 1979), pp. 140-51.
[144]

R. Robinson, *Clinical Chemistry and Automation: A Study in Laboratory Proficiency* (Baltimore, MD, Williams and Wilkins, 1971).
[49]

P. Robitaille, J. G. Mongeau, L. Lortie, P. Sinnassamy, "Long-Term Follow-Up of Patients Who Underwent Unilateral Nephrectomy in Childhood," *Lancet,* 2 (1985): 1297-99.
[173]

G. Rockswold, B. Sharma, E. Rutz, et al., "Follow-up of 514 Consecutive Patients with Cardiopulmonary Arrest Outside the Hospital," *J. Am. Coll. Emerg. Phys.,* 8 (1979): 216-20.
[185]

M. Rodstein, L. Wolloch, "The Determination of Aortic Size by Use of the Sheridan Index in the Elderly — A Study of 300 Individuals 65 years of Age and Older," *Trans. Assoc. Life Insur. Med. Dir. Amer.,* 51 (1967): 341-49.
[269]

J. M. Romeder, J. McWhinnie, "Potential Years of Life Lost Between Ages 1 and 70: An Indicator of Premature Mortality for Health Planning," *Int. J. of Epidemiol.,* 6 (1977): 143-50.
[144]

R. Rothenburg, M. Woefel, R. Stoneburner, et al., "Survival with the Acquired Immunodeficiency Syndrome," *N. Engl. J. Med.,* 317 (1987): 1297-302.
[145]

J. W. Rowe, J. R. Wards, "Familial Hemochromatosis: Characteristics of the Precirrhotic Stage in a Large Kindred," *Medicine,* 56, no. 3 (1977): 197-211.
[260]

A. Rozanski, D. S. Berman, "The Efficacy of Cardiovascular Nuclear Medicine Studies," *Semin. Nucl. Med.,* 17 (1987): 104-20.
[232]

J. Rozenman, R. Pausner, Y. Lieberman, G. Gamsu, "Bronchial Adenoma," *Chest,* 92, no. 1 (1987): 145-47.
[163]

M. H. Rudov, et al., "Medical Malpractice Insurance Claim Files Closed in 1970," in Appendix, *Report of the Secretary's Commission on Medical Malpractice* (D.H.E.W. Publication No. [OS] 73-89, 1973).
[144]

S

D. L. Sackett, R. B. Haynes, P. Tugwell, "How to Read a Clinical Journal," *Clinical Epidemiology: A Basic Science for Clinical Medicine* (Boston, Little Brown and Company, 1985), p. 285-319.
[43, 49, 64, 81]

M. H. Schreiber, "The Volume of the Heart — A Roentgenographic Determination," *Ariz. Med.*, 21 (1964): 551.
[269]

J. S. Schroeder, I. H. Lamb, M. Hu, "Do Patients in Whom Myocardial Infarction Has Been Ruled Out Have a Better Prognosis After Hospitalization Than Those Surviving Infarction?" *N. Engl. J. Med.*, 303 (1980): 1-5.
[207]

J. S. Schwartz, "Understanding Laboratory Test Results," *Med. Clin. North Am.*, 71 (1987): 639-52.
[49]

W. B. Schwartz, R. S. Patil, P. Szolovits, "Artificial Intelligence in Medicine: Where Do We Stand? (Editorial)," *N. Engl. J. Med.*, 316 (1987): 685-88.
[44]

G. B. Scott, C. Hutto, R. W. Makuch, et al., "Survival in Children with Prenatally Acquired Human Immunodeficiency Virus Type I Infection," *N.Engl. J. Med.*, 321 (1989): 1791-96.
[145]

W. C. Sheldon, F. D. Loop, "Coronary Artery Bypass Surgery: The Cleveland Clinic Experience, 1967-1982," *Postgrad. Med.*, 75 (1984): 108-21.
[233]

J. T. Sheridan, "The Transverse Diameter of the Cardiac Silhouette," *Trans. Assoc. Life Insur. Med. Dir. Amer.*, 28 (1941): 49-73.
[269, 274]

S. Sherlock, "Hemochromatosis: Course and Treatment," *Annu. Rev. Med.*, 27 (1976): 143-49.
[260]

E. H. Shortliffe, "Computer Programs to Support Clinical Decision Making," *JAMA*, 258 (1987): 61-66.
[44]

F. J. Siber, A. E. Brown, R. B. Singer, F. I. Pitkin, "A Cardiovascular Survey of the Chest X-ray in Nearly 5,000 Life Insurance Applicants: Normal Standards and Distribution Curves for Relative Heart Diameter," *Trans. Assoc. Life Insur. Med. Dir. Amer.*, 63 (1979): 159-74.
[274, 281]

G. Siest, et al., *Interpretation of Clinical Laboratory Tests* (Foster City, CA, Biomedical Publications, 1985).
[64]

J. Singer, H. S. Sacks, F. Lucente, et al., "Physician's Attitudes Toward Applications of Computer Data Base Systems," *JAMA*, 249 (1983): 1610-14.
[44]

R. B. Singer, L. Levinson, eds., *Medical Risks: Patterns of Mortality and Survival* (Lexington, MA, Lexington Books, 1976).
[3, 49, 69, 88, 99, 103, 121]

R. B. Singer, "Mortality Follow-up Studies and Risk Selection: Retrospect and Prospect," *Trans. Assoc. Life Insur. Med. Dir. Amer.*, 62 (1978): 215-38.
[88, 185]

R. B. Singer, J. R. Avery, M. W. Kita, "A Classification System for Mortality and Morbidity Abstracts and Related Data," *J. Ins. Med.*, 23 (1991): 94-96.
[99]

R. B. Singer, L. Levinson, eds., *Medical Risks: Patterns of Mortality and Survival* (Lexington, MA, Lexington Books, 1976). See Cancer Mortality Abstracts (100), pp. 1-1 to 1-5, 1-30 and 1-48 to 1-51. Source of data: life table computer output for End Results Group Report No. 4, M.H. Myers, personal communication to the editors.
[164]

R. B. Singer, "An Analysis of Electrocardiographic Abnormalities in Insurance Applicants: Bundle Branch Block and Related Defects," *Proc. Medical Section. Am. Life Convention*, 50th Annual Meeting, (1962), pp. 114-44.
[269]

R. B. Singer, Unpublished Study of New England Life Mortality Experience, 1958-74 Standard and Rated Policy Issues with Impairment Code, Followed to 1975 Policy Anniversary (various reports 1978).
[274]

Data from "New York Life Single Impairment Study — 1972" in Mortality Abstract 399, in *Medical Risks: Patterns of Mortality and Survival*, R. B. Singer, L. Levinson, eds. (Lexington, MA, Lexington Books, 1976).
[274]

P. Skolnik, B. Kosloff, L. Bechtel, K. Huskins, T. Flynn, N. Karthas, K. McIntosh, M. Hirsch, "Absence of Infectious HIV-1 in the Urine of Seropositive Viremic Subjects," *J. Infect. Dis.,* 160 (1989): 1056-60.
[248]

W. V. Slack, "A History of Computerized Medical Interviews," *MD Comp.,* 1 (1984): 52-59.
[43]

G. L. Snider, *Clinical Pulmonary Medicine,* 1st ed. (Boston, Little Brown and Company, 1981), p. 415.
[163]

N. Sohon, R. D. Robbins, "Computer-Assisted Surgery (Letter)," *N. Engl. J. Med.,* 312 (1985): 924.
[44]

R. W. Solazzi , R. J. Ward, "The Spectrum of Medical Liability Cases," *Inter. Anesthesiol. Clin.,* 22 (1984): 43-59.
[144]

P. Sorlie, *Section 32. Cardiovascular Diseases and Death Following Myocardial Infarction and Angina Pectoris: Framingham Study, 20-year Follow-up* (Bethesda, MD, National Institutes of Health, DHEW Publication No. [NIH] 77-1247, 1977).
[88, 208]

H. C. Sox, "Probability Theory in the Use of Diagnostic Tests," *Ann. Intern. Med.,* 104 (1986): 60-66.
[49]

H. C. Sox, Jr., "Noninvasive Testing in Coronary Artery Disease," *Postgrad. Med.,* 74 (1983): 319-36.
[232]

C. E. Speicher, J. W. Smith, *Choosing Effective Laboratory Tests* (Philadelphia, Saunders, 1983).
[64]

H. F. Starr, Jr., Moderator, "Panel Discussion: The Mortality Monograph, a Medico-Actuarial Milestone," *Trans. Assoc. Life Insur. Med. Dir. Am.,* 60 (1976): 142-70.
[69]

D. Steinhertz, C. Tan, L. Murphy, "Cardiac Toxicity 4-20 Years After Completing Anthrocycline Therapy," *Proceedings of the ASCO,* 8 (1989): 296.
[173]

L. C. Strong, "Genetics of Wilms' Tumor," *Dialogues Pediatr. Urol.,* 6 (1983): 2.
[173]

T

C. H. Tator, V. E. Edmonds, "Acute Spinal Cord Injury: Analysis of Epidemiologic Factors," *Can. J. Surg.,* 22 (1979): 575-78.
[144]

C. H. Tator, et al., "Diving: A Frequent and Potentially Preventable Cause of Spinal Cord Injury," *Can. Med. Assoc. J.,* 124 (1981): 1323-24.
[144]

L. G. Tesler, "Programming Languages," *Sci. Am.,* 251 (1984): 70-78.
[43]

J. E. Thompson, R. D. Patman, C. M. Talkington, "Asymptomatic Carotid Bruit," *Ann. Surg.,* 188 (1978): 308-16.
[99]

W. M. Tierney, C. J. McDonald, D. K. Martin, S. L. Hui, M. P. Rogers, "Computerized Display of Past Test Results," *Ann. Intern. Med.,* 107 (1987): 569-74.
[44]

T. R. Todd, J. D. Cooper, D. Weissberg, N. C. Delarue, F. G. Pearson, "Bronchial Carcinoid Tumors," *J. Thorac. Cardiovasc. Surg.,* 79 (1980): 532-36.
[163]

G. A. Tolis, W. A. Fry, L. Head, T. W. Shield, "Bronchial Adenomas," *Surg. Gynecol. Obstet.,* 134 (1972): 605-10.
[163]

J. S. Torg, et al., "The National Football Head and Neck Injury Registry: 14-Year Report on Cervical Quadriplegia, 1971 through 1984," *JAMA,* 254 (1985): 3439-42.
[144]

M. A. Tucker, G. A. D'Angio, J. D. Boice, Jr., et al., "Bone Sarcomas Linked to Radiotherapy and Chemotherapy in Children," *N. Engl. J. Med.,* 317 (1987): 588-93.
[88]

M. A. Tucker, A. T. Meadows, J. D. Boice, et al., "Cancer Risk Following Treatment of Childhood Cancer," in J. D. Boice, J. F. Fraumeni, Jr., eds., *Radiation Carcinogenesis: Epidemiology and Biological Significance* (New York, Raven Press, 1984), pp. 211-24.
[173]

U

H. E. Ungerleider, C. P. Clark, "A Study of the Transverse Diameter of the Heart Silhouette and Prediction Table Based on the Teleoroentgenogram," *Trans. Assoc. Life Insur. Med. Dir. Amer.*, 25 (1938): 84-103.
[121, 269, 274]

H. E. Ungerleider, C. P. Clark, "A Study of the Transverse Diameter of the Heart Silhouette and Prediction Table Based on the Teleoroentgenogram," *Am. Heart J.*, 17 (1939): 92-102.
[121, 269]

V

G. E. Vaillant, *The Natural History of Alcoholism* (Cambridge, MA, Harvard University Press, 1983).
[50]

W

F. J. T. Wackers, D. J. Russo, D. Russo, J. P. Clements, "Prognostic Significance of Normal Quantitative Planer Thallium-201 Stress Scintigraphy in Patients with Chest Pain," *J. Am. Coll. Cardiol.*, 6 (1985): 27-30.
[232]

J. Wallach, *Interpretation of Diagnostic Tests: A Synopsis of Laboratory Medicine* (Boston, Little Brown and Company, 1986).
[50, 64]

M. C. Weinstein, H. V. Fineberg, *Clinical Decision Analysis* (Philadelphia, W. B. Saunders Company, 1980).
[49, 64]

R. S. Weinstein, K. J. Bloom, L. S. Rozek, "Telepathology and the Networking of Pathology Diagnostic Services," *Arch. Pathol. Lab. Med.*, 111 (1987): 646-52.
[44]

L. R. Weintraub, M. E. Conrad, W. H. Crosby, "The Treatment of Hematochromatosis by Phlebotomy," *Med. Clin. North Am.*, 50 (1966): 1579-90.
[260]

T. R. Welch, A. J. McAdams, "Focal Glomerulosclereosis as a Late Sequela of Wilms' Tumor," *J. Pediatr.*, 108 (1986): 105-9.
[173]

J. E. Wennberg, N. Roos, L. Sola, A. Schori, R. Jaffe, "Use of Claims Data Systems to Evaluate Health Care Outcomes," *JAMA*, 257 (1987): 933-36.
[44]

R. K. Wertz, "CD-ROM, A New Advance in Medical Information Retrieval," *JAMA*, 256 (1986): 3376-78.
[43]

B. M. White, C. E. Swanson, D. A. Cooper, "Survival of Patients with the Acquired Immunodeficiency Snydrome in Australia," *Med. J. Austral.*, 150 (1989): 358-362.
[145]

Q. E. Whiting-O'Keefe, D. W. Simborg, W. V. Epstein, A. Warger, "A Computerized Summary Medical Record System Can Provide More Information Than the Standard Medical Record," *JAMA*, 254 (1985): 1185-92.
[44]

S. Whitman, et al., "Comparative Head Trauma Experiences in Two Socioeconomically Different Chicago-Area Communities. A Population Study," *Am. J. Epidemiol.*, 119 (1984): 570-80.
[144]

T. M. Wicker, M. Samuelson, "Using Claims Data to Set Health Promotion Goals," *Bus. and Health*, 4 (1987): 28-31.
[44]

P. H. Wiernink, "Hodgkin's Disease," *Clinical Medicine, Vol. 5*, edited by John O. Spittell, Jr., (Philadelphia, Harper & Row, 1986).
[157]

E. W. Wilkins, H. C. Grillo, A. C. Moncure, J. G. Scannell, "Changing Times in Surgical Management of Bronchopulmonary Carcinoid Tumor," *Ann. Thorac. Surg.*, 38, no. 4 (1984): 339-44.
[163]

M. Williamson, *Artificial Intelligence for Microcomputers* (New York, Brady Communications Company, Inc., 1986).
[43]

P. W. F. Wilson, R. J. Garrison, W. P. Castelli, "Postmenopausal Estrogen Use, Cigarette Smoking, and Cardiovascular Morbidity in Women Over 50 — The Framingham Study," *N. Engl. J. Med.*, 313 (1985): 1038-43.
[88]

M. D. Wittenborg, M. C. Sossman, "Heart Measurements by X-Ray," *Mod. Concepts Cardiovasc. Dis.*, 16 (1947).
[269]

P. A. Wolf, R. B. D'Agostino, W. B. Kannel, et al., "Cigarette Smoking as a Risk Factor for Stroke — The Framingham Study," *JAMA*, 259 (1988): 1025-29. [88]

J. L. Young, Jr., R. W. Miller, "Incidence of Malignant Tumors in U.S. Children," *J. Pediatr.*, 86 (1975): 254. [173]

Z

Y

J. P. Zettas, et al., "Injury Patterns in Motorcycle Accidents," *J. Trauma*, 19 (1979): 833-36. [144]

J. S. Young, et al., *Spinal Cord Injury Statistics* (Phoenix, Good Samaritan Medical Center, 1982). [144]

J. Zylke, "Medical Libraries Undergoing Dramatic Changes (Medical News)," *JAMA*, 258 (1987): 3216. [44]

ISBN 0-275-94553-7